Third Edition

# INTEGRATED SCIENCE
for
Health Students

**Third Edition**

# INTEGRATED SCIENCE
for
Health Students

T. Randall Lankford
*Galveston College*

RESTON PUBLISHING COMPANY, INC
*A Prentice-Hall Subsidiary*
Reston, Virginia

*Library of Congress Cataloging in Publication Data*

Lankford, T. Randall
   Integrated science for health students.

   Includes index.
   1. Human physiology.  2. Anatomy, Human.  I. Title.
QP34.5.L37  1984      612      83–17702
ISBN  0-8359-3106-4

*Editorial/production supervision and
interior design by Camelia Townsend*

© 1976, 1979, 1984 by Reston Publishing Company, Inc.
*A Prentice-Hall Company*
Reston, Virginia 22090

10  9  8  7  6  5  4  3  2  1

PRINTED IN THE UNITED STATES OF AMERICA

*To Billie Jo, Christopher, and Nicholas*

# CONTENTS

# PREFACE

This text presents in an integrated manner anatomy–physiology, chemistry, and microbiology. The purpose of integrating these three entities is to present to health science students a more complete picture of how the body normally functions and the diseases that cause the body to malfunction. The level of writing assumes that the student has had no previous chemistry, anatomy–physiology, or microbiology. The text has been written for students majoring in nursing, allied health-science programs, mortuary science, medical records, biological sciences, predental, premedical, and physical education.

In order to learn physiology, a student must have some chemistry background. The chemistry in the text is only enough to help a student learn basic physiology and microbiology. It is oriented toward the human body and integrated into all of the subsequent units. The microbiology material also is oriented toward the human body and integrated into each succeeding unit.

In addition to the integration of chemistry and microbiology, various organ systems are presented and integrated into the following units. For example, Chapters 5 and 6 present the coordinating systems—nervous and endocrine systems—prior to any of the other systems. Many of the drawings integrate more than one organ system and illustrate how microorganisms interact with them.

Some student-oriented features of the text are study objectives, glossary, index, multiple choice questions, chapter summaries, and many drawings that clarify difficult physiological concepts. The entire text is written so that physiological functions, chemical reactions, and diseases can be easily understood by a student. A separate study guide and lab manual is coordinated with the text. Numerous lab exercises, study questions, and drawings reinforce and broaden concepts presented in the text.

Finally, I wish especially to thank Camelia Townsend, production editor at Reston Publishing Company, for invaluable help in editing this text.

# Chapter 1

# UNITS AND METHODS OF MEASUREMENT

After reading and studying this chapter, a student should be able to:

1. Give the metric unit of measurement and abbreviation for weight, length, and volume.
2. Make conversions between the metric and British units of weight, length, and volume.
3. Write and apply the density formula in calculating the density of a fluid.
4. Write and apply the specific gravity formula in calculating the specific gravity of a fluid.
5. Give the temperature values for freezing and boiling points of water on the Celsius and Fahrenheit temperature scales.
6. Make the conversions between the Fahrenheit and Celsius temperature scales.

*Making accurate and precise measurements is essential in the various areas of science. To understand life and its characteristics, we must make measurements, interpret their importance, and communicate them. An example of the fundamental importance of measurements can be made by asking the question "How does a physician know whether you are sick?" Once a physician determines you are sick, how does he or she determine where the root of the problem is and how bad it is? Specific, accurate, and precise measurements must be made and interpreted before these questions can be answered.*

# 1  THE METRIC SYSTEM

The metric system was adopted in the eighteenth century by scientists all over the world. This system is used also in commerce by all major countries in the world except the United States. The United States is presently engaged in the long-term process of converting from the British system to the metric system in the areas of commerce.

The metric system is easy to use since the subdivisions or multiples of its basic units are all factors of 10. The size of each subunit is indicated by a prefix. The prefixes commonly used in the metric system are shown in Table 1–1.

There are three commonly used fundamental types of measurement: weight, length, and volume. Each type will be discussed as to its characteristic metric units, subdivisions, and conversion equations.

## LENGTH

The **meter** (m) is the metric unit of length (Figure 1–1). Most of the measurements you will be making will be considerably smaller than a meter. Some of the common subdivisions and multiples of the meter are:

| 1 meter (m) | = 100 centimeters (cm) |
| | = 1000 millimeters (mm) |
| 1 centimeter (cm) | = 10 millimeters (mm) |
| 10 millimeters (mm) | = 1 centimeter (cm) |
| 10 decimeters (dm) | = 1 meter (m) |
| 1,000,000 microns ($\mu$) | = 1 meter (m) |
| 1 kilometer (km) | = 1000 meters (m) |

Most people are familiar with the British units for length; therefore, it will often be necessary to convert British units to metric units, and vice versa.

### TABLE 1–1.  *Metric Prefixes*

| Prefix | Abbreviation | Value | Example |
|---|---|---|---|
| micro- | $\mu$ (micron) | one one-millionth 1/1,000,000 or 0.000001 | *micro*meter ($\mu$m) 1/1,000,000 of a meter or 0.000001 of a meter |
| milli- | m | one one-thousandth 1/1000 or 0.001 | *milli*meter (mm) 1/1000 of a meter or 0.001 of a meter |
| centi- | c | one one-hundredth 1/100 or 0.01 | *centi*meter (cm) 1/100 of a meter of 0.01 of a meter |
| deci- | d | one one-tenth 1/10 or 0.1 | *deci*meter (dm) 1/10 of a meter or 0.1 of a meter |
| kilo- | k | one thousand 1000 | *kilo*meter (km) 1000 meters |

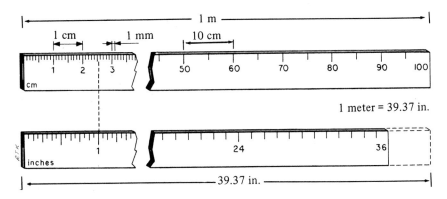

**Figure 1-1.** The meter stick (metric system) with its subdivisions is compared to the yardstick (British system).

Conversion equations for length are as follows:

| | |
|---|---|
| 1 inch (in.) = 2.5 cm | 1 meter = 39.4 in |
| 1 foot (ft) = 30.5 cm | 1 meter (m) = 3.3 ft |
| 1 mile (mi) = 1.6 km | 1 kilometer (km) = 0.6 mi |

## Examples

A patient is 5 ft 9 in. (69 in.) tall. Convert this to centimeters (cm). (This first example will be explained step by step.)

1. Write down what you are converting on the left-hand side of a page and make a fraction out of it by writing it over 1.

$$\frac{69 \text{ in.}}{1}$$

2. Find the appropriate conversion equation: 1 in. = 2.5 cm. Change the conversion equation into a conversion factor so that the unwanted unit or the one you are converting is in the denominator.

$$1 \text{ in.} = 2.5 \text{ cm}$$
$$\frac{2.5 \text{ cm}}{1 \text{ in.}}$$

One inch is the unwanted unit, or the one being converted in this problem.

3. Write the conversion factor to the right of the number you are converting and multiply the two fractions.

$$\frac{69 \text{ in.}}{1} \times \frac{2.5 \text{ cm}}{1 \text{ in.}} = \frac{69 \times 2.5 \text{ cm}}{1} = 172.5 \text{ cm}$$

4. If you set the problem up correctly and multiply the numbers properly, the unwanted units will cancel out and your numerical answer and unit will be correct.

A patient is 176.0 cm long. Convert this to inches.

$$\frac{176.0 \text{ cm}}{1} \times \frac{1 \text{ in.}}{2.5 \text{ cm}} = \frac{176.0 \times 1 \text{ in.}}{2.5} = 70.4 \text{ in.}$$

## VOLUME

The **liter** (l) is the metric unit of volume. The common subdivisions and multiples of the liter are as follows:

| | |
|---|---|
| 1000 milliliters (ml) | = 1 liter (l) |
| 1000 cubic centimeters (cc)* | = 1 liter (l) |
| 1000 cubic centimeters (cc) | = 1000 milliliters (ml) |
| 1 cubic centimeter (cc) | = 1 milliliter (ml) |

Conversion equations for volume are as follows:

| | |
|---|---|
| 1 liter (l) | = 1.1 quart (qt) |
| 1 fluid ounce (fl oz) | = 30 milliliters (ml) |
| | or cubic centimeters (cc) |
| 1 gallon (gal) | = 3.8 liters (l) |

## Example

A syringe containing 1/3 (0.33 oz) of a fluid ounce of a medication would be equal to how many milliliters (ml) or cubic centimeters (cc)?

$$1 \text{ fl oz} = 30 \text{ ml (or cc)} \quad \text{or} \quad 30 \text{ ml (cc)/fl oz}$$
$$\frac{0.33 \text{ oz}}{1} \times \frac{30 \text{ ml (cc)}}{1 \text{ oz}} = \frac{0.33 \times 30 \text{ ml (cc)}}{1} = 9.9 \text{ ml (cc)}$$

---

* Also abbreviated $cm^3$.

## WEIGHT OR MASS

The metric unit of weight or mass is the **kilogram** (kg). Most of the weight measurements you will encounter will be considerably smaller than a kilogram. The common subdivisions and conversion factors for the kilogram are as follows:

$$1 \text{ kilogram (kg)} = 1000 \text{ grams (g)}$$
$$1 \text{ gram (g)} \quad = 1000 \text{ milligrams (mg)}$$

Conversion equations for weight or mass:

$$1 \text{ pound (lb)} \quad = 454 \text{ grams (g)}$$
$$1 \text{ kilogram (kg)} = 2.2 \text{ pounds (lb)}$$
$$1 \text{ gram (g)} \quad = 15 \text{ grains}$$

### Example

A patient's weight was measured as 165 lb. Convert this weight to kilograms (kg).

$$1 \text{ kilogram (kg)} = 2.2 \text{ lb} \quad \text{or} \quad 2.2 \text{ lb/kg}$$
$$\frac{165 \text{ lb}}{1} \times \frac{1 \text{ kg}}{2.2 \text{ lb}} = \frac{165 \times 1 \text{ kg}}{2.2} = 75.0 \text{ kg.}$$

## 2   DENSITY

**Density** is the mass (quantity) of a substance contained in a certain volume.

$$\text{Density} = \frac{\text{mass}}{\text{volume}} \quad \text{or} \quad D = \frac{M}{V}$$

From this formula, one can manipulate the symbols and calculate the following equations:

$$M = D \times V \quad \text{and} \quad V = \frac{M}{D}$$

A dense substance is one that has a large amount of mass in a small volume. The units that accompany density measurements are a combination of weight and volume: g/ml, lb/ft³, mg/liter.

### Examples

1.  What is the density of water* if 15 ml weighs 15 g?
$$D = \frac{M}{V} = \frac{15 \text{ g}}{15 \text{ ml}} = \frac{1 \text{ g}}{\text{ml}}$$

---

* The density of water is important to know, especially for calculating specific gravity.

2.  What is the density of blood if 10 ml (cc) weighs 10.54 g?
$$D = \frac{M}{V} = \frac{10.54 \text{ g}}{10.00 \text{ ml}} = 1.054 \frac{\text{g}}{\text{ml}}$$

3.  What is the density of urine if 15 cc weighs 15.150 g?
$$D = \frac{M}{V} = \frac{15.150 \text{ g}}{15.000 \text{ cc}} = 1.010 \frac{\text{g}}{\text{cc}}$$

## 3   SPECIFIC GRAVITY: CALCULATIONS AND EXAMPLES

**Specific gravity** is a measurement that is used to compare the weights and densities of different substances. Specific gravity is a measurement that expresses the relative mass of one liquid compared to that of another. Specific gravity can be calculated in two ways. One way is to measure the mass of a given volume of a substance and divide it by the mass of an equal volume of water. Another way is to measure the density of a substance and divide it by the density of water. To illustrate this, we will compare the specific gravity of whole blood, urine, and cerebrospinal fluid. Figure 1–2 shows water

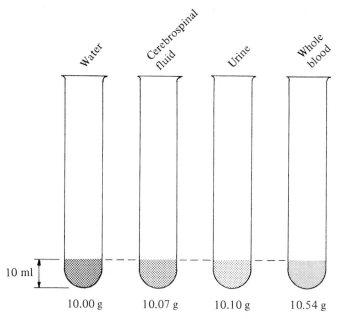

**Figure 1-2.** The weights of 10 ml of cerebrospinal fluid, urine, and whole blood are compared to the weight of 10 ml of water. The specific gravity of these body fluids can be calculated by the formula: specific gravity (S.G.) = mass of substance/mass of equal volume of water.

and three important body fluids upon which specific gravity tests are performed to help in diagnosing certain diseases. Notice that each tube contains an equal volume (10 ml) of fluid, and the weight and the density of each fluid are given. The method for calculating the specific gravity of each fluid is as follows:

$$\text{Specific gravity (S.G.)} = \frac{\text{mass of substance}}{\text{mass of equal volume of water}}$$

$$\text{Specific gravity (S.G.)} = \frac{\text{density of substance}}{\text{density of water}}$$

### FOR WHOLE BLOOD

$$\frac{10.54 \text{ g}}{10.00 \text{ g}} = 1.054 \text{ specific gravity (S.G.)}$$

$$\frac{1.054 \frac{\text{g}}{\text{cc}}}{1.000 \frac{\text{g}}{\text{cc}}} = 1.054 \text{ specific gravity (S.G.)}$$

### FOR URINE

$$\frac{10.10 \text{ g}}{10.00 \text{ g}} = 1.010 \text{ specific gravity (S.G.)}$$

$$\frac{1.010 \frac{\text{g}}{\text{cc}}}{1.000 \frac{\text{g}}{\text{cc}}} = 1.010 \text{ specific gravity (S.G.)}$$

### FOR CEREBROSPINAL FLUID

$$\frac{10.07 \text{ g}}{10.00 \text{ g}} = 1.007 \text{ specific gravity (S.G.)}$$

$$\frac{1.007 \frac{\text{g}}{\text{cc}}}{1.000 \frac{\text{g}}{\text{cc}}} = 1.007 \text{ specific gravity (S.G.)}$$

Notice two things about these examples of specific gravity. First, specific gravity is a number without a unit. The units cancel when specific gravity is calculated. The number is indicative of how much heavier or lighter a substance is than water. In other words, whole blood, urine, and cerebrospinal fluid are all slightly heavier than water. Second, since the density of water (1.000 g/cc or g/ml) is a constant, then *the density of a liquid is numerically equal to its specific gravity.*

# 4 TEMPERATURE SCALES, MEASUREMENTS, AND CONVERSIONS

## TEMPERATURE SCALES

Temperature measurements that are used in normal daily activities are in terms of degrees Fahrenheit (°F) even though the °F are often not stated. In scientific areas, temperature measurements must specify the unit since several temperature units may be used. In chemistry, the **Celsius**\* (centigrade) (°C) temperature scale is most commonly used.

If you were to place Celsius and Fahrenheit thermometers into a container of ice and water, the temperature reading on each thermometer would be different. Almost everyone knows that the freezing point of water is 32°F, but on the Celsius thermometer the temperature would be 0°C. A difference in temperature readings also would be evident if these thermometers were placed in boiling water, 212°F and 100°C (Figure 1–3). The boiling and freezing points of water are used as points of reference on these thermometers. On the Celsius scale there are 100 degrees (0°C to 100°C) between the freezing and boiling points. There are 180 degrees (32°F to 212°F) between the freezing and boiling points on the Fahrenheit scale (Figure 1–3). There is a 32° (32°F and 0°C) difference between the freezing points on the Fahrenheit and Celsius scales.

## TEMPERATURE CONVERSIONS

Converting Fahrenheit temperatures to Celsius, and vice versa, is based on the ratio of 180 divisions on the Fahrenheit scale and 100 divisions on the Celsius scale.

$$\frac{180}{100} = \frac{9}{5} = 1.8$$
$$1°C = 1.8°F$$

The relationship between these two scales is 9/5 or 1.8. In other words, 1°C equals 1.8°F. Remember also that the difference between freezing points on the scales is 32°. Using these figures, one now can make conversions between the scales. Conversion formulas and examples are as follows:

---

\* Celsius is the accepted official international scientific temperature scale, but it is frequently called the centigrade scale.

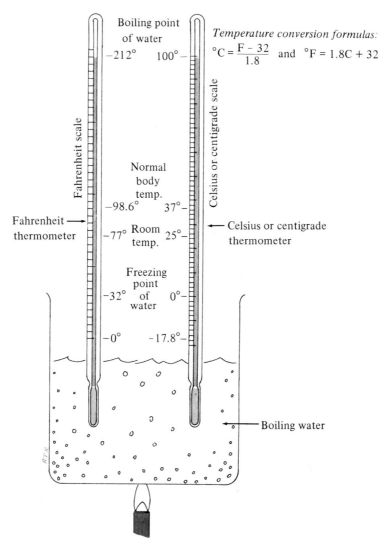

**Figure 1-3.** The temperature of boiling water varies on the Fahrenheit and Celsius thermometers as do other temperatures we commonly measure.

$$^\circ C = \frac{^\circ F - 32}{1.8} \quad \text{or} \quad ^\circ C = \frac{5(^\circ F - 32)}{9}$$

$$^\circ F = 1.8^\circ C + 32 \quad \text{or} \quad ^\circ F = \frac{9}{5}^\circ C + 32$$

### Examples

1. The normal body temperature is 98.6°F. Convert this to normal body temperature on the Celsius scale.

$$^\circ C = \frac{^\circ F - 32}{1.8} \qquad ^\circ C = \frac{5(^\circ F - 32)}{9}$$

$$= \frac{98.6 - 32.0}{1.8} \quad \text{OR} \quad = \frac{5(98.6 - 32.0)}{9}$$

$$^\circ C = \frac{66.6}{1.8} = 37.0^\circ C \qquad ^\circ C = \frac{5(66.6)}{9} = \frac{333.0}{9} = 37^\circ C$$

$$98.6^\circ F = 37^\circ C$$

2. The normal boiling point of water on the Celsius scale is 100°C. Convert this to the proper temperature on the Fahrenheit scale.

$$^\circ F = 1.8^\circ C + 32 \qquad\qquad ^\circ F = \frac{9}{5}^\circ C + 32$$

$$= 1.8(100^\circ) + 32 \quad \text{OR} \quad = \frac{9}{5}(100) + 32$$

$$^\circ F = 180 + 32 = 212^\circ F \qquad ^\circ F = 180 + 32 = 212^\circ F$$

$$100^\circ C = 212^\circ F$$

# SUMMARY

**The Metric System**
A. Length: meter (m) is the metric unit of length.
B. Volume: liter (l) is the metric unit of volume.
C. Weight or mass: kilogram (kg) is the unit of weight or mass.

**Density:** mass (quantity) of a substance contained in a certain volume.

$$\text{Density} = \frac{\text{mass}}{\text{volume}} \quad \text{or} \quad D = \frac{M}{V}$$

**Specific Gravity:** Calculations and Examples
Specific gravity is the measurement used to compare the weights and densities of different substances.

$$\text{Specific gravity (S.G.)} = \frac{\text{mass of substance}}{\text{mass of equal volume of } H_2O}$$

**Temperature Scales, Measurements, and Conversions**
A. Temperature scales: Fahrenheit (°F)  32°    to    212°
                                        freezing      boiling
           Celsius (°C)          0°    to    100°
                                        freezing      boiling

B. Temperature conversions:

$$\frac{180}{100} = \frac{9}{5} = 1.8 \qquad °C = \frac{5(°F\ 1\ 32)}{9} \quad \text{or} \quad \frac{°F\ 1\ 32}{1.8}$$

$$1°C = 1.8°F \qquad °F = \frac{9}{5}°C + 32 \quad \text{or} \quad 1.8°C + 32$$

## Units and Methods of Measurement

Matching: Questions 1 to 5; each answer may be used only once.

1. metric unit of length                                  **A.** density
2. unit of weight or mass                                 **B.** liter (l)
3. metric unit of volume                                  **C.** specific gravity
4. mass of substance contained in a certain volume        **D.** gram (g)
5. compares weights and densities of different substances **E.** meter (m)

6. A patient is 5 ft 9 in. tall. Convert this to centimeters (1 in. = 2.5 cm).

    (a) 174.5 cm    (b) 192.5 cm    (c) 172.5 cm    (d) 150 cm    (e) None of these

7. An adult weighing 70 kg weighs _____ lb (1 kg = 2.2 lb).

    (a) 174         (b) 145         (c) 164         (d) 140 lb.       (e) None of these

8. A person contains 5 quarts of blood. This is _____ liters (l) of blood (1 l = 1.1 qt).

    (a) 5.5         (b) 4.5         (c) 3.5         (d) 5.0           (e) None of these

9. When calculating the density of a fluid, the formula is

    (a) $m = D \times V$    (b) $D = \dfrac{M}{V}$    (c) $V = \dfrac{m}{D}$    (d) $\dfrac{\text{density of substance}}{\text{density of water}}$

    (e) None of these

10. A patient's temperature is 98.6°F. This is equal to _____ °C [°C $= \dfrac{5 \ (^\circ F - 32)}{9}$ or $\dfrac{^\circ F - 32}{1.8}$ ].

    (a) 37.0        (b) 39.3        (c) 38.5        (d) 0             (e) None of these

11. A 10-ml tube of blood has a density of 1.054 g/cc. The specific gravity of the blood is _____ (density of water = 1.000 g/cc).

    (a) 1.010       (b) 1.007       (c) 10.54       (d) 1.054        (e) None of these

12. Mrs. G. gave birth to a child that weighed $7\frac{1}{2}$ lb or 7 lb 8 oz. How many kilograms does the child weigh? (16 oz = 1 lb and 1 lb = 454 g.)

    (a) 34          (b) 3405        (c) 3.4         (d) 68           (e) None of these

13. A patient has a temperature of 38.2°C. This temperature in °F is _____ .

    (a) 100.8       (b) 108.0       (c) 101.8       (d) 68.8         (e) None of these

14. A patient has a temperature of 102.5°F. This temperature in °C is _____ .

    (a) 37.2        (b) 38.5        (c) 38.8        (d) 39.2         (e) None of these

# Chapter 2

# CHEMISTRY OF THE BODY

After reading and studying this chapter, a student should be able to:

1. Differentiate between mass and weight.
2. Name and describe the three physical states of matter.
3. Name and describe the three subatomic particles composing an atom.
4. Identify the energy levels of an atom (starting at nucleus) and number of electrons each one holds.
5. Write the chemical symbol and specific atomic weight, atomic number, and mass number for oxygen, carbon, nitrogen, and hydrogen atoms.
6. Define an isotope.
7. Define energy and give an example of each form.
8. Define and differentiate between a calorie and a kcalorie.
9. Describe the structure of an ATP molecule.
10. Define and differentiate among element, compound, and mixture, and give an example of each.
11. Describe and recognize an ionic and covalent chemical bond.
12. Describe and recognize an endergonic and exergonic chemical reaction.
13. Describe and recognize synthesis, decomposition, exchange, and oxidation–reduction reactions.
14. Describe the four factors that determine the speed of chemical reactions.
15. Define and recognize examples of an acid and a base.   Describe a pH scale.
16. Describe the components of a buffer system and how they work.
17. Define and recognize an example of a salt.
18. Identify and give functions of each of the four inorganic compounds described in this chapter.
19. Identify the basic chemical building blocks and the functions of carbohydrates, lipids, proteins, and nucleic acids.

*Often one hears students say, "Why do I need to learn chemistry and how will it help me if I am going to study nursing or some paramedical area?" This question can be answered by stating that all living material in the body is composed of various chemicals such as elements, compounds, and mixtures. The ability to read the words on this page is made possible partly because of chemical reactions. All the activities necessary to maintain the body in a normal state involve chemical reactions. Chemistry knowledge is vital to understand the normal and abnormal structure and functions of the body.* **Chemistry can be defined as a science concerned with the composition and properties of substances, the changes they undergo, and the energy relationships involved in these changes.**

# 1  LIVING MATTER

**Matter** is anything that occupies space and has weight. Everything that we can see or feel is matter. All the obvious organs and parts of the body such as the heart, kidneys, liver, and stomach are composed of matter. Even things we cannot see, such as oxygen and carbon dioxide gases, are composed of matter. To better understand matter, the term weight and the way it relates to mass will be discussed next.

## MASS AND WEIGHT

**Mass** is a term that designates the quantity of matter. Mass is expressed in terms of grams, pounds, and ounces, but the meaning of mass is slightly different from weight. The quantity in an object—or its mass—is constant, and does not vary even if the location of the object is changed. **Weight** is the amount of attraction between two objects, and it varies with the position of the two objects. If you stepped on a scale, and it registered 105 lb, this weight is actually a measure of the gravitational attraction between your body and the earth. If you were an astronaut on the moon, your weight would be slightly over 20 lb, since the moon's gravitational attraction is about one-fifth that of the earth's. However, the quantity of matter (mass) making up your body is the same on earth as on the moon. Scientists usually are interested in the mass of objects; however, the terms mass and weight are often used interchangeably.

## PHYSICAL STATES OF MATTER

Matter exists in three states: solid, liquid, and gas. All three of these can be found everywhere in the environment, as well as in the human body.

### Solid

Solids (Figure 2-1) have a definite shape and volume. The particles making up a solid are held together firmly and closely. *Examples:* protein structure of cell membranes, bone tissue, ice.

### Liquid

Liquids (Figure 2-1) have a definite volume but take on the shape of the container into which they flow. In a liquid, the particles are farther apart and more active than in a solid. *Examples:* blood (the liquid part or the plasma), tissue fluids, water.

Blood, tissue fluids, and water are maintained in fairly constant volumes in the body, but their shape depends on the container (blood vessels, stomach, or cells) they are in.

### Gas

Gases (Figure 2-1) have an indefinite shape and volume. The particles are farther apart and are moving more rapidly compared to particles in a liquid or a solid. *Examples:* oxygen in blood and lungs, carbon dioxide in blood and lungs, water vapor. Gases have another

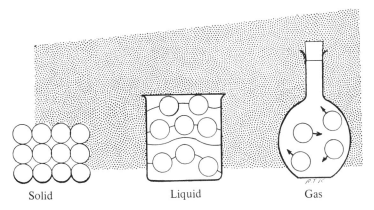

**Figure 2-1.** Physical states of matter. The characteristics of each physical state are determined by how close together the atoms are and by their activity.

feature, and that is compressibility. They can be compressed into a smaller area, resulting in gas pressure. The pressures exerted by $O_2$ and $CO_2$ gases are very important for respiration.

## STRUCTURE OF MATTER

Matter is made up of many, many small particles called atoms. An atom is the basic building block of all types of matter. Each atom is composed of a central nucleus and three fundamental types of subatomic particles: protons, neutrons, and electrons (Figure 2–2). There are other subatomic particles that result from nuclear reactions.

The nucleus is the dense central core of an atom.

Almost all the mass of an atom is contained in the nucleus.

Two types of particles are found in the nucleus and one type outside the nucleus.

1. *Protons.* Particles with a positive electrical charge of + 1. The weight of a proton is one atomic mass unit, and the number of protons in an atom equals the number of electrons.
2. *Neutrons.* Particles lacking an electrical charge or having a charge of zero (0). The weight of a neutron is about one atomic mass unit.
3. *Electrons.* Electrons are located outside the nucleus and have an electrical charge of minus one (– 1). The weight is 1/1836 of an atomic mass unit. In the normal stable atom, the number of electrons (– charge)

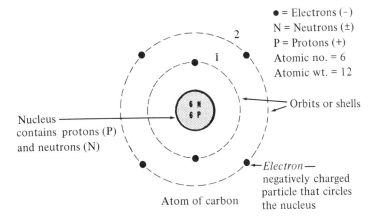

**Figure 2-2.** Structure of atoms. This is a model of an atom and not intended to represent what atoms actually look like.

is equal to the number of protons (+ charge) in the nucleus.

The nucleus has a positive (+) electrical charge because of the protons. The electrons with a negative electrical charge are attracted to and circle around the positively charged nucleus. Positive and negative electrically charged particles are attracted to each other, whereas like charges (+ and + or − and −) repel each other. The total charge on an atom is zero since the number of positive charges in the nucleus is balanced by the number of negative charges surrounding the nucleus. Chemical reactions between atoms involve interaction of outer energy level electrons in separate atoms.

### Energy Levels and Locations of Electrons in Atoms

Electrons circle around the nucleus (Figure 2-2) in various **energy levels** (also called orbits or shells). The energy levels (shells) are numbered starting at the nucleus and working outward. Each shell holds only a specific number of electrons, as shown in Figure 2-2. When the necessary number is present to fill a shell, it is complete and stable. The shell nearest the nucleus is filled with electrons first, then the second shell, and so forth. This sequence occurs because the attraction between the positively charged nucleus and the negatively charged electrons is greatest at the first energy level and gradually decreases in the more distant levels. Each or-

bit strives for stability, which means acquiring its maximum number of electrons; however, each orbit is considered stable (except for the first) when it contains eight electrons, even though its maximum number may be higher (Figure 2-3). If the outer orbit of atoms contains less than eight electrons, the outer orbit electrons of separate atoms interact to achieve stability.

This interaction of outer orbit electrons is called a **chemical reaction.** All the preceding can probably be better understood by comparing the four most common atoms in the human body (Figure 2-3). Notice that carbon has four electrons in its outer orbit, oxygen has six, nitrogen has five, and hydrogen has one. Eight electrons in the outer orbit make an atom stable with the exception of the first orbit, which needs only two. Carbon needs four electrons in its outer shell, oxygen two, nitrogen three, and hydrogen one to be stable.

### Valence

**Valence** (bonding capacity) is the number of electrons an atom needs to share, acquire, or give up to have a stable outer orbit. It also is the number of bonds that an atom can form with other atoms. For example, Table 2-1 shows that sodium (Na) has a valence of + 1, and that chlorine (Cl) has a valence of − 1. This means that Na will lose one electron from its outer orbit, whereas Cl will gain one. When you look at Figure 2-7 you can see that these losses and gains will make the outer electron orbits of Na and Cl stable. More importantly, a bond is formed between Na and Cl as described in Chapter 3.

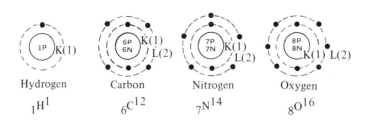

Hydrogen $_1H^1$    Carbon $_6C^{12}$    Nitrogen $_7N^{14}$    Oxygen $_8O^{16}$

Note: The upper number indicates the atomic mass and the lower one the atomic number.

| Energy Levels | Electron Distribution in Atoms | | | | | | |
|---|---|---|---|---|---|---|---|
| Level number | 1 | 2 | 3 | 4 | 5 | 6 | 7 |
| Shell number | K | L | M | N | O | P | Q |
| Maximum number of electrons | 2 | 8 | 18 | 32 | 32 | 18 | 2 |

**Figure 2-3.** The four most common atoms in the human body. Under each atom is its symbol with its atomic number and atomic mass number. The energy levels are indicated by numbers and shell letters with maximum numbers of electrons that can be found in each.

## TABLE 2-1. Important Elements Found in the Human Body

| Element | Symbol | Atomic Number | Atomic Weight* | Valence |
|---------|--------|---------------|----------------|---------|
| Barium | Ba | 56 | 137.3 | +2 |
| Carbon | C | 6 | 12.0 | +4, −4 |
| Calcium | Ca | 20 | 40.1 | +2 |
| Chlorine | Cl | 17 | 35.5 | −1 |
| Cobalt | Co | 27 | 58.9 | +2 |
| Copper | Cu | 29 | 63.5 | +1, +2 |
| Fluorine | F | 9 | 19.0 | −1 |
| Iron | Fe | 26 | 55.8 | +2, +3 |
| Hydrogen | H | 1 | 1.0 | +1 |
| Iodine | I | 53 | 126.9 | −1 |
| Potassium | K | 19 | 39.1 | +1 |
| Lithium | Li | 3 | 6.9 | +1 |
| Molybdenum | Mo | 42 | 95.9 | +6 |
| Magnesium | Mg | 12 | 24.3 | +2, +4 |
| Manganese | Mn | 25 | 54.9 | +2 |
| Nitrogen | N | 7 | 14.0 | +5, +3, −3 |
| Sodium | Na | 11 | 23.0 | +1 |
| Nickel | Ni | 28 | 58.7 | +2 |
| Oxygen | O | 8 | 16.0 | −2 |
| Phosphorus | P | 15 | 31.0 | −3 |
| Sulfur | S | 16 | 32.1 | +6, +4, −2 |
| Silicon | Si | 14 | 28.1 | +4 |
| Vanadium | V | 23 | 50.9 | +5 |
| Zinc | Zn | 30 | 65.4 | +2 |

* These atomic weights are rounded values.

### Identification of Atoms: Symbols, Atomic Weight, Atomic Number, Mass Number, and Formula

How is one atom identified from another? We distinguish people from each other by their names or initials, weight, and age. Atoms can be distinguished from each other using similar criteria.

**SYMBOLS OF ATOMS AND ELEMENTS.** Writing the full name of atoms or elements (matter that contains only one kind of an atom) is very time consuming. Symbols are used as a shorthand way to refer to atoms and elements. Symbols are often the first letter of the name of an atom or element; carbon, hydrogen, oxygen, and nitrogen atoms are represented by the symbols C, H, O, and N, respectively. Since there are about 106 elements and only 26 letters in our alphabet, most elements are identified by two-letter symbols with only the first letter being capitalized. Sodium (Na) and Calcium (Ca) are two examples.

**ATOMIC NUMBERS OF ATOMS.** Another method used to distinguish atoms from one another is their atomic number (Table 2-1). *The atomic number of an atom is the number of protons in the nucleus.* Since a stable, neutral atom has as many electrons as protons, the atomic number indicates the number of protons and electrons present in a stable atom.

**ATOMIC MASS NUMBER.** Atomic mass number is the *total number of protons and neutrons in an atom.* The proton and neutron are assigned equal masses of 1 and, due to its small mass, the electron is ignored in calculating the atomic mass number of an atom. The mass number and atomic number of an atom can be represented as follows:

$_6C^{12}$ (6 = atomic number and 12 = atomic mass number)

$_8O^{16}$

$_7N^{14}$

**ATOMIC WEIGHT AND MOLECULAR WEIGHT.** **Atomic weight** is the relative weight of an atom compared to a standard, carbon 12 ($C^{12}$). This relative weight means that the weight of all atoms is not an actual weight but rather a weight that is relative to the weight of $C^{12}$, which has been arbitrarily set at 12. The atomic weights of atoms composing the 23 important elements found in the human body are given in Table 2-1.

Oxygen has an atomic weight of 16, which means that one oxygen atom is slightly heavier than a carbon atom but is 16 times heavier than a hydrogen atom, which has an atomic weight of 1. A sodium atom is almost twice as heavy as a carbon atom, and a carbon atom is 12 times heavier than a hydrogen atom.

The atomic mass number and atomic weight for an atom are very nearly the same and *unless great accuracy is required the atomic weight and atomic mass numbers may be considered identical.*

Molecular weight is the total weight of all the atoms that compose a molecule. $C_6H_{12}O_6$ is a molecule of glucose. This formula for glucose shows that one molecule is composed of 6 carbon, 12 hydrogen, and 6 oxygen atoms. When the weights of all these atoms are added up, the molecular weight of glucose is equal to 180.

### Isotopes

The number of protons and electrons within atoms of an element is always the same; therefore, the atomic number is always constant. The number of neutrons within atoms of an element can vary, resulting in dif-

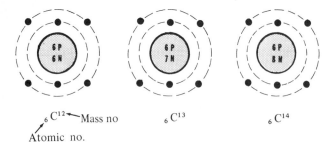

$_6C^{12}$—Mass no          $_6C^{13}$          $_6C^{14}$
Atomic no.

Figure 2-4.   Isotopes of carbon. The atomic number (number of protons) does not change in isotopes, but the number of neutrons and the mass number (number of protons + number of neutrons) do vary.

ferent mass numbers for an element. **Isotopes** are atoms of the same element that have a different number of neutrons; however, their number of protons and electrons remains the same. This means that an element can have varying mass numbers (number of protons plus number of neutrons). The element carbon, for example, is made up of three isotopes (Figure 2-4): $C^{12}$, $C^{13}$, $C^{14}$. Notice that the difference in mass number reflects the different number of neutrons that each isotope contains.

**STABLE AND RADIOACTIVE ISOTOPES.** Some isotopes are stable and their nuclei do not disintegrate or decay. This means that their nuclei do not give off radiation (energy) either in the form of particles or in energy waves. Other isotopes, called **radioactive isotopes** (radioisotopes), emit radioactive particles and energy waves.

As particles are given off the radioactive isotopes gradually change or decay into another element. The rate at which isotopes decay varies. The rate at which an isotope decays determines its **half-life**. *The half-life of an isotope is the amount of time required for half of the atoms in a given sample to decay.* Table 2-2 gives the half-life for some common and medically important isotopes. The radioisotope $^{131}I$, for example, has a half-life of about 8 days. A 50-mg sample, at the end of 8 days (one half-life period), would have decayed to where 25 mg are left. At the end of 16 days, two half-life periods,

half of the 25 mg or 12.5 mg would be left. Radioactive isotopes have half-lives of seconds, hours, days, and even thousands of years.

**MEDICAL IMPORTANCE OF RADIOACTIVE ISOTOPES.** Radioactive isotopes play an important role in medicine as *tagged atoms.* Two criteria for a good medical radioactive isotope are, *first,* a half-life that allows it to remain in the body long enough to be traced, but not long enough to be damaging, and *second,* it must be an element that the body normally uses. Table 2-2 lists some important medical radioactive isotopes and their medical importance. These radioactive atoms are important medically because their passage through the body can be followed by sensitive instruments such as a scanner or Geiger counter. These tagged atoms are used in the diagnosis and treatment of various disorders in the human body. The anatomic sites and physiologic processes in which these isotopes are important will be discussed later.

## 2   ENERGY

Up to now our discussion has dealt with matter and the various aspects of it. Although it is true that in the body everything that occupies space and has mass is composed of matter, the normal body functions could not take place if matter were not acted upon to produce energy. We stated previously that "all the activities necessary to maintain the body in a normal state involve chemical reactions." We can summarize these statements into word equations:

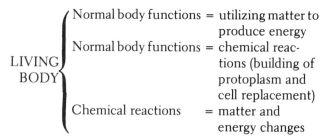

LIVING BODY { Normal body functions = utilizing matter to produce energy
Normal body functions = chemical reactions (building of protoplasm and cell replacement)
Chemical reactions = matter and energy changes }

TABLE 2-2.   *Medically Important Isotopes*

| Name | Half-Life | Medical Importance |
|---|---|---|
| $^{131}I$ (iodine 131) | 8.04 days | Used to diagnose and treat thyroid gland disorders |
| $^{60}Co$ (cobalt 60) | 5.2 years | Used in treatment of different kinds of cancer |
| $^{32}P$ (phosphorus 32) | 14.3 days | Used to help locate brain tumors |
| $^{24}Na$ (sodium 24) | 14.9 hours | Used to locate blood clots and determine whether amputation of a limb is necessary |

It is obvious that a "living body" involves two fundamental components: matter and energy. Death occurs when the body is no longer able to utilize matter to produce energy. What actually is energy? What does utilizing matter to produce energy actually mean? How is energy measured?

*Energy* is defined as the capacity for doing work. Unlike matter, energy neither occupies space nor has mass; therefore, it is an elusive concept since it lacks structure, physical characteristics, and mass. Energy can be classified into two kinds and five forms, four of which are important to the human body.

## KINDS OF ENERGY

**Potential energy** is stored or inactive energy. When released it is capable of causing an effect on matter. Food and the high-energy compound ATP (adenosine triphosphate) are examples of potential energy. Chemical reactions release the potential energy of these compounds, which is utilized by the body.

**Kinetic energy** is energy in action or energy that performs work. When potential energy is released it becomes kinetic energy. Examples of kinetic energy are muscles contracting, synthesis of chemical molecules, and transmission of nerve impulses.

## FORMS OF ENERGY

**Chemical energy** is energy that is present in chemical substances (Figure 2–5). The energy is present in the bonds making up the compounds. Food, such as carbohydrates, lipids, and proteins, contains potential chemical energy. Various bodily processes transform food substances from potential chemical energy to kinetic energy. This chemical kinetic energy is used by the body for muscle movement, nerve impulse transmission, and all activities in the human body. Chemical energy is the most basic form taken in and utilized by the body. Chemical energy is transformed or changed into the other three forms.

**Electrical energy** results from the flow of electrons (negatively charged particles) along a conductor or in the body from a negative wave of depolarization. Everyone uses electrical energy in everyday activities such as turning on a light, heating hair rollers, and toasting bread. In each of these examples electrons flow along a conductor—the electrical wire. In the human body the conductors are the nerves, and a wave of depolarization flows along the nerves (Figure 2–5). The normal functioning of the brain and nervous system is made possible only by the conduction of the wave of depolarization.

**Mechanical energy** is directly involved in moving

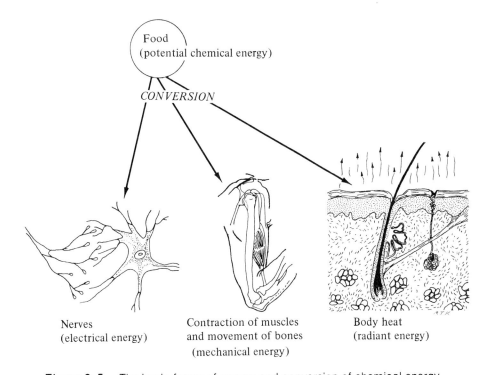

Nerves
(electrical energy)

Contraction of muscles
and movement of bones
(mechanical energy)

Body heat
(radiant energy)

**Figure 2-5.** The basic forms of energy and conversion of chemical energy.

matter. In the body, mechanical energy is utilized to contract muscles (Figure 2–5) that move the levers (bones) of the body. This total movement of muscles and bones is mechanical energy.

**Radiant energy** travels in waves. Heat and visible light are examples of radiant energy. Inside the body, heat is constantly given off from chemical reactions (Figure 2–5). Heat energy speeds up the particles composing matter. Speeding up the movements of particles is vital to chemical reactions in the body. Light energy enters the eye of an individual and starts a chemical process that initiates an electrical energy wave along the optic nerve to the brain.

### Transformation (Conversion) of Energy

Energy is constantly transformed from one form to another. The body primarily takes in potential chemical energy in the form of food of chemical energy; but as stated previously body activities require electrical, mechanical, and radiant energy. As a result of various chemical reactions, potential chemical energy in chemical bonds is transformed into radiant, mechanical, and electrical energy (Figure 2–5). This transformation process is vital if all the activities necessary to maintain life are to continue.

### Conservation of Energy and Matter

When potential chemical energy is converted into mechanical and electrical energy, not all the original energy is converted to these two forms. To an unsuspecting person it would appear that some of the energy is simply lost. What is the reason? Numerous studies on this concept have shown that the transformation of energy is never 100 percent efficient; some is always lost as heat. These studies led to the formulation of the laws of conservation of energy and matter:

---

*The first law of conservation or first law of thermodynamics* states that energy and matter can be neither created nor destroyed, but can be transformed from one form to another. Earlier we said that it appears as if energy is often lost. Energy is lost as a usable form, but it is not destroyed.

*The second law of conservation or second law of thermodynamics* states that an energy or matter transformation is never 100 percent efficient. Whenever energy or matter is transformed from one form to another some energy is dispersed into unusable heat. Normal body temperature of

---

98.6°F (37 °C) is maintained because of the loss of heat from chemical transformations.

---

## MEASUREMENT OF ENERGY

Chemical energy is the basic form of energy in the body, and it usually appears as heat energy. We use heat energy units to measure chemical energy. The metric unit of heat energy is called a joule (J). A joule is the amount of heat required to raise the temperature of one gram of water one degree Celsius.

The **kilocalorie** (food calorie or large calorie) is used when measuring the heat energy of the body and the nutritional value of foods. It is abbreviated Cal. with a capital "C." *The kilocalorie is equal to 1000 gram calories (cal).*

One gram calorie (cal) or small calorie is the amount of heat required to raise the temperature of one gram of water one degree Celsius.

The kilocalorie (Cal) or food calorie or large calorie is used when measuring the heat energy of the body and the nutritional value of foods. One kilocalorie is defined as the amount of heat required to raise the temperature of 1000 grams of water one degree on the Celsius scale.

Almost any food you eat contains calories (Cal). These calories are large calories or food calories and are the calories that you count when you are on a diet. Three basic food categories produce calories in the body: lipids (fat), carbohydrates, and proteins. Lipids produce 9 Cal/g, carbohydrates 4 Cal/g, and proteins 4 Cal/g.

## ATP (ENERGY CURRENCY OF CELLS)

An important high-energy compound found in the human body is **ATP** (adenosine triphosphate). This compound is found in all body cells and releases stored energy for various cellular activities (muscle contractions, nerve impulses). ATP consists of adenosine with three phosphate groups attached to it. The two end phosphate groups are called high-energy phosphate groups. The bonds between these phosphate groups release four to six times more energy when broken than any other chemical bonds. Wavy bond lines ( ~ ) are used to indicate the high-energy content of these bonds.

adenosine-$PO_4 \sim PO_4 \sim PO_4 \rightleftharpoons$
(ATP)

adenosine-$PO_4 \sim PO_4 \sim + PO_4 +$ energy
(ADP)

As indicated, when one $PO_4$ is broken off, energy is released. Each cell has a limited amount of ATP; therefore, each cell must manufacture ATP. This is possible by combining adenosine diphosphate (ADP) + $PO_4 \rightarrow$ ATP. The energy necessary for this remanufacture comes from various sources inside cells.

# 3 CHEMICAL CHANGE

Before we can discuss chemical changes or reactions, we must first describe the classification of matter or the three categories of matter: elements, compounds, and mixtures. Previously, we discussed the three physical states of matter: solid, liquid, and gas. Each of these states can be a pure combination of only one type of atom or a combination of various atoms. To truly understand chemical changes, one must know what classification of matter is undergoing the chemical change.

## PROPERTIES OF ELEMENTS, COMPOUNDS, AND MIXTURES

### Elements

An **element** is matter that is composed of only one type of atom (Figure 2-6). Atoms are the basic building blocks of elements.

There are 92 naturally occurring elements on earth and 14 synthetic elements. Only 23 of these 106 elements are normally found in the body. Four elements (oxygen, hydrogen, nitrogen, and carbon) make up 96 percent of the body. Only oxygen and nitrogen gases are found in any appreciable quantity as pure uncombined elements. The other elements in the body are combined in various ways to form compounds. Compounds are the second classification of matter and will be discussed next.

### Compounds

A *compound* is a substance made up of two or more elements chemically bonded together (Figure 2-6). Any compound may be broken down into simpler substances. Another feature of a compound is that the elements are combined in a fixed ratio. Some of the important compounds found in the body are as follows:

| | |
|---|---|
| $H_2O$ (water) | Two hydrogen atoms combined with one oxygen atom |
| $C_6H_{12}O_6$ (glucose sugar) | Six carbon atoms, 12 hydrogen atoms, and 6 oxygen atoms combined |
| NaCl (sodium chloride) | Salt |
| $CO_2$ (carbon dioxide) | |

The basic "building block" of a compound is the molecule. A compound is made up of many, many building blocks (molecules). A **molecule** is the smallest particle of a compound that exhibits the chemical characteristics of that compound. For example, water is composed of molecules that are made up of two hydrogen atoms and one oxygen atom. The molecules

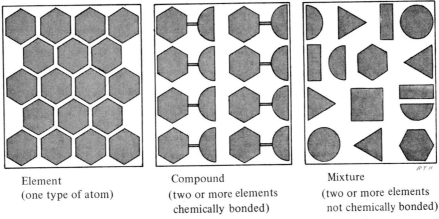

| Element | Compound | Mixture |
|---|---|---|
| (one type of atom) | (two or more elements chemically bonded) | (two or more elements not chemically bonded) |

Figure 2-6. These diagrams show the types of atoms that compose the three classes of matter (each symbol represents a different atom).

of compounds and atoms of elements are related since both are basic building blocks.

## Mixtures

The third classification of matter is the mixture. A **mixture** is two or more elements or compounds not chemically combined (Figure 2–6). The elements or compounds are dispersed together.

There are two types of mixtures, solutions and suspensions.

1. **Solution** A homogeneous mixture of two or more elements or compounds. In a solution, the substance present in the largest amount is called the **solvent.** The substances dissolved in the solvent are called the **solutes.** In the body the most common solvent is water. *Examples:* blood and urine
2. **Suspension** A nonhomogeneous mixture of two or more elements or compounds. A colloidal suspension is one that is composed of colloids suspended in a solvent. *Example:* protoplasm

## CHEMICAL BONDS

The atoms composing a molecule are joined together by chemical bonds. Previously, we stated that chemical bonds are formed when outer orbit electrons of atoms interact in their attempt to achieve stability. The continual attempt of atoms to achieve stability in their outer orbits is probably the main theme of chemistry. The methods by which atoms interact and form bonds are very important. Two major types of chemical bonds that bind atoms of molecules together are **ionic** and **covalent.**

### Ionic Bonds or Electrovalent Bonds

*An ionic bond is a bond formed between atoms when they lose and accept electrons.* The atoms that lose and gain electrons no longer have a neutral charge, but rather possess positive and negative charges respectively.

*These charged atoms are called positive and negative ions.* A simpler way to refer to these charged atoms is to call them **cations** ( + charge) and **anions** ( − charge). Oppositely charged ions are attracted to each other, resulting in a bond being formed between the cation and anion. An example showing the formation of an ionic bond is Figure 2–7. Notice that the sodium (Na) atom has one electron in its third and outer orbit, and the chlorine (Cl) atom has seven electrons in its third and outer orbit. Eight outer-orbit electrons give an atom stability; therefore, Na needs seven and Cl needs one electron to be stable. It is impossible for Na to pick up seven electrons for the third orbit, but it is possible for Na to lose the one outer orbit electron, making the second orbit stable. The Na atom is now a cation (positively charged) since it has one more proton that it has electrons. The Cl atom receives the electron lost by Na. It is now an anion (negatively charged) since it has one more electron than it has protons. The $Na^+$ (sodium ion) and $Cl^-$ (chloride ion) are attracted to each other because of their opposite electrical charges and form an electrovalent bond.

**IONIZATION OF IONIC COMPOUNDS.** When ionic compounds are placed in water they dissociate or break apart into cations and anions (Figure 2–8). This dissociation of ionic compounds is called **ionization.** A water solution with oppositely charged ions (electrolytes) is able to conduct an electrical current. This ionization process is one of the basic characteristics of ionic compounds and is shown in Equation 1.

Water molecules are actually responsible for pulling the ions apart. The characteristic of water that allows it to do this will be discussed later. An important point about ionization is that water molecules do not permanently break the ionic bonds. This can be demonstrated by removing the water molecules. The ions will reform ionic bonds once water is removed.

The ionization of ionic compounds is essential since the individual ions rather than the intact ionic compounds are important to the body (muscle contractions, nerve impulse transmissions, and development of bones). In other words, it is the sodium and chlorine

$$H_2O + NaCl \rightarrow Na^+ + Cl^- + H_2O$$

         (sodium          (sodium ion)     (chlorine ion)
         chloride)

$$H_2O + HCl \rightarrow H^+ + Cl^- + H_2O$$

        (hydrochloric     (hydrogen ion)   (chlorine ion)
        acid)

**Equation 1**   Ionization of NaCl and HCl are shown.

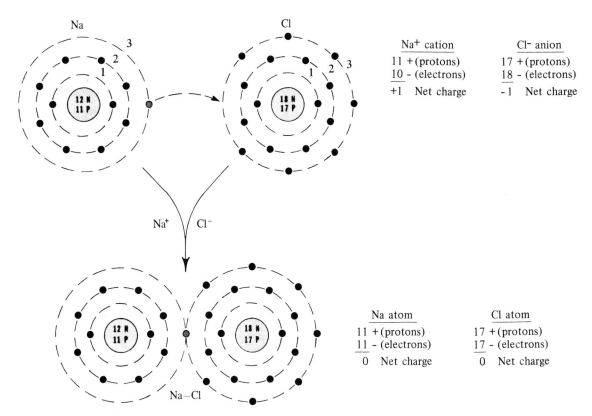

Na

Cl

Na⁺ cation

| 11 + (protons) |
| 10 - (electrons) |
| +1 Net charge |

Cl⁻ anion

| 17 + (protons) |
| 18 - (electrons) |
| - 1 Net charge |

Na⁺ Cl⁻

Na atom

| 11 + (protons) |
| 11 - (electrons) |
| 0 Net charge |

Cl atom

| 17 + (protons) |
| 17 - (electrons) |
| 0 Net charge |

Na—Cl

**Figure 2-7.** An ionic bond is formed when positively ( + ) and negatively ( − ) charged ions are attracted to each other.

ions that are important to the body and not the compound NaCl. Some common cations and anions important in the body, their quantities, and functions are listed in Table 2–3.

**ATOMS THAT LOSE ELECTRONS AND GAIN ELECTRONS.** In forming an ionic bond, one atom will always lose electrons (electron donor), and one atom will always take or accept electrons (electron acceptor). But which atoms lose electrons and which atoms accept them? Atoms with fewer than four electrons in the outer energy level tend to lose electrons, and those with more than four accept electrons. Some electron donors and acceptors are the following:

| Donors (Cations) | Acceptors (Anions) |
| --- | --- |
| (sodium) $Na \rightarrow Na^{1+}$ | (oxygen) $O \rightarrow O^{2-}$ |
| (potassium) $K \rightarrow K^{1+}$ | (chlorine) $Cl \rightarrow Cl^{1-}$ |
| (hydrogen) $H \rightarrow H^{1+}$ | (sulfur) $S \rightarrow S^{2-}$ |
| (calcium) $Ca \rightarrow Ca^{2+}$ | (iodine) $I \rightarrow I^{1-}$ |
| (iron) $Fe \rightarrow Fe^{3+}$ | |

**CATIONS, ANIONS, AND HOMEOSTASIS (STEADY STATE).** Homeostasis (steady state) is a dynamic state

of equilibrium of bodily processes. All body processes are controlled within certain limits or death will result. The term dynamic means that bodily processes can fluctuate within upper and lower limits. Table 2–3 indicates that cations and anions are involved in many bodily processes. As long as the blood levels of cations and anions are maintained within their normal ranges (Table 2–3), these respective processes will tend to be in homeostasis. An example of how the concentration of a cation can affect the homeostasis of a bodily process is $Ca^{2+}$ and muscle contractions. Table 2–3 shows that the normal range of $Ca^{2+}$ is

5.5 mEq*/liter—upper limit
4.7 mEq/liter— lower limit } normal range

As long as the level of blood $Ca^{2+}$ is maintained within this range (assuming everything else is also normal), muscle contractions will tend to be normal. However, if something happens to cause the $Ca^{2+}$ level to drop below 4.7 mEq/liter (say to 4.5 mEq/liter), then the $Ca^{2+}$ homeostasis is upset, which can cause certain muscles to abnormally contract. In other words, the af-

---

* Milliequivalent (mEq).

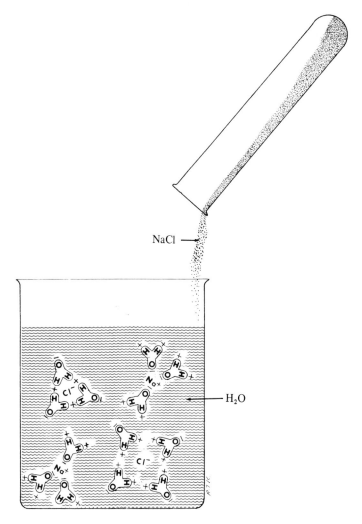

**Figure 2-8.** Ionic compounds ionize or dissociate when mixed with water molecules. The polarized water molecules surround the ions and prevent them from reestablishing ionic bonds.

fected muscles are not in homeostasis and muscle spasms result. These muscle spasms are common in facial and larynx muscles.

Maintaining homeostasis of body processes is very dependent upon the concentrations of the cations and anions in Table 2–3. Likewise, various body processes are important in maintaining the normal ranges of the cations and anions. **The concept of homeostasis is quite important in understanding the normal and abnormal functions of cells, tissues, and organs. As you proceed in studying this chapter and the following chapters, you will find homeostasis to be a recurring and unifying concept in your study of body processes.**

**POLYATOMIC IONS (RADICALS; COMPLEX IONS).** When some ionic compounds ionize, they ionize into **monoatomic** and **polyatomic** ions.

| | | Monoatomic ion | | Polyatomic ion |
|---|---|---|---|---|
| $H_2Co_3$ | $\longrightarrow$ | $H^+$ | $+$ | $HCO_3^-$ |
| Carbonic acid | | Hydrogen ion | | Bicarbonate ion |

In this example, carbonic acid ionizes into $H^+$ and $HCO_3^-$. $H^+$ is a monoatomic ion (one charged atom), whereas $HCO_3^-$ is a polyatomic ion (two or more charged atoms). **Radicals and complex ions are syn-**

### TABLE 2-3. Important Cations and Anions in the Body

| | Name | Concentration in Blood (mEq/liter) | Functions |
|---|---|---|---|
| Cations: | Na + Sodium | 133-146 | Normal functioning of nerves and muscles; maintenance of body fluid osmolarity |
| | K + Potassium | 3.8-5.6 | Maintenance of body fluid osmolarity; heart contractions; promotes cellular growth; skeletal muscle function |
| | $Ca^{2+}$ Calcium | 4.7-5.5 | Bone and teeth formation; muscle contraction; clotting of blood; maintenance of body fluid osmolarity |
| | $Mg^{2+}$ Magnesium | 1.0-3.0 | Body fluid osmolarity; activates some enzymes important for carbohydrate metabolism |
| Anions: | $HCO_3^-$ Bicarbonate | 21-31 | Helps to regulate acid-base balance |
| | $Cl^-$ Chloride | 98-108 | Maintenance of body fluid osmolarity |
| | $HPO_4^{2-}$ Phosphate (organic) | 1-3 | Maintenance of body fluid osmolarity; helps to regulate acid-base balance |
| | $SO_4^{2-}$ Sulfate | 0.5-2.0 | Maintenance of body fluid osmolarity |
| | Protein | 16-20 | Conduction of nerve impulses; maintenance of body fluid osmolarity |
| | Organic Acids | 2-6 | Maintenance of body of fluid osmolarity |

The concentrations of the cations and anions are expressed in terms of ranges rather than mean (average) values. These ranges may vary from source to source.

onyms for polyatomic ions. Table 2-3 lists five polyatomic ions (all of the anions except $Cl^-$) important in the body. Each example results from ionization of ionic compounds.

### Covalent Bonds

Many compounds, in fact most compounds, do not consist of ions. Covalent bonds are formed without the complete transfer of electrons from one atom to another. A **covalent bond** is a bond formed by the sharing of one or more pairs of electrons between compatible atoms. Every covalent bond involves the sharing of one electron by each of the reacting atoms. The electrons involved in covalent bonds are shared by the atoms and tend to circle the nucleus of each atom in the molecule.

Figure 2-9 shows the formation of water molecules by covalent bonds. Notice that the unbonded oxygen atom has six electrons in its outer orbit and therefore needs two more electrons to have eight and a stable outer orbit. Each hydrogen atom needs one more electron to be stable. The one oxygen atom and two hydrogen atoms share electrons, or form covalent bonds. The two hydrogen atoms each share their one electron with oxygen's six electrons, giving oxygen eight electrons and a stable outer orbit. Oxygen also shares two of its electrons (one with each of the hydrogen atoms). Notice that the shared electrons circulate around both the oxygen and hydrogen atoms. This sharing of electrons forms covalent bonds, which are much stronger than the ionic bonds discussed previously.

Not all covalent bonds involve only a single bond, sharing of one electron pair between two atoms. Many covalent compounds possess double or triple bonds. A double bond involves the sharing of two pairs of electrons between atoms (Figure 2-10). A triple bond involves the sharing of three pairs of electrons. Oxygen and nitrogen gas are examples of compounds possessing double and triple bonds. Nitrogen atoms need three

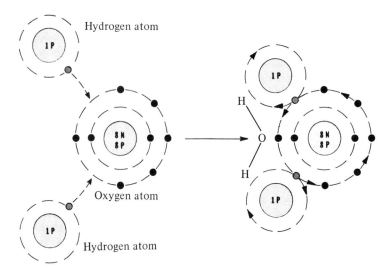

**Figure 2-9.** Covalent bonds are formed when some outer-orbit electrons are shared between atoms.

electrons to fill their outer shells; therefore, as shown in Figure 2–10, each nitrogen atom shares three of its electrons with the other nitrogen atom or forms a triple bond. For the sake of simplicity, a bond generally is represented by a line between two atoms. Two lines indicate a double bond and three lines indicate a triple bond.

### *Endergonic (Endothermic) and Exergonic (Exothermic) Reactions*

All the following types of chemical reactions involve an exchange of **free energy ($\Delta G$)**. The symbol $\Delta$ represents change and **G** represents free energy. The form of energy involved in chemical reactions is heat (radiant energy). On the basis of free energy exchange, there are two classes of chemical reactions, **endergonic** and **exergonic**.

**ENDERGONIC.** Endergonic reactions are energy-absorbing reactions. In other words, for the reactants to be able to interact and form products, heat must be added to the reactants. Normally, the reactants are able to absorb free energy from the surroundings, resulting in a

drop in temperature of the solution. At the completion of an endergonic reaction the amount of free energy in the solution is greater than it was at the beginning. This increase in free energy is represented by $+\Delta G$. An example is

$$6CO_2 + 12H_2O + 686\frac{kcal}{mole} \rightarrow C_6H_{12}O_6 +$$

$$6H_2O + 6O_2 \uparrow \quad \Delta G = +686\frac{kcal}{mole}$$

This example is photosynthesis in which green plants must take in large amounts of radiant energy (heat) in order to convert $CO_2$ and $H_2O$ to carbohydrates.

Notice in the endergonic example that the amount of heat required is written on the left side of the equation. In other words, heat is another reactant. Another endergonic example is shown in Equation 2.

This example shows that when the salt, ammonium nitrate, dissolves it absorbs energy. This compound is used in hospitals or first-aid stations to form a cold pack. A cold pack can be used to reduce swelling, remove heat from inflammation, and lessen the effect of hemorrhaging.

$$NH_4NO_{3\,(solid)} + Heat \xrightarrow{\;H_2O\;} NH_4^+{}_{(aqueous)} + NO_3^-{}_{(aqueous)} + \Delta G$$

Ammonium                Ammonium    Nitrate
nitrate                    ion         ion

**Equation 2** An endergonic reaction with heat as a reactant.

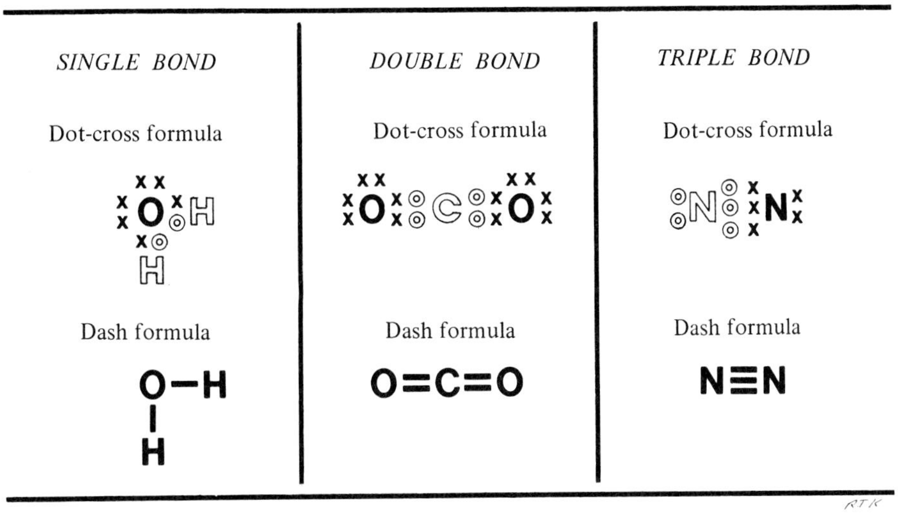

| SINGLE BOND | DOUBLE BOND | TRIPLE BOND |
|---|---|---|
| Dot-cross formula | Dot-cross formula | Dot-cross formula |
| | | |
| Dash formula | Dash formula | Dash formula |
| $O{-}H$ <br> $\mid$ <br> $H$ | $O{=}C{=}O$ | $N{\equiv}N$ |

Figure 2-10.  Single, double, and triple covalent bonds are represented by both the dot-cross and the dash formulas. Each dash in a covalent compound represents a shared pair of electrons.

**EXERGONIC.** Exergonic reactions release more energy than they absorb. At the completion of an exergonic reaction the amount of free energy in the solution is less than it was at the beginning. This decrease in free energy is represented by $-\Delta G$. An example of an exergonic reaction is

$$C_6H_{12}O_6 + 6O_2 \rightarrow 6CO_2 + H_2O + 686\,\frac{kcal}{mole}\quad \Delta G =$$

$$-686\,\frac{kcal}{mole}$$

This example is a summary of the reactions involved in breaking down glucose to form energy, which is a vital reaction for maintaining homeostasis of bodily functions. Notice in this example that heat is written on the right-hand side of the equation. This means that heat is a product of the reaction.

Another exergonic example is

$$\text{Ca Cl}_{2(solid)} \xrightarrow{H_2O} Ca^{+2}_{(aqueous)} + 2Cl^-_{(aqueous)} + \text{heat} - \Delta G$$
Calcium
chloride

Calcium chloride gives off much energy when dissolved in water and therefore can be used by hospitals in hot packs. The heat from the hot pack is effective in lessening aches and cramps, relaxing muscles, and increasing blood circulation.

## TYPES OF CHEMICAL REACTIONS

Chemical reactions are numerous and complex. They can be classified into four basic types: synthesis, decomposition, exchange, and oxidation–reduction.

### Synthesis (Combination)

**Synthesis** reactions involve two or more elements or an element and a compound chemically bonding together to form a more complex single compound.

$$\begin{array}{ccc} A & B & AB \\ ADP & + \; PO_4 & \rightarrow \; ATP \end{array}$$

Many synthesis reactions in the body (especially the synthesis of carbohydrates, lipids, and proteins) involve chemical removal of $H_2O$ from the reactants before the synthesis reaction can be completed. This type of synthesis reaction is called **dehydration synthesis.**

$$\begin{array}{ccc} A & B & AB \\ \text{Glucose} & + \; \text{Glucose} & \rightarrow \; \text{Maltose} + H_2O \end{array}$$

Synthesis reactions frequently take place inside cells and are the major type of reaction involved in anabolism (buildup phase of metabolism). Anabolic reactions frequently require more energy to be completed than they release and therefore are said to be **endergonic (endothermic).**

## Decomposition

**Decomposition** reactions are characterized by a compound decomposing into the elements that make it up, or into simpler compounds.

$$AB \longrightarrow A + B$$
$$ATP \longrightarrow ADP + PO_4$$

The decomposition of carbohydrates, lipids, and proteins in the digestive tract often is called **digestion** or **hydrolytic reaction**, since $H_2O$ plays a role in the decomposition.

$$\begin{array}{ccc} AB & _{+H_2O} & A & B \\ \text{Maltose} & \longrightarrow & \text{Glucose} + \text{Glucose} \\ \text{(Carbohydrate)} \end{array}$$

Absorbed molecules such as glucose, amino acids, and fats are decomposed into simpler compounds inside cells. This is the major type of reaction involved in catabolism (breakdown phase of metabolism). Catabolic reactions frequently release more energy than they absorb and therefore are said to be **exergonic (exothermic).**

## Exchange

An **exchange** reaction involves two compounds exchanging their positive and negative parts.

$$A^+ B^- + C^+ D^- \rightarrow A^+ D^- + C^+ B^-$$

Being able to predict which parts will exchange and combine with parts from another compound is not too difficult. As you can see, the positively charged (+) part will exchange and combine with the negatively (−) charged part, and vice versa. This type of reaction is typical of how ionic compounds react with each other. Another example of an exchange reaction in the body is the reaction of the carbonic acid–sodium bicarbonate buffer system with acids and bases as shown in Equation 3.

## Oxidation–Reduction (Redox)

**Oxidation** is the loss of electrons or acceptance of oxygen. **Reduction** is the gain of electrons or loss of oxygen. Oxidation–reduction reactions always occur together. If a compound is oxidized (loss of electrons), then another compound is reduced. Oxidation–reduction can take place in three different ways (Figure 2–11).

**Oxidation–reduction reactions in the body normally involve the loss of hydrogen atoms rather than individual electrons.** The loss of hydrogen atoms from one compound is often referred to as **dehydrogenation.**

Oxidation–reduction reactions are very important in the body because they result in the formation of the high-energy compound ATP in the cells.

| $A^+$ | $B^-$ | $C^+D^-$ | | $A^+D^-$ | $C^+B^-$ |
|---|---|---|---|---|---|
| $Na^+HCO_3^-$ | | $+ H^+Cl^-$ | $\rightleftharpoons$ | $Na^+Cl^-$ | $+ H^+HCO_3^-$ |
| Sodium bicarbonate | | Hydrochloric acid | | Sodium chloride | Carbonic acid |

| $A^+$ | $B^-$ | $C^+D^-$ | | $A^+D^-$ | $C^+B^-$ |
|---|---|---|---|---|---|
| $H^+HCO_3^-$ | | $+ Na^+OH^-$ | $\rightleftharpoons$ | $H^+OH^-$ | $- Na^+HCO_3^1$ |
| Carbonic acid | | Sodium hydroxide | | Water | Sodium bicarbonate |

**Equation 3**  Exchange reactions involving sodium bicarbonate and carbonic acid with hydrochloric acid and sodium hydroxide.

$$\begin{array}{l} \qquad\qquad \text{Molecule B} \\ \qquad\qquad \text{COOH} \\ \text{Molecule A} \qquad | \qquad\qquad\qquad\qquad \text{Molecule A} \quad \text{Molecule B} \\ \text{NADH}_2 \quad + \quad \text{C} = \text{O} \longrightarrow \text{NAD} \qquad \text{COOH} \\ \qquad\qquad | \qquad\qquad\qquad\qquad \text{(Oxidized)} \quad + \quad \text{H*}-\text{C}-\text{OH*} \\ \qquad\qquad \text{CH}_3 \qquad\qquad\qquad\qquad \text{(Lost 2 H} \qquad\qquad \text{CH}_3 \\ \qquad\qquad \text{Pyruvic acid} \qquad\qquad\quad \text{atoms)} \qquad\qquad \text{Lactic Acid} \\ \qquad\qquad\qquad\qquad\qquad\qquad\qquad\qquad\qquad\qquad \text{(Reduced) (Gained 2 H atoms)} \end{array}$$

**Equation 4**  The oxidation of $NADH_2$ to NAD and reduction of pyruvic acid to lactic acid.

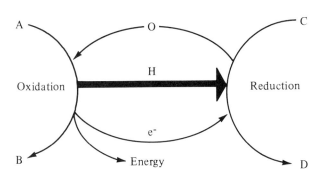

**Figure 2-11.** The characteristics of oxidation–reduction.

Equation 4 is an example of an oxidation-reduction reaction.

Oxidation–reduction reactions in the body tend to be *exergonic* (exothermic) with the release of energy. An example of this is the previous example of

$$C_6H_{12}O_6 + 6O_2 \rightarrow 6CO_2 + 6H_2O + energy \quad \Delta G =$$
$$-680\frac{kcal}{mole}$$

This example is a summarization of the many oxidation–reduction reactions that result in the release of 680 kcal/mole of energy. This series of oxidation–reduction reactions continuously occurs in the cells of the body and is frequently referred to as **cellular respiration. These oxidation–reduction reactions are absolutely vital since they result in the release of energy that is essential for maintaining the homeostasis of bodily processes.**

SUMMARY OF IMPORTANT POINTS ABOUT OXIDATION–REDUCTION

1. *Oxidation.* Loss of electrons, H atoms, or gain in O atoms

2. *Reduction.* A gain in electrons, H atoms, or loss of O atoms

3. *Compound oxidized.* Loses H atoms and becomes + charged (most common method of oxidation in body)

4. *Compound reduced.* Gains H atoms and becomes − charged (most common method of reduction in body)

5. *Exergonic (exothermic) reactions* (−ΔG). Oxidation–reduction reactions in body tend to release energy

6. *Vital reactions.* Oxidation-reduction reactions frequently occur in cells (often called cell respiration) and release energy vital for maintaining homeostasis of bodily processes.

# 4 FACTORS DETERMINING THE SPEED OF CHEMICAL REACTIONS

## FACTORS INFLUENCING THE SPEED OF CHEMICAL REACTIONS

Some chemical reactions, for example the natural destruction (decay) of wood, proceed very slowly. The body produces new tissues very slowly. Other reactions occur quite rapidly. The destruction of wood is speeded up by burning it. The neutralization of acids and bases in water solutions occurs almost simultaneously in the body. Four factors influence the speed of chemical reactions: (1) temperature of the reactants, (2) concentration of the reactants, (3) effect of catalysts (enzymes), and (4) amount of surface area exposed.

### Temperature of the Reactants

Chemical reactions are greatly affected by the temperature of reactants and temperature changes. There is a direct relationship between the temperature changes of solutions and the rates of chemical reactions. As the temperature increases, the speed of a reaction increases, and as the temperature decreases, the speed of a reaction decreases. It has been proven that the speed of a reaction doubles for every 10°C increase in temperature up to a certain temperature. A reaction rate takes place about eight times faster at 30°C than at 0°C.

Molecules in a chemical system are activated by an increase in temperature, which results in more effective collisions. The increase in effective collisions increases the speed of chemical reactions.

A slight change in body temperature can greatly increase activity of chemical molecules, thereby increasing the activity of chemical reactions throughout the body. The warmup period is vital to an athlete since it increases the rate of chemical reactions in the body and allows her or him to perform more effectively. When a patient has fever, the increase in temperature is followed by increases in pulse rate, respiration rate, and other body activities.

### Effect of Enzymes

Without enzymes, many vital chemical reactions in the body would occur so slowly that a person would probably die. An enzyme cannot cause a reaction to occur that would not normally occur, but it does bring normally occurring reactions to completion faster. In a chemical system, molecules with the right charge and electron needs will eventually collide and interact. An enzyme speeds up the interaction and lowers the energy of activation.

Many chemical reactions in the body have specific enzymes involved with the reaction. Some examples are the following:

$$Carbohydrates \xrightarrow[Amylases]{Enzymes} Simple\ sugars$$

$$Proteins \xrightarrow[Proteinases]{Enzymes} Amino\ acids$$

Enzymes will be discussed in more detail later.

### Amount of Surface Area Exposed

The rate of a chemical reaction is also dependent on the amount of surface area the reactants expose for reactions. A single large particle has little surface area available for reactions compared to the surface area that would be available if this single particle were broken into many small particles. The increased surface area increases the number of reactions; therefore, the reaction rate is speeded up.

Medications are often given in small-particle form to increase their rate of absorption and reaction rate in the body. Fats, taken into the body, often appear in large globular form with little surface area. Fat globules are broken into many small particles by bile, which is secreted from the gallbladder. The increased surface area allows enzymes to digest fat particles faster.

## 5   ACIDS–BASES, BUFFERS, AND SALTS

Some examples of chemical reactions that are quite prevalent and important in the body include the reactions of acids–bases, buffers, and salts.

## ACIDS AND BASES

### Acids

An **acid** is a substance that releases hydrogen ions in water solutions. A hydrogen ion ($H^+$) is a proton; therefore, an acid can also be defined as a substance that releases protons ($H^+$) in a water solution. This ability of an acid is diagrammed as follows:

$$HA \xrightarrow{H_2O} H^+ + A^-$$

Some specific examples of acids are

$$\underset{\substack{(Hydrochloric \\ acid)}}{HCl} \xrightarrow{H_2O} H^+ + \underset{(Chloride\ ion)}{Cl^-}$$

$$\underset{(Sulfuric\ acid)}{H_2SO_4} \xrightarrow{H_2O} H^+ + HSO_4 \rightarrow 2H^+ + \underset{(Sulfate\ ion)}{SO_4^{2-}}$$

Notice that every acid dissociates or forms ions (charged particles) in water solutions. The hydrogen ion ($H+$) combines with a water molecule to form a hydronium ion ($H_3O^+$).

### Bases

A **base** is a substance that gives up hydroxide ions ($OH^-$) or accepts hydrogen ions ($H^+$) in water solutions. The $H^+$ or proton is common to all acids, whereas bases either give up $OH^-$ or receive $H^+$ in water solutions. Diagrams and examples of these reactions are

$$\underset{(Base)}{B\!-\!OH} \xrightarrow{H_2O} B^+ + \underset{\substack{(Hydroxide \\ ion)}}{OH^-}$$

$$\underset{(Proton)}{H^+} + \underset{(Base)}{A^-} \longrightarrow HA$$

$$\underset{(Proton)}{H^+} + \underset{(Bicarbonate)}{HCO_3} \longrightarrow H_2CO_3$$

### pH Scale Measurement of $H^+$ and $OH^-$ Concentration

Previously, comments were made about the effects of dilute and concentrated acids and bases on the body. The numerical scale used to measure the degree of acidity and alkalinity is the **pH scale**.

The pH scale runs from 0 to 14 (Figure 2–12). The numbers below seven refer to acid solutions and those above seven to alkaline solutions. Notice in Figure 2–12

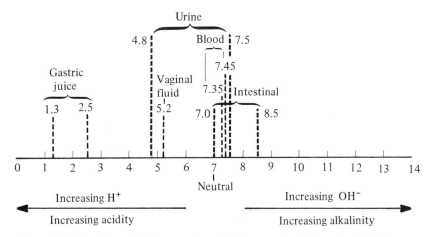

**Figure 2–12.** pH scale. Decreasing pH is increasing H$^+$ and acidity. Increasing pH is increasing OH$^-$ and alkalinity. Notice that several body fluids have a sizable pH range except blood, which has several mechanisms to maintain its narrow range.

that the concentration of H$^+$ progressively increases from 7 to 0. The concentration of OH$^-$ increases from 7 to 14. The concentration of H$^+$ and OH$^-$ at 7 is equal; therefore, this is the *neutral* point.

The pH scale is actually based on the concentration of H$^+$ in a solution. The actual measurements of the H$^+$ are logarithmic measurements, and pH = −log (H$^+$). This means that the scale is a **logarithmic progression** and not an arithmetic progression. If the pH scale were an arithmetic progression, pH = 2 would indicate twice the concentration of H$^+$ compared to pH = 1, and pH = 3 would be three times the concentration of H$^+$ compared to pH = 1. Since it is a logarithmic progression, a pH change of one unit is actually a tenfold change in H$^+$ concentration. For example, a solution of pH = 2 (H$^+$ = 0.01 mole/liter) has ten times fewer H$^+$ than does a solution of pH = 1 (H$^+$ = 0.1 mole/liter). A pH = 3 (H$^+$ = 0.001 mole/liter) has 100 times fewer H$^+$ than pH = 1. The point being emphasized here is that **a change of one pH unit is actually a tenfold change in hydrogen ion concentration.**

Notice in Figure 2–12 that as pH values decrease the acidity level increases. This always is a confusing point; however, just remember that

> Increasing acidity
> ───────────────────
> 0 1 2 3 4 5 6 7
> ───────────────────
> Decreasing pH values

and

> Decreasing acidity
> ───────────────────
> 0 1 2 3 4 5 6 7
> ───────────────────
> Increasing pH values

The alkaline part of the scale is logical in that as the alkalinity increases, the pH increases.

**MEASUREMENT OF pH.** The pH of a solution can be measured by a pH meter. A solution of known pH is placed under the electrodes, and the instrument is standardized. Then a solution of unknown pH is placed under the electrodes, and the pH registers on the scale of the instrument. Another method involves putting a drop of solution on special colorimetric indicator paper. The color of the paper is then matched with a set of permanent color standards to determine the pH of the unknown.

More than 75 compounds can be used as acid–base indicators; that is, they change colors depending on whether they are in an acidic or basic solution. Many of these are used in the liquid form. One very common indicator is phenolphthalein, which is pink in basic solutions and colorless in acidic solutions.

**pH VALUES OF BODY FLUIDS.** Hydrogen (H$^+$) and hydroxide (OH$^-$) ions are involved in various chemical reactions in living cells. Acids are constantly being formed in the body by metabolic activity. Substances that produce bases are constantly brought into the body in our food. H$^+$ and OH$^-$ are present in all the body fluids, giving them a characteristic pH value. Figure 2–12 shows the wide pH variation of body fluids. Cells are sensitive to changes in pH; in fact, if blood deviates only slightly from the narrow range of pH 7.3 to 7.5, all body functions can be affected and therefore the body will no longer be in a state of homeostasis.

**HYPERACIDITY, HYPOACIDITY, ACIDOSIS, AND ALKALOSIS.** Gastric juice in the stomach always contains hydrochloric acid (HCl) with a pH = 1.3 to 2.5. This pH varies during diseases, causing hyperacidity and hypoacidity. Hyperacidity is a condition in which the $H^+$ concentration is above normal, and the pH drops below 1.3. (Remember that an increase in $H^+$ is accompanied by a decrease in pH.) If hyperacidity persists in the stomach, ulcers can result. Hypoacidity is a condition in which the $H^+$ is below normal, and the pH rises above 2.5.

Acidosis is a condition in which the level of $H^+$ in body tissues and fluids is above normal. Acidosis is different from hyperacidity in that hyperacidity is limited to gastric juices, and acidosis can exist in all tissues of the body. Acidosis can result from intake of too much acidic material, faulty metabolism, or respiratory obstruction. Blood acidosis is indicated when the blood pH drops below 7.3. If the blood pH drops to 6.8, a person will die. Alkalosis is a condition in which the concentration of $H^+$ decreases and $OH^-$ increases. Alkalosis of the blood is characterized by an increase in pH above 7.5, and at 7.8 death occurs. These conditions, if persistent, can cause damage to body tissues and in extreme cases even death. The body has several ways of keeping the pH of body fluids in homeostasis. The buffer systems found in the blood help to maintain the narrow pH range.

## Buffers

A **buffer system** is a pair of compounds that resist changes in pH with addition of acids or bases. A buffer system is composed of a weak acid and a weak base (weak acid/weak base). The weak acid will react with a base, neutralizing it. The base neutralizes an acid. It does not matter whether an acid or base is added to a solution with a buffer in it; one member of the pair will react with either the acid or the base to neutralize it. The ultimate result will be that the buffer system will prevent the fluid from becoming more acid or base.

## Buffers Found in the Blood

The blood maintains a very narrow pH range, 7.3 to 7.5; therefore, it has several buffer pairs to maintain this range. Some of the buffers present in the blood are as follows.

**BUFFERS IN THE PLASMA (LIQUID PORTION OF THE BLOOD)**

$$\frac{H_2CO_3}{NaHCO_3} \quad \frac{\text{Carbonic acid (weak acid)}}{\text{Sodium bicarbonate (weak base)}}$$

$$\frac{NaH_2PO_4}{Na_2HPO_4} \quad \frac{\text{Monosodium phosphate (weak acid)}}{\text{Disodium phosphate (weak base)}}$$

$$\frac{\begin{matrix} R \\ | \\ {}^+H_3N-C-COOH \\ | \\ H \end{matrix}}{\begin{matrix} R \\ | \\ H_2N-C-COO^- \\ | \\ H \end{matrix}} \quad \begin{matrix} \text{Acid protein} \\ \\ \text{Base protein} \end{matrix}$$

**BUFFERS IN RED BLOOD CELLS**

$$\frac{HHbO_2}{KHbO_2} \quad \frac{\text{Acid oxyhemoglobin}}{\text{Alkaline oxyhemoglobin}}$$

$$\frac{KH_2PO_4}{K_2HPO_4} \quad \frac{\text{Acid potassium phosphate}}{\text{Alkaline potassium phosphate}}$$

## HOW DO BUFFER SYSTEMS WORK TO MAINTAIN OR RESTORE HOMEOSTASIS?

As an example of buffer action, let us look at what happens when hydrochloric acid (HCl) and sodium hydroxide (NaOH) are added to blood plasma. If a fairly large amount of HCl were added to the blood to where the pH dropped below 7.3, the pH would be below the normal homeostasis range. The following reaction would occur to restore the normal pH range.

$$\underset{\substack{\text{Sodium} \\ \text{bicarbonate} \\ \text{(base)}}}{H^+Cl^- + Na^+HCO_3} \longrightarrow \underset{\substack{\text{Sodium} \\ \text{chloride} \\ \text{(neutral} \\ \text{compound)}}}{Na^+Cl^-} + \underset{\substack{\text{Carbonic} \\ \text{acid} \\ \text{(weak acid} \\ \text{buffer)}}}{H_2CO_3}$$

Notice in this reaction that the base reacts with the acid, producing sodium chloride, which is neutral, and $H_2CO_3$. In effect, the sodium bicarbonate neutralizes the HCl so that the pH of the blood quits dropping into the acid range. The end result is that the pH of the blood will climb into the normal 7.35 to 7.45 range.

$$\text{NaOH} \quad + \quad \text{H}_2\text{CO}_3 \quad \longrightarrow \quad \text{NaHCO}_3 \quad + \quad \text{H}_2\text{O}$$

| | | | |
|---|---|---|---|
| Sodium hydroxide | Carbonic acid | Sodium bicarbonate | |
| (base) | (acid) | (buffer) | |

This reaction illustrates what happens when a basic compound enters the plasma so that the blood pH increases above 7.45. The weak acid of a buffer pair neutralizes the base, forming more buffer and water. These products have no effect on the blood pH, and again the buffer has resisted a change in the pH of the blood plasma. In all buffer reactions the weak acid reacts with a base to form more buffer and water; the base reacts with an acid to form more buffer and a salt.

The metabolic processes produce various acids such as hydrochloric, lactic, phosphoric, and sulfuric, which tend to cause the pH of the blood to drop into the acid range. To maintain and restore homeostasis of the blood, the base will constantly neutralize these acids and raise the pH into the normal range.

The bicarbonate buffer tends to play a minor role in regulating pH of the plasma, with phosphate buffers being more important and the protein buffers playing the largest role. The $\dfrac{\text{HHbO}_2 \text{ acid oxyhemoglobin}}{\text{KHbO}_2 \text{ base oxyhemoglobin}}$ buffer pair is the most important buffer in the red blood cells; in fact, it accounts for approximately 60 percent of the buffering done by the blood.

## SALTS

A **salt** is a compound often formed by the reaction of an acid with a base. A salt does not have a common ion like the $\text{H}^+$ and $\text{OH}^-$ of acids and bases; rather, it contains the negative ion of an acid linked to the positive ion of a base. Examples of salt formation are

| Acid | Base | Salt | Water |
|---|---|---|---|
| $\text{H}^+\text{Cl}^-$ + | $\text{K}^+\text{OH}^- \longrightarrow$ | $\text{KCl}$ | + $\text{H}_2\text{O}$ |
| | Potassium hydroxide | Potassium chloride | |
| $\text{HCl}$ + | $\text{NaOH} \longrightarrow$ | $\text{NaCl}$ | + $\text{H}_2\text{O}$ |
| | Sodium hydroxide | Sodium chloride | |

### Salts Are Ionic Compounds

A salt possesses ionic bonds binding the atoms together. The body cannot utilize salts in the ionic bonded ($\text{NaCl}$, $\text{KCl}$) form. The body utilizes ions (cations and anions) making up salts. For example, $\text{Na}^+$, $\text{K}^+$, $\text{Cl}^-$, $\text{Ca}^{2+}$, and $\text{PO}_4^-$ are what the body actually utilizes, to coordinate such activities as muscle contractions and nerve impulse transmissions.

The ions composing salts pull apart as salts dissolve in water. The water molecules are responsible for the initial and continual separation of ions.

## 6 INORGANIC COMPOUNDS IMPORTANT IN THE BODY

Chemistry is traditionally divided into inorganic and organic compounds. **Inorganic compounds** are all compounds that lack carbon atoms, bonded to hydrogens.

Several inorganic compounds important in the body have already been discussed—$\text{HCl}$, $\text{NaCl}$, $\text{H}_2\text{SO}_4$, and $\text{KCl}$. Some other important inorganic compounds that play major roles in the body are $\text{H}_2\text{O}$, $\text{CO}_2$, $\text{O}_2$, and $\text{NH}_3$.

### WATER ($H_2O$)

#### Water in the Body

Water is the most prevalent inorganic compound in the body. Water makes up 65 to 75 percent of our body weight. In other words, a person weighing 100 pounds actually contains about 65 to 75 pounds of water. From a quantity standpoint, water is obviously important. It is also involved in essential body processes, such as digestion, elimination, circulation, and regulation of body temperature.

#### Functions of Water Molecules in the Body

Water molecules are actively involved in several important roles in the body.

REACTANT.  A reactant is a substance that interacts with other substances to produce products. Water molecules are involved in various chemical reactions in the body. Ionic compounds are broken apart by water molecules. An example of this is

$$\text{NaCl} + \text{H}_2\text{O} \longrightarrow \text{Na}^+ + \text{Cl}^- + \text{H}_2\text{O}$$

The structure of the water molecule is responsible for pulling the NaCl molecule apart and for ionization of all ionic compounds.

The four major kinds of organic compounds (carbohydrates, lipids, proteins, and nucleic acids) are broken into their building blocks by water breaking their bonds or hydrolytic reactions. This process is illustrated later.

**SOLVENT.** A **solvent** is a fluid that causes a compound (solute) to dissolve, forming a solution. A **solute** is a substance that dissolves in a solvent. Water serves as the solvent for most chemical reactions in the body.

The success of water as a solvent is related to the chemical structure of water molecules. The oxygen atom of the water molecule tends to be negatively charged and the hydrogen atoms tend to be positively charged (Figure 2–13). The reason the oxygen atom in $H_2O$ is negatively charged can be seen in Figure 2–13. Oxygen has four unpaired electrons circling around it in addition to the electrons shared with the two hydrogen atoms. This quantity of negative charges circling the oxygen atom gives it a negative charge. Since the hydrogen atoms have fewer electrons they tend to be positively charged. The water molecule then can be described as having positive and negative poles, or it is a **dipole.** Any chemical molecule that has positive and negative regions is said to exhibit **polarity** or it is a **polar molecule.**

This polar characteristic of water is what makes it such a good solvent. An example of how $H_2O$ operates as a solvent is shown in Figure 2–8. Notice that the $Na^+$ ions are surrounded by $H_2O$ molecules with the negative end oriented toward the $Na^+$. The $Cl^-$ ions are surrounded by $H_2O$ molecules with the positive end oriented toward the $Cl^-$. The $Na^+$ and $Cl^-$ are now prevented from bonding together since they are insulated from one another by the water molecules.

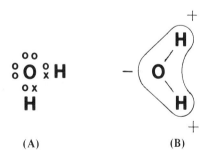

**Figure 2–13.** Water as a polar molecule: (A) the four unpaired negative electrons that circle the oxygen atom; (B) the oxygen atom is negatively charged relative to the hydrogen atoms.

**EXCELLENT TRANSPORT AGENT.** Blood is primarily made up of water and it serves to transport nutrient materials to cells and waste materials away from the cells to the lungs and kidneys. Urine is primarily water with various other compounds dissolved in it. Urine transports waste products out of the body. Sweat is primarily water with dissolved salts. It is transported out of the body from the sweat glands.

**RESISTS CHANGES IN TEMPERATURE.** Water requires more heat than any other liquid to raise 1 gram of it 1°C. This amount of heat is called **specific heat.** This characteristic is responsible for water being slow to change from cold to hot or from hot to cold. In other words, water does not change temperature very readily and this is the reason why water is used in hot water bottles and cold compresses. Hot water bottles release heat slowly, and cold water compresses absorb heat slowly. The high specific heat of water benefits the body by preventing rapid cooling or rapid heating. This tends to maintain the fairly stable body temperature that is necessary for the many chemical reactions occurring in the body.

**GOOD TISSUE LUBRICANT.** Bones, ligaments, tendons, body walls, and organs constantly rub against each other. Water is the major constituent of synovial and serous fluids. Synovial fluid is found in joint cavities and serves to reduce the friction between the bones articulating at the joint. Serous fluid is secreted by serous membranes and serves to reduce friction between the body walls and organs that come in contact.

The roles of water just discussed should help one to see why neither animals (humans included) nor plants can exist without it.

### Carbon Dioxide ($CO_2$: O=C=O)

This small inorganic molecule is composed of one carbon atom double bonded to two oxygen atoms. $CO_2$ results from cell respiration. It moves from the cells into the blood and some combines with $H_2O$ to form carbonic acid and the rest is exhaled from the body. The concentration of $CO_2$ in the blood affects the rate of heart contractions and respiration, as will be discussed later.

### Oxygen ($O_2$: O=O)

Oxygen gas is essential for cell respiration. This process occurs in body cells and involves the breakdown of glucose, ultimately producing $H_2O$, $CO_2$, and releasing energy. The energy released by this process is in the form of ATP and heat. ATP is a high-energy compound required for the occurrence of all activities. Heat is given off from the cells and ultimately from the body.

It is important to realize that the real significance of breathing is to bring $O_2$ to the cells of the body where it helps to release necessary energy (ATP).

### Ammonia ($NH_3$: H—N—H)

$$\underset{\underset{H}{|}}{}$$

Ammonia results from the deamination of proteins. This inorganic molecule is poisonous to the cells and tissues; therefore, usually two $NH_3$ molecules join with $>$C—O to form nonpoisonous urea, $H_2N$—C—$NH_2$.

$$\underset{\overset{\|}{O}}{}$$

This compound is then removed from the body in urine. $NH_3$ can be utilized in the synthesis of amino acids, which are the building blocks of proteins.

## 7 CHARACTERISTICS OF ORGANIC COMPOUNDS

Organic compounds consist of compounds that contain the element carbon.

### Bonding in Organic Compounds

The atoms making up organic compounds are joined together by covalent bonds. Covalent bonds are formed by atoms sharing electrons (Figure 2–9). Carbon has four electrons in its outer orbit, which it shares with other atoms (carbon, hydrogen, oxygen, and nitrogen). The bonds carbon forms with other atoms can be represented as

$$-\overset{|}{\underset{|}{C}}-\quad -\overset{|}{C}=\quad -C\equiv\quad =C=$$

## IMPORTANT ORGANIC COMPOUNDS FOUND IN THE BODY

There are probably over 1 million organic compounds, and of these, four classes are important in the body— carbohydrates, lipids, proteins and nucleic acids. These classes include compounds whose structures can be

quite large and complex; however, study of these compounds is simplified because they are made up of "basic building blocks." Carbohydrates, lipids, proteins, and nucleic acids each have their own characteristic basic building block. The characteristic building block of each group is connected together in a repeating manner to form a complex compound.

### Carbohydrates

This important class includes sugars, starches, and cellulose. **Carbohydrates** are organic compounds composed of carbon, hydrogen, and oxygen with a 2:1 ratio of hydrogen to oxygen atoms. Plants produce carbohydrates by reacting $CO_2$, $H_2O$, chlorophyll, and energy from the sun. This reaction is as follows:

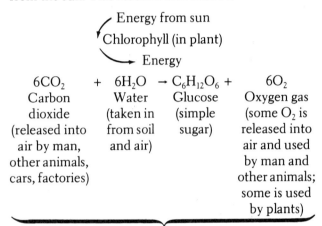

| $6CO_2$ | + | $6H_2O$ | → | $C_6H_{12}O_6$ | + | $6O_2$ |
|---|---|---|---|---|---|---|
| Carbon dioxide (released into air by man, other animals, cars, factories) | | Water (taken in from soil and air) | | Glucose (simple sugar) | | Oxygen gas (some $O_2$ is released into air and used by man and other animals; some is used by plants) |

This entire chemical reaction is **photosynthesis.**

This chemical reaction is a good example of how symbols and numbers can say a lot without words. The reaction in effect says that 6 molecules of $CO_2$ + 6 molecules of $H_2O$ + energy that chlorophyll releases due to stimulation of sun *yield* 1 molecule of glucose + 6 molecules of $O_2$. The number of $CO_2$ and $H_2O$ molecules (6 each) needed to produce 1 molecule of glucose + 6 molecules of $O_2$ would not really be clear if the equation were not balanced. Also, the balanced equation demonstrates the first law of conservation of matter. This is demonstrated by the fact that the numbers of carbon, hydrogen, and oxygen atoms are equal on both sides of the equation.

**BUILDING BLOCKS OF CARBOHYDRATES.** **Monosaccharides** (mono—single; saccharide—sugar) or simple sugars are the basic building blocks of carbohydrates. There are three monosaccharides that are nutritionally important in the body—galactose, glucose, and fructose. (See Figure 2–14.)

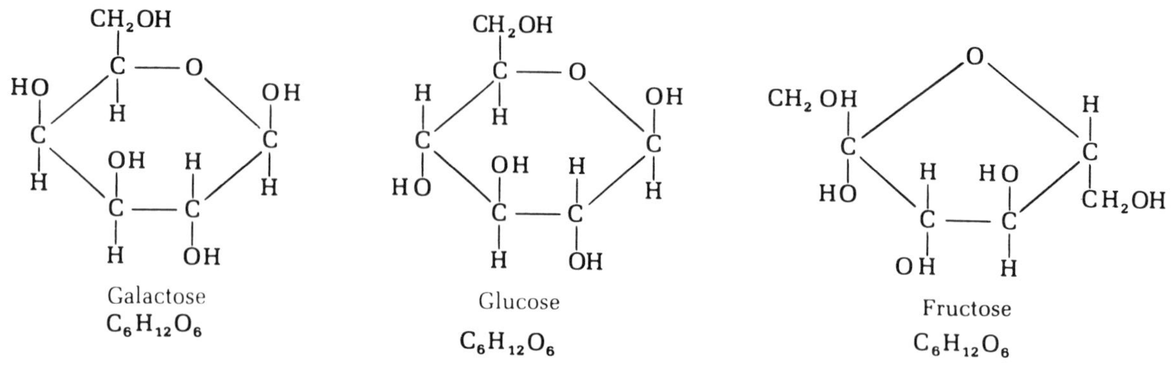

Figure 2-14.   Structural formulas for the monosaccharides.

Notice that the molecular formula for all three is the same, but their structural formulas vary slightly.

**CLASSIFICATION OF CARBOHYDRATES.** One way to classify carbohydrates is by the number of saccharide units they contain. Table 2-4 gives the various classes of carbohydrates, examples, and their importance.

A portion of a polysaccharide such as glycogen is shown diagrammatically as follows:

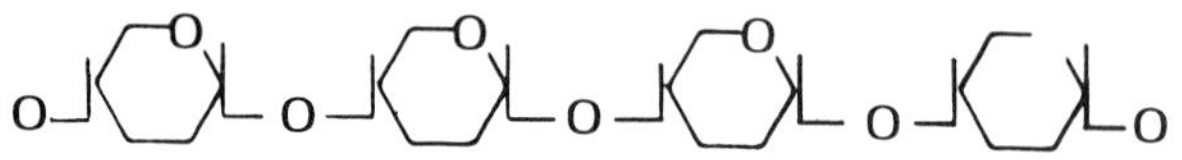

**Glycogen**

Glycogen is composed of many glucose units. In Table 2-4, polysaccharides are represented by $(C_6H_{10}O_5)_n$. The $n$ represents the total number of saccharide units.

The structural formulas for the disaccharides are as shown in Figure 2-15.

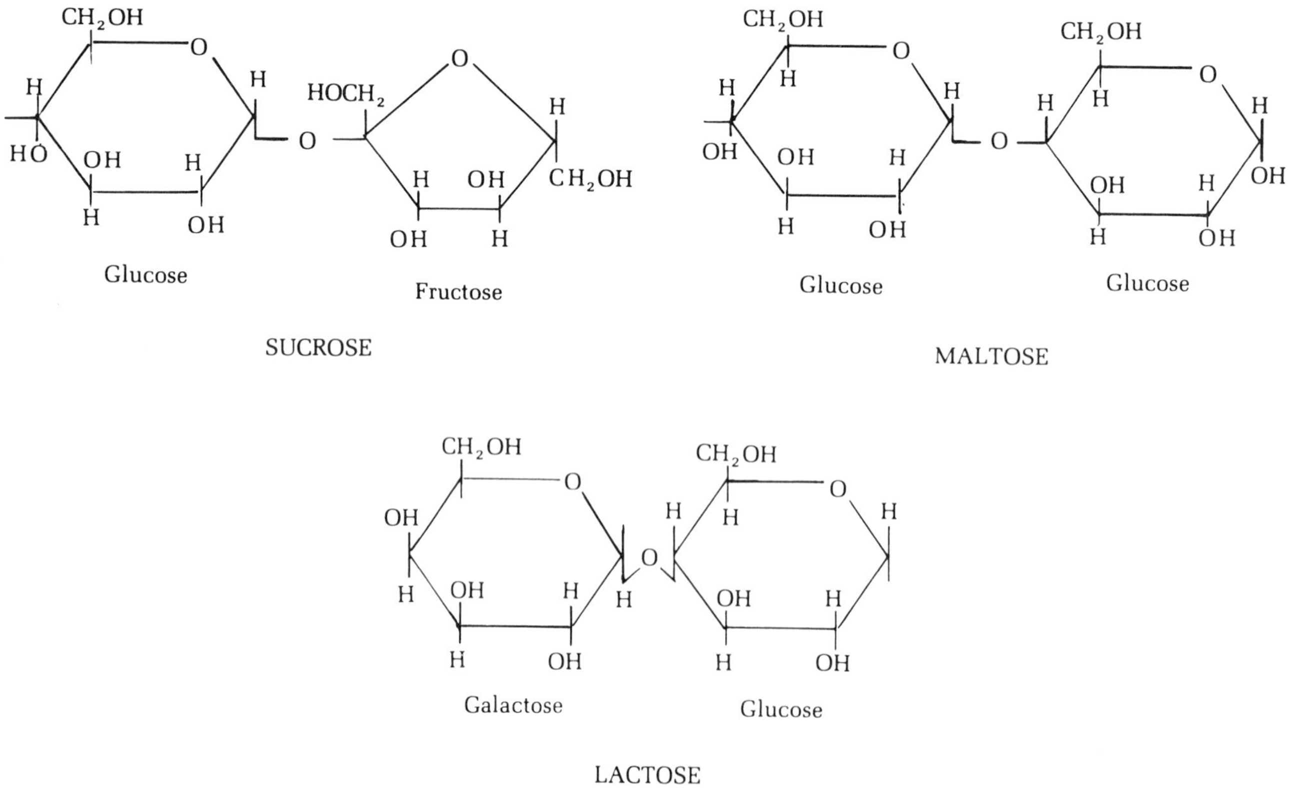

Figure 2-15.   Structural formulas for the disaccharides.

### TABLE 2-4. Classes of Carbohydrates

| CLASS | EXAMPLES | IMPORTANCE |
| --- | --- | --- |
| Monosaccharides | Glucose (dextrose; grape sugar) Fructose (fruit sugar) Galactose | The form in which carbohydrates are absorbed into blood and carried to the cells. Glucose is the most important monosaccharide and can be given intravenously. |
| Disaccharides | Sucrose (common table sugar) Lactose (milk sugar) Maltose | Cannot be absorbed directly into blood; therefore, broken down into their respective monosaccharides in digestive tract. Cells can build disaccharides. |
| Polysaccharides $(C_6H_{10}O_5)_n$* | Starch Cellulose Glycogen (animal starch) | Also cannot be absorbed directly into bloodstream and must be broken down. Glycogen is the form in which excess glucose molecules are stored in the body (liver and muscles). |

*$n$ = number of monosaccharides

**FORMATION OF DISACCHARIDES AND POLYSACCHARIDES.** Monosaccharides combine chemically to form disaccharides and polysaccharides. The actual site of the bonds and the way they combine are shown in the previous structural formulas.

Notice that the bond between the two glucose molecules is initially formed by the OH or hydroxyl group of one glucose pulling off a hydrogen atom from the other glucose molecule, forming an $H_2O$ molecule. The carbon that lost its OH group and the oxygen that lost its hydrogen are both free to form new bonds. The carbon atom forms a new bond with the oxygen atom, satisfying the need of both atoms and forming the disaccharide maltose. This same process is repeated many times to form a polysaccharide.

---

*Important Point*

This process of chemically uniting the building blocks of carbohydrates is made possible by the loss of $H_2O$ molecules from the monosaccharides. Dehydration synthesis is the chemical name of this process. The formation of disaccharides and polysaccharides occurs inside cells of the body. This intracellular (intra—within; cellular—cell) synthesis of carbohydrates is important for the production of reserve fuel molecules (glycogen).

---

**DECOMPOSITION OF DISACCHARIDES AND POLYSACCHARIDES.** The formation of disaccharides and polysaccharides involves the loss of $H_2O$ molecules or **dehydration synthesis**. The destruction of these molecules is just the opposite; $H_2O$ molecules break the bonds between the building blocks, as shown in Figure 2-16.

Each bond connecting the monosaccharides is broken by an $H_2O$ molecule. This is a **hydrolytic** (*hydro*—water; *lysis*—break) **reaction** or a **digestion reaction** and is what happens during digestion in the small intestine. Note that water is essential for digestion to occur.

These hydrolytic reactions take place with disaccharides and polysaccharides because they are too large to be absorbed into the blood from the small intestine. Once absorbed, they can be carried to the cells of the body.

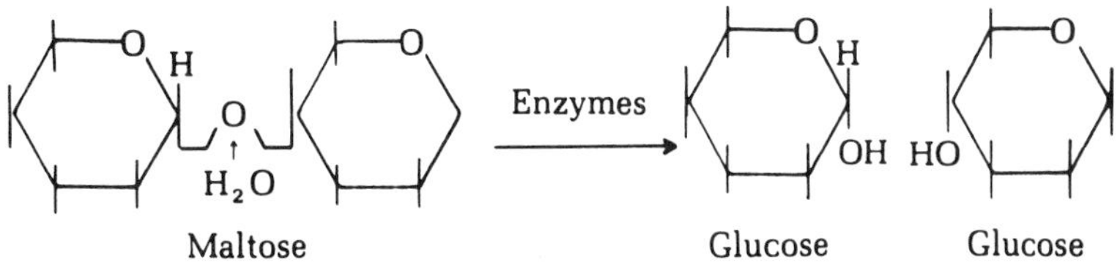

Maltose → Enzymes → Glucose    Glucose

Figure 2-16.

In summary, hydrolytic or digestion reactions break large carbohydrate molecules into their building blocks. The building blocks can then be absorbed into the blood and transported to the cells of the body.

The destruction and formation of disaccharides and polysaccharides can be diagrammed as follows:

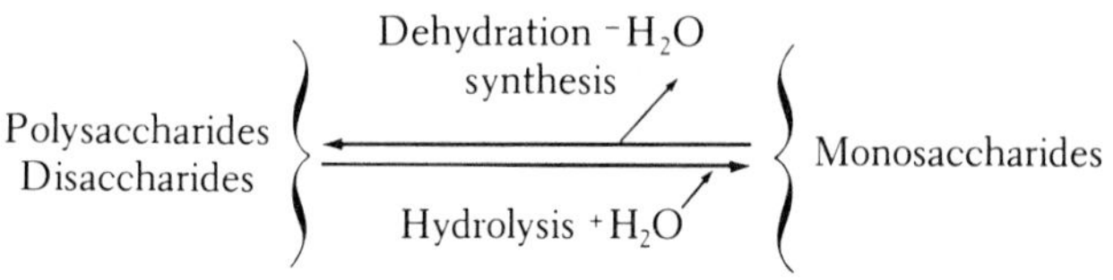

$$\text{Polysaccharides} \atop \text{Disaccharides} \left\{ \underset{\text{Hydrolysis }^+\text{H}_2\text{O}}{\overset{\text{Dehydration }^-\text{H}_2\text{O} \atop \text{synthesis}}{\rightleftharpoons}} \right\} \text{Monosaccharides}$$

The diagram shows that hydrolysis reactions breakdown complex carbohydrates into their basic building blocks, which can be absorbed. Dehydration synthesis reactions combine the basic building blocks into more complex molecules, which will be stored for future use.

These characteristics of carbohydrate hydrolysis and dehydration reactions also apply to lipids, proteins, and nucleic acids. We will discuss these shortly.

**FUNCTIONS OF CARBOHYDRATES IN HUMANS.** Carbohydrates are the primary source of energy for the various body processes. Glucose is the main carbohydrate that is borken down to release energy. The formula for the chemical breakdown of glucose is shown in Equation 5.

### Lipids*

This group includes triglycerides, phospholipids, and steroids. **Fats** are organic compounds that contain carbon, hydrogn, and oxygen with a greater than 2:1 ratio of hydrogen to oxygen atoms.

**BUILDING BLOCKS OF TRIGLYCERIDES.** The basic building block of triglycerides consists of one molecule of glycerol combined with three molecules of fatty acids. The synthesis of these component parts to form the basic building block is shown in Figure 2–17.

$$\text{C}_6\text{H}_{12}\text{O}_6 + 6\text{O}_2 + 6\text{H}_2\text{O} \rightarrow 6\text{CO}_2 + 12\text{H}_2\text{O} + \text{Energy}$$

Taken in by breathing — Given off from cells into blood and then exhaled from lungs — Used for various body processes: muscle contractions, transmission of nerve impulses, etc.; each gram of glucose that is broken down releases four calories of heat energy

Equation 5

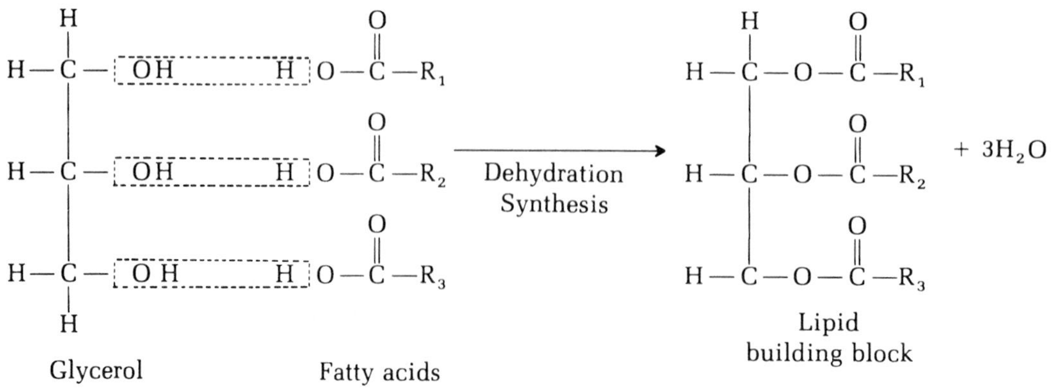

Figure 2–17.   Synthesis of a triglyceride molecule is shown.

---

* The terms "lipids" and "fats" are often used interchangeably. They are not identical, however. Fats (triglycerides) are a specific class of lipids, with the other classes being phospholipids, steroids, and porphyrins.

Notice that each fatty acid donates a hydrogen to each hydroxyl group of the glycerol. Three water molecules split off and now the free glycerol carbons combine with the free oxygens of the fatty acids. This is a dehydration synthesis reaction with three molecules of $H_2O$ formed. The $R_1$, $R_2$, and $R_3$ represent chains composed primarily of carbon atoms with attached hydrogens. Each chain can vary in length and contain other atoms in addition to carbon and hydrogen.

**EXAMPLES OF IMPORTANT LIPIDS.** Some other important classes of lipids are phospholipids, steroids, and porphyrins.

1. *Phospholipids.* These are lipids that contain a phosphate group and a nitrogen-containing base in place of one of the three fatty acids.

Cephalins

Lecithin

Cephalins, lecithins, and other phospholipids occur in the greatest amount in the brain and nerves. Phospholipids are important constituents of cell membranes and play a role in blood clotting.

2. *Steroids.* The structure of the lipids in this group is much different from the structure of lipids in the other groups.

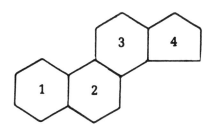

Notice that this group does not have the typical fatty acid chains that the other lipid groups have. Steroids typically have four interlocking rings of carbon atoms. The difference between steroid compounds is the side groups that come off the rings.

Some important examples of steroids are:

- *Cholesterol.* A structural component of cell membranes. A high concentration of cholesterol in the blood can contribute to, if not cause, atherosclerosis and hardening of the arteries.
- *Testosterone.* The male hormone secreted from the testes. It is responsible for development of secondary sex characteristics (beard and muscle configuration). The male sex drive and behavior are dependent upon testosterone also.
- *Estrogen.* A female hormone that affects development of secondary female characteristics (breasts, hips).
- *Bile salts.* A compound secreted from the liver into the small intestine that aids in the digestion and absorption of fats.

Vitamins E and K also are steroids.

3. *Porphyrins.* These are lipid portions of organic molecules. Hemoglobin is an example.

**ESSENTIAL FATTY ACIDS.** There are three essential fatty acids—linoleic, linolenic, and arachidonic. These fatty acids are essential in the diet of an infant. If they are absent, the child can lose weight and develop eczema (inflammation of the skin).

**BREAKDOWN OF FATS.** Fat molecules, like carbohydrates, are much too large to be absorbed into the blood from the small intestine and must be broken down to their basic building blocks. Fats are an excellent reserve source of energy. (See Figure 2–18.)

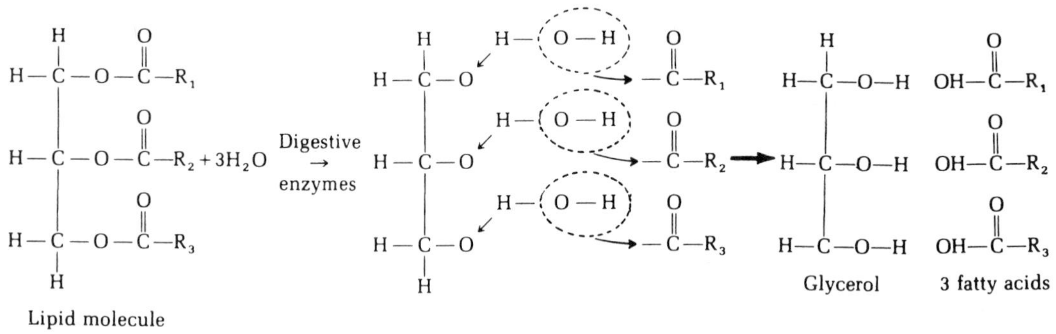

**Figure 2-18.** Hydrolysis of a triglyceride.

Notice that the hydrogen atoms of the water molecules attach to the oxygen atoms of glycerol, and the hydroxyl (OH) groups attach to the fatty acids.

The **dehydration synthesis** and **hydrolytic breakdown** of fats can be summarized as follows:

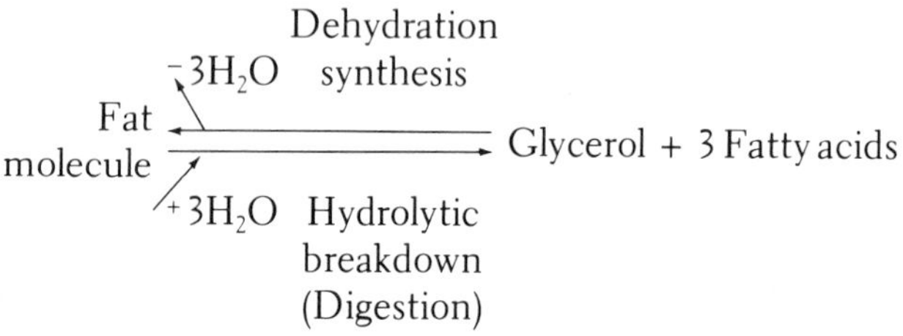

$$
\text{Fat molecule} \underset{\substack{+3H_2O \\ \text{Hydrolytic} \\ \text{breakdown} \\ \text{(Digestion)}}}{\overset{\substack{\text{Dehydration} \\ \text{synthesis} \\ -3H_2O}}{\rightleftharpoons}} \text{Glycerol} + 3 \text{ Fatty acids}
$$

**FUNCTIONS OF LIPIDS.** Lipids have several important functions in the body:

• *Reserve energy source.* Fats actually release twice as much energy per gram as do carbohydrates (fats, 9 Cal/g; carbohydrates, 4 Cal/g). Why, then, are they a reserve energy source rather than the primary energy source? The answer is that the efficiency of fats in releasing energy is 10 to 12 percent less than carbohydrates. Fats are stored in fat depots and are utilized as a source of energy when a person's carbohydrate intake is low.

• *Heat insulation.* Fat does not conduct heat very well; therefore, layers of fat help the body to retain heat.

• *Structural component of cell membranes.* The plasma membrane of cells is composed of both lipids and proteins. The lipids help regulate what compounds can enter and exit a cell through the plasma membrane.

• *Padding for organs.* All organs in the body have a certain amount of fat surrounding them to help absorb any blows or mechanical injuries. For example, the inner surface of each eyeball is covered with fat tissue that absorbs the impact of any blows to the eyes.

• *Aid absorption of fat-soluble vitamins.* There are two major groups of vitamins, fat-soluble and water-soluble. Fat-soluble vitamins dissolve and are absorbed only with fats.

## Proteins

This is the most important group of compounds in the body. **Proteins** are the most fundamental constituent of living matter. Examples of important proteins are hair, blood, enzymes, muscles, antibodies, and hormones. Proteins are organic compounds that contain hydrogen, carbon, oxygen, and nitrogen. Sulfur and iodine are found in some proteins, as are phosphorus and iron.

**BUILDING BLOCKS OF PROTEINS.** Amino acids are the building blocks of proteins. There are about 20 different amino acids that commonly make up proteins. An amino acid is represented as follows:

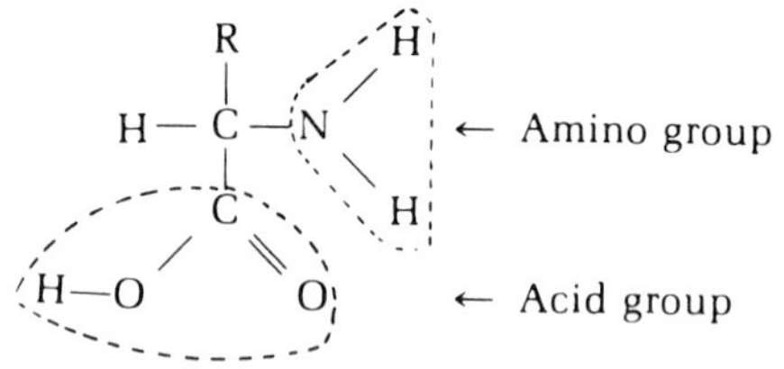

The $-N\begin{smallmatrix}H\\H\end{smallmatrix}$ group is the source of the amino part of the name. The $H-O$ $C$ $O$ carboxyl group is the source of the acid part of the name, since the hydrogen of the carboxyl group can be given off in aqueous solution. The R part of the molecule varies from one hydrogen atom to a group of carbon atoms with hydrogens and other atoms attached. Each of the 20 different amino acids is different because of the R groups. Three of the eight essential amino acids in the body are shown in Figure 2-19.

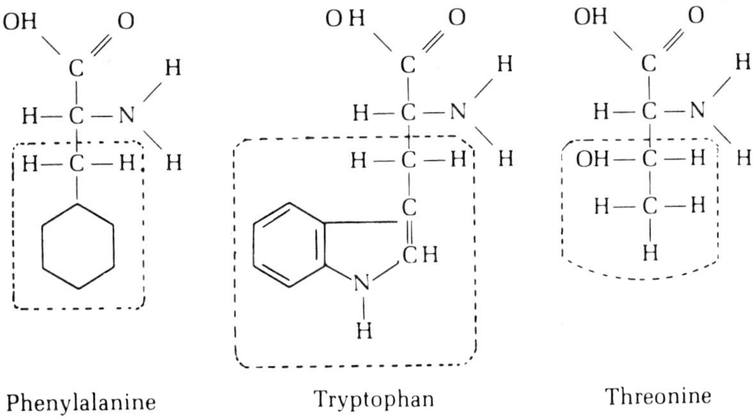

Phenylalanine          Tryptophan          Threonine

**Figure 2-19.**   Three amino acids with different R-groups (within dotted lines).

Notice that the area within the dotted lines, which represents the R group, is the only part of each amino acid that is different from the other two.

**PEPTIDE BONDS: JOINING TOGETHER OF AMINO ACIDS.**   Protein molecules are extremely large. Before a protein is formed, many, many, many amino acids are connected together. The bonds formed between amino acids are called peptide bonds. A typical peptide bond is formed as follows:

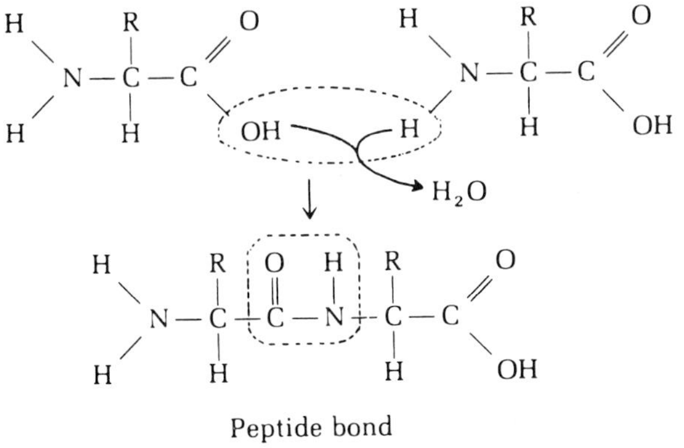

$H_2O$

Peptide bond

Notice that formation of a peptide bond initially involves loss of a water molecule between two amino acids. The bond is finally formed when the free carbon atom of one amino acid bonds with the free nitrogen atom of another amino acid. Two amino acids bonded together form a dipeptide, three a tripeptide, and four or more amino acids bonded together form a polypeptide. All are single structures composed of several amino acids bonded together. A protein is finally formed when several polypeptides are joined together.

As stated previously, proteins are very large molecules and often consist of several hundred to over a thousand amino acids. (See Figure 2-20.)

**SEQUENCE OF AMINO ACIDS IN PROTEINS.** Every protein is made up of many, many amino acids and the sequence in which they are arranged is vital. A good analogy of the importance of the sequence of amino acids in a protein is the sequence of letters that compose a word. Look at the word protein as an example. The letters P–R–O–T–E–I–N in this sequence make up a known word with meaning; however, if the position of the letters O and T is changed,

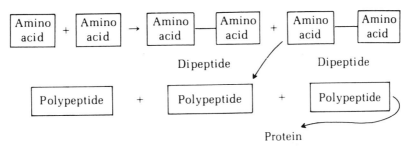

**Figure 2-20.**   Bonding of amino acids together to form dipeptides, polypeptides and a protein molecule.

P–R–T–O–E–I–N, the word is not recognizable and has no meaning. In a protein that is composed of a hundred or more amino acids, changing the sequence of just two amino acids can completely change a protein. Later we will discuss how cells synthesize proteins and the mechanism that guarantees the amino acids will be hooked together in the proper sequence.

### Enzymes: Important Protein Compounds

A very important group of proteins are the ones that act as catalysts. These are called enzymes. They are globular proteins.

**DEFINITION OF AN ENZYME.** A biological organic catalyst that affects the speed of chemical reactions but is not itself chemically changed is an **enzyme.** Enzymes cannot cause reactions to occur that would not normally occur. They are generally very specific in that each enzyme can generally affect only one specific compound (substrate).

**GENERAL FUNCTIONS OF ENZYMES.** Generally, enzymes function to speed up chemical reactions and lower the amount of energy needed to initiate chemical reactions. Many chemical reactions that take place in the body will take place outside the body also; however, in the absence of enzymes, they usually take place much slower and require higher temperatures. The higher temperatures are needed outside the body to increase the amount of energy required to break chemical bonds.

Many chemical reactions in the body could not occur rapidly enough at body temperature (98.6°F or 37°C) if it were not for enzymes. It has been theorized that, if all enzymes were removed from the body, chemical reactions would still occur, but so slowly that vital body functions (respiration and contraction of heart) could not maintain homeostasis.

**ENZYMES AND ENERGY REQUIREMENTS FOR CHEMICAL REACTIONS.** Previously, we said that energy is needed to cause chemical reactions. This energy is referred to as **energy of activation ($E_a$).** Enzymes tend to lower the amount of energy needed to cause a chemical reaction, as shown in Figure 2–21. The amount of energy needed to initiate a reaction is compared with enzymes present and without enzymes. The energy of activation ($E_a$) is lower with enzymes present and higher without enzymes. The change in potential energy ($\Delta G$) is the same for the initial compound and the product compound in both the enzyme and nonenzyme reactions; therefore, enzymes do not cause more energy to be released from reactants. This ability of enzymes to lower the $E_a$ of chemical reactions is important. It is significant because the body does not have to use as much energy to initiate chemical reactions as it would if enzymes were absent.

**ENZYME LOCK AND KEY THEORY.** One theory that attempts to explain enzyme activity is the lock and key theory. The enzyme corresponds to a key and the substance upon which an enzyme acts corresponds to a lock. The substance acted upon is also called a **substrate.** The basis for this theory is that enzymes are very specific for certain substrates and seem to have a specific surface shape. This theory is diagrammatically shown in Figure 2–22. The point at which the enzyme and substrate combine is the **active site.** A key has a specific shape that will fit only into locks with a complementary shape. This concept is how enzymes and substrates supposedly operate. An enzyme with its specific shape can combine only with a substrate having a complementary shape. The point at which they combine is the active site of the enzyme.

All enzyme reactions involve the three steps shown in Figure 2–23. The first step involves the enzyme combining with the substrate. The second step is the formation of the enzyme–substrate complex. The third step is the formation of the product(s).

#### Important Point

Notice that the arrows go in both directions. This means that the reactions are reversible or, in other words, two or more substrates can be chemically joined, as well as one substrate can be broken into two or more products. Notice also that the shape of the enzyme is not changed by these reactions.

**SPECIFIC EXAMPLES OF ENZYME REACTIONS AND NAMING OF ENZYMES.** An enzyme usually can be recognized by the -ase ending on a word. The -ase is usually attached to the substrate. Some examples of this and specific enzyme reactions are shown in Table 2–5.

### Nucleic Acids

This is the last major group of organic compounds found in the body that will be discussed. Nucleic acids are interesting because they are responsible for hooking

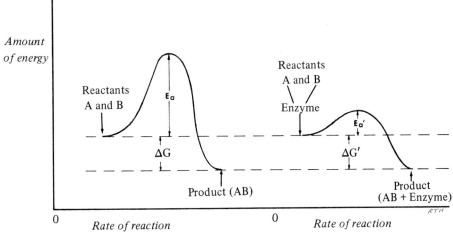

$E_a$ = Energy of activation without enzymes

$E_a'$ = Energy of activation with enzymes present

$\Delta G$ = Change in potential energy without enzymes

$\Delta G'$ = Change in potential energy with enzymes present

**Figure 2-21.** The $E_a$ for chemical reactions without enzymes is higher than the $E_a$ for chemical reactions with enzymes present. The change in potential energy of reactants and products for enzyme and nonenzyme reactions is the same.

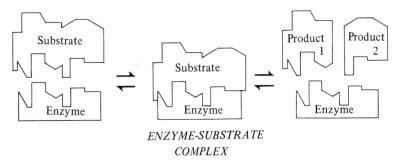

*ENZYME-SUBSTRATE
COMPLEX*

**Figure 2-22.** Enzymes have very specific chemical shapes and can chemically bond with substances (substrates) that have a complementary shape. Enzymes can either combine compounds to form one new product or break apart a compound to form two or more products.

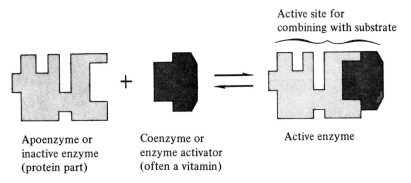

**Figure 2-23.** Some enzymes are composed of an apoenzyme (protein) part and a coenzyme part (often a vitamin). The enzyme is inactive unless both parts are present.

**TABLE 2-5.**

| SUBSTRATE | | ENZYME | | ENZYME-SUBSTRATE COMPLEX | | PRODUCT(S) | | |
|---|---|---|---|---|---|---|---|---|
| Lactose | + | Lactase | → | Lactose–Lactase | → | Galactose | + | Glucose |
| Sucrose | + | Sucrase | → | Sucrose–Sucrase | → | Glucose | + | Fructose |
| Maltose | + | Maltase | → | Maltose–Maltase | → | Glucose | + | Glucose |

amino acids together in specific sequences to make the various proteins. Nucleic acids are very large complex structures and are the major component of chromosomes. Chromosomes contain the genetic information that every person inherits from his parents. This inherited genetic information is responsible for all of the various traits that each person possesses—hair color, eye color, skin color, height, and many more.

**DEFINITION OF NUCLEIC ACIDS.** Nucleic acids are large organic molecules that are primarily responsible for hooking amino acids together in specific sequences to form proteins.

**NUCLEIC ACID BUILDING BLOCK: NUCLEOTIDE.** Every nucleic acid is made up of many nucleotides. A nucleotide is made up of three parts: an organic base, a sugar, and a phosphate. These parts are connected together in a specific manner as shown in Figure 2-24. There are four different nucleotides. Each contains the same phosphate and sugar molecules, but the four differ in the base they contain. The four bases that nucleotides contain are adenine, thymine, cytosine, and guanine. The chemical structure and a diagrammatic picture of the bases are shown in Figure 2-25. Nucleic acids are the same as carbohydrates, lipids, and proteins in that the building blocks are chemically bonded together.

**STRUCTURE OF A NUCLEIC ACID.** A nucleic acid is composed of a long chain of nucleotides connected together as shown in Figure 2-26. One nucleotide is connected to another by the sugar bonding to a phosphate, sugar to phosphate, and so on.

Some of the nucleic acids messenger RNA (m-RNA) and transfer RNA (t-RNA) are composed of a single chain of nucleotides. Deoxyribonucleic acid (DNA) is composed of a double chain of nucleotides bonded together so that it is similar to a winding stairway (Figure 2-27). The two nucleotide chains are connected by hydrogen bonds between complementary bases (A–T, G–C). Adenine–thymine and guanine–cytosine are called complementary bases because each can bond only with a base that has a complementary chemical structure. This complementary structure of the bases and the joining of the nucleotide chains are very important in at least two ways:

- The joining together of amino acids in a specific sequence to form certain proteins.
- Determines the genetic code of each person.

These two points and others will be discussed in more detail in Chapter 4.

**DEHYDRATION SYNTHESIS AND HYDROLYTIC BREAKDOWN OF NUCLEIC ACIDS.** The process for the synthesizing (composing) and breaking down of nucleic acids is shown as follows:

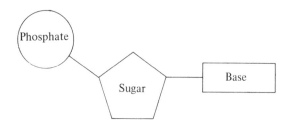

Figure 2-24.   Nucleotide, the building block of nucleic acids. A nucleotide molecule is composed of a phosphate bonded to a 5-carbon sugar that is bonded to a base.

$$\text{Nucleotides} \; \underset{\substack{\nearrow \\ \text{Hydrolytic} \\ \text{breakdown}}}{\overset{\substack{\text{Dehydration synthesis} \\ -H_2O \; \nearrow}}{\rightleftharpoons}} \; \text{Nucleic acids}$$

$$+ H_2O$$

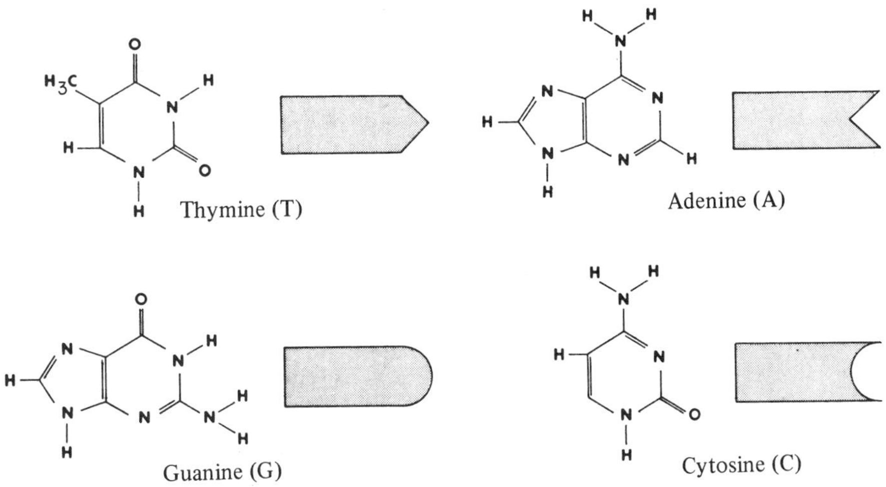

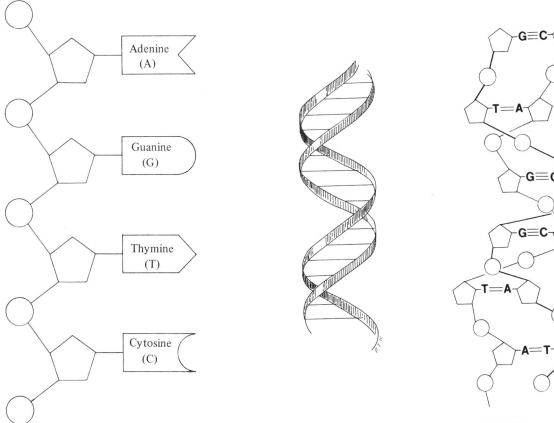

**Figure 2-25.** The chemical structure for the four bases found in nucleotides. The diagrams show that T–A and G–C have complementary shapes.

**Figure 2-26.** A nucleic acid is composed of many nucleotides. Each nucleotide is connected to the next by a bond between phosphate and sugar groups.

**Figure 2-27.** Deoxyribonucleic acid (DNA) composed of two strands of nucleic acids twisted around each other. The two strands are connected by bonds between complementary bases.

# SUMMARY

**Living Matter**

Matter: anything that occupies space and has weight
A. Mass and Weight
    1. Mass: designates quantity of matter; a constant value that does not vary as location of object changes.
    2. Weight: amount of attraction between two objects; it varies according to the gravitational attraction of two objects.
    *Ex.*    Weight of an object on the moon is one-fifth that on earth due to less gravitational attraction.
B. Physical States of Matter
    1. Solids: have a definite shape and volume.
    2. Liquids: have a definite volume but shape varies according to container that it is in.
    3. Gases: have indefinite shape and volume.
C. Structure of Matter
    1. Atom: basic building block of all types of matter; composed of three subatomic particles:
        a. Protons: positive charge ($+1$); located in nucleus and number equals the number of electrons.
        b. Neutrons: located in nucleus; electrical charge is zero.
        c. Electrons: located outside nucleus in orbits or shells; electrical charge is negative ($-$).
    2. Energy Levels and Locations of Electrons in Atoms
        a. Energy level (orbits and shells): electrons circle around nucleus; each holds a certain number; eight electrons in outer orbit (except first, only 2) make atom stable.
        b. Valence (bonding capacity): number of electrons an atom needs to share, acquire, or give up to have a stable outer orbit.
    3. Identification of atoms: symbols, atomic weight, atomic number, mass number, and formula.
        a. Symbols of atoms and elements; shorthand way to identify elements; often first letter of name of atom; most elements identified by two-letter symbols with only the first letter capitalized.
        b. Atomic numbers of atoms: number of protons in the nucleus.
        c. Atomic mass number: total number of protons and neutrons in an atom;

$$\text{(atomic number)} \quad {}_6C^{12} \quad \text{(atomic mass)}$$

        d. Atomic weight: relative weight of an atom compared to a standard, carbon 12.
        e. Molecular weight: total weight of all atoms that compose a molecule.
    4. Isotopes: atoms of the same element that have a different number of neutrons; some are stable and give off no radiation; radioactive isotopes give off radiation that can be detected; half-life is amount of time required for half of atoms in a sample to decay.

**Energy:** Capacity for Doing Work
A. Kinds of energy: potential, stored, or inactive energy; kinetic, energy in action.
B. Forms of energy: Chemical, present in chemical substances. Electrical, energy flows along a conductor; nervous system utilizes electrical energy. Mechanical, moves matter; contraction of muscles is an example. Radiant, travels in waves; heat and light are examples.
    1. Transformation (conversion) of energy: body changes chemical energy in food into the other three forms.
    2. Conservation of energy and matter: the conversion of energy and matter obeys the first and second laws of conservation or thermodynamics.

C. Measurement of energy: small calorie (cal) the amount of heat required to raise the temperature of one gram of water one degree Celsius; kilocalorie (Kcal.) measures heat energy of body and nutritional value of foods.

D. ATP and stored energy: ATP (adenosine triphosphate) is the energy currency of the cell; energy is released when one of the phosphate groups is broken off; energy is utilized for cell activities.

**Chemical Change**

A. Properties of Elements, Compounds, and Mixtures
   1. Elements: matter composed of only one type of atom; oxygen, hydrogen, nitrogen, and carbon elements make up 96 percent of body; atom is building block.
   2. Compound: made up of two or more elements chemically bonded together; molecule is building block.
   3. Mixtures: two or more elements or compounds not chemically combined.
      a. Solution: homogenous mixture of two or more elements.
         *Ex.*    blood or urine.
      b. Suspension: a nonhomogenous mixture of two or more elements or compounds.
         *Ex.*    protoplasm.

B. Chemical Bonds
   1. Ionic bonds or electrovalent bonds: bond formed between atoms when they lose or accept electrons; cations (+ charge) are attracted to anions (− charge).
   2. Covalent bonds: bond formed by sharing one or more pairs of electrons between compatible atoms.

C. Endergonic (Endothermic) and Exergonic (Exothermic) Reactions
   1. Endergonic (endothermic): energy-absorbing reactions; $+\Delta G$.
   2. Exergonic (exothermic): energy-releasing reactions; $-\Delta G$.

D. Types of Chemical Reactions
   1. Synthesis (combination): two or more elements or an element and a compound chemically bonded together.
      *Ex.*    $A + B \rightarrow AB$; $ADP + P \rightarrow ATP$.
   2. Decomposition: compound decomposes into elements or simpler compounds.
      *Ex.*    $AB \rightarrow A + B$; $ATP \rightarrow ADP + P$.
   3. Exchange: two compounds exchange negative and positve parts.
      *Ex.*    $A^+B^- + C^+D^- \rightarrow A^+D^- + C^+B^-$; $Na^+HCO_3^- + H^+Cl^- \rightarrow Na^+Cl^- + H^+HCO_3^-$.
   4. Oxidation–reduction (redox): oxidation, the loss of electrons, hydrogens, or acceptance of oxygen; reduction, gain of electrons or loss of oxygen; oxidation–reduction in the human body normally involves the loss of hydrogen atoms or the loss and gain of electrons from hydrogen atoms.

$$
Ex. \quad NADH_2 + \underset{\substack{\displaystyle CH_3 \\ \text{Pyruvic} \\ \text{acid}}}{\overset{\substack{COOH \\ | \\ }}{C=O}} \quad \longrightarrow \quad NAD \atop \text{(oxidized)} \quad + \underset{\substack{\displaystyle CH_3 \\ \text{Lactic acid} \\ \text{(reduced)}}}{\overset{\substack{COOH \\ | \\ }}{H-C-OH}}
$$

**Factors Determining the Speed of Chemical Reactions**

A. Temperature of the reactants: increase in temperature increases rate of reaction, and vice versa.

B. Concentration of reactants: increasing the concentration of reactants in a reaction increases the rate of the reaction.

C. Effect of enzymes (catalysts): enzymes increase the rate of chemical reactions; each reaction has a specific enzyme or enzymes that increase its rate of reaction.

D. Amount of surface area: rate of a reaction is dependent on the amount of surface area exposed by the reactants.

## Acids–Bases, Buffers, and Salts

A. Acids and Bases

1. Acid: a substance that forms hydrogen ions in water solutions.

   Ex.      $HCl \xrightarrow{H_2O} H^+ + Cl^-$.

   Acidosis is a high level of acids in blood and can damage tissues if not lowered.

2. Base: a substance that gives up hydroxide ions ($OH^-$) or accepts hydrogen ions in water solution.

   Ex.      $NaOH \xrightarrow{H_2O} Na^+ + OH^-; H^+ + NH_3 \xrightarrow{H_2O} NH_4^+$.

   A high level of bases in blood, alkalosis, can be quite damaging to body tissues.

3. pH scale measurement of $H^+$ and $OH^-$ concentrations; extends numerically from 0 to 14; numbers below 7 refer to acids and numbers above 7 refer to alkaline (base) solution.

B. Buffers

1. Buffer system: pair of compounds that resists changes in pH with addition of acids or bases; composed of a weak acid and a base.

2. How do buffer systems work to maintain or restore homeostasis: either the acid or base member of the buffer system neutralizes the acid or base that is added to the tissues.

$$Ex. \qquad HCl \quad + NaHCO_3 \longrightarrow NaCl + H_2CO_3$$
   (Hydrochloric   (Weak
   acid)           acid
                   buffer)

C. Salts

1. A salt is a compound composed of a negative ion of an acid linked to the positive ion of a base.

   Ex.      $K^+Cl^-$          and   $Na^+Cl^-$
            (Potassium              (Sodium
               chloride)               chloride)

2. Salts are ionic compounds: salts ionize or separate into the ions that compose them when dissolved in water.

   Ex.      $K^+Cl^- + H_2O \rightarrow K^+ + Cl^- + H_2O$.

## Inorganic Compounds Important in the Body

Compounds that lack carbon are inorganic.

A. Water ($H_2O$): most prevalent substance in body; composes 65 to 75 percent of body weight. Functions: (1) reactant, involved in chemical reactions; (2) solvent, causes most compounds in body to dissolve; (3) transport agent, transports materials throughout body; (4) tissue lubricant, functions to reduce friction where body parts rub against each other.

B. Carbon dioxide ($CO_2$): produced in cells and exhaled; concentration in blood affects rate of respiration and heart contractions.

C. Oxygen ($O_2$): essential to cell respiration, producing the energy compound ATP.

D. Ammonia ($NH_3$): results from deamination of proteins; poisonous to cells and tissues; therefore, two molecules join together to form urea, which is excreted in urine.

**Characteristics of Organic Compounds**

Organic compounds are composed of many carbon atoms bonded to hydrogens.

A. Bonding in organic compounds: atoms in organic compounds are bonded together by covalent bonds.

B. Important Organic Compounds Found in the Body

Four classes of organic compounds are important in the body: carbohydrates, lipids, proteins, and nucleic acids.

1. Carbohydrates: basic building block, monosaccharides or simple sugars; three monosaccharides found in the body are galactose, glucose, and fructose. Functions, primary source of energy.

2. Lipids: fats are most common type lipid in body; building block, glycerol, and three fatty acids. Functions: (1) reserve energy source, (2) heat insulation, (3) structural component of cell membrane, (4) padding for organs, (5) aid absorption of fat-soluble vitamins.

3. Proteins: composed of hydrogen, carbon, oxygen, and nitrogen. Building block, amino acids (there are twenty different ones). Functions: (1) structure, compose structure of various tissues; (2) enzyme, increase rate of reactions; (3) immunity, protection against infection; (4) hormonal, some hormones that regulate rate of reactions are proteins; (5) transport, hemoglobin and certain other proteins transport materials in body.

4. Nucleic acids: major component of chromosomes; building block, nucleotide is composed of a phosphate, sugar, and base. Function, responsible for synthesis of proteins and determines genetic code of each person.

## Chemistry of the Body

1. Mass is a term that designates_____ and weight is _____.
   (a) amount of attraction between two objects—quantity of matter
   (b) quantity of matter—amount of attraction between two objects
   (c) weight of an object—gravitational attraction between two objects
   (d) None of these

2. The name and correct accompanying description of the three physical states of matter are given in _____.
   (a) solids—definite shape but indefinite volume
       liquids—indefinite shape and volume
       gases—definite volume but shape varies
   (b) solids—definite shape and volume
       liquids—definite volume but variable shape
       gases—indefinite shape and volume

3. The three subatomic particles composing an atom are:
   (a) protons—positive charge and located in nucleus
       neutrons—located outside nucleus with a negative charge
       electrons—located outside nucleus with a negative charge
   (b) protons—zero charge and located in nucleus
       neutrons—located outside nucleus with negative charge
       electrons—located in nucleus with positive charge

4. The three forms of energy and an example of each are:
   (a) chemical—chemical substances
       electrical—contraction of muscles
       mechanical—conduction of nerve impulses in nervous system
   (b) chemical—chemical substances
       electrical—conduction of nerve impulses in nervous system
       mechanical—contraction of muscles

Matching, Questions 5 to 9.

5. element            A. two or more elements or compounds not chemically com-
                         bined
6. compound           B. matter composed of only one type of atom
7. mixture            C. made up of two or more elements chemically bonded to-
                         gether
8. solution           D. a non-homogenous mixture of two or more elements or
                         compounds
9. suspension         E. None of these

Questions 10–20 are to be answered true (A) or false (B).

10. An ionic bond is formed between atoms where they lose or accept electrons.

11. A covalent bond is formed when an anion is attracted to a cation.

12. A cation is positively charged.

13. Anions are attracted to anions in forming ionic bonds.

14. $C_6H_{12}O_6 + 6O_2 \rightarrow 6CO_2 + H_2O + 686$ Kcal/mole; $\Delta G = -686$ Kcal/mole. This is an exergonic reaction.

15. Endergonic reactions absorb more energy than they release.

16. ADP + P→ATP; this is a synthesis reaction.

17. NaCl $\overset{H_2O}{\rightleftharpoons}$ Na+ + Cl−; this is a decomposition reaction.

18. Exchange reactions involve addition of smaller atoms to form a larger product.

19. An oxidation reaction involves gain of electrons or hydrogens.

20. A reduction reaction involves loss of electrons or hydrogens.

21. Factors that determine the speed of chemical reactions are:
    - (a) temperature of reactants
    - (b) concentration of reactants
    - (c) effect of enzymes
    - (d) all of these
    - (e) none of these

Matching, Questions 22 to 26.

22. acid

23. base

24. pH scale

25. buffer system

26. salt

   **A.** substance that gives up hydroxide ions (OH −)

   **B.** KCl

   **C.** composed of a weak acid and base

   **D.** numbers below 7 refer to acids and numbers above 7 refer to alkaline (base)

   **E.** none of these

Matching, Questions 27 to 30.

27. water ($H_2O$)

28. carbon dioxide ($CO_2$)

29. oxygen ($O_2$)

30. ammonia ($NH_3$)

   **A.** poisonous to cells and forms urea

   **B.** essential to cell respiration

   **C.** produced in cells and exhaled

   **D.** most prevalent inorganic compound in body

Questions 31 to 35 are to be answered true (A) or false (B).

31. The basic building block of carbohydrates is a monosaccharide.

32. Lipids aid absorption of fat-soluble vitamins.

33. Proteins are composed of nucleotides.

34. A nucleic acid functions to transport materials in the body.

35. Nucleic acids determine the genetic code of a person.

# Chapter 3

# MICROBIOLOGY

After reading and studying this chapter, a student should be able to:

1. Describe the contributions of Louis Pasteur and Robert Koch.
2. Name the components of a two-word name given microbes.
3. Contrast procaryotic and eucaryotic cells.
4. Describe bacterial cellular structure, morphology, and reproduction.
5. Name the general types of bacteria and where they are found on and in the body.

*What is microbiology? A careful analysis of the word will answer the question. The first part of the word, **micro,** means small or it refers to something invisible to the un-aided eye. The root word, **bio,** refers to living organisms. The last part of the word, **logy,** means study of. When one puts all the parts together the result is micro—small, mi-croscopic; bio—living organisms; logy—study of. A working definition of microbiol-ogy is then the study of microscopic living systems. The microorganisms studied are often referred to as microbes. In some cases microbiology may involve using micro-scopic methods to detect the presence of larger organisms like parasitic worms.*

*Microorganisms are living systems that maintain a constant homeostatic internal environment. They affect their external environment and changes in their external en-vironment may often affect them. A drastic external change may threaten their life.*

*Most microbes are important contributors to the overall quality of our environment, and many play vital ecological roles. However, a significant number cause disease in humans and other animals because they upset the animal's homeostasis. These medically important microorganisms receive most of the emphasis in this text.*

*The broad scope of microbiology, therefore, includes the occurrence of microor-ganisms in nature and the environment of the body, their physiologic and reproductive processes, the harmful and beneficial roles they play in the body and in nature, and their cause and effect relationships to disease.*

# 1  HISTORICAL ASPECTS OF MICROBIOLOGY, SOME IMPORTANT CONTRIBUTIONS OF MICROBIOLOGY

The development of microbiology as a science received its first stimulus through the work and publications of one person. Antonj van Leeuwenhoek (1632–1723) was a Dutch linen merchant who ground lenses for a hobby. He developed a simple microscope that allowed him to see and describe "wee animalcules" in many different materials. His accurate and precise observations still amaze modern-day microbiologists.

Many individuals made significant contributions that led to the development of medical microbiology. The two most important contributors were probably Louis Pasteur (1822–1895) and Robert Koch (1843–1910).

Louis Pasteur was a French chemist and bacteriolo-gist whose serious scientific inquiries were essential in aiding several French industries. He came to the aid of the wine industry by showing that microorganisms were the cause of desirable and undesirable fermentations. Pasteur developed the process known today as pasteur-ization in his research on problems in wine production. He helped the silk industry of France by demonstrating the microbial cause of "pebrine," a silkworm disease. Pasteur is also credited with dealing the death blow to

the theory of spontaneous generation by showing that life always comes from preexisting life. Pasteur and his coworkers developed the first successful treatment for humans bitten by rabid animals.

Robert Koch also made giant steps in the early years of medical microbiology. His early work revolved around the development and improvement of microbi-ological culture methods. The development of a suit-able semisolid culture medium using agar was a major innovation. This agar medium provided the necessary surface for isolation of pure bacterial cultures. Koch also proposed four rules (Koch's postulates) for estab-lishing the microbial causative agents of disease. These rules are still used by researchers today.

### Koch's Postulates

1. The same organisms must be associated with every case of the disease.
2. The specific organism must be isolated in pure cul-ture.
3. The specific organism must always produce the dis-ease in a susceptible host animal.
4. The organism must be reisolated from the diseased test animal.

Because of the great effort of men like Pasteur, Koch, and many others, the science of medical microbi-ology progressed rapidly. The **"germ theory"** of disease became widely accepted. This theory proposes that diseases in man and other animals are often caused by microorganisms, and these diseases are transmitted from one animal to another through a variety of methods that will be discussed later. Other contributions of microbiology include:

1. Containment of diseases and prevention of their spread by initiating isolation and quarantine procedures.
2. The need for development of aseptic (free from germs) and antiseptic (prevention of development of microorganisms) techniques in medicine and nursing procedures.
3. Development of techniques for properly treating water and food for human consumption.
4. Tests for assaying and developing medicines.
5. Development of vaccines and various immunization procedures.

We are too often guilty of thinking that microbes (germs) are harmful and dangerous. Even though it is true that some microbes are harmful, most microbes are helpful to man and other life forms in the environment. The following list gives just a few beneficial roles that microorganisms play in our lives.

1. Commercial antibiotic and vitamin production.
2. Yeast activities in baking and brewing.
3. Vitamin K production in man's intestine.
4. Microbial decomposition in soil fertility.

## 2   NAMING OF MICROBES

Microorganisms are named systematically using a system originally developed by the Swedish scientist Linnaeus. In this system every organism is given a two-word name; thus it is a binomial system of nomenclature. The two names together represent the species of the organism. The medically important bacterium *Staphylococcus aureus* is a species example. The first word (*Staphylococcus*) is the specific genus that the organism is classified under. The second name (*aureus*) is the species of that particular organism. Since scientific names are given from foreign language derivatives, the name must be either italicized or underlined. Also, the first letter of the genus is always capitalized and the first letter of the species is never capitalized.

A microbe's name often indicates to the reader some particular characteristic of that organism. The name *Staphylococcus aureus*, for example, indicates several morphological characteristics. The word "coccus" means round; the word "Staphylo" means irregular; and the word "aureus" means gold. Thus, *Staphylococcus aureus* is a round-shaped bacterium that normally is seen in irregular clusters, and it produces a gold-colored colony.

The genus and species scientific name for all microbes is quite important since it can be accurately communicated between people in the United States and throughout the world. This scientific nomenclature will be adhered to throughout this text.

## 3   THE CELL: THE SMALLEST AND SIMPLEST UNIT OF LIVING MATTER

### THE CELL THEORY

Early in the history of biology as a science, the simplest living units were identified as cells. The cell theory states that the smallest and simplest unit of living matter that is capable of maintaining and reproducing itself is the cell. All organisms from the tiniest bacterium to the largest mammals possess cells as their basic structural and functional units. The only exceptions to this generalization are the viruses, which are **acellular.**

Each small cell is a complete life system maintaining a constant uniformity in its internal environment (homeostasis). This internal physiological equilibrium is important for each individual cell, whether the organism is a simple unicellular microbe or just one cell in the trillions that may make up a macroorganism.

### TYPES OF CELLS

Two basic types of cells are encountered among living systems. Both kinds of cells are represented in the microorganisms, and an understanding of the similarities and differences of these cell types is essential. The two types of cells differ primarily in degrees of complexity. The **procaryotic** cells are very simple with little internal complexity. The **eucaryotic cells** possess a striking degree of internal complexity that definitely sets them apart from procaryotic cells (Figure 3–1).

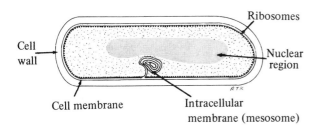

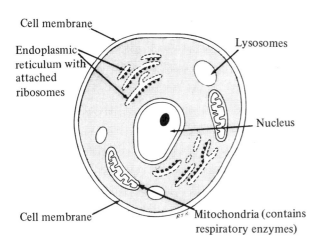

**Figure 3-1.** Procaryotic cell (top) and eucaryotic cell (bottom).

**PROCARYOTIC CELLS.** Procaryotic cells, which lack a true nucleus and other internal cellular compartments, are the simple cell type seen only in the bacteria and blue-green algae. These two groups of microorganisms are always unicellular and undifferentiated. Every cell within a species is always like every other cell. They nearly always exhibit a rigid outer cell wall with a cell membrane adhering closely to it. The internal cytoplasm is generally homogeneous with some inclusions evident. No nuclear compartment is ever seen, though special stains show a nuclear area. The only true working organelles are the ribosome units. The precise structure and function of each cell part will be discussed later in specific conjunction with bacteria.

**EUCARYOTIC CELLS.** (*Eu*—true, *caryotic*—nucleus). The striking difference between procaryotic and eucaryotic cells is the presence of membrane-defined cellular compartments such as the nucleus, mitochondria, and lysosomes. Figure 3-1 shows that the eucaryotic cells are more highly organized, with specific functions being localized in specific cellular compartments.

The nuclear compartment contains the genetic machinery necessary for operating the cell. The mitochondria contain the enzymes necessary for energy production within the cell. The lysosomes contain powerful digestive enzymes for hydrolysis of organic molecules. Each compartment then has only one specific job. In procaryotes, all the same general cellular jobs must be accomplished in an undifferentiated cellular cytoplasm.

# 4 GROUPS OF MICROORGANISMS

The microorganisms are separated into several different groups based on their degree of internal cellular organization. The procaryotic microbes are the bacteria, blue-green algae, rickettsias, and chlamydias. Eucaryotic microbes are the fungi (yeasts and molds) and the protozoans. One group of organisms, the viruses, have not been presented in the procaryote or eucaryote group because they are *acellular* (lacking a cellular organization).

Each group of microorganisms will be discussed in order to give a working knowledge of the important roles these microbes play in our bodies and in the environment. Even though many of these microbes are **pathogenic** (disease causing), most are not harmful and, in fact, many are beneficial to human life.

## *BACTERIA*

The bacteria are unicellular procaryotes. This group has more pathogenic types of microorganisms than any of the other groups.

### *Bacterial Cellular Structure*

Bacteria typically have an outer cell wall, a cell membrane beneath the cell wall, a limited amount of internal cellular membranes, ribosomes, and a nuclear region not contained within a nuclear membrane.

**CELL WALL.** The rigid outer cell wall of bacteria supports the cell and determines the cell's specific shape. A cell wall may play a protective role in bacteria when harmful external changes, such as changes in osmotic pressure, threaten their life. Without a cell wall a cell may rupture.

The bacterial cell wall is unique in that it is composed of a special chemical combination called a mucocomplex or **murien** layer. Murien is found nowhere else in nature except in the procaryotic unicellular microorganisms. The murien layer is one large macromolecule composed of carbohydrate and polypeptide units linked together in such a way as to produce a saclike envelope completely surrounding the cell.

Figure 3–2 shows the carbohydrate component to be repeating units of the two amino sugars N-acetylglucose amine (NAGA) and N-acetylmuramic acid (NAMA) linked together in infinitely long chains. The polypeptide component of the cell wall is illustrated as a chain of specific amino acids that cross-link the chains of amino sugars. The bacterial cell wall is sometimes compared with a barrel where the carbohydrate chains represent the wooden staves of the barrel and the polypeptides represent the metal hoops that hold the barrel together.

The bacterial cell wall is also the site of action of some drugs important in medical microbiology. Figure 3–2 shows that penicillin (an antibiotic) affects the cross-linking of the carbohydrate chains and thus prevents biosynthesis of the cell wall in growing organisms. Bacitracin, vanomycin, cycloserine, and other drugs also affect cell wall synthesis.

The cell wall of bacteria can be affected by enzymes. The bacteriolytic enzyme **lysozyme** found in tears, saliva, and gastric juices, ruptures the cell wall by cleaving the chemical bond between the amino sugars NAMA and NAGA.

Bacteria are divided into two basic groups using the gram-staining procedure outlined in your laboratory manual. A bacterium is gram-positive if it retains the primary dye of the stain (crystal violet) and is colored blue or purple. A gram-negative bacterium loses the primary dye during the decolorizing step and is counterstained red with safranin. The gram stain reaction of an organism is primarily due to the chemical constituents of its cell wall. The gram-staining procedure is one of

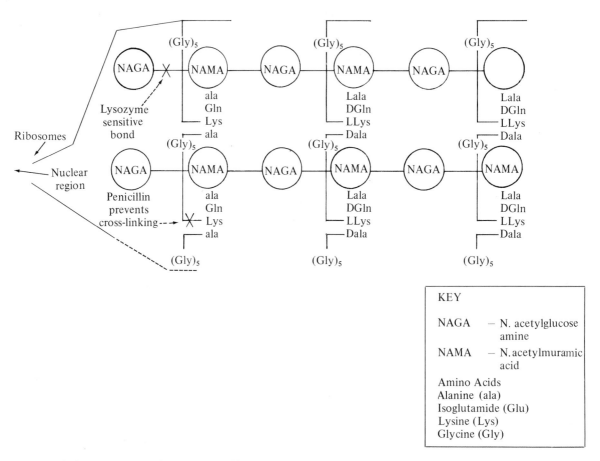

KEY

NAGA — N. acetylglucose amine

NAMA — N.acetylmuramic acid

Amino Acids
Alanine (ala)
Isoglutamide (Glu)
Lysine (Lys)
Glycine (Gly)

**Figure 3–2.** Bacterial cell wall murien. The bacterial cell wall is a unique combination of molecules. Carbohydrate and polypeptide units are cross-linked to produce a rigid saclike envelope around the cell. The sites of action of an enzyme (lysozyme) and an antibiotic (penicillin) are shown.

the most widely used staining procedures employed by bacteriologists.

Gram-positive bacteria have a thick cell wall composed almost entirely of mucocomplex. The cell wall is usually one layer thick, and most gram-positive bacteria are sensitive to penicillin and lysozyme.

Gram-negative bacteria have a much more complicated cell wall. The cell wall is generally composed of two layers of material, the internal mucous complex and the outer membranous structure. The outer membrane contains protein and lipopolysaccharide (fatty acids linked to polysaccharide). The lipopolysaccharide of some gram-negatives is called **endotoxin** and has been shown to be responsible for certain disease symptoms such as high fevers seen in infections by these organisms.

**CELL MEMBRANE.** The cell or cytoplasmic membrane is the actual physiological barrier between the bacterium and its environment. It is a thin-layered structure composed primarily of protein and lipid (its exact composition will be given in Chapter 4). The cell membrane controls precisely what enters and exits the cell. This important cellular structure plays a dynamic regulatory role essential for maintaining microbial cellular homeostasis.

Bacteria have specialized transport systems associated with their cytoplasmic membrane. These energy-requiring systems involve specific permeases or carrier proteins for many specific nutrients. For example, one permease transports glucose, another lactose, another sulfate ions. These specialized transport systems enable the bacterium to accumulate the required molecules inside the cell to provide the proper concentration of nutrients needed for rapid growth.

Connected to the cellular membrane and extending inward are intracellular membranes. These intracellular membranes furnish a large surface area on which chemical reactions take place. The respiratory enzymes for generating cellular energy are associated with such intracellular membranes. In gram-positive organisms these membranes are more prominent and are a specialized differentiated invagination of the cell membrane termed a **mesosome** ("middle body"). There is evidence that mesosomes may have certain specialized functions in cell division (cell wall formation and DNA replication) and endospore formation (may have a role analogous to that of the Golgi apparatus in eucaryotic cells).

**RIBOSOMES.** These are small intracellular particles found free in the cytoplasm or attached to the membrane system. They function as the physical site for biosynthesis of protein from amino acid subunits. DNA and other nucleic acids are involved in the direction of protein synthesis. The number of ribosomes present in a bacterial cell vary with several factors. Actively growing cells in a rich medium possess numerous ribosomes, whereas static cells in a poor medium have few ribosomes. Some antibiotics affect protein synthesis by stopping chemical activity at ribosomes.

**NUCLEAR REGION.** Bacteria lack the membrane-defined nucleus of eucaryotic cells. They do possess "bodies" within their cytoplasm that can be regarded as a nuclear region. The nuclear region is sometimes called a **nucleoid.** Only one chromosome of DNA is demonstrated in bacteria and it is usually circular. The DNA is a double-stranded macromolecule composed of nucleotides. This bacterial chromosome, occupying only about 10 percent of the cell volume, contains all the genetic information responsible for the protein synthesis within the cell.

**ACCESSORY CELLULAR STRUCTURES.** The following structures are not present on all bacteria. Some of the structures can be produced by bacteria under certain conditions and some are permanently present.

1. *Flagellum* (sing.), *flagella* (pl.) (Figure 3–3). A bacterium cell utilizes **flagella** as its organs of motility; they propel the cell through fluid. They are found on motile bacilli (rod-shaped bacteria) and spirilla (coiled bacteria), but they are never found on cocci (round bacteria) because cocci are nonmotile. Flagella are thin, hairlike appendages that protrude through the cell wall, and they originate from a granular structure just beneath the cell membrane. Flagella are composed of a protein called **flagellin.** Flagellar proteins are antigenic, and their presence can be detected with specific antisera; thus there are good diagnostic tests for certain pathogens that possess flagella (*Salmonella typhi*).

Flagella are very thin and cannot be seen with the light microscope unless a special stain is used. Microscopic studies show distinct patterns of flagellar arrangement on motile bacteria. The particular patterns of flagellation are shown in Figure 3–3. Bacteria that lack flagella are called **atrichous;** those with one polar flagellum are **monotrichous;** those with one flagellum from both poles are **amphitrichous;** those with a tuft of flagella from one or both poles are **lophotrichous;** those with many flagella over their entire surface are **peritrichous.**

2. *Pilus* (sing.), *pili* (pl.) (also called *fimbriae*). Gram-negative bacteria have shorter, straighter, filamentous cellular appendages called **pili.** They are composed of proteinlike flagella, but they do not impart cellular motility. One specialized type of pilus is important in the

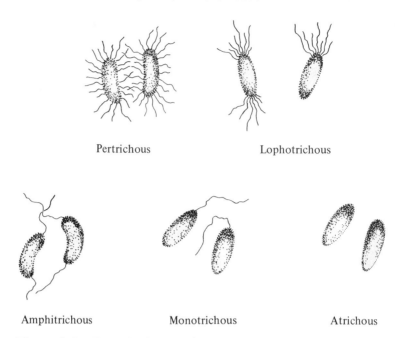

Pertrichous                    Lophotrichous

Amphitrichous          Monotrichous          Atrichous

**Figure 3-3.** Bacterial flagella. Some bacteria produce flagella, thin proteinaceous organs of motility. Patterns of flagellation are shown.

process of conjugation in certain bacteria. Other functions include the attachment of the cells to objects and the formation of scums or pellicles on the surfaces of liquids.

3. *Capsules* (Figure 3-4). Some bacteria possess the ability to secrete a slimy mucuslike layer called a **capsule.** It is excreted through the cell wall and forms a slimy coat on the outside of the cell. The capsule is composed of polysaccharide, polypeptide, or polysaccharide–protein complexes. These materials have low affinity for routine dyes, and a special stain or an India-ink mount is used to visualize them.

The capsule provides a protective, structural cover-

ing for the bacterium, and this covering may serve as a nutrient reservoir as well as a site for disposal of waste products. In the case of *Streptococcus mutans*, the primary causative agent of dental caries (tooth decay), the capsule enables the bacterium to adhere to the surface of the teeth.

Capsules are important from a medical standpoint because they increase the virulence (ability to cause disease) of an organism since they enable the microbe to resist **phagocytosis** ("cell eating") by white blood cells. *Diplococcus (Streptococcus) pneumoniae* (causative agent for lobar pneumonia) is pathogenic for man only when it is encapsulated. The nonencapsulated cells are

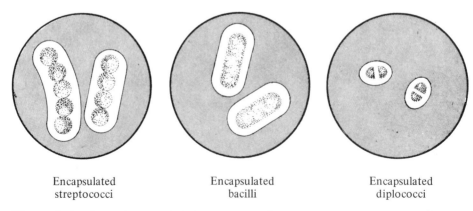

Encapsulated          Encapsulated          Encapsulated
streptococci          bacilli               diplococci

**Figure 3-4.** Bacterial capsules. Some bacteria form a capsule that is a mucuslike layer outside the cell wall. Illustrated are capsules on streptococci, bacilli, and diplococci.

**avirulent** (not capable of producing disease). The chemical constituents of the capsule are very specific for each species, and they are antigenic. This allows precise immunological typing of pathogenic bacteria that have a capsule.

4. *Bacterial endospores* (Figure 3–5). Certain bacteria (genera *Bacillus* and *Clostridium*) produce special dormant resting cells when the environment becomes unfavorable for normal growth and reproduction. These special cells are classified as **endospores** because they are formed inside the cytoplasm of the cell that produces them. Endospore formation is not a means of reproduction, but it is specifically a survival mechanism when conditions are not suitable for normal life.

The endospore is a unique cell in that it has very thick spore coats, a dehydrated cytoplasm, unusual cytoplasmic chemicals, and no metabolic activity. These unusual physical and chemical properties have been related to the resistance of the endospore to harsh physical and chemical treatments. Endospores remain viable after desiccation (drying), inanition (starvation, lack of nutrients), and radiation exposure. Their most striking property of resistance is their ability to survive extreme heat treatments. Boiling spores in water has little or no effect on them even though the same treatment readily kills **vegetative forms** (actively growing form of bacteria).

Because of their high resistance, the procedures in hospitals for sterilzation must be designed to result in the ultimate destruction of endospores. A treatment must then be **sporicidal** in order to ensure the required surgical and bacteriologic sterilization. Similar harsh treatments are also necessary in the home and industrial food canning procedures to ensure destruction of spores. Figure 3–5 shows that spores may be found in various regions within the maternal cell's cytoplasm. Spores may be located centrally, terminally, or subterminally. Position of the spore may be an aid in identification of a particular type of spore-forming bacteria.

### Bacterial Morphology

Bacterial morphology (Figure 3–6) is the study of the form and structure of bacteria. Examination of bacteria reveals three basic forms of bacteria based on the shape of their cells.

**COCCUS (SING.), COCCI (PL.).** Cocci are round (berry-shaped) spherical bacteria. Sometimes oval cocci or cocci slightly flattened on one side may be seen. The cocci display distinct patterns or groupings of cells depending on their type of cell division, and these patterns are an aid in identifying the bacteria.

- *Diplococci* These cocci are found in pairs. Figure 3–6 shows an encapsulated diplococci group. Diplococci are responsible for bacterial meningitis, gonorrhea, and other diseases.
- *Streptococci* These cocci exist in chains. Encapsulated streptococci are also shown. Streptococci are responsible for the "strep throat" disease.
- *Gaffykya* These cocci occur in a regular pattern of four cells.
- *Sarcina* These cocci exist in regular cuboidal packets of eight cells.
- *Staphylococci* These cocci are found in irregular clusters (grapelike). Staphylococci are responsible for a variety of diseases, but they are the notorious causative agents of the "hospital staph" infections.

**BACILLUS (SING.), BACILLI (PL.).** In Figure 3–6 the bacilli are illustrated as rod-shaped bacteria. They ex-

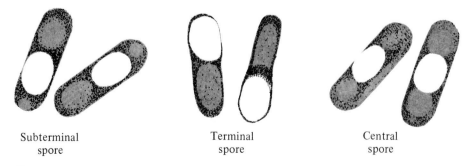

Subterminal spore          Terminal spore          Central spore

**Figure 3–5.** Bacterial endospores. Bacterial spores are produced inside cells at various points (subterminal, terminal, central). They contain cellular material and enable a microbe to resist unfavorable conditions.

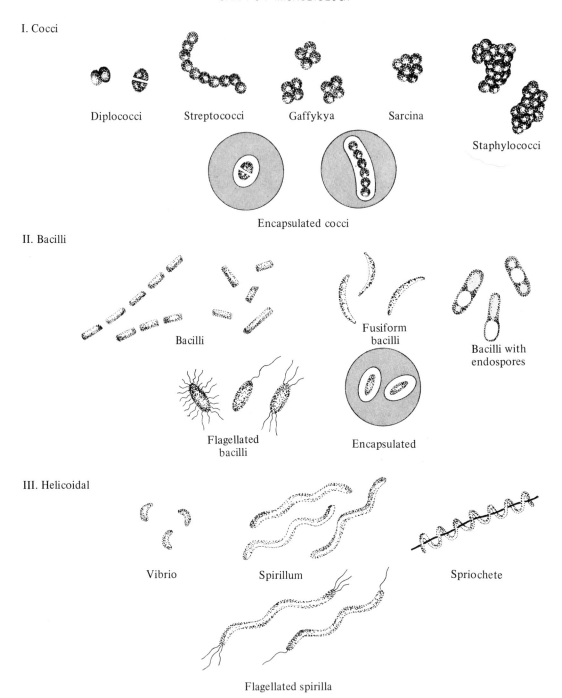

I. Cocci

Diplococci     Streptococci     Gaffykya     Sarcina

Staphylococci

Encapsulated cocci

II. Bacilli

Bacilli

Fusiform
bacilli

Bacilli with
endospores

Flagellated
bacilli

Encapsulated

III. Helicoidal

Vibrio          Spirillum          Spriochete

Flagellated spirilla

**Figure 3-6.** Bacterial morphology. Bacteria have three basic forms: cocci (round), bacilli (rod-shaped), helicoidal (spiral).

hibit some variety in shape as some are long and slender, others are short and plump, and others are even slightly curved with pointed ends. Flagellate bacilli, which are motile, are also shown. Endospores are seen in the bacilli, and sometimes bacilli form a capsule. The spore-forming organism *Bacillus anthracis* causes anthrax, whereas the non-spore-forming flagellated bacillus *Salmonella typhi* causes typhoid fever. Other diseases caused by bacilli are tetanus, diphtheria, and tuberculosis.

**HELICOIDAL (SPIRAL-SHAPED).** Figure 3-6 shows this group to contain three basic spiral organisms: vibrio, spirillum, and spirochete.

- *Vibrio* The vibrio bacteria are comma-shaped, slightly curved bacteria. Cholera is caused by a vibrio.
- *Spirillum* (*spirilla,* pl.) Spirilla are long, corkscrew-shaped spirals that are rigid. Figure 3–6 shows non-motile spirilla that lack flagella and motile spirilla with flagella. These organisms are common inhabitants of the mouth.
- *Spirochete* The spirochetes are flexible spiral-shaped organisms. Figure 3–6 shows the spirochete to possess an axial filament that spirals around the organism between the cell wall and the cell membrane. This axial filament confers both the spiral shape and flexibility to the organism. Syphilis is caused by the spirochete organism *Treponema pallidum.*

## Reproduction of Bacteria

Bacteria reproduce primarily by the asexual process called **transverse binary fission.** A single cell divides into two cells by forming a transverse cell wall between the developing daughter cells. Each daughter cell is identical to the original parent cell, and under favorable conditions the daughter cells will rapidly divide again to form even more new cells. Several events occur during cell division. First, the parent cell increases in size (elongation) and reproduces its DNA to supply two exact copies of genetic information. Second, there is an invagination of cell wall and cell membrane at the center of the cell, and usually the duplicated DNA is distributed to either side of the cell. Third, the transverse cell wall between the two cells is completed and the cells often separate. This cell-division cycle is similar to the process of **mitosis** in eucaryotic cells.

Bacteria can divide very rapidly under optimum conditions. Some newly formed bacterial cells can reach full size and divide in 15 to 30 minutes. This explains how a bacterial infection can spread so rapidly in the body, and why the proper handling of specimens for microbiological cultures is so important. For example, suppose a urine specimen is not refrigerated as it should be if it is not to be cultured immediately, but is left at room temperature. This will provide the proper conditions for bacterial reproduction. If the urine specimen is contaminated with approximately 100 gram-negative organisms that are dividing every 20 minutes, there will be over 6000 organisms in 2 hours, over 50,000 organisms in 3 hours, and over 400,000 organisms in 4 hours. What began as a small contamination could now be incorrectly interpreted as a severe urinary tract infection in the patient.

Occasionally, one may observe a special type of mating in gram-negative bacilli called **conjugation.** Conjugation allows the transfer of genetic information through a bridge formed by a special pilus. This process is very important to the microbiologist who studies bacterial genetics and recombination of genes in gram-negative microorganisms.

**REPRODUCTION CURVE OF BACTERIA.** Bacteria grow and reproduce rapidly in favorable environments, and population changes in cultures are interesting to study. Increases of cells in cultures follow a geometric progression:

$$1 \xrightarrow{\text{cell division}} 2 \rightarrow 2^2 \rightarrow 2^3 \rightarrow 2^4 \ldots 2^n$$

If one follows the changes in a bacterial culture, four definite phases can be observed (Figure 3–7).

The **lag phase** is a period where no growth occurs. The graph may even show a decrease in cell number. Lag-phase bacterial cells are not inactive, but rather the

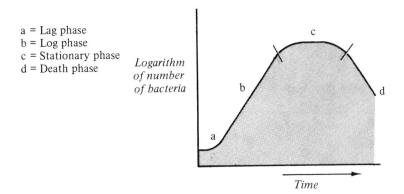

a = Lag phase
b = Log phase
c = Stationary phase
d = Death phase

*Logarithm of number of bacteria*

*Time*

**Figure 3–7.** The reproduction curve of bacteria exhibits four phases. This process is so rapid for some microbes that they can complete all four stages and produce a new generation in 30 minutes.

cells are becoming adapted to their environment and many chemical adjustments are occurring within each cell's cytoplasm. The lag phase may last for several hours to several days depending on the type and age of the organisms and the culture medium. The **incubation period** of some diseases (time between the entrance of microbes and appearance of disease symptoms) results from various factors but probably corresponds to the lag phase of bacterial reproduction.

The **log phase** (growth phase) is a period of most rapid cell division, and the typical characteristics of the organism can be observed. This phase is called the log phase because if one plots the logarithm of the number of cells against time, the graph is a straight line. Data from the log phase can be used to calculate the exact generation time (time for doubling of number of cells) for an organism under specific conditions. Since there is such a rapid increase in cell numbers during the growth phase, one may associate this phase with the appearance and spread of the symptoms of disease in a bacterial infection.

The log phase occurs when the nutrients for growth and reproduction are plentiful and the microbes have adapted to their surroundings. Growth can be so rapid that if one cell divides every 30 minutes, in 10 hours there may be 1 million cells. This rapid increase in cell number cannot continue indefinitely because nutrients will quickly be depleted and a slowing of the growth rate will occur.

The **stationary phase** follows the log phase and is characterized by a leveling off of the graph (Figure 3–7). The rate of cell division slows to a rate equal to that of cell death. This leveling off is primarily due to changes in the environment, such as depletion of essential nutrients and the buildup of toxic waste products in the medium. These changes toward more unfavorable conditions may stimulate spore-forming bacteria (*Bacillus* and *Clostridium*) to undergo sporulation.

The **death phase** follows the stationary phase and is characterized by a decline in number of cells because more cells are dying than are produced by cell division. High concentrations of toxic waste products and severe depletion of nutrients cause the rapid decline. Death of cells may be rapid at first, but it may take weeks to months before all the cells in a culture are dead. Spore-forming bacteria may not demonstrate a death phase because every cell may produce a resistant endospore to survive the harsh environments.

**APPLICATION OF THE REPRODUCTION CURVE OF BACTERIA.** In comparing the growth of bacteria in the body and on artificial culture media, a parallel could be drawn between the development of a general-ized or systemic infection in the human body and the growth of bacteria in a liquid medium. Likewise, the growth of a bacterial colony on solid medium corresponds to the development of a localized infection.

The isolated bacterial colony growing and developing on solid media demonstrates the characteristics of the bacterial reproduction curve. There must be a lag phase before the initial cell—which will ultimately produce the colony—begins to divide. Then the cells will begin to divide at a constant rate during the growth phase as nutrients are plentiful. However, after a few divisions, the cells will become crowded and the competition for the available nutrients will increase. As toxic products build up and nutrients decrease, the cells in the center will enter the stationary phase and then the death phase as conditions worsen, while cells on the periphery of the colony may still be in the growth phase. Therefore, within a single colony there will be cells in the growth phase, the stationary phase, or the death phase, depending on their location in the colony.

### Requirements for Growth of Bacteria

Microbes require specific conditions before they can grow in the body or before they can be grown on artificial media in a laboratory. Microbes often are cultured or grown on specially prepared media in laboratories. Our discussion and comments in this area, in general, refer to the requirements for microbial growth both on artificial media and in the body.

**NUTRITION.** Bacteria, like humans, have certain nutritional requirements that are essential for their life. Bacteria require a source of carbon, hydrogen, oxygen, nitrogen, and various other inorganic compounds. Some require vitamins and amino acids that have been preformed because they lack synthesis systems to make their own. These nutritional requirements are necessary for the microbe to synthesize its carbohydrate, protein, lipid, and nucleic acid cytoplasmic constituents. The bacteria, as a group, exhibit tremendous versatility in nutritional requirements. Some bacteria are capable of using $CO_2$ as their sole carbon source for synthesizing organic compounds. These bacteria are called **autotrophic** (*auto*—self, *trophic*—feed) or self-feeding bacteria. Bacterial autotrophs may utilize radiant energy and are called **phototrophic bacteria.** Other bacterial autotrophs oxidize inorganic substrates to generate cellular energy for life (**chemotrophs**). There are few if any pathogenic autotrophic bacteria because the external environment supplies the nutrients and living conditions they need; therefore, they do not need to break down living cells to obtain nutrients.

Most bacteria are nutritionally classified as **heterotrophic** (*hetero*—other, *trophic*—feed) because they require a preformed organic carbon source. This means they must utilize organic material that has already been synthesized by others. They literally must rely on the "feeding of others" for their nutritional needs. Most heterotrophic bacteria play an important decay role in the environment by breaking down the tissue material of dead plants and animals. These heterotrophic bacteria are called **saprophytes** (*sapro*—rot, *phyte*—plant). Saprophytes may be able to cause disease in our bodies if given the opportunity and therefore are potentially pathogenic microorganisms. The pathogenic saprophytes do not usually invade healthy tissues. For example, *Clostridium tetani*, the organism that causes tetanus, invades deep puncture wounds where the $O_2$ concentration is low and some dead tissue is present. The Clostridium bacteria grow and excrete toxic waste products. The waste products cause the disease symptoms because the bacteria are not invasive. *Clostridium botulinum*, the causative agent of botulism food poisoning, normally lives in the soil. Its spores may be carried by air and contaminate foods. Vegetative cells may grow if there is no air and their toxic metabolic waste products may cause a serious (usually fatal) food poisoning.

Some pathogenic organisms are classified as **parasites** (live on a host at the expense of the host). Parasites can only live and reproduce in the tissue of a host organism. Examples of strict human parasites are the bacteria *Neisseria gonorrhea* (causes gonorrhea) and *Treponema pallidum* (causes syphilis). A pathogenic bacteria, whether saprophyte or parasite, is a heterotrophic microorganism living on human tissue that either invades living tissue or grows on dead tissue. They may excrete toxic metabolic products that cause disease and malfunction in the human body.

**WATER.** Water is vital for the survival of most microbes. Water is utilized for chemical reactions and as a component for various essential chemical compounds. Dry conditions are fatal to microbes; however, spore-forming bacteria and encapsulated bacteria are more resistant to dry conditions than are other microbes. Spores are formed specifically when conditions exist that are detrimental to vegetative cell growth and reproduction.

**OXYGEN ($O_2$).** Many microorganisms as well as macroorganisms, like humans, require oxygen gas for energy production. Organisms that utilize oxygen are called **aerobes** (*aero*—air). Most of the time the $O_2$ is supplied by air, which is about 21 percent $O_2$.

Oxygen is utilized in the final step of producing chemical energy (ATP) in cells. This energy is used by the organism for various chemical processes such as transporting nutrients across the cell membrane (active transport) and the biosynthesis of needed cellular components and compounds.

Some microbes cannot exist in the presence of atmospheric oxygen. These organisms are called **anaerobes** (*an*—without, *aero*—air). Oxygen may be toxic to strict anaerobes such as the Clostridia. Anaerobes obtain cellular energy by oxidizing glucose without oxygen through a process like fermentation. Anaerobic glucose oxidation is very energy inefficient. Few pathogenic bacteria are strict anaerobes. Two anaerobic bacteria are *Clostridium tetani*, which causes tetanus, and *Clostridium perfringen*, one organism responsible for gas gangrene.

Many bacteria grow in the presence or absence of free atmospheric oxygen and are called **facultative** bacteria. These bacteria are versatile and manage very well in either an anaerobic or aerobic environment. *Salmonella typhi*, which causes typhoid fever, is a facultative bacterium.

**TEMPERATURE.** All microbes have a temperature range within which they are able to live and reproduce. At one end of the range is the *minimum* and at the other end is the *maximum* temperature at which these organisms are able to function. Somewhere between the two extremes is their optimum temperature. Bacteria that normally inhabit the body and pathogenic ones usually have an optimum temperature of 37°C. However, their temperature range is 20° to 45°C. These organisms are termed **mesophiles** (*meso*—middle, *phil*—loving). **Psychrophiles** are another important group of organisms, which have their optimum temperature below 15°C and may still multiply at 2 to 3°C. These organisms grow slowly in refrigerators and may cause the spoilage of food or the contamination of microbiologic cultures. The third group of organisms delineated by optimum growth temperature is the **thermophiles,** which grow at temperatures above 45° to 50°C. These organisms do not present any health problem and are found in nature in hot springs.

High temperatures are much more damaging to microbes than are low temperatures and, therefore, are used to sterilize and disinfect instruments and other objects used in hospitals. Essentially, this same technique is used in the kitchen in preparing food and washing eating utensils.

**pH OR HYDROGEN ION CONCENTRATION.**
The medium or area of the body in which bacteria grow

must not be too acid or alkaline or certain bacteria will be unable to survive. Most pathogenic organisms grow best at a neutral pH (pH 7) or that of the blood (pH 7.3 to 7.5). However, some pathogenic bacteria found in the body grow better at an alkaline pH (for example, the cholera bacillus, *Vibrio cholerae*), and some grow only at an acid pH (for example, the lactobacilli in the female vagina, pH 4 to 6).

## VIRUSES

Viruses are acellular particles much smaller than bacteria. They only exhibit characteristics of life when parasitizing a specific host cell, and the host cell is usually killed during viral reproduction inside the host cell. Viruses are too small to be seen with a light microscope, but the electron microscope reveals much about their structure. Four basic types of viruses are based on the host organism: they infect animals, plants, bacteria, and insects. Viruses are specific disease agents; a bacterial virus will not infect plant cells.

### Structure of a Virus Particle

Virus particles (**virions**) are very simple structures. They are generally composed of an outer coat made of protein called a **capsid** (Figure 3–8). The capsid surrounds the core nucleic acid (either DNA or RNA, never both). Repeating protein units called **capsomeres** aggregate to form the capsid. The capsid is often seen to form a faceted **icosahedron** composed of 20 facets, each facet being an equilateral triangle. Figure 3–8 shows one such polyhedral viral capsid. Outer protein capsid material protects the inner nucleic acid and aids in attaching the virus particle to the appropriate host cells. Some virions may be surrounded by a lipid envelope, and these enveloped viruses derive the membrane (composing the envelope) from the host cells. The envelope may aid the entrance of virus into new host cells.

### Virus Life Cycle

Since viruses cannot replicate outside of living host cells, and they require specific host cell systems for reproduction, it is important to understand the events involved in viral infection and reproduction. The life cycle of the T phage bacterial virus (a virus that infects bacteria) will be illustrated and discussed (Figure 3–9). The T phage first must contact a susceptible host bacterium cell and attach at specific receptor sites on its cell wall. Attachment is followed by a forceful injection of the core DNA into the bacterium, with the protein coat material remaining outside. Viral DNA, once inside the host cell, takes over the cell metabolism. Viral DNA is reproduced repeatedly, followed quickly by the synthesis of specific viral proteins. Once the synthesis phase is complete, the viral protein and DNA are assembled into separate virion packages. Lysis of the bacterium releases the newly formed virions into the environment. Each virion can potentially infect a new susceptible host cell.

Animal viruses also infect specific cells. Hepatitis viruses infect chiefly liver cells; intestinal viruses infect intestinal cells; and cold viruses primarily infect cells of the upper respiratory tract. Animal cells have specific receptor sites for their contact with specific animal viruses. Infection of the animal cell occurs somewhat differently from that of bacterial cells. Once the virus contacts the animal cell, the whole virion is taken in either by phagocytosis ("cell eating") or by pinocytosis ("cell drinking"). The uptake of an enveloped animal virus by a host cell may be facilitated by the fusion of the lipid viral envelope with the host cell membrane. Viral reproduction is very similar in bacterial hosts and animal hosts. Animal cells are not necessarily lysed at the end of animal viral reproduction.

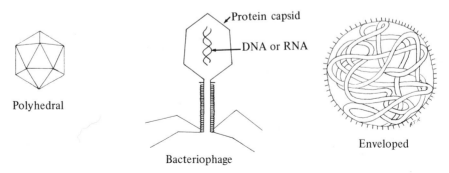

Polyhedral

Protein capsid

DNA or RNA

Bacteriophage

Enveloped

**Figure 3–8.**   Three different types of viruses.

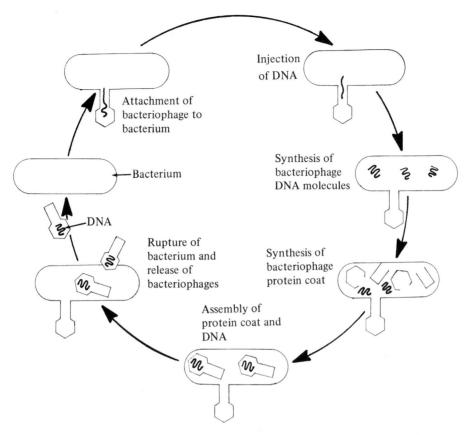

**Figure 3-9.** Life cycle of a bacteriophage virus. (Adapted from *Life Cycle of a Virus*, copyright by CEBCO Standard Publishing)

## FUNGI

Fungi are eucaryotic organisms much larger than bacteria. Some fungi, the mushrooms and toadstools, are actually large multicellular plantlike organisms. The other fungi, the yeasts and molds, are generally considered to be microorganisms. Yeasts and molds cause several important human diseases, which will be discussed later. In general a fungal disease is called a **mycoses,** and the study of these diseases is medical mycology. **Dermatomycoses** are fungal infections of the skin and superficial tissues; **systemic mycoses** are deep infections involving many different body tissues.

### Molds

Molds are filamentous fungi. The cells form long and short filaments called **hyphae.** Patches of mold growth may be visible, but magnification is necessary to see single hyphae and the individual cells that comprise them. Cell size ranges from 1 micrometer to 10 to 20 microme-

ters in diameter. As the hyphae grow, they mesh together, forming a mass of hyphae called **mycelium.**

Molds reproduce by forming special spores. A mold spore is like the seed of a plant. Spores in a favorable (moist and warm) environment will germinate and produce new hyphae and mycelia. After spore germination is complete, an asexual method of cell reproduction similar to bacterial binary fission occurs to increase the length of growing filaments. Filaments elongate and undergo differentiation to produce spores.

The spores of molds are classified into two general groups, **asexual** and **sexual.** Sexual spores are formed by the fusion of nuclear material from separate cells (fertilization). Asexual spores require no fertilization and are produced by the differentiation of the cytoplasm in one cell. Spores can be picked up by and transported to new environments by agents such as water or air currents.

### Yeasts

**Yeasts** are unicellular microorganisms with typical round to oval cell forms. The usually reproduce by the

asexual process known as **budding** (blastospore formation). On a growing cell, a small bulge will develop that
increases in size until it pinches off to be completely se-
vered from the maternal cell. Some yeasts are ascospore
formers. One such yeast genus, *Saccharomyles,* is widely
used in the brewing industry for making wine, beer, and
ales.

*Candida albicans* causes a mycotic infection of the
mouth, vagina, and skin. Infection of the mouth by
*Candida* is called thrush. *Candida (Monilia)* infections
are not uncommon following prolonged broad-spec-
trum antibiotic treatments where the normal microbial
flora is upset. *Cryptococcus neoformans* is the causative
agent of a severe meningitis. Humans contract the disease in inhaling dust containing the organism. The
yeast may infect the lungs or other body tissues, but
meningitis is the most frequently observed manifesta-
tion.

## PROTOZOA

Protozoa are large unicellular eucaryotic microbes that
differ from the other microorganisms in that they ingest
their food material as particles. They also differ from
bacteria and fungi because they lack a cell wall. Many
persons consider the protozoans to be simple animals.
Four general groups of protozoans are classified according to their particular type of motility (method of move-

ment). Each group will be discussed, and medically significant examples will be given.

### Sarcodina

This class of protozoans contains the amoebas (Figure
3–10) and related organisms. Motility in the amoebas is
seen as flowing extensions of their cytoplasm known as
**pseudopods.** Pseudopods (false feet) are used to surround food particles, and the particles are said to have
been ingested by phagocytosis (cell eating). Many of the
sarcodinan species are common inhabitants of soil and
water environments. Several species are found in the
human intestine. *Entamoeba coli* is a nonpathogenic
amoeba seen routinely in human stool specimens. *Entamoeba histolytica* is a pathogenic amoeba; it is probably
the most severe pathogen of all the intestinal protozoan
parasites. It causes acute amoebic dysentery that can be
fatal if left untreated.

### Ciliates

Figure 3–10 shows these protozoans to possess short
hairlike cellular appendages called cilia as organs of motility. Ciliates are common inhabitants of soil and water
habitats. *Paramecium* species are routinely used in laboratories to demonstrate to students the morphology
of protozoans. Only one ciliate species is of particular
medical importance. *Balantidium coli,* the largest of all

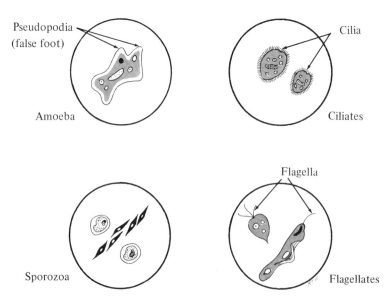

**Figure 3–10.**   The various types of protozoa are named according to
their means of locomotion (motility).

intestinal protozoans, causes a severe dysentery; it is normally found in pigs and is passed to humans when cysts (dormant, resistant protozoan forms) gain access to the digestive tract.

### Flagellates

These protozoans are motile by long whiplike cellular appendages called flagella. The flagellates comprise a diverse group of microbes ranging from autotrophic (photosynthetic) to strict parasites of people and animals. *Trichomonas vaginalis* causes a vaginitis primarily contracted through sexual intercourse (VD). Several species of the genus *Trypanosoma* cause the African sleeping sickness disease transmitted to people by the bite of the tsetse fly. *Leishmania donouani* causes the Leishmaniasis (kala-azar) disease in South America and Mexico. Leishmania is transmitted to humans by the bite of the sandfly *Phlebotomus*. Both *Trypanosoma* and *Leishmania* are known as **hemoflagellate protozoans** because they travel in the bloodstream. These hemoflagellate diseases can be fatal if they are not treated.

### Sporozoa

Sporozoans are all parasites of some host animal. They differ from the other protozoans in several ways. Sporozoans do not ingest particulate food; they are not motile as adult forms; and they demonstrate a very complex life cycle involving asexual and sexual reproduction. The sporozoan genus *Plasmodium* contains the species that causes malaria in people. Plasmodia are transmitted to humans by the bite of an infected female Anopheles mosquito. Even though malaria is rare in the United States, it still is a serious health problem in tropical areas of our world.

# 5 MICROORGANISMS NORMALLY FOUND ON AND IN THE BODY

Microorganisms on and in the body are referred to as the **resident** or **normal flora** (flora refers to plant life). Bacteria often are classified as plants and since most of the resident organisms are bacteria, therefore the name flora. Organisms present on the body for a short time only are termed **transient flora**. As stated previously,

many microorganisms are helpful to humans. These normal inhabitants play various roles on the skin and in the mouth, respiratory tract, intestinal tract, and genitourinary tract. Some of the normal inhabitants are harmless **commensals** and some are potentially harmful **opportunists**. However, the three groups, symbionts, commensals, and opportunists, are not mutually exclusive, and under certain conditions a symbiont or a commensal may act as a pathogen producing a diseased state. Therefore, the bacteria are categorized by their normal role in the human body only. We will look at organisms found in each of these areas and the roles they play.

## SKIN

Most of the skin is too dry, lacks nutrients, and has a pH that is too acidic (pH 5.6) for bacteria to grow. Many bacteria live in hair follicles and sweat glands. Skin areas where bacteria are able to live include the underarm (axillary) region, urinary and perineal areas, between the toes, in the scalp, and in the ears. The moisture level is high enough in these areas to support bacteria.

The majority of the bacteria are *Staphylococcus* species and some species of *Corynebacterium* that can survive in the "adverse" conditions of the skin. These bacteria seem to interact and compete with foreign pathogenic bacteria to prevent their colonization on the skin. The anatomic structure of the skin plus the oil and sweat that are normally present serve as very effective barriers to the entrance of bacteria. However, *Staphylococcus aureus*, found on normal skin, may also act as an opportunist and invade the skin when it is traumatized by cuts or burns.

## MOUTH AND RESPIRATORY TRACT

Various species of cocci, spirochetes, and bacilli are found in the mouth. The surface of the teeth is an especially favorable area for bacterial growth. **Dental plaque,** or the material on the teeth that is brushed off, consists of bacteria and organic material. Tooth decay (dental caries) can be initiated by waste products from these bacteria that weaken the calcium content of teeth. Bacteria then can move into the inner tissues of the teeth and cause further decay.

Various cocci, including species of staphylococci, streptococci, and *Neisseria*, are also found in the nose, mouth, and throat. Many of these organisms are opportunists, and it is for that reason that surgical masks are worn in dealing with patients who are particularly susceptible to infection. The bacteria in these regions tend to compete with pathogenic bacteria, molds, and yeasts. This is emphasized by the fact that in a newborn child the normal organisms have not been established yet; however, within a few hours after birth colonization begins. Often yeast (*Candida albicans*) will localize in an infant's mouth and cause a condition called "thrush." These yeasts are contracted during infant's passage through the birth canal.

## LARGE AND SMALL INTESTINES

Mircoorganisms are not usually present in the stomach because they are susceptible to the high acidic level (pH about 1.3 to 2.5) of the gastric juices. The pH in the small and large intestines is alkaline, and bacteria are prevalent in these areas. The large intestine contains both aerobic and anaerobic bacteria. Approximately 75 percent of the normal bacteria are species related to *Escherichia coli* (bacilli called coliforms). These bacteria are responsible for the gases produced and expelled from the large intestine. Vitamin K and the B-complex vitamins are produced by bacteria in the large intestine and are absorbed into the bloodstream. Antibiotics taken in large quantities often destroy these bacteria, allowing others to colonize, and diarrhea may result.

The intestinal tract of the newborn infant is sterile, but soon a characteristic flora develops from the milk taken in by the infant.

## GENITOURINARY TRACT

The urinary tract (urethra) is the urinary passageway from the bladder to the outside. The male and female urinary tract is usually sterile except for the lower area at the opening to the outside. Various groups of bacteria are present in the vagina, with lactobacilli being the prominent group between puberty and menopause. The lactobacilli contribute to the acidic pH of the vagina by the production of lactic acid, which helps prevent the colonization of pathogens such as *Neisseria gonorrhoeae* (causative agent of gonorrhea). Before puberty and after menopause the vagina is alkaline and the normal flora are different, being composed of various cocci and coliforms (gram-negative bacilli).

## BLOOD

Generally, the blood of a healthy individual is sterile (free from contamination by microorganisms). Bacteria may get into the blood through cuts, after a dental extraction, or by absorption with food from the intestinal tract, but they are readily eliminated by white blood cells. However, viruses and other organisms may be present in the blood during their incubation period (time interval between when the infection is contracted and the appearance of disease symptoms) and even after the person has recovered from the disease (for example, serum hepatitis). For this reason, blood banks will refuse blood from donors who have had hepatitis, malaria, syphilis, and other diseases because these organisms may still be present in the bloodstream.

---

# SUMMARY

---

**Historical Aspects of Microbiology,**
Some Important Contributions of Microbiology

A. Louis Pasteur. Developed pasteurization process; demonstrated cause of pebrine; showed that life came from preexisting life; developed first treatment for rabid animal bite.

B. Robert Koch. Developed and improved microbiological culture methods; proposed Koch's postulates for establishing the microbial causative agents of disease.

**Naming of Microbes**

A. Microbes are given a two-word name, genus first, followed by a species name; *Staphylococcus* (genus) *aureus* (species) is an example.

**The Cell:** The Smallest and Simplest Unit of Living Matter

A. Cell theory. Smallest and simplest unit of living matter that is capable of maintaining and reproducing itself is a cell.

B. Types of Cells
 1. Procaryotic: lack a true nucleus and other internal cellular compartments.
 *Ex.*    blue–green algae and bacteria.
 2. Eucaryotic: have defined cellular compartments such as nucleus, mitochondria, and lysosomes.

**Groups of Microorganisms**

A. Bacteria
 1. Bacterial cellular structure: have an outer cell wall, membrane, limited amount of internal cellular membranes, ribosomes, and a nuclear region not contained within a nuclear membrane.
  a. Cell wall: outer protective layer; protects bacterium against external changes.
  b. Cell membrane: physiological barrier between bacterium and environment; controls what enters and exits the bacterium.
  c. Ribosomes: small particles in cytoplasm that are site of protein synthesis.
  d. Nuclear region: bacteria lack membrane-defined nucleus; do have a nuclear region; responsible for protein synthesis within a bacterium.
  e. Accessory cellular structures: (1) *flagella,* hairlike appendages; function to propel a bacterium; (2) *pilus,* short appendages on gram-negative bacteria, propel bacterium; (3) *capsules,* mucuslike layer on outside of cell wall in some bacteria; (4) *endospores,* special dormant, resting cells produced by some bacteria (*Bacillus* and *Clostridium*) when environment becomes unfavorable for normal growth and reproduction.
 2. Bacterial Morphology
  a. Three basic forms of bacteria: (1) cocci (round), (2) bacilli (rod-shaped), (3) helicoidal (spiral).
 3. Reproduction of Bacteria
  a. Reproduce by asexual process called transverse binary fission.
  b. Reproduction curve of bacteria. Consists of four phases (1) lag phase, period where no growth occurs; (2) log phase (growth phase), period of most rapid cell division; (3) stationary phase, population is stable; (4) death phase, decline in number of cells due to high concentration of toxic wastes.
 4. Requirements for Growth of Bacteria
  a. Autotrophic: use $CO_2$ as carbon source for synthesizing organic compounds.
  b. Heterotrophic: require a preformed organic carbon source.
  c. Parasites: live and reproduce in tissues of a host.

B. Viruses
 1. Acellular particles, smaller than bacteria; cannot be seen except with electron microscope.
 2. Structure of virus particle: virus particle (virion) has an outer protein coat, capsid; inner core composed of either DNA or RNA.
 3. Virus life cycle: cannot reproduce outside of living cells; steps are shown in Figure 3–9.
 4. Cause a variety of human diseases.

C. Fungi
 Eucaryotic organisms much larger than bacteria; a fungal disease is called a *mycoses*.
 1. Molds: filamentous fungi; reproduce by forming special spores, which are either asexual or sexual.

2. Yeasts
   a. Unicellular microorganisms with typical round to oval cell forms; reproduce asexually by budding.
   b. *Candida albicans* causes mycotic infection of the mouth, vagina, and skin; *Cryptococcus neoformans* causes meningitis.

D. Protozoa
   Large unicellular eucaryotic microbes; differ from bacteria and fungi since they lack a cell wall; simple animals; four groups are found in humans.
   1. Sarcodina: contains amoebas; *Entamoeba histolytica* causes acute amoebic dysentery.
   2. Ciliates: have many cilia; *Balantidium coli* causes severe dysentery.
   3. Flagellates: have long flagella; *Trichomonas vaginalis* causes vaginitis.
   4. Sporozoa: parasites found in animals; *Plasmodium* genus causes malaria in man.

## Microorganisms Normally Found on and in the Body
Bacteria found on and in the body are called normal flora.

A. Skin: bacteria are found in hair follicles, sweat glands, axillary and urinary areas, toes, scalp, and in ears; staphylococcus is most common.

B. Mouth and respiratory tract: cocci, spirochetes, and bacilli are found in mouth and respiratory tract.

C. Large and small intestines: approximately 75 percent of bacteria are *Escherichia coli*; produce gas in large intestine and vitamin K and B-complex.

D. Genitourinary tract: lactobacilli are most common in vagina; before puberty and after menopause, the bacteria tend to be various cocci and coliforms.

E. Blood: generally sterile in a healthy individual; viruses and bacteria may be present in blood during their incubation period.

## Microbiology

True (A) or False (B).

1. The term Microbiology means study of small bacteria.

2. The scientific name of organisms includes genus and species.

3. The two basic types of cells found in living organisms are eucaryotic and true nuclear organisms.

4. If some bacteria were able to survive a dry high temperature condition then this would be possible as a result of a cell wall and formation of spores.

5. Bacteria are found in three basic shapes—cocci, bacilli, and helicoidal.

6. Bacteria reproduce by mitosis.

7. The reproduction curve of bacteria includes a lag phase when bacteria reproduce at a very rapid rate.

8. Autotrophic bacteria require preformed food whereas heterotrophic bacteria can synthesize their own.

9. Pathogenic saprophytic bacteria include *Clostridium tetani* and *Clostridium botulinum.*

10. Viruses are acellular particles that only exhibit characteristics of life when parasitizing a specific host.

11. Fungi are eucaryotic organisms that do not cause human diseases.

12. Yeasts are unicellular organisms and *Candida albicans* causes infection in the mouth, vagina, and skin.

13. Bacteria often found on the body are called *resident* or *normal flora.*

14. Bacteria are not normally found in the stomach due to acidic pH, whereas the large intestine contains many bacteria that produce vitamin K and B complex vitamins.

# Chapter 4

# INTRODUCTION TO ANATOMY–PHYSIOLOGY OF THE BODY

After reading and studying this chapter, a student should be able to:

1. Identify the anatomical positions of the body.
2. Identify the planes or sections of the body.
3. Describe the two major body cavities and their subdivisions.
4. Define a cell, tissue, organ, and system.
5. Describe the structure and function of each cell organelle.
6. Define, describe, and give an example of diffusion, active transport, phagocytosis, pinocytosis, and filtration.
7. Define and describe osmosis, osmolality, hyperosmolar, isosmolar, and hypoosmolar.
8. Describe the transcription and translation steps of protein synthesis.
9. Name and describe the steps of mitosis.
10. Describe the anatomic features and functions of the types of epithelial, connective, muscular, and nerve tissues.
11. Describe the structure and function and give an example of a serous, mucous, synovial, fascial, and miscellaneous membrane.

*In this unit we will begin to study the structure (anatomy) of the body parts and their functions (physiology). Studying the anatomy of the various parts of the body is essential before one can effectively understand the physiology of the body parts and how they interact to produce normal body functions or homeostasis. We will begin to integrate the chemistry and microbiology facts and principles (covered in Chapters 2 and 3) into our discussions of anatomy–physiology. Physiologic processes primarily involve chemical reactions.*

*A disease involves pathogenic microbes penetrating the anatomic barriers of the body and interfering with the normal physiologic processes. Infections and diseases of the body will be discussed in an integrated manner along with the anatomy–physiology of the body.*

# 1  DIRECTION TERMS

Various terms will be used to describe the location and position of the various body parts. These terms are very important and will be used extensively throughout this text. The terms are always used when the body is in the normal anatomic position (Figure 4–1). This position consists of the body being erect, facing forward, the arms down at the sides with the palms of the hands facing forward (anteriorly).

1. **Superior**   above or in a higher position. *Example:* The stomach is superior to the small intestines.
2. **Inferior**   below or in a lower position. *Example:* The chest is inferior to the neck.
3. **Anterior (ventral)**   located near the belly surface or front of the body. *Example:* The bladder is anterior to the rectum. The penis is anterior to the scrotum.
4. **Posterior (dorsal)**   located near the back side of the body. *Example:* The esophagus is posterior to the trachea. The spinal cord is dorsal to the stomach.
5. **Lateral**   farther away from midline or toward the side.* *Example:* The eyes are lateral to the nose. The thumb is lateral to the hand in the normal anatomical position.
6. **Medial**   nearer the midline of the body. *Example:* The heart is medial to the lungs. The nose is medial to the eyes.

7. **Internal**   deeper within the body. *Example:* The heart is internal to the breasts.
8. **External**   nearer the outer surface of the body or any part of the body. *Example:* The breasts are external to the heart.
9. **Distal**   farther from the point of origin or attachment. This term is used in reference to appendages. *Example:* The upper arm attaches or originates at the shoulder; therefore, the hand is distal to the upper arm.
10. **Proximal**   nearer the point of origin or attachment. *Example:* The upper leg attaches to the body at the pelvic area or hipbone; therefore, the knee is proximal to the foot.
11. **Peripheral**   extensions from the center of the body or midline. *Example:* The peripheral nervous system consists of nerves that go to or away from the brain and spinal cord.
12. **Parietal**   refers to the walls of a cavity. *Example:* The membrane that lines the wall of the abdominal pelvic cavity is called the **parietal peritoneum membrane**. The membrane that lines the wall of the thoracic cavity is called the **parietal pleura membrane**.
13. **Visceral**   this term pertains to the organs within a cavity, but does not mean the organs themselves. The term viscera is used to refer to the internal organs collectively as a group. *Example:* The membrane that covers the organs (viscera) in the abdominopelvic cavity is the **visceral peritoneum membrane**. The membrane that covers the organs (viscera) within the thoracic cavity is the **visceral pleura membrane**.

You should become so familiar with these terms that you do not even have to think about their meaning.

---

* This term can be used in reference to structures located on the torso or trunk, as well as any of the individual parts of the body.

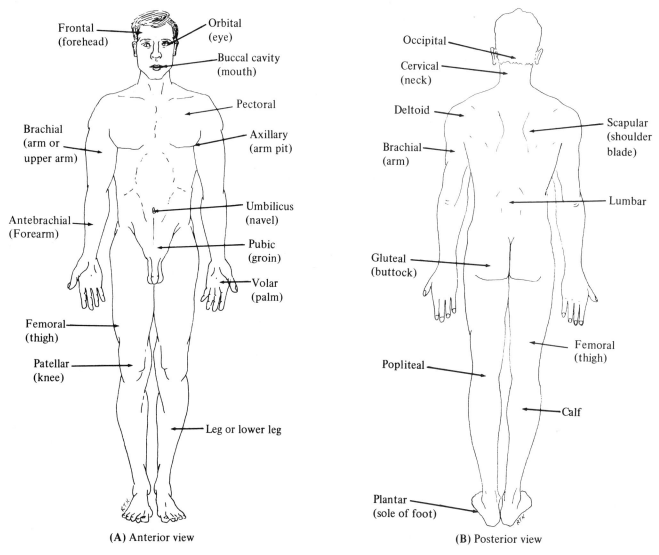

**Figure 4–1.**    Anatomical positions of the body. The proper anatomical terms are given first and the common terms are given in parentheses.

## 2    PLANES OR SECTIONS OF THE BODY

To see and visualize parts of the body better, cuts are made through the body in different planes.* Figure 4–2 illustrates planes and the points at which they pass through the body.

_____

* These planes not only are used in reference to a cut through the body but also through any small part of the body or an organ.

1. **Sagittal plane**   any cut that passes lengthwise through the body, dividing it into right and left sections.

2. **Midsagittal plane**   any cut that passes lengthwise through the midline of the body, dividing it into equal right and left halves.

3. **Transverse or horizontal plane**   any cut that passes through the body in a horizontal or transverse direction, dividing it into lower and upper sections.

4. **Frontal or coronal plane**   any cut that passes through the body from head to foot, dividing it into anterior and posterior portions.

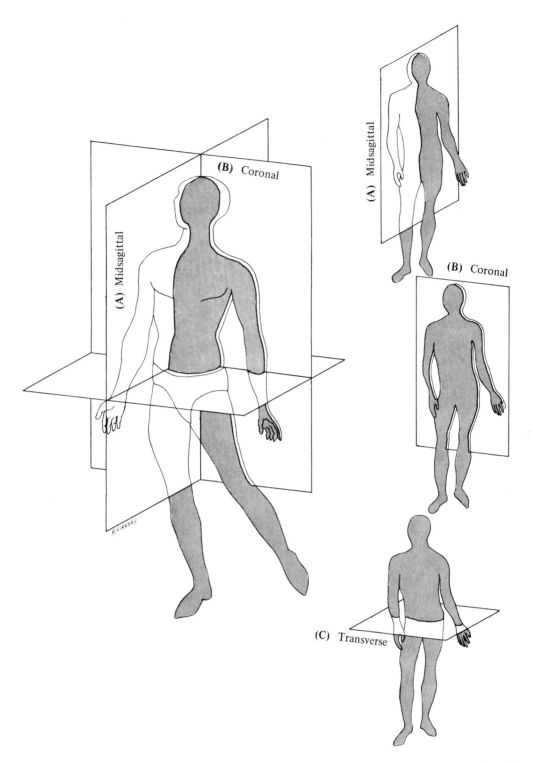

**Figure 4-2.** The planes of the body. Note that a sagittal section is a plane that passes lengthwise through the body, dividing it into right and left sections.

# 3  BODY CAVITIES

The organs of the body are found in two large body cavities, which are then subdivided into smaller cavities (Figure 4–3).

## DORSAL CAVITY

The **dorsal** cavity contains two smaller cavities:

1. Cranial cavity, which contains the brain
2. Vertebral (spinal) cavity, which contains the spinal cord

### Functions of the Dorsal Cavity

The **dorsal cavity** houses the brain and spinal cord that coordinate the activities of the organs located lower in the body. The spinal cord conducts impulses to and from the brain. It is like a major freeway in that most nerves either carry their sensory information to the spinal cord or the motor nerves carry command impulses away from the spinal cord. The brain receives the sensory impulses and integrates them, then sends out a command or motor impulse to the various areas of the body. This dorsal cavity is like the headquarters since it is responsible for coordinating the functions of the organs in the ventral cavity to maintain homeostasis.

## VENTRAL CAVITY

The **ventral cavity** (Figure 4–3) is much larger than the dorsal cavity and is divided into thoracic and abdominopelvic cavities.

The **thoracic cavity** contains the heart, lungs, and great blood vessels. The diaphragm muscle lies inferior to the lungs and heart and is the division point between the thoracic and abdominopelvic cavities.

In the **abdominopelvic cavity** the **abdominal area** contains the stomach, small intestine, large intestine,

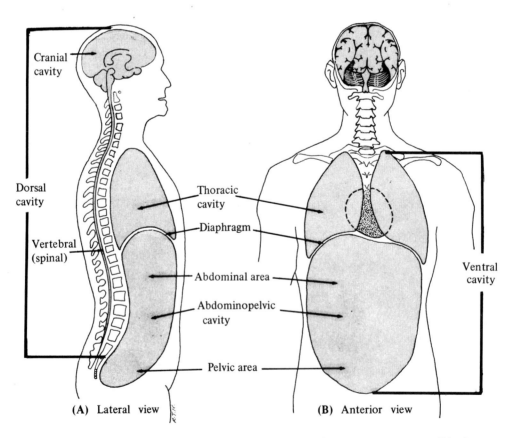

**Figure 4–3.**   Body cavities. (A) primarily shows the dorsal cavity and subdivisions. (B) primarily shows the ventral cavity and subdivisions.

liver, gallbladder, pancreas, spleen, kidneys, adrenal gland, and ureters. The **pelvic area** is inferior to the abdominal area and contains the urinary bladder, end of the large intestine, and certain reproductive organs.

The abdominal area is so large that it is necessary to divide it into nine regions (Figure 4-4). These regions make it convenient to locate the various abdominal organs. Notice in Figure 4-4 that the top horizontal line crosses the body at the level of the ninth rib cartilages. The lower horizontal line crosses the body at the level of the iliac crests.

### Functions of the Ventral Cavity

The ventral cavity contains all the organs responsible for maintaining homeostasis of body functions. The brain receives and sends out impulses that coordinate the functions of all the organs in the ventral cavity.

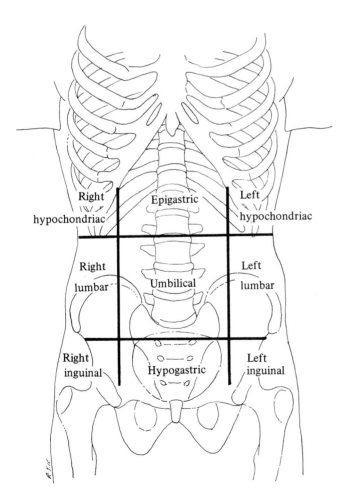

**Figure 4-4.** The nine regions that subdivide the abdomen.

# 4  STRUCTURAL UNITS

The body is like the large organic molecules (lipids, proteins, carbohydrates, and nucleic acids) in the sense that it is composed of building blocks or structural units. The simple structural units are combined together to form more complex structural units, and so on.

## CELLS

**Cells** are the simplest structural and functional unit of the body. They are capable of functioning independently and reproducing themselves. The structure of a cell and its functions are interdependent of each other. In other words, the structure of a cell is related to its function, and vice versa.

Cells are very important, and in reality all physiologic functions are intracellular (within cells) chemical reactions or intercellular (between cells) chemical reactions.

A more complex structural unit is formed by combining cells with similar structure and functions. This unit is called a tissue.

## TISSUES

A **tissue** is composed of cells with similar structure and function. The tissue, therefore, has a characteristic structure and function. Muscle tissue is an example; it is composed of many, many muscle cells each with the same characteristic structure and function. All the muscle cells function as a group by contracting and moving a part of the body.

An even more complex structural unit is formed when two or more tissues combine to form a structure that has certain functions. This structure is called an organ.

## ORGANS

An **organ** is a structure that is composed of two or more different tissues. The tissues combine their individual functions, which enable the organ to accomplish more important functions. The heart is a good example of an organ. It is composed of cardiac muscle tissue, but it is also composed of blood, nervous, and connective tissues. All of these tissues combine their functions, which enables the heart to receive and pump blood to all parts of the body.

The activities of two or more organs can be combined together to perform major body functions. The grouping of organs to combine their functions results in the formation of a system.

## SYSTEMS

A **system** is a group of organs. The individual functions of the organs combine to accomplish a major body task. An example of an organ system is the circulatory system. The heart is an organ that pumps blood to the body, but the heart needs the help of other organs to circulate the blood. The other organs that help the heart are the arteries, veins, and capillary beds. The arteries, veins, and capillaries are organs by definition, since they are composed of more than two different tissues. The heart, arteries, veins, and capillaries are the organs that make up the circulatory system.

There are nine organ systems in the body: (1) skeletal system; (2) muscular system; (3) nervous system; (4) circulatory system; (5) respiratory system; (6) digestive system; (7) urinary system; (8) endocrine system; and (9) reproductive system.

We will be studying these systems in an integrated manner to show how they interact to accomplish complicated body functions. After discussing the integration of these organ systems, we will then discuss how bacteria, viruses, protozoa, and fungi interfere with these systems, resulting in diseases.

# 5 THE CELL AND HOMEOSTASIS

In Chapter 2 the concept of homeostasis was described. It was also stated that homeostasis would be a recurring and unifying concept in your study of body processes. At the beginning of this unit the concept of physiology was discussed. **The main importance of physiologic reactions is to maintain or restore homeostasis of cells. Since homeostasis has to be sustained in order for life to continue, we can conclude then that cells are the smallest unit that can sustain life.**

Not only are cells the site of normal homeostatic activities but also the site of disease and sickness. In Chapter 3 you studied various microorganisms (bacteria and viruses, for example) that cause various diseases and in-

fections. These pathogens frequently cause diseases by invading cells and interfering with the normal activities of the organelles.

## CHEMICAL COMPOSITION OF PROTOPLASM

The chemical material inside cells is called **protoplasm.** Often it is called the "living substance" since it has to be present for a cell to sustain life.

Protoplasm is a thick, viscous, colloidal suspension of organic and inorganic materials. Table 4–1 gives the percentages of the various organic and inorganic compounds that make up protoplasm. A brief discussion of the functions of the various chemical components follows.

### Organic Compounds (Proteins, Lipids, and Carbohydrates)

These substances compose almost 30 percent of the total protoplasm. They have a variety of functions. The overall structure of the cell is one of the most important functions of organic compounds.

### Inorganic Compounds

**WATER.** This inorganic compound is absolutely vital for the physiologic reactions in the cell. This is evidenced by the fact that 55 to 70 percent of the protoplasm is water. The various functions of water were discussed in Chapter 2. The two most important functions that occur within the cell are that water takes part in some reactions and that water serves as a **solvent** for some reactions. These two functions of water are very important in order to have normal physiologic and homeostatic reactions. Later in this unit the process of osmosis and how water is pulled into and out of cells will be discussed.

### TABLE 4–1. Composition of Protoplasm

| Organic Compounds | Percentage |
| --- | --- |
| Proteins | 16.0 |
| Lipids | 13.0 |
| Carbohydrates | 0.6 |
| Inorganic Compounds | |
| Water | 55.0–70.0 |
| Inorganic salts | 4.4 |

**INORGANIC SALTS.** Although they compose only 4.4 percent of the total protoplasm composition, they are very important for the normal functions of the cell. In Chapter 2 the fact that salts actually ionize in water into cations and anions was discussed. The concentrations and functions of various cations and anions were given in Chapter 2. These cations and anions result from water acting as a **solvent.** The polar characteristics of water molecules are responsible for ionizing salts into their respective cations and anions. Later in this unit we will discuss how the normal concentrations of cations and anions in the protoplasm are maintained by osmosis, diffusion, active transport, and pinocytosis.

## CELL MEMBRANE OR PLASMA MEMBRANE

The protoplasm is surrounded by a membrane called the **cell membrane** or **plasma membrane.** One should not think of the plasma membrane as a solid, inert object. Electron microscope studies plus many experiments reveal that actually the plasma membrane is composed of organic chemical molecules that constantly change shape and chemically interact with other molecules. Actually, the plasma membrane is a dynamic, living, ever-changing fluid layer. As you will see, the ability of the cell to maintain homeostasis is quite dependent upon the plasma membrane.

### Chemical Composition of Plasma Membrane

The organic molecules in the membrane are proteins and lipids. The proteins are **globular proteins** and the lipids are **phospholipids.** As Chapter 2 shows, phospholipids (lecithin and cephalin, for example) contain a charged phosphate group in place of one fatty acid; therefore, phospholipids are polar molecules. The polar end of the phospholipid is **hydrophilic** or water soluble, whereas the two fatty acid chains are **hydrophobic** or water insoluble. The shape of each phospholipid molecule can be compared to a tuning fork (Figure 4–5). The two prongs are the two fatty acid chains. The polar group occupies the handle of the tuning fork. In the cell membrane the phospholipids are arranged so that the prongs or **hydrophobic** ends are pointing toward each other in the center of the membrane. The polar or **hydrophilic** ends point toward the inside and outside of a cell. Possibly, the reason the hydrophilic ends are arranged the way they are is due to the amount of water both in the protoplasm of the cell and outside the cell.

The double layer of lipids and their arrangement play an important role in determining what enters and leaves the cell. Molecules that are lipid soluble easily pass through the membrane, whereas lipid-insoluble molecules have a more difficult time passing through the plasma membrane.

The globular proteins in the plasma membrane fall into two types, **external** and **internal.** Figure 4–5 shows that the external proteins do not penetrate into the double layer of lipids. They sort of float along the inside and outside of a plasma membrane. The internal proteins penetrate into the lipid bilayer. Some internal proteins penetrate partially through the lipid layers and some penetrate totally through the lipid layers.

### Function of Proteins in a Plasma Membrane

The proteins in a plasma membrane are theorized to function in three ways: maintain structural integrity of plasma membrane, bind enzymes, and facilitate transport of materials through membrane. Previously (Chapter 2), it was stated that proteins have many charged side groups and therefore actually exist as polar groups in a pH around 7. The electrically charged sites on the proteins react readily with chemicals in the interior and exterior of the cell. **The charged (polar) characteristics of both proteins and lipids are important in the overall functioning of a plasma membrane.**

### Functions of Plasma Membrane

- *Limits protoplasm to a confined region.* The protoplasm and organelles contained in the cell are limited to a confined region due to the plasma membrane. This ensures that cellular activities will be more consistent and efficient.

- *Controls movement of materials into and out of cells.* Due to the lipid bilayer, many substances cannot pass through the plasma membrane due to their lipid insolubility. Compounds such as $O_2$, $CO_2$, and certain anesthetics are lipid soluble and readily pass through a plasma membrane.

- *Creates an osmolarity (osmotic pressure) difference between the inside and outside of a cell.* Later in this unit the mechanisms by which a plasma membrane actively transports $Na^+$ and $K^+$ into and out of cells will be discussed. This process is important because the osmolarity difference that is created directly affects the volume of fluid in a cell.

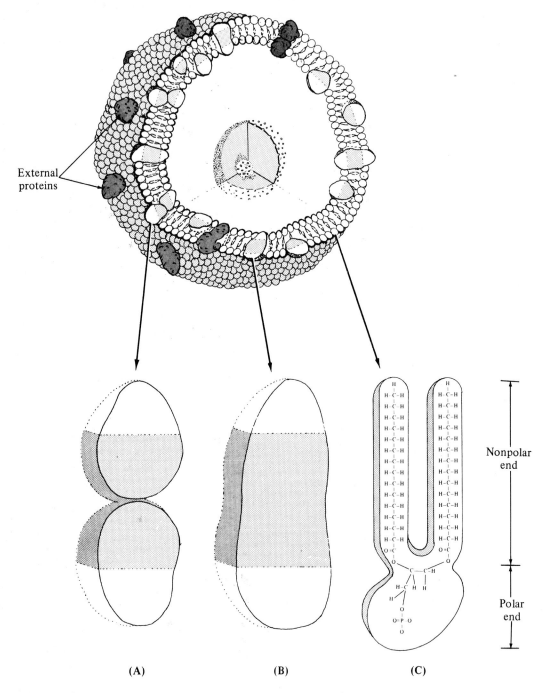

External proteins

Nonpolar end

Polar end

(A)                    (B)                    (C)

**Figure 4-5.** Chemical composition of a plasma membrane. The proteins in the plasma membrane are globular in shape. Some proteins penetrate partially the double layer of lipids. Some proteins penetrate totally the double layer of lipids; some of these are composed of two units as shown in (A), and some are composed of a single unit as shown in (B). The lipids are phospholipids and (C) shows the polar phosphate end and two nonpolar fatty acid chains of a phospholipid molecule.

# 6  SPECIALIZED ORGANS (ORGANELLES) OF A CELL

A cell can be thought of as a miniature factory. Factories usually take in raw materials and chemically and physically change them to produce products for their own use and for others. Waste products resulting from these actions are disposed of in various ways. A factory has various areas that perform specialized functions on the raw materials, eventually producing finished products. All these comments also apply to cells in the body. The specialized areas that perform specialized functions in a cell are called **cell organelles.** These cell organelles are composed of chemical molecules arranged in such a way that they have definite shapes and functions. Organelles are suspended in the cytoplasm, which is all the protoplasm surrounding the nucleus. The structure and function of the cell organelles will be discussed next.

## *Endoplasmic Reticulum*

The **endoplasmic reticulum** (ER) (Figures 4-6, 4-7, and 4-8) is an extensively branched interconnected system of membranes. This system of membranes extends from the nucleus out to the cell membrane (Figure 4-8). Since an endoplasmic reticulum membrane is con-

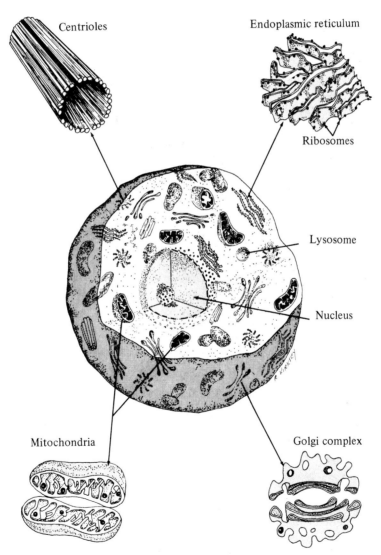

**Figure 4-6.**  Each cell contains specialized structures, called organelles, that carry out certain functions.

Endoplasmic
reticulum

Connects to
golgi complex

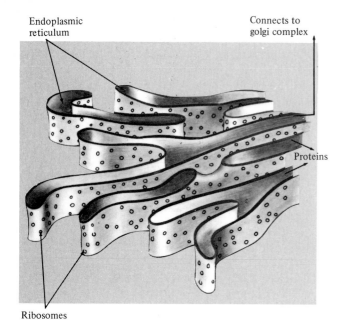

Proteins

Ribosomes

**Figure 4-7.** A rough endoplasmic reticulum (ER) with ribosomes. The point where an ER might attach to a Golgi complex and the pathway that proteins follow as they are transported within and out of a cell are also shown.

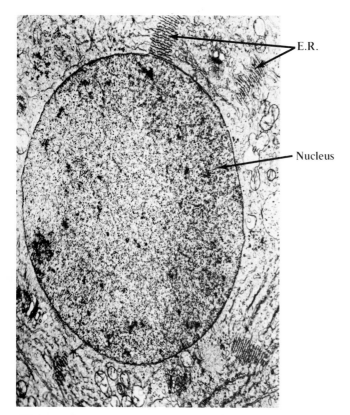

E.R.

Nucleus

**Figure 4-8.** The electron micrograph shows a nucleus and an endoplasmic reticulum (ER) attached (3000×) to it in a grasshopper spermatocyte. *(Courtesy of Dr. James N. Lindsey, University of Texas Medical Branch, Galveston, Texas.)*

tinuous with a plasma membrane, the ER membrane also is composed of phospholipids and globular proteins.

There are two forms of ER, **granular (rough)** and agranular (smooth). The granular ER (Figure 4–7) is so named because it has many small granules called **ribosomes** attached to it. Each granular ER is interconnected to others and to a **Golgi complex.** The smooth (or agranular) ER lacks the ribosomes; therefore, it has a smooth appearance.

**FUNCTIONS OF GRANULAR ENDOPLASMIC RETICULUM (GER).** The GER transports proteins, produced by ribosomes that are attached to it, within the cell and out of the cell.

**FUNCTIONS OF AGRANULAR ENDOPLASMIC RETICULUM (AER).** AER is thought to perform the following functions:

- *Synthesis of steroids.* The cells that compose endocrine glands, which secrete steroid hormones, have well-developed agranular endoplasmic reticular (AER). The AER are thought to be responsible for the synthesis of steroid hormones, such as testosterone in testes and sex hormones in adrenal cortex.
- *Glycogen metabolism.* In liver cells (hepatocytes) AER play a role in glycogen metabolism.
- *$Ca^{2+}$ release and storage.* Skeletal muscle cells that contain AER are referred to as **sarcoplasmic reticula.** They function to release and store $Ca^{2+}$, which is involved in the contraction of the muscle fibers.

### Ribosomes

Ribosomes are spherical and granular in appearance (Figure 4–6) and are composed of RNA (ribonucleic acid). Ribosomes can be found attached to a granular ER and floating freely in the cytoplasm. Ribosomes often are found in large clusters called **polysomes** or **polyribosomes.**

*Function:* Ribosomes are called "protein factories" because they are the site at which proteins are synthesized. The attached ribosomes synthesize proteins that are exported out of the cell by the ER. Free-floating ribosomes synthesize proteins that are used by the cell itself. In other words, free-floating ribosomes synthesize proteins important to the structure of the cell and for intracellular enzymes.

### Golgi Complex (Dictysome)

This organelle consists of many small flattened membranes (Figure 4–9 and 4–10) stacked on top of each other. It interconnects with the granular ER membranes. **Golgi complexes** are quite numerous in secretory cells (goblet, liver, and plasma cells).

*Functions:* In reference to a cell being similar to a factory, the **Golgi complex** corresponds to the storage and shipping area of a factory:

- *Storage of materials.* Proteins, lipids, and carbohydrates are packaged and stored here before being secreted.
- *Synthesis of carbohydrates and attachment of proteins.* The Golgi complex synthesizes carbohydrates and attaches them to proteins. An example is **glycoproteins.**

### Mitochondria

The size and shape of mitochondria (mitochondrion, sing.) (Figures 4–11 and 4–12) vary considerably, as does the number per cell. The shape of mitochondria vary from a sausage to a round shape. They have an outer and an inner membrane. Notice in Figure 4–11 that the inner membrane is extremely branched and forms shelf-like structures called **cristae.** The presence of the cristae increases the total surface area of the inner membrane. Attached to the inner membrane are oxidative enzymes and with the increased surface area more enzymes can attach to the membrane. Each mitochondrion is self-producing. Each one contains its own DNA, RNA, ribosomes, and other material necessary for reproduction. This is very unusual since the nucleus contains the genetic material necessary for reproduction of the other organelles and the rest of the cell. Later in this unit the process of cell reproduction will be discussed in greater detail.

*Function:* Continuing our comparison of a cell to a factory, a mitochondrion corresponds to the "power plant" of a factory. Mitochondria release energy that is utilized by cells to carry out cellular functions. In Chapter 2 we briefly discussed the following chemical reaction:

$$C_6H_{12}O_6 + 6O_2 + 6H_2O \xrightarrow[\text{enzymes}]{\text{Oxidative}} 6CO_2 + 12H_2O + \text{energy (ATP)}$$

This reaction is an oxidation–reduction reaction that releases energy, which is utilized to synthesize ATP. In the mitochondria, essentially this same reaction occurs with one exception:

$$2 \text{ Pyruvic acid} + 6O_2 + 6H_2O \xrightarrow[\text{enzymes}]{\text{Oxidative}} 6CO_2 + 12H_2O + \text{energy (ATP)}$$

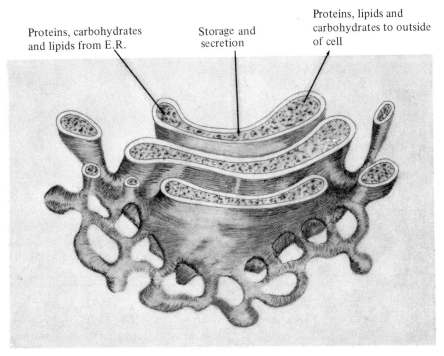

Proteins, carbohydrates and lipids from E.R.

Storage and secretion

Proteins, lipids and carbohydrates to outside of cell

**Figure 4-9.** Golgi complex (dictysome). This group of flattened membranes acts as a warehouse, since it stores, secretes, and synthesizes various organic materials.

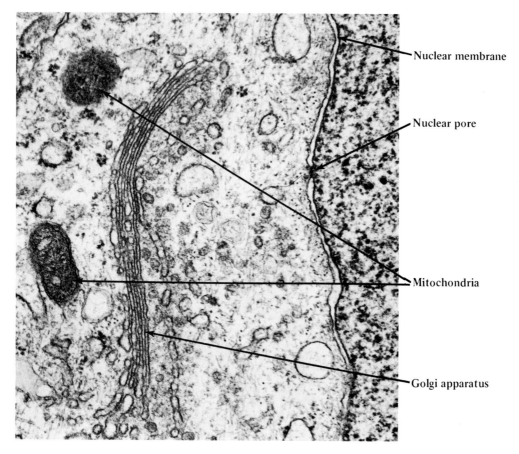

Nuclear membrane

Nuclear pore

Mitochondria

Golgi apparatus

**Figure 4–10.** An electron micrograph (28,500 ×) of a Golgi apparatus from a rat sertoli cell. *(Courtesy of Dr. James N. Lindsey, University of Texas Medical Branch, Galveston, Texas.)*

Notice in Figure 4–11 that glucose is broken into two pyruvic acid molecules in the cytoplasm, which moves into the mitochondria. Oxygen molecules move into the mitochondria along with the pyruvic acid. These two nutrients interact with **oxidative enzymes** on the surface of the cristae to produce ATP (a high-energy compound), heat, $CO_2$, and $H_2O$. ATP (adenosine triphosphate) moves out of the mitochondria throughout the cell and releases its energy wherever it is needed. All physiologic activities such as muscle contractions and conduction of nerve impulses require energy released from ATP. Very active cells require large amounts of energy compared to inactive cells. Likewise, active cells contain large numbers of mitochondria compared to inactive cells. For example, nerve cells are more active than cells in the dermis of the skin; therefore, nerve cells contain more mitochondria than do cells in the dermis.

## Lysosomes

**Lysosomes** (Figure 4–6 and 4–13) are small, somewhat rounded structures containing large numbers of digestive enzymes. The membrane that surrounds the lysosome is effective in preventing the enzymes from escaping.

Lysosomes are very abundant in white blood cells (WBCs), which function to phagocytize bacteria and other foreign material that may enter the body. After a WBC takes in a bacterium cell, the lysosomes release their hydrolytic and proteolytic enzymes. Remember that a bacterium cell is a procaryote and is composed of proteins, lipids, and carbohydrates. Therefore, the digestive enzymes function to break down the cell wall and inner contents of a bacterium, resulting in its destruction.

*Function:* The digestive or hydrolytic enzymes break

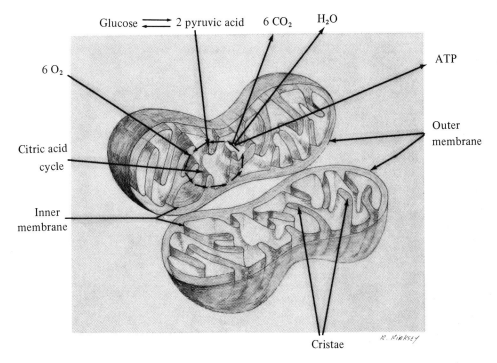

Glucose ⇌ 2 pyruvic acid   6 $CO_2$   $H_2O$

6 $O_2$

ATP

Citric acid
cycle

Outer
membrane

Inner
membrane

Cristae

R. Kirksey

**Figure 4-11.** Mitochondrion, the "power plant" of a cell. The inner membrane is extensively branched to form cristae. Oxidative enzymes attached to the cristae act to oxidize pyruvic acid and produce ATP (high energy compound), $Co_2$, and $H_2O$.

complex molecules into smaller ones for the cell's use (Chapter 2). When complex molecules enter a cell, the lysosomes release their digestive enzymes, which break down the complex molecules. They also break down worn-out organelles within a cell. They can destroy the entire contents of a healthy cell if all the lysosomes were to release their digestive enzymes.

## Centrioles

A **centriole** is a small cylindrical structure located near the nucleus. Usually there are two per cell (Figures 4-14, 4-15, and 4-16). A centriole is composed of nine longitudinal bundles. The centrioles are active during the division stages of a cell or mitosis. In human cells the two centrioles often are positioned at right angles to each other, as shown in Figure 4-15.

## INCLUSIONS

**Inclusions** are clusters or clumps of materials in the cytoplasm of a cell. They are not organelles. Usually an inclusion is some type of organic compound.

## Types of Inclusions

**PERMANENTLY RETAINED INCLUSIONS.** Some inclusions are permanently retained within a cell's cytoplasm. Two examples are **melanin** and **hemoglobin**. Melanin is a protein pigment substance that gives the skin its color. It is produced by melanocytes, which are located in the epidermis of the skin. **Hemoglobin**, as previously described, is a quaternary, globular protein. It is synthesized and permanently retained within red blood cells (RBCs). It is a vital inclusion since $O_2$ and $CO_2$ attach to it and are transported by the RBCs to and from tissues.

**TEMPORARILY RETAINED INCLUSIONS.** Some inclusions are finished products, as a result of that cell's activities, but are exported whole or broken down prior to being exported. **Glycogen,** a polysaccharide, is a finished product found in liver (hepatocyte) cells and skeletal muscle cells. Remember that glycogen is composed of many glucose molecules. As the body needs more energy, the hepatocytes and skeletal muscle cells will break down glycogen to glucose and release it into the blood.

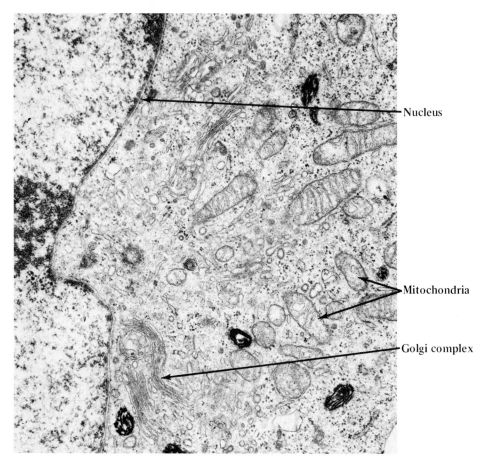

Nucleus

Mitochondria

Golgi complex

**Figure 4-12.** An electron micrograph of a human melanoma cell (18,000×) shows several mitochondria of various shapes. Golgi complexes and the nucleus also are shown. *(Courtesy of Dr. Jeffrey P. Chang, University of Texas Medical Branch, Galveston, Texas.)*

*Lipid droplets* are stored in adipose cells often temporarily. When the body needs more energy, the lipids will move out of adipose cells to the liver, where they will be broken down to release energy. **Mucus** is an example of an inclusion that is continuously produced by cells in mucous membranes. Mucus functions to protect passageways that open to the outside of the body against invasion of bacteria.

## NUCLEUS

The **nucleus** (Figure 4-6) sends directions into the cytoplasm and these directions guide the production of proteins. They are vital finished products that are involved in the structure and functions of the cell. Since the pro-

duction of proteins is a major function of cells, it must be carefully controlled; therefore, the nucleus is the control center of the cell.

A **nuclear membrane** surrounds the internal contents of the nucleus. This membrane is double layered and is perforated by pores. The fluid surrounded by the nuclear membrane is called **nucleoplasm.** It contains **nucleoli** and **chromatin material.** The nucleoli are small, rounded, dark-staining structures that contain proteins and nucleic acids. They appear to function in protein synthesis. Chromatin material is granular, dark-staining, and scattered throughout the nucleoplasm. The chromatin granules are composed of DNA and proteins and are the genetic material of the cell. As a cell begins to undergo division (mitosis), the loosely organized chromatin material organizes itself into elongate chromosomes. The chromosomes contain genes, which actually determine the hereditary traits of the body.

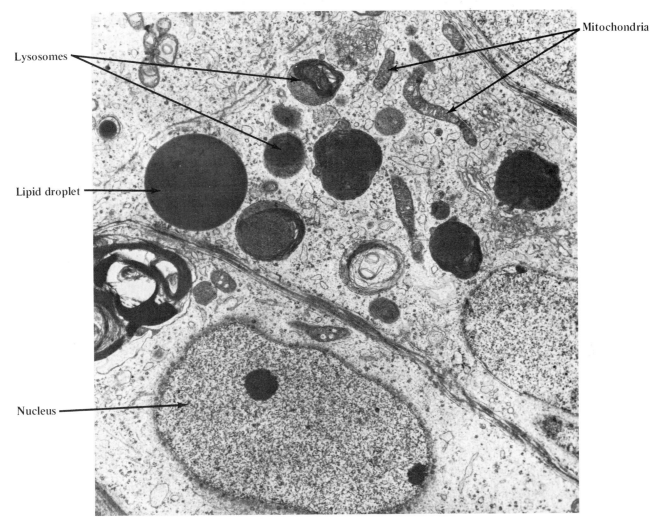

Lysosomes

Mitochondria

Lipid droplet

Nucleus

**Figure 4-13.** Several lysosomes as seen in a rat sertoli cell with an electron microscope (4623 ×). *(Courtesy of Dr. James N. Lindsey, University of Texas Medical Branch, Galveston, Texas.)*

# 7 MOVEMENT OF SUBSTANCES ACROSS CELL MEMBRANES

Chemical substances must move into and out of cells for them to function properly. Several processes are involved in moving substances through the cell membrane, because of its selective permeability. Five main processes by which substances pass through a cell membrane are diffusion, osmosis, active transport, bulk transport, and filtration.

## Diffusion

**Diffusion is the movement of particles from an area of high concentration to an area of lower concentration of the particles.** This process continues until the concentration of particles is equally distributed between the two areas or until equilibrium is established.

The molecules present in any matter (solid, liquid, and gas) are constantly in motion. These particles constantly are bouncing off each other and the walls of the compartment or container in which they are contained. The number of collisions is greatest in the area where the particles are most concentrated. The collisions

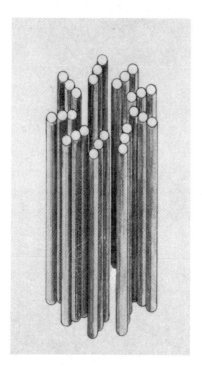

**Figure 4-14.**   A centriole is a small, round structure composed of nine longitudinal bundles. A centriole is active only during cell division or mitosis.

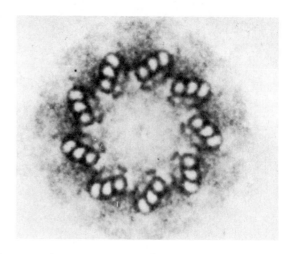

**Figure 4-16.**   A higher magnification (97,500 ×) of a cross-sectional view of a centriole in a Chinese hamster cell. [Reprinted by permission from Elton Stubblefield and B. R. Brinkley, *Symposium of the International Society for Cell Biology,* Vol. 6. New York: Academic Press, Inc., 1978), pp. 175–218.]

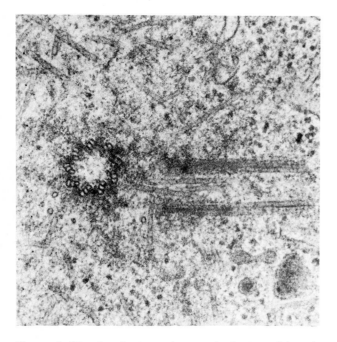

**Figure 4-15.**   An electron micrograph of a centriole pair (45,000 ×) in a Chinese hamster cell. *(Courtesy of Dr. B. R. Brinkley, University of Texas Medical Branch, Galveston, Texas.)*

force the particles to move gradually into a less concentrated area until they are equally distributed throughout the container. This constant motion of molecules is called **brownian motion.**

Figure 4–17 illustrates diffusion using a sugar cube as an example. Notice the movement of the sugar molecules in the bottom of the container. The molecules gradually diffuse up into the areas of less sugar concentration, until they are distributed equally throughout the container. The molecules moved along a concentration gradient (separation of concentrations), which in diffusion is from high concentration to low concentration.

As an example of diffusion in the body, $CO_2$ molecules are more concentrated in the blood than in the lung alveoli. The brownian motion of the $CO_2$ molecules causes them to diffuse from the blood into the less concentrated areas of the alveoli. This movement continues until the $CO_2$ molecules are evenly distributed between the blood and alveoli. Other examples of compounds that diffuse through cell membranes are oxygen molecules and ions.

## Osmosis

In cell physiology, **osmosis** is the movement of water from a region of low solute concentration to a high solute concentration through a membrane permeable to

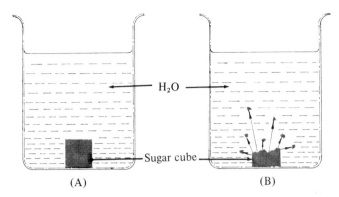

**Figure 4-17.** Diffusion. (A) Sugar cube in water. (B) Diffusion of sugar molecules from a high concentrated region to lower concentrated regions.

water only.* This definition means that for osmosis to occur the membrane must be permeable to water (solvent), but impermeable to materials (solutes) dissolved in water. If both water and solutes pass through a membrane, then this is not osmosis but diffusion.

The force responsible for pulling water through a membrane is osmotic pressure, which is a pulling pressure. **Osmotic pressure** is defined as pressure that results from dissolved solutes that cannot pass through a membrane. This pressure directly varies with the amount of dissolved solute. In other words, the greater the concentration of the solutes the higher the osmotic pressure, and the lower the concentration of solutes the lower the osmotic pressure. See Figure 4-18 for the word equation that expresses this relationship. The concentration of a solution likewise is the result of the concentration of solutes. Water always is pulled from a weaker solution into a stronger solution and therefore to the highest osmotic pressure. Water will be pulled into the strongest solution, diluting it until the concentrations of the two solutions are equal.

Notice in Figure 4-19 that a 0.5 percent NaCl solution is separated from a 0.9 percent solution by a membrane permeable to water but impermeable to NaCl. The 0.9 percent NaCl solution is the strongest solution and also has the highest osmotic pressure. The osmotic pressure of the 0.9 percent NaCl solution pulls water into it until the concentrations of the two solutions are equal at 0.7 percent NaCl. The osmotic pressures of the

---

* Another definition of osmosis is, **movement of $H_2O$ from a region of high water concentration to low water concentration through a membrane permeable to water only.** The definition based on solute concentration will be used throughout the text because it makes it easier to figure out which way water moves, since strengths of solutions are always expressed in terms of solute concentration rather than water.

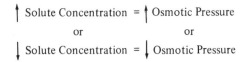

**Figure 4-18.** This word equation is a shorthand way of expressing the relationship between two phenomena. What it says is that ↑ (increased) solute concentration = (results in) ↑ (increased) osmotic pressure, or vice versa. This is a direct relationship in that as one phenomenon (solute) changes, it results in a related phenomenon changing in the same way, that is, either up or down.

two solutions also are equal when the concentrations are equal.

In Figure 4-18 the reason why the concentration of NaCl inside the cell dropped from 0.9 percent to 0.7 percent is that as water moves inside the cell the concentration of salt is diluted, and therefore it goes down. In the fluid outside the cell, Figure 4-18, the concentration of NaCl rose from 0.5 percent to 0.7 percent. This occurred because as water was lost from outside the cell the concentration of salt rose due to the same number of salt particles being present in a smaller amount of water, and leading to an increase from 0.5 percent to 0.7 percent of the NaCl. When both concentrations reached 0.7 percent, an equilibrium between the inside and outside of the cell had been established and osmosis ceased. In effect, then, homeostasis, as regards concentration of NaCl and $H_2O$ inside and outside of the cell, has been established.

**OSMOLALITY.**   The concentration of a solute can be expressed in terms of osmolality, which is defined as **the number of osmoles of the particles (solute) per kilogram of solvent.** The greater the number of dissolved particles per liter of solution then the greater the osmolality of the solution. As an example, in Figure 4-18 the cell contains 0.9 percent NaCl, whereas outside the cell there is 0.5 percent NaCl. The 0.9 percent NaCl has more particles per liter of solution than 0.5 percent NaCl. Therefore, the 0.9 percent NaCl has a greater osmolarity than the 0.5 percent NaCl.

**OSMOL AND MILLIOSMOL.**   The ability of solutes to cause osmosis and osmotic pressure is measured in terms of **osmols.** Generally, the **osmol** is too large a unit for satisfactory use in expressing osmotic activity of a solution in the body. Therefore, the term **millismol** (mOsm), which equals 1/1000 osmol, is commonly used. The osmotic pressure of a solution, at body temperature, can be calculated by the following formula:

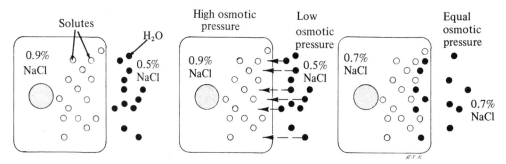

**Figure 4-19.** Osmosis. A membrane impermeable to solutes separates a 0.9% NaCl solution from a 0.5% NaCl solution. The 0.9% NaCl solution has a higher concentration of solutes and therefore a higher osmotic pressure. Water is pulled into the higher osmotic pressure region until the two solutions are equal in concentration (in this case 0.7% and 0.7%).

Osmotic pressure (mm of Hg) = 19.3 + concentration in milliosmols

All the cations and anions (as a group) in blood plasma create an osmolality of approximately 290 mOsm/liter. Hospitals can measure the osmotic pressure of a fluid with an osmometer. However, in regard to measuring osmolality in the body, hospitals measure the level of Na⁺ in the blood. Normally, the level of Na⁺ in blood plasma is 133 to 146 mEq/liter. As long as the normal range of blood plasma Na⁺ is maintained, the osmolality and osmotic process of the blood is in homeostasis (steady state). Previously we stated that homeostasis is a dynamic equilibrium and is characterized by a normal range of values with an upper limit of 133 mEq and a lower limit of 146 mEq. Various problems, conditions, and changes in body functions can cause the Na⁺ level in plasma to exceed the upper limit or go below the lower limit. These changes in plasma can affect the RBCs circulating in blood and ultimately the tissue cells. The names of these conditions and effects on cells will be discussed next.

**ISOOSMOLAR OR ISOTONIC.** (0.9% NaCl, 133 to 146 mEq Na⁺/liter, 0.5 percent glucose). The term *isoosmolar* (*iso*—equal, *osmolar*—concentration of solutes) **refers to body fluids and fluids within cells having equal osmolalities and equal osmotic pressures.** Figure 4-20A shows that when plasma and RBCs have equal osmolalities the osmotic pressure inside RBCs equals the osmotic pressure outside RBCs. Since the two osmotic pressures are equal, there is no net movement of water in or out of RBCs. This condition in the body is desirable since the fluid volume of all body cells is not changed; therefore, homeostasis of cellular functions can be maintained.

*Physiological Solutions.* When people are ill or hurt, solutions often have to be introduced into their bodies for help to recover. Solutions that are identical in osmotic pressure to those of body fluids are called **physiological solutions.** Two examples are 0.9 percent NaCl **(physiological saline)** and 5 percent glucose **(dextrose). It should be emphasized that body fluids are not composed of 0.9 percent NaCl and 5 percent glucose; but instead the body fluids have osmotic pressures that are equal to the 0.9 percent NaCl and 5 percent glucose solutions.** In terms of mOsm/liter, physiological solutions exert an osmotic pressure of about 290 mOsm/liter. Generally, injections, intravenous solutions (IVs), and others are prepared from these physiological solutions so that osmotic pressures and cellular volumes are not disturbed.

As described previously, hospital laboratories use the plasma sodium level as an indication of osmolality. If a person's sodium level is 133 to 146 mEq/liter, the medical personnel know that the body fluids are isoosmolar to each other; and, therefore, homeostasis of water volume within cells and fluid compartments is being maintained.

**HYPEROSMOLAR OR HYPERTONIC.** This term means that **an intercellular solution has a greater osmolality than an intracellular one.** In the body, whenever the osmolality of plasma exceeds 0.9 percent NaCl, 146 mEq Na⁺ /liter, or 5 percent glucose, plasma is hypertonic to fluids within cells. Figure 4-20C shows that whenever this condition exists in blood plasma the osmotic pressure outside the RBCs is greater than that inside. As a result the net movement of water will be out of the RBCs (remember water moves from low to high solute concentration). As a result the RBCs become shrunken or **crenated.** This condition destroys the functions of the RBCs. A hyperosmolar condition within the plasma and other body fluids will cause all

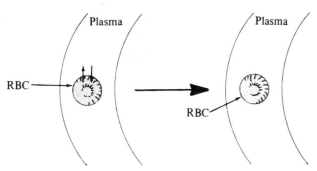

**(A)** Isoosmolar. The osmolality of the plasma and RBC are equal. As a result, the movement of water into and out of the RBC is equal and no net change occurs to the RBC.

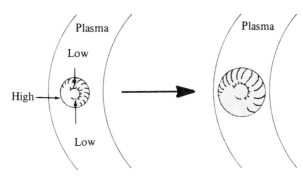

**(B)** Hypoosmolar. The osmolality of the plasma is lower than the RBC. The result is a net movement of water into RBC as indicated by the arrows.

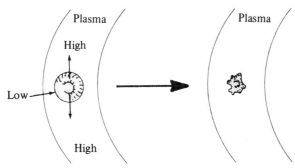

**(C)** Hyperosmolar. The osmolality of the plasma is higher than the RBC. The result is a net movement of water out of the RBC, causing the RBC to shrink or become crenated.

**Figure 4-20.** Isoosmolar, hypoosmolar, and hyperosmolar conditions are shown, along with the effects on RBCs.

cells to lose water or become dehydrated and therefore be destroyed.

*Decreasing Water or Increasing Sodium.* Hyperosmolar imbalances frequently result from either a decrease in $H_2O$ ($\downarrow H_2O$ or an increase in sodium ions ($\uparrow Na^+$). If a decrese in water occurs, the number of $Na^+$ are normal, but they are dissolved in too little water thereby increasing osmolarity. In $Na^+$ excess there are too many $Na^+$ per liter of water. Causes of water deficit and $Na^+$ excess will be discussed in Chapter 16.

**HYPOOSMOLAR OR HYPOTONIC.** This term means that **an intercellular solution has a lower osmolality than an intracellular one.** In the body, whenever the os-

**TABLE 4–2.   *Summary of Isoosmolar, Hyperosmolar, and Hypoosmolar Conditions***

| | OSMOLARITY (CONCENTRATION OF SOLUTES) | | | |
|---|---|---|---|---|
| CONDITION | FLUID INSIDE CELLS | PLASMA AND FLUIDS OUTSIDE CELLS | NET MOVEMENT OF $H_2O$ | EFFECT ON CELL(S) |
| Isoosmolar | Normal | Normal | No net movement | No change |
| Hyperosmolar | Normal | Higher than normal | Out of Cell | Crenation or dehydration |
| Hypoosmolar | Normal | Lower than normal | Into cell | Swell(s) or hemolysis of RBCs |

molality of plasma drops below 0.9 percent NaCl, 133 mEq $Na^+$/liter, or 5 percent glucose, the plasma is **hypotonic** to fluids within cells. Figure 4–20B shows that whenever this condition exists in blood plasma the osmotic pressure inside the RBCs is greater than that outside. As a result the net movement of water will be into RBCs (remember water moves from low to high solute concentration). Often so much water is pulled into cells that they rupture. The rupturing of RBCs is called **hemolysis.** Table 4–2 summarizes **isoosmolar, hyperosmolar,** and **hypoosmolar** conditions.

## Active Transport

**Active transport** (Figure 4–21) **is the movement of substances through a membrane from a low concentration to a high concentration.** This process is different from diffusion and osmosis in that energy is required to move the substances against the concentration gradient (low to high concentration). The energy necessary for this process is produced in the cell membrane. Figure 4–21 shows that active transport involves **carrier systems.**

The carriers that transport materials through the plasma membrane are thought to be internal proteins located in the membrane. Figure 4–21 shows a model or theory as to how certain compounds are actively transported through a plasma membrane. Figure 4–21 shows that the concentration of $Na^+$ in RBCs is low (26 mEq /liter) and high (144 mEq/liter) outside RBCs in plasma. $Na^+$ will diffuse inside RBCs from a high to low concentration. To move the $Na^+$ through the plasma membrane to the outside, energy is required as the $Na^+$ are being moved against a concentration gradient. ATP furnishes the energy required for the process. Another example of active transport shown in Figure 4–21 is that of potassium ions ($K^+$). The concentration of $K^+$ in RBCs is 150 mEq/liter and 5 mEq/liter in blood plasma. $K^+$ naturally diffuse out of RBCs, from high to low concentration. For the $K^+$ to be moved back inside RBCs, energy is required to move them against a concentration gradient. Figure 4–21 shows that the protein

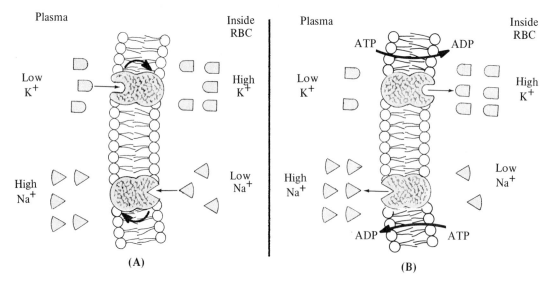

**Figure 4–21.** Active transport: (A) $Na^+$ and $K^+$ to attach to the protein carriers; (B) protein carriers flip-flop or transport $Na^+$ and $K^+$ through RBC membrane from low to high concentration.

carriers sort of flip-flop or make a 180° change in position in order to transport the Na+ and K+ through the plasma membrane. It should be emphasized that this flip-flop mechanism of the protein carriers is strictly a theory, and various researchers have differing theories from this one.

Na+ AND K+ PUMP AND ITS IMPORTANCE. Active transport often is described as a "pumping mechanism." The reason for this is that ions and molecules are being moved against a concentration gradient. This requires energy, and therefore one could say the ions and molecules are being pumped. Cells in the body pump Na+ and K+ back to their respective positions; therefore, the term Na+–K+ pump is frequently used.

The importance of the Na+–K+ pump is to maintain normal osmolality of cells, and therefore maintain homeostasis of fluid volume in cells. For example, if RBCs did not pump Na+ out of cells into plasma, then the osmolality inside the RBCs would become higher than plasma and excessive amounts of water would be pulled inside RBCs. One problem with certain diseases and abnormal conditions is that the Na+–K+ pump stops working, which could result in dehydration or swelling of cells. In certain cells, nerve, and muscle, the Na+–K+ pump is vital for the conduction of nerve impulses, which will be discussed in Chapter 5.

## Bulk Transport

This process involves moving large particles, such as proteins and bacteria, inside cells. There are two types of bulk transport occurring in the body, **phagocytosis** and **pinocytosis**.

Figure 4–22 shows a white blood cell (WBC) taking in some bacteria by **phagocytosis**. The cell membrane of the WBC literally reaches out and surrounds the bacterium until it is inside. The bacterium contained in a vacuole in the cytoplasm, is broken down by enzymes released from lysosomes inside the white blood cells.

White blood cells actively carry out phagocytosis against various foreign substances such as bacteria, protozoa, and dust. A **phagocyte** is a cell that actively carries out phagocytosis. They are found in various places in the body, such as the lymph nodes, liver, and reticulo-endothelial system.

Figure 4–23 shows **pinocytosis**. This process is very similar to phagocytosis in that the cell membrane invaginates, carrying particles inside the cell. A portion of the membrane breaks off, carrying the particles into the cy-

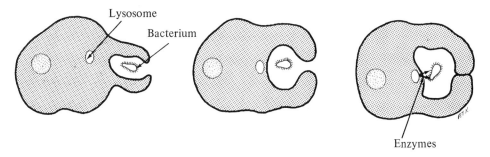

**Figure 4-22.** Phagocytosis. A white blood cell (WBC) is shown surrounding a bacterial cell. A lysosome releasing enzymes that break down the bacterial cell also is shown.

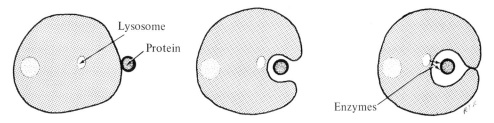

**Figure 4-23.** Pinocytosis. A cell membrane invaginating and moving a protein molecule inside the cell is shown. A lysosome releasing enzymes to break down the protein is also shown.

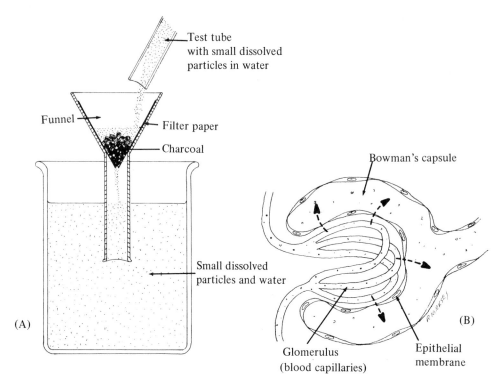

**Figure 4–24.** Filtration. (A) A higher pressure in the funnel than in the beaker below it forces water and small molecules through the filter paper into the beaker. (B) A higher pressure in the glomerulus than in the Bowman's capsule forces water and small molecules through the glomerulus into the Bowman's capsule.

toplasm. Proteins often are moved into a cell by this process. Enzymes released by lysosomes act to break down proteins that are brought in by pinocytosis.

Phagocytosis involves bulk transport of solids and pinocytosis transport of liquids. These processes are similar to active transport since energy is required for both.*

### Filtration

**Filtration** (Figure 4–24) **is a process that pushes water and substances from a higher pressure to a lower pressure through a membrane.** Hydrostatic pressure or blood pressure is responsible for pushing water and materials through a membrane.

Filtration is responsible for the formation of tissue fluids found between cells in the body. Figure 4–24 shows this process in a laboratory funnel and in a glomerulus of a Bowman's capsule in a kidney. The blood pressure in the capillaries of the Bowman's capsule is much higher than the pressure outside them; therefore, water and small dissolved materials (called filtrate) are pushed through the membrane of the Bowman's cap-

sule toward the lower pressure. Urine in the kidneys, cerebrospinal fluid (CSF) in the brain, and aqueous humor fluid in the eye are all formed by filtration. Blood pressure is responsible for the filtration process; therefore, the amount of fluid pushed out of blood capillaries is directly affected by how high or low the blood pressure is. The word equation for this direct relationship is:

$$\updownarrow \text{Blood pressure (BP)} = \updownarrow \text{filtration}$$

## 8   CHARACTERISTICS THAT ENABLE THE CELL MEMBRANE TO BE SELECTIVELY PERMEABLE

A cell membrane is selectively permeable; therefore, it does not allow all compounds to enter the cell and is selective as to what leaves. This selective permeability is made possible by chemical and structural features. An important chemical feature is the double layer of lipids.

---

* Some authorities disagree as to energy being required for pinocytosis and phagocytosis.

Compounds that are lipid soluble (dissolve in lipids) can pass through this layer into the cytoplasm; however, many compounds are not lipid soluble and are prevented from entering the cell.

Another chemical feature is the total charge on the cell membrane, which can be either positive (+) or negative (−). Ions that have a charge opposite to that of the membrane are able to enter or leave the cell; ions with the same charge as the membrane are repelled. For example, if both the ion and membrane are negatively charged (−), the ion is repelled. If the ion is positively charged (+) and the membrane negatively charged (−), the ion can enter the cell.

An important structural feature is the size of the pores in the cell membrane. These pores help regulate what compounds can enter and leave the cells. Small molecules such as water, urea, and chloride ions easily pass through the pores. Molecules too large for the pores must pass through by other means.

A cell membrane must be selective as to what it allows to enter and leave a cell. The lipid solubility, total membrane charge, and size of pores are what allow the membrane to be selectively permeable.

# 9 PROTEIN SYNTHESIS

The building blocks of proteins are amino acids, and they move into the cytoplasm from the blood by active transport (Figure 4-25). The amino acids have to be connected in specific sequences to synthesize certain proteins. These specific proteins fall into two groups: **structural** and **genetic proteins.** The structural proteins help maintain the structure of cells. Genetic proteins result in the hereditary traits of each individual, such as eye color, hair color, skin color, and many others. The information necessary to synthesize the specific sequences of the amino acids is contained in the DNA molecules.

DNA molecules are composed of two long strands of *nucleotides* connected together by bases. The sequence of these bases along a DNA molecule determines the genetic code for each person. DNA is too important to leave the nucleus; therefore, the genetic code information must be copied by a messenger and carried into the cytoplasm.

## Formation of m-RNA (Transcription)

*Messenger RNA (m-RNA)* is a single-stranded nucleic acid that copies one-half of the genetic code (or it is transcribed) along the DNA molecule. In Figure 4-25,

showing how m-RNA copies one-half of the genetic code, uracil base is substituted for thymine on m-RNA. m-RNA moves from the nucleus to ribosomes in the cytoplasm. A second RNA molecule, transfer RNA (t-RNA), is located in the cytoplasm. t-RNA is a single-stranded chain of many nucleotides. It is cloverleaf–shaped, and three of the nucleotides are very important as they are complementary to three nucleotides on the m-RNA molecule. There are at least 20 different t-RNA molecules. Each t-RNA attaches to one of the 20 different amino acids by means of an ATP-activated reaction.

## Attachment of t-RNA to m-RNA (Translation)

Each t-RNA molecule carries its amino acid to a ribosome attached to the m-RNA. The ribosomes actually are composed of a large and small subunit (Figure 4-26), and the m-RNA threads itself through many ribosomes, forming a **polysome.** After two t-RNAs are attached to a ribosome, the ribosome moves along the m-RNA, lining up the complementary bases of each t-RNA with those on the m-RNA. When the complementary bases of the two t-RNAs are properly aligned with those on m-RNA, a peptide bond is formed between their amino acids. The t-RNAs then leave the ribosome, and more t-RNAs with their attached amino acids move in to take their place. The ribosome continues to move along the m-RNA molecule, aligning complementary m-RNA and t-RNA bases, which results in the joining together of amino acids. The ribosome gradually forms a polypeptide or protein tail (Figure 4-25) in this manner until it reaches the end of the m-RNA molecule. Then the ribosome and polypeptide or protein separate. As complex as this process seems, it is possible for 25 amino acids a second to be added to a polypeptide chain.

The m-RNA leaves the ribosomes after the protein is synthesized and moves back into the nucleus. The newly formed protein will be utilized in various ways.

## Base Specificity and Triplet Coding

The nucleotide bases attached to DNA and RNA can bond with other bases that have a complementary chemical structure (Chapter 2). The base pairing is adenine (A)–thymine (T) and guanine (G)–cytosine (C). This complementary base pairing is very important in protein synthesis. When m-RNA copies one-half of the genetic code, it is copying the sequence of bases along a portion of the DNA molecule. The base, uracil (U), replaces thymine (T) in the base sequence along RNA. Uracil is found only in m-RNA and t-RNA molecules.

m-RNA copies only one-half of the genetic code of a portion of a DNA molecule. The other half of the code

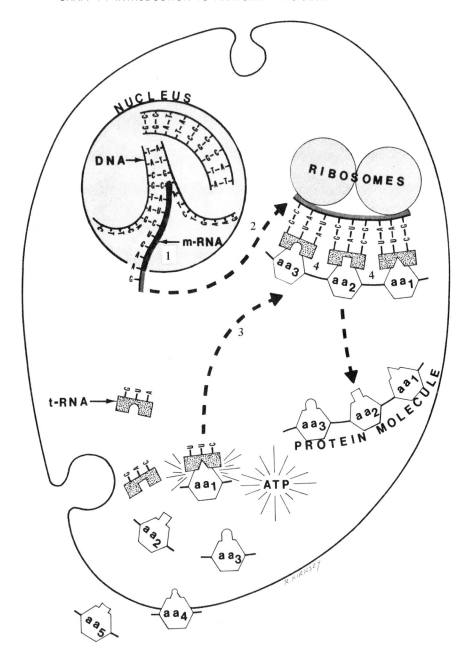

**Figure 4–25.** Protein synthesis. Before a protein can be synthesized, amino acids (aa) have to be moved into the cell cytoplasm by active transport. The process then involves (1) m-RNA copying half of the genetic code on DNA, (2) m-RNA moving out of the nucleus to ribosomes, (3) t-RNAs transferring their specific amino acids to the m-RNA, and (4) m-RNA and t-RNA bases bonding together and amino acids bonding together in the proper sequence to form a protein.

is produced when the bases attached to t-RNA bond to their complementary bases on m-RNA. It is important that the genetic code on DNA be reproduced exactly in the cytoplasm to produce the proper protein. This exact duplication of the genetic code is possible only because the bases are specifically complementary for each

other. Amino acids will be bonded together in the proper sequence since the t-RNA molecules have to bond to m-RNA in a proper sequence, due to complementary base pairing between m-RNA and t-RNA.

Each t-RNA molecule contains three nucleotides that are complementary for three nucleotides on

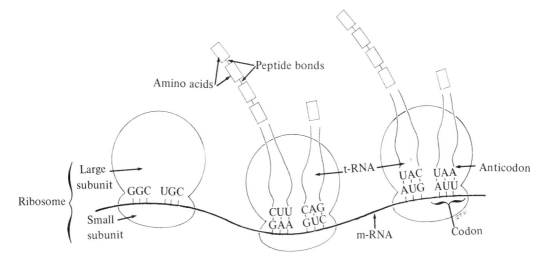

**Figure 4–26.** The connection of m-RNA to three ribosomes to form a polysome is shown. Codons (three nucleotides attached to m-RNA), complementary anticodons (three nucleotides attached to t-RNA), and growing polypeptide chains attached to t-RNAs are also shown.

m-RNA. This triplet of nucleotides on the m-RNA molecule is called a **codon** (Figure 4–26) and the triplet on the t-RNA molecule is called an **anticodon.** Since each codon and anticodon that align with each other involve triplets of complementary bases, this is called **triplet coding.** This means that, for every triplet of bases along m-RNA and t-RNA, a certain amino acid will be positioned. For example, if a genetic code for protein involves 900 complementary bases, then 300 amino acids are required to synthesize that particular protein. These amino acids will be connected in the proper sequence because of the triplet coding and bonding between complementary bases on m-RNA and t-RNA. If the sequence of bases on m-RNA is altered compared to the proper sequence on DNA, an abnormal genetic code will be produced. This improper code results in synthesis of an abnormal protein, which ultimately results in an unusual trait called a **mutation.** A mutation often is quite visible.

Table 4–3 provides a summary of protein synthesis.

# 10  CELL MITOSIS OR SOMATIC CELLULAR REPRODUCTION

The adult body is composed of many millions of cells; however, the body developed from a single cell. This single cell is the fertilized egg that results from the

**TABLE 4–3.  Summary of Protein Synthesis**

1. One-half of the genetic code on DNA is copied (transcribed) onto m-RNA.
2. The m-RNA molecules move out of the nucleus to ribosomes.
3. Each t-RNA molecule attaches to and transfers the amino acid, for which it is coded, to the m-RNA (translation).
4. Ribosomes move along m-RNA, aligning anticodon of t-RNA with proper codon of m-RNA.
5. Amino acids brought by t-RNA are attached to each other to form a polypeptide chain.
6. The t-RNAs separate from m-RNA and move back into the cytoplasm.
7. The m-RNA separates from the ribosomes and moves back into the nucleus.

union of the female egg (ovum) and the male sperm. The cell contains genetic information from both the mother and the father, which is needed to ultimately produce a mature adult body. This fertilized cell, with its important genetic information, obviously must give rise to many new cells to produce a new human being. A newborn child must grow and produce many new cells before a mature adult body finally results.

These processes by which a fertilized cell produces new generations are called **mitosis** and **cytokinesis. Mitosis** is a sequence of stages during which a nucleus divides, forming two genetically identical nuclei. The two new nuclei are identical to the parent nucleus in that they each contain the same DNA and genetic information. The cytoplasm of the parent cell is divided into half by cytokinesis. Each half of the cytoplasm

Parent Cell

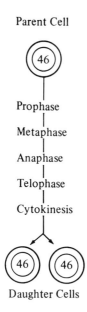

Figure 4-27.   Summary of cell mitosis.

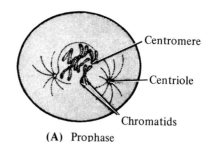

(A)  Prophase

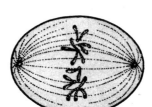

(B)  Metaphase

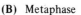

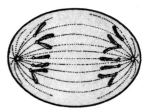

(C)  Anaphase

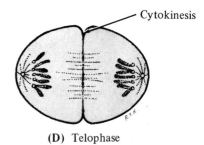

(D)  Telophase

along with the nucleus compose two new cells. This process is summarized by Figure 4-27.

## Interphase

If a cell is not undergoing mitosis, it is in **interphase.** A cell increases in size and carries out all its normal physiologic activities during interphase. Interphase (between phase) is not one of the four stages of mitosis; however, a very important event occurs during interphase; the DNA content doubles. If a parent cell (with 46 chromosomes) is to divide and form two cells, each with 46 chromosomes, then the parent cell must double its DNA content. This doubling of DNA material is absolutely essential if mitosis is to occur properly. It involves first a separation of two nucleotide strands. Free-floating nucleotides move in and bond with their complementary base on the single strands. This finally results in two exact replicas of the original DNA molecule, and the entire amount of DNA has been doubled. Now that a cell has two identical sets of DNA molecules, it can divide and send an identical set to each new cell.

## Prophase

Distinct chromosomes now become visible. The number of chromosomes doubles, to transport double the normal amount of DNA. Figure 4-28 shows double chromosomes, each part of which is called a **chromatid.** The 92 chromatids ultimately are split between two

Figure 4-28.   Mitosis is a process where a parent cell undergoes a series of division stages forming two daughter cells, each identical to the original parent cell.

cells in which they are called chromosomes. Three other features of this stage are as follows: the nuclear membrane disappears; centrioles move to opposite ends of the cell; and spindle fibers radiate out from the centrioles and attach to the centromere of each double chromosome.

## Metaphase

The double chromosomes move to the center of the cell where they line up in a single line. Each centromere splits, resulting in 92 chromatids or chromosomes across the center of the cell (Figure 4–28).

### Anaphase

The spindle fibers contract toward their respective centriole. As they contract they pull the chromatids to the centrioles. The end result is that 46 chromatids (chromosomes) are pulled to each centriole (Figure 4–28).

### Telophase

The chromosomes elongate until they are no longer distinguishable, or chromatin material is re-formed. Each new daughter nucleus now has DNA with the same genetic information as the parent cell. Another important occurrence during telophase is the division of cytoplasm (Figure 4–28). This process occurs when the cell membrane extends inward from each side of the cell until the two extensions meet. When the extensions meet, the cytoplasm has been divided; this process is called **cytokinesis.** Two new daughter cells are formed at the completion of telophase.

Table 4–4 provides a summary of mitosis.

### Time Required for Mitosis

The length of time required for mitosis varies considerably. The mitosis rate depends on the type of cell, environment, and temperature. Mitosis may be as short as 30 minutes or as long as several hours. Most cells undergo mitosis often during the time that a person is growing; however, when a part of the body has reached its ultimate size and development, mitosis stops. The cells of a particular part of the body will never undergo mitosis again except to replace cells destroyed by disease or injury.

## 11 ABNORMAL GROWTHS, ABNORMAL MITOSIS, AND TYPES OF CANCER

As indicated, cell mitosis continues to a certain point and then ceases. If mitosis occurs in an abnormal manner, then abnormal growths, cancers, and tumors often

**TABLE 4–4.  *Summary of Stages of Mitosis***

PROPHASE

- Doubling of chromosome number to 92.
- Nuclear membrane disappears.
- Centrioles move to opposite ends of the cell.
- Attachment of spindle fibers to centromere of each double chromosome

METAPHASE

- Double chromosomes line up along center of cell.
- Each centromere splits, resulting in 92 chromatids, single chromosomes now being present.

ANAPHASE

- Contraction of spindle fibers toward their respective centriole.
- Pulling of 46 single chromosomes (chromatids) toward each pole.

TELOPHASE

- Chromosomes unravel back to their chromatin state.
- Nuclear membrane reappears.

CYTOKINESIS

- The cytoplasm is split in half when the membrane on each side extends toward center until they meet.

result. We know much about the phases of mitosis, but we still know little about the mechanisms that initiate and control mitosis.

**CANCER.**  Cancer is a cellular disease that is characterized by malignant **neoplasms** (a mass of new, abnormal tissue or a tumor). Neoplasms are either **malignant** or **benign.** The term malignant means that the neoplasm forms secondary growths that originate from the primary tumor and are growing elsewhere in the body. A secondary growth is often referred to as a **metastasis,** and therefore malignant tumors are said to **metastasize.** A benign neoplasm or tumor does not **metastasize.**

**NAMING OF NEOPLASMS.**  Several nomenclature systems are used for naming cancers worldwide. In the United States, nomenclature has evolved around the suffix **-oma,** which literally means tumor. With a few exceptions, words with this suffix refer to neoplasms.

**BENIGN NEOPLASMS (TUMORS).**  Benign tumors are named with a prefix that designates the tissue in which they arose combined with the suffix **-oma.**

## Examples

| Fibroma | Adenoma |
|---|---|
| Fibrous — Tumor | Gland — Tumor |
| A benign tumor of fibrous tissue. A common example is fibroma of the uterus. | A benign tumor of glandular tissue. |

**CANCEROUS NEOPLASMS (TUMORS).** Cancerous tumors are named by the previous method combined with a name that gives their embryologic origin, for example, **sarcoma** and **carcinoma**. A sarcoma is a cancer that arises from **mesodermal** tissue. A **carcinoma** is a cancer that arises from **ectodermal** or **endodermal** tissue. During the development of an embryo the cells all become arranged into three layers—ectoderm, mesoderm, and endoderm (detail concerning these germ layers is given in Chapter 21). From these germ layers all organs and tissues of the body are formed.

Ectoderm—skin and appendages, nerve tissue
Mesoderm—bone, muscle, cartilage, and related tissues
Endoderm—intestinal system and its associated organs

Let's now look at some examples of these two nomenclature systems combined.

| ADENOCARCINOMA | | FIBROSARCOMA | |
|---|---|---|---|
| Glandular | Arising from ectodermal or endodermal embryonic origin | Fibrous tissue | Arising from mesodermal tissue |
| Common locations of this type are stomach, pancreas, and breast | | Common location is smooth muscle tissue of uterus | |

### Common Examples of Benign Tumors

Three very common benign tumors are fibroma, lipoma, and leiomyoma.

**FIBROMA.** This is a tumor of fibrous tissue and is very often found in the uterus. These tumors usually are small and encapsulated. They usually do not cause any symptoms unless their location results in pressure on a bone or nerve. Usually they can be easily removed by surgery.

**LIPOMA.** As the name indicates, this tumor is found in adipose tissue. Like the fibroma it rarely causes any symptoms but can put pressure on surrounding tissues as they expand.

**LEIOMYOMA.** This tumor originates in smooth muscle tissue and is the most common benign tumor in women. They can develop in smooth muscle tissue anywhere in the body, but they frequently are located in the walls of the uterus.

### Common Examples of Malignant Neoplasms

Three common examples of malignant neoplasms are carcinoma in situ, fibrosarcoma, and bronchiogenic sarcoma.

**CARCINOMA IN SITU.** (*In situ*—confined to the site of origin). A carcinoma originates in the ectodermal or endodermal tissues. This type quite often develops in the squamous epithelium of the uterus. As the name indicates, it usually remains localized, but it can invade surrounding tissues.

**FIBROSARCOMA.** This name tells us that this malignant neoplasm is in fibrous tissue that arose from mesodermal tissue. A common site is the walls of the uterus.

**BRONCHIOGENIC CARCINOMA.** This malignant neoplasm arises in the lower trachea and lower bronchi. It tends to metastasize easily and is the cause of about 90 percent of all cases of lung cancer.

## 12   TISSUES

A tissue is composed of cells with similar structure and function. Tissues are one of the four basic structural units that make up the body. Each tissue has a characteristic shape and carries out certain functions that help to maintain homeostasis of the body. The shapes of tissues and their characteristic functions are an excellent example of the structure–function concept. There are four main types of tissues: epithelial (lining), connective (supporting), muscular, and nervous.

## EPITHELIAL TISSUE

This tissue covers both the surface of the body and organs and lines body cavities and organs. Varous glands are formed from epithelial tissue that has grown into the body.

### Anatomic Features of Epithelial Tissue

Epithelial cells can vary considerably in their shape, depending on the specific type of epithelial tissue. All epithelial cells fit together very closely with no true intercellular material (matrix) present. The various types of epithelial tissue typically occur in thin membranes or sheets. They are not very strong membranes and rely upon support from connective tissues. A permeable, adhesive **basement membrane** (Figure 4–29) connects epithelial tissue to the deeper connective tissue.

An important characteristic of epithelial tissue is the lack of blood vessels. Since epithelial tissue lacks blood vessels, it obtains nutrients and gives off wastes to blood capillaries in the underlying connective tissues.

### Types of Epithelial Tissue

The names of the different types of epithelial tissue depend upon the shape and arrangement of the epithelial cells.

**Simple squamous epithelium** (Figure 4–29) is characterized by one layer of thin, flattened cells. Passage of materials can occur easily through this tissue since it is so thin. It is not surprising then to find simple squamous tissue lining regions of the body where diffusion and filtration materials commonly occur. The inner lining of blood vessels, lymphatic vessels, and the walls of capillaries are composed of simple squamous tissue.

*Function:* Simple squamous tissue facilitates diffusion and filtration of materials into and out of certain regions of the body, such as blood capillaries. $O_2$ and $CO_2$ diffuse into and out of capillaries.

**Simple Cuboidal Epithelium** (Figure 4–29) consists of cube-shaped cells arranged in a single layer. This tissue is located in certain endocrine glands such as the thyroid and the ovaries.

*Function:* The simple cuboidal tissue functions in secretion of materials. The thyroid and ovaries secrete various hormones.

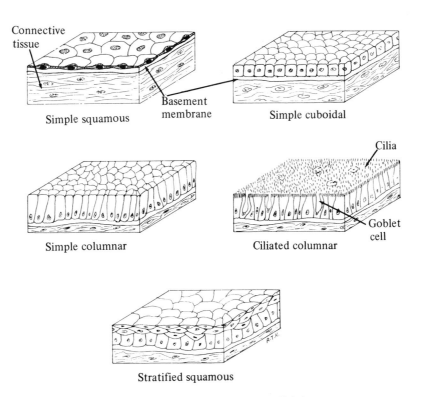

Connective tissue

Basement membrane

Simple squamous

Simple cuboidal

Simple columnar

Cilia

Goblet cell

Ciliated columnar

Stratified squamous

**Figure 4-29.** The common types of epithelial tissue.

**Simple columnar epithelium** (Figure 4–29) is characterized by tall, columnar cells. Interspersed through the columnar cells are specialized cells called **goblet cells,** which resemble inverted goblets. These cells secrete mucus to the surface of the simple columnar tissue. This tissue lines the small intestine.

*Function:* The large surface area of these cells enables them to absorb large amounts of materials in the small intestine. The secretion of mucus acts to protect the walls of the small intestine from concentrated HCl and bacteria. The mucus also acts to keep the lining moist to reduce friction.

**Ciliated columnar epithelium** (Figure 4–29) is like simple columnar epithelium, except that hairlike processes called **cilia** protrude from the cells. Goblet cells also are found in ciliated columnar tissue, just as in simple columnar tissue. This tissue lines some of the respiratory passages and uterine tubes and also is found in the uterus.

*Function:* The cilia combined with mucus in the respiratory tract act to protect the deeper parts of the body. The mucus traps bacteria and foreign material that may get into the respiratory tract. The cilia act to remove the trapped material from the respiratory tract by waves of contractions. The cilia in the uterine tubes act to propel or move ova (eggs) from ovaries into the uterus.

**Stratified squamous epithelium** (Figure 4–29) is characterized by seveal layers of epithelial tissue. The layers of cells act to protect the deeper tissues and the surface cells often are lost because of friction. There are two types of stratified squamous tissue, **keratinized** and **nonkeratinized.** The stratified keratinized squamous tissue is composed of dead cells that contain tough, waterproof keratin material. This keratinized stratified tissue composes the epidermis of the skin. The stratified nonkeratinized tissue is composed of living cells. It lines the mouth and the upper portion of the esophagus where the tissue is constantly moist.

**Transitional** tissue resembles nonkeratinized stratified squamous epithelial tissue in that there are several strata of cells. It differs from the previous though in that the superficial cells are larger and more rounded, compared to the flattened cells in the stratified tissue. There are some cells that are transitional in shape, or they can be pulled out of shape during certain body functions.

*Function:* This tissue permits distention or stretches. The walls of the urinary bladder are composed of this tissue, and when the urinary bladder fills with urine, the walls distend due to the transitional epithelium.

Table 4–5 summarizes the types of epithelial tissue.

## CONNECTIVE (SUPPORTING) TISSUE

This tissue is very abundant and widely distributed throughout the body. As the name indicates, the main function of this tissue is to connect and support the various parts of the body.

**TABLE 4-5.** *Summary of Types of Epthelial Tissue*

| Tissue | Description | Location | Function(s) |
|---|---|---|---|
| Simple squamous | One layer of thin, flattened cells | Inner lining of blood vessels Lymphatic vessels Capillary walls | Facilitates diffusion and filtration |
| Simple cuboidal | Cube-shaped cell in single layer | Thyroid gland Ovaries | Secretion |
| Simple columnar | Tall columnar cells; goblet cells interspersed, which secrete mucus | Lining small intestine | Absorption Secretion |
| Ciliated columnar | Tall columnar cells with cilia protuding; contains goblet cells, which secrete mucus | Respiratory passages Uterine tubes | Traps and removes bacteria and foreign material |
| Stratified squamous | Several layers of epithelial tissue; can be keratinized or nonkeratinized. | Epidermis of skin Lines mouth | Protects deeper tissues from friction |
| Transitional | Several strata cells like stratified cells; can change shape when pulled or stretched | Walls of urinary bladder | Permits distension or stretching |

### Anatomic Features of Connective Tissue

Connective tissue, in direct contrast to epithelial tissue, is richly supplied with blood vessels and intercellular material called **matrix.** The type and amount of intercellular material is a very important characteristic of connective tissue. The number of cells is few compared to the amount of intercellular material. The consistency of intercellular material varies from liquid in blood, to jellylike in areolar tissue, to very hard in bone tissue.

### Types of Connective Tissue

The important types of connective tissue are as follows:

**Adipose tissue** (Figure 4–30) is composed of adipose cells, which contain a large amount of fat. This fat pushes the nucleus to one side. Adipose tissue is found under the skin, around all body organs, around joints, and in the yellow marrow of long bones.

*Function:* Fat or lipid tissue is the body's primary reserve food supply. It acts as an insulator to prevent excess loss of heat through the skin and as a shock absorber to protect organs from hard blows.

**Blood (hemopoietic) tissue** (Figure 4–31) is primarily fluid intercellular material with cells floating in it. It circulates in the blood vessels throughout the body.

*Function:* Blood is a connective tissue in that it connects nutrient sources and excretory organs to all the body cells.

**Tendons and ligaments** contain jellylike intercellular material with a large amount of fibers. These fibers are very resistant to a pulling force in one direction. Tendons are an extremely strong attachment between muscles and bones. Ligaments attach bones together at joints.

*Function:* Tendons and ligaments connect muscles to bones and bones to bones. They give greater strength to these particular areas during movement.

**Cartilage** is characterized by its elasticity and pliabil-

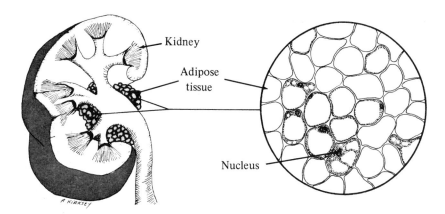

**Figure 4–30.** Lipid molecules compose adipose tissue. The amount of fat in each cell is so great that the nucleus is pushed off to the side.

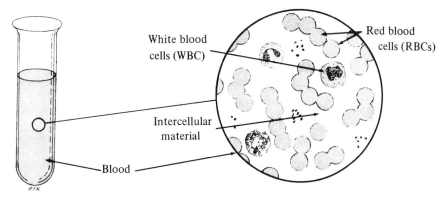

**Figure 4–31.** Blood (hemopoietic) tissue is a connective tissue composed primarily of intercellular material with red and white blood cells floating in it.

ity. The intercellular material is composed of jelly or gel-like material through which many fibers course. The cartilage tissue is surrounded by a fibrous membrane called the **perichondrium,** which furnishes nutrients and picks up wastes from the cartilage cells. Blood vessels are not present in the tissue itself. The cartilage cells are called **chondrocytes,** and they tend to be clumped together in groups of two and four.

There are three types of cartilage, and each varies in the kind of fibers that are found in the intercellular material:

**Hyaline cartilage** is white and glassy (hyaline) in appearance. It is composed of collagenic fibers that are randomly distributed throughout the intercellular material (Figure 4–31). Hyaline cartilage is located on the articulating surfaces of all bones and in the larynx, and makes up the skeleton in the developing fetus.

**Chondrocytes** are located in hollow cavities called **lacunae.** Hyaline cartilage is the most abundant cartilage in the body. Figure 4–32 shows that hyaline cartilage on the articulating surfaces of bones is called articular cartilage. In addition to the previously mentioned locations, hyaline cartilage also is located in the bronchi and bronchial tubes that carry air to and from the lungs.

*Function:* Hyaline cartilage furnishes firm but flexible support.

**Elastic cartilage** is composed of yellow elastic fibers in the matrix (Figure 4–33). The elastic fibers give this cartilage a lot of elasticity and therefore the cartilage is adapted to bending and then returning to its normal shape. The normal locations of this cartilage are the external ear, the epiglottis, and portions of the larynx.

*Function:* Elastic cartilage allows some degree of

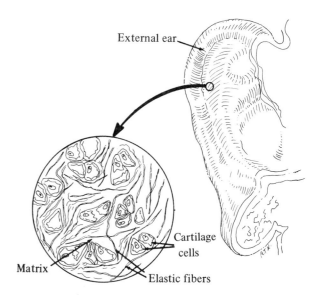

Figure 4–33.   Elastic cartilage tissue.

stretch and change but then returns the part of the body to its normal shape.

**Fibrous cartilage** is similar to hyaline cartilage in that it is composed of collagenic fibers; however, the collagenic fibers in the fibrous tissue are arranged in a regular manner (Figure 4–34) compared to that of hyaline cartilage. The regular arrangement of the fibers gives this tissue great strength. This cartilage is found in the intervertebral disks (round disklike structures located between the vertebrae of the vertebral column), semilunar disks in the knee joint, and the pubic symphysis.

*Function:* Fibrous cartilage furnishes firm but flexible support, such as the vertebral column and the knee joint. These cartilaginous disks act to absorb jolts and blows, while at the same time furnishing support to these regions of the body.

**Loose (areolar) connective tissue** is characterized by a large amount of fibers intermixed in a soft, jelly matrix. There are various collagen and elastic fibers that are loosely distributed among the soft matrix. This is the most abundant connective tissue of the body and typically is found beneath the skin, in most epithelial tissues (Figure 4–35), and around blood vessels and nerves. It serves to support and maintain the position of these structures. This tissue is well endowed with blood vessels and various types of cells.

1. **Fibroblasts** are the majority of the cells. It is believed that fibroblasts form collagen fibers when an injury occurs to this tissue. These cells are large and flat with branching processes.

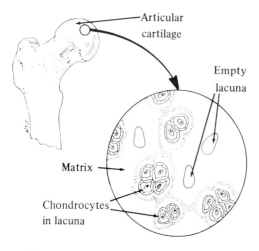

Figure 4–32.   Hyaline cartilage tissue.

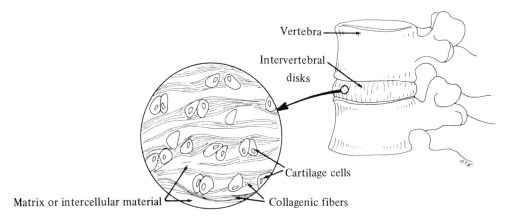

Figure 4-34.   Fibrous cartilage tissue.

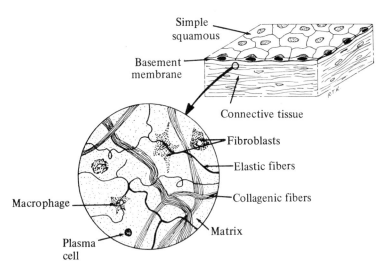

Figure 4-35.   Loose (areolar) connective tissue.

2. **Macrophages (histiocytes)** are more irregular than fibroblasts, with short branching processes. Macrophages carry out phagocytosis or they take in bacteria and destroy them. The presence of these cells enables loose areolar connective tissue to function as an important defense for the body against bacteria.

3. **Plasma cells** are small and usually irregularly shaped. They function to provide immunity to a person by producing antibodies when stimulated by foreign antigens. These cells are found most frequently in loose areolar connective tissue around the digestive tract.

4. **Mast cells** function to produce **histamine** and **heparin. Histamine** is released when injury to this tissue occurs. It functions to dilate (enlarge) small blood vessels or initiates inflammation of tissues. **Heparin** is a natural anticoagulant and prevents blood from clotting within blood vessels.

**Bone (osseous) tissue** (Figure 4–36) is found in all bones in the body. Bones are rigid levers in that they give strength and support to parts that are moved. Their intercellular material is quite dense and hard due to calcium and phosphate salts. Bone cells (**osteocytes**) are imprisoned in minute hollow cavities (**lacunae**). Osteocytes are responsible for producing the intercellular material. Bone tissue is located in all 206 bones of the body.

*Function:* Bone tissue helps to support and protect

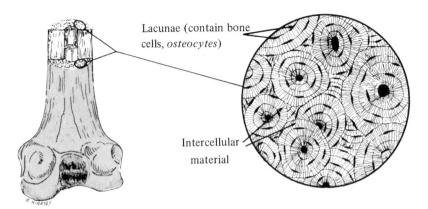

Lacunae (contain bone cells, *osteocytes*)

Intercellular material

**Figure 4-36.** Bone (osseous) tissue is composed of bone cells (osteocytes) contained in lacunae. The intercellular material is very dense and hard due to calcium and magnesium salts.

all areas of the body. It also acts as a storage area for calcium and magnesium ions until they are needed by the body. Bones act as levers and in coordination with muscles are responsible for moving various parts of the body.

Table 4-6 summarizes the types of connective tissue.

## MUSCLE TISSUE

Muscle tissue has the ability to shorten or contract, and thus is responsible for body movement. There are three types of muscle tissue: visceral, skeletal, and cardiac.

### Visceral (Smooth, Involuntary) Muscle Tissue

This tissue is a muscular tissue composing the walls of the visceral organs (Figure 4-37). It is called involuntary

muscle tissue because a person cannot voluntarily contract it. It contracts automatically or involuntarily. Some examples of where it is found are the stomach, intestines, and blood vessels.

Visceral muscle tissue contracts slowly and automatically. This results in gradual, continual movement of materials through the digestive tract, blood vessels, and other areas. Details concerning the anatomic structure of this tissue will be discussed later.

### Skeletal (Striated, Voluntary) Muscle Tissue

This tissue derives its name from the fact that it connects to bones (skeletal system) by means of tendons (Figure 4-38). It is the skeletal muscles that act in coordination with bones (levers) to move parts of the body. These muscles are voluntary in that they can be contracted at will. Details concerning the anatomic structure of this tissue will be discussed in Chapter 13.

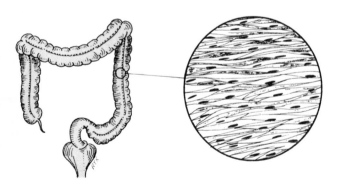

**Figure 4-37.** Visceral (smooth) muscle tissue is characterized by no striations and a single nucleus per cell.

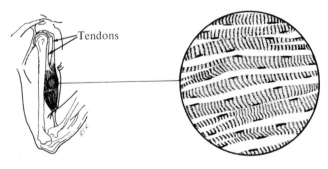

Tendons

**Figure 4-38.** Skeletal muscle tissue is characterized by long cells with striations. Each cell has many nuclei or is multinucleated.

### TABLE 4-6.  Summary of Connective (Supporting) Tissue

| TISSUE | DESCRIPTION | LOCATION | FUNCTION(S) |
|---|---|---|---|
| Adipose | Composed of adipose cells that contain fat | Under skin and around all body organs | Reserve food supply, heat insulator, shock absorber |
| Blood (hemopoietic) | Primarily a fluid tissue with cells floating in it | Blood vessels | Circulates nutrients to all cells and wastes away |
| Tendons and ligaments | Contain jellylike intercellular material; contain large amount of fibers | Tendons connect muscles to bones. Ligaments attach bones together at joints | Connect bones and muscles together with great strength |
| Cartilage Hyaline | White and glassy in appearance; composed of collagenic fibers | Articulating surfaces of long bones, larynx, fetal skeleton | Firm, flexible support |
| Elastic | Yellow elastic fibers in matrix | External ear, epiglottis, larynx | Allows stretch and change |
| Fibrous | Composed of collagenic fibers | Intervertebral disks, semilunar disk | Firm, flexible support |
| Loose (areolar) | Soft jelly matrix with fibers loosely arranged. Well-endowed with blood vessels and different types of cells | Beneath skin and beneath most epithelial tissues | Forms collagen fibers; phagocytosis; produces antibodies, histamine, and heparin |
| Bone (osseous) | Intercellular material is quite hard and dense due to presence of calcium and magnesium salts | In all 206 bones | Support and protect all areas of body; stores calcium and magnesium ions |

## Cardiac Muscle Tissue

This tissue is found only in the heart. It is similar to involuntary muscles in that it cannot be voluntarily contracted. It is also similar to skeletal or striated muscle tissue in that each muscle cell is long and has striations (stripes) (Figure 4-39) across the cell. Cardiac muscle tissue is responsible for movement of blood through the heart when it contracts. More details concerning the anatomic structure of this tissue will be discussed later.

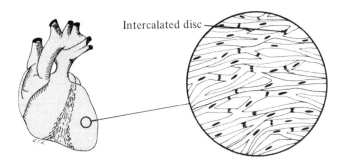

**Figure 4-39.** Cardiac muscle tissue is characterized by striated cells that interconnect to form a syncytium or network. The ends of each cardiac cell are thickened to form an intercalated disk.

Intercalated disc

## NERVE TISSUE

Each tissue contributes in some way to the total coordinated action of the whole body. This coordinated action of the tissues is controlled by the brain and the spinal cord. Nerve tissue conducts impulses from all parts of the body to the spinal cord and brain and also from the brain out to all parts of the body. Nerve tissue is composed of many, many neurons. Most neurons are long, cylindrical cells. Their cytoplasm is drawn out into stringlike processes that can be microscopic or quite long. Chapter 5 presents a detailed discussion of nervous tissue.

## HOW TISSUES HELP TO MAINTAIN HOMEOSTASIS

Previously in this unit it was stated that cells are the site of normal homeostatic activity. Since tissues are composed of cells similar in shape and function, then obviously tissues function to maintain homeostasis. Some examples of body functions involved in maintaining homeostasis and the tissues involved are discussed next.

**PROTECTION.**    Stratified squamous epithelial tissue, adipose, and loose areolar connective.

**SUPPORT.**    All the connective tissues function in support in one way or another.

**FILTRATION.**    Simple squamous epithelium allows diffusion and filtration of materials across its surface. This process is very important in the normal functioning of blood capillaries and also in the kidneys.

**ABSORPTION.**    Once carbohydrates, lipids, and proteins have been broken down to their basic building blocks, they must be absorbed into the bloodstream before being carried to the cells for their use. Simple columnar epithelium carries out this important function.

**SECRETION.**    Epithelial tissue that composes glands like sweat, sebaceous, thyroid, and adrenal glands that function to secrete materials that play very important roles in maintaining homeostasis.

**MOVEMENT.**    All muscle tissues produce important movements, such as heart contractions and movement of food along digestive tract.

**TRANSPORTATION.**    The blood connective tissue functions to transport nutrients and wastes to and from all cells.

# 13   MEMBRANES

Membranes were discussed previously as being important in the structure of the ER, mitochondria, and Golgi complex. The cell membrane and nuclear membrane are important since they select which materials will pass into and out of the cytoplasm and nucleus. These were chemical membranes in that they were composed of layers of chemical molecules. There are tissue membranes in the body that are composed of layers of a combination of tissues. They are actually the simplest combination of tissues. Tissue membranes cover and line the body surfaces and divide organs into sections. The main membranes of the body are serous, mucous, synovial, fascial, and miscellaneous fibrous membranes.

## SEROUS MEMBRANE

The **serous membrane** derives it name from the fact that it exudes (slow oozing out) a thin watery serous fluid. Serous fluid acts as a lubricant and prevents friction when organs rub against each other and the body wall. This membrane always lines closed cavities and covers the organs within it. Two examples of large serous membranes are the **pleural** and **peritoneal** membranes. Each has two layers. The parietal layer lines the walls of a cavity and the visceral layer covers the surface of organs.

The pleural membrane is located within the thoracic cavity. The parietal pleura layer lines the walls of the thoracic cavity. The visceral pleura layer covers the surface of lungs. When the lungs increase and decrease in size (during breathing), the visceral pleura slides against the parietal pleura with little friction.

The peritoneal membrane is located within the abdominal pelvic cavity. The parietal peritoneum layer lines the wall of the abdominal pelvic cavity. The visceral peritoneum layer covers the surface of organs within the abdominal pelvic cavity.

Serous membranes are composed of an outer layer of epithelial tissue that secretes the serous fluid and a deeper layer of connective tissue. The connective tissue layer gives the membrane strength.

## MUCOUS MEMBRANE

The **mucous membrane** has an outer layer of epithelial tissue and an inner layer of connective tissue. The goblet cells within the epithelial tissue secrete mucus. Mucous membranes line all body cavities that open to the outside of the body, such as respiratory, digestive, urinary, and reproductive tracts. These tracts are the prime entrance points for microbes, dirt, and foreign materials. The mucus helps to trap and remove these foreign substances. The mucus that lines the stomach protects the deeper tissues from powerful HCl (hydrochloric acid) and digestive juices. The mucous membrane that lines the small intestine functions to absorb digested food.

## SYNOVIAL MEMBRANES

**Synovial membranes** are composed entirely of connective tissue. They exude a very thick viscous fluid, called synovial fluid. The synovial membranes line freely movable joints. The membrane, along with the synovial fluid, acts as a lubricant. The ends of bones in a freely movable joint must be lubricated to prevent damage by friction.

## FASCIAL MEMBRANES

The **fascial membranes** are composed entirely of connective tissue. Fascial membranes differ from the previous three in that fascial membranes do not secrete a fluid. They primarily act to retain and support stuctures. The two types of fascial membranes are superficial and deep fascia membranes.

### Superficial Fascia Membrane (Subcutaneous Tissue)

The **superficial fascia membrane** is composed of adipose and loose connective tissues. Superficial fascia is attached to the deep layer of the skin (dermis), and it functions to connect the skin to deeper structures—bone, cartilage, and deep fascia.

### Deep Fascia Membrane

**Deep fascia** is composed of dense connective tissue and no fat. This membrane tends to form a capsulelike structure around the visceral organs and glands. It also forms a sheathlike structure around muscles, nerves, blood vessels, and the brain.

## MISCELLANEOUS FIBROUS MEMBRANES

These membranes are found throughout the body and are composed entirely of fibrous connective tissue.

### Periosteum

The **periosteum** covers the surface of bones. Ligaments attach muscles to the periosteum, and arteries and veins pass through it into and out of the bone tissue.

### Sclera

The **sclera** is the outer white layer of the eye. This fibrous connective tissue layer protects the deeper sensitive layers.

### Dura Mater

The **dura mater** is the outer covering of the brain and the spinal cord. It is one of three membranes that cover the brain and the spinal cord.

## 14 DISEASES AND THEIR RELATIONSHIP TO MEMBRANES

Membranes are located extensively throughout the body and are obvious sites for microorganisms to both localize and spread. Mucous membranes are prime sites for microorganisms since they line tracts and passageways that open to the outside. The mucous fluid secreted by the membrane is normally effective in preventing microorganisms from spreading and penetrating into deeper tissue.

Some examples of diseases localized in membranes are the common cold (**rhinitis**), **peritonitis**, and **gonorrhea**. Cold viruses localize in the nasal mucosa, causing inflammation. **Peritonitis** is inflammation of the peritoneal membrane that lines the walls of the abdominopelvic cavity. This often results from the appendix rupturing and releasing bacteria into the abdominopelvic cavity. **Gonorrhea** is a disease of the mucous membranes that line the reproductive tracts. It is caused by gonococcus organisms.

## SUMMARY

Direction Terms
A. Superior: above or higher in position.
B. Inferior: Below or in a lower position.
C. Anterior: located near belly surface or front of body.
D. Posterior: located near back side of body.
E. Lateral: farther from midline or toward side.
F. Medial: nearer midline of body.

G. Internal: deeper within body.

H. External: near the outer surface of body.

I. Distal: farther from point of attachment.

J. Proximal: nearer point of origin.

K. Peripheral: extensions from center of body.

L. Parietal: refers to walls of a cavity.

M. Visceral: pertains to the organs within a cavity.

## Planes or Sections of the Body

Cuts made through the body in different planes:

A. Sagittal: cut that divides body into right and left sections.

B. Midsagittal: cut that divides body into equal right and left halves.

C. Horizontal: cut that divides body into upper and lower sections.

D. Frontal: cut that passes through body, dividing it into anterior and posterior portions.

## Body Cavities

A. Dorsal cavity: contains the organs that coordinate activities of organs located lower in the body.
   1. Cranial cavity: contains the brain.
   2. Vertebral: contains the spinal cord.

B. Ventral cavity: divided into thoracic and abdominopelvic cavities.
   1. Thoracic: contains heart, lungs, and great blood vessels.
   2. Abdominopelvic: abdominal area contains stomach, small intestine, large intestine, liver, gallbladder, pancreas, spleen, and so on. Pelvic area contains urinary bladder, end of large intestine, and certain reproductive organs.

## Structural Units

A. Cells: simplest structural and functional unit of body; physiologic functions are intracellular or intercellular.

B. Tissue: composed of cells with similar structure and function.

C. Organ: composed of two or more different tissues.

D. System: a group of organs that combine to accomplish a major body task.

## The Cell and Homeostasis

A. Chemical composition of protoplasm: composed of organic and inorganic materials
   1. Organic compounds: proteins, lipids, and carbohydrates make up about 30 percent of protoplasm.
   2. Inorganic compounds
      a. Water: 55 to 70 percent of protoplasm; takes part in some reactions; serves as a solvent for some reactions.
      b. Inorganic salts: ionize into anions and cations that have a wide variety of functions.

B. Cell Membrane or Plasma Membrane
   1. Chemical composition of plasma membrane: composed of globular proteins and phospholipids; double layer of phospholipids important in determining what enters and leaves cell.
   2. Function of proteins in plasma membrane: maintain structural integrity of plasma membrane, bind enzymes, and facilitate transport of materials.
   3. Functions of plasma membrane:
      a. Limits protoplasm.
      b. Controls movement of materials into and out of cells.
      c. Creates an osmolarity difference between inside and outside of a cell.

## Specialized Organs (Organelles) of a Cell

A. Endoplasmic reticulum (ER): extensively branched interconnected system of membranes; granular endoplasmic reticulum (GER) transports proteins attached to it; agranular endoplasmic reticulum (AER) involved in synthesis of steroids, glycogen metabolism, $Ca^{2+}$ release, and storage.

B. Ribosomes: spherical; contain RNA; attach to ER or float free; the site of protein synthesis.

C. Golgi complex (dictysome): small, flattened membranes stacked on top of one another. Functions: storage of proteins, lipids, and carbohydrates; synthesis of carbohydrates and attachment of proteins.

D. Mitochondria: contains outer and inner branched membrane that forms cristae. Function: releases energy utilized by all cells.

E. Lysosomes: rounded membranous structure. Function: releases digestive or hydrolytic enzymes to break down large molecules.

F. Centriole: cylindrical structure composed of nine longitudinal bundles; two in a cell and lie at right angles to each other. Function: mitotic division of cell.

G. Inclusions: clusters or clumps of material in a cell; permanent are melanin and hemoglobin; temporary are glycogen and fat.

H. Nucleus: composed of outer nuclear membrane and fluid called nucleoplasm. Function: directs synthesis of proteins.

## Movement of Substances across Cell Membrane

A. Diffusion: movement of particles from an area of high concentration to an area of lower concentration.
    *Ex.*    $O_2$ and $CO_2$ diffusing into and out of lung alveoli.

B. Osmosis: movement of water from a region of low solute concentration to a high solute concentration through a membrane permeable to water only; osmotic pressure functions to pull water through membrane. Isoosmolar or isotonic: body fluids and fluids within cells have equal osmolalities and equal osmotic pressures. Hyperosmolar or hypertonic: an intercellular solution has a greater osmolality than an intracellular one. Hypoosmolar or hypotonic: an intercellular solution has a lower osmolality than an intracellular one.

C. Active transport: substances move through a membrane from a lower concentration to a higher concentration; energy is required to move the substances against a concentration gradient; carrier molecules in cell membrane move substances.
    *Ex.*    $Na^+$ and $K^+$.

D. Bulk transport. (1) Phagocytosis: cell membrane reaches out and surrounds a particle until it is inside the cell; WBCs commonly carry out this process. (2) Pinocytosis: cell membrane invaginates until a large particle is inside, whereby a vacuole breaks off with the particle inside.

E. Filtration: a process that pushes water and substances from a higher pressure to a lower pressure through a membrane.

## Characteristics that Enable the Cell Membrane to Be Selectively Permeable

Three basic features enable a membrane to be selectively permeable: (1) double layer of lipids; compounds insoluble in lipids do not pass through; (2) total charge on membrane; ions with same charge as membrane are rejected, whereas opposite charges are attracted through membrane; (3) size of pores in membrane.

## Protein Synthesis

A. Formation of m-RNA (transcription): messenger RNA (m-RNA) is a single-stranded nucleotide that results from copying (transcription) of one-half of DNA genetic code. Moves from nucleus to ribosomes.

B. Attachment of t-RNA to m-RNA (translation): t-RNAs bring amino acids to ribosomes, which then move along an m-RNA and link up complementary bases; a t-RNA releases its amino acid to a polypeptide chain after a linking up of the complementary bases.

C. Base specificity and triplet coding: codon is a triplet of nucleotides on m-RNA; anticodon is a triplet of nucleotides on t-RNA; each triplet codes for a specific amino acid; amino acids will be connected in proper sequence for a protein because of the triplet coding and bonding between complementary bases on m-RNA and t-RNA.

### Cell Mitosis or Somatic Cellular Reproduction

A. Mitosis: division of parent nucleus into two daughter nuclei that are identical to parent nucleus in DNA and genetic information.
1. Interphase: between phase of mitosis; not a stage of mitosis; DNA content of a nucleus doubles so that in effect it has two exact replicas of each DNA molecule.
2. Prophase: distinct double chromosomes now visible; each chromosome composed of two chromatids; nuclear membrane disappears, centrioles move to opposite ends of cell, and spindle fibers radiate out from centrioles and attach to centromeres.
3. Metaphase: double chromosomes move to center of cell and line up in a single line.
4. Anaphase: spindle fibers contract toward their respective centrioles; chromatids (single chromosomes) are pulled toward centrioles.
5. Telophase: chromosome elongates until no longer distinguishable; nuclear membrane reappears; cytokinesis or division of cytoplasm occurs.

### Abnormal Growths, Abnormal Mitosis, and Types of Cancer

A. Cancer: cellular disease; characterized by malignant neoplasms that metastasize or spread.
B. Benign tumors: tumors that do not spread or metastasize. Three common examples of benign tumors: fibroma—tumor of fibrous tissue, *Ex.*—uterus; lipoma—tumor in adipose tissue; Leiomyoma—originates in smooth muscle tissue, *Ex.*—uterus.

### Tissues

A. Epithelial: anatomic features are (1) cells fit together tightly with no intercellular (matrix) present, (2) no blood vessels, (3) basement membrane connects epithelial tissue to deeper connective tissues.
1. Simple squamous epithelium: one layer flattened cells; located in lining of blood vessels, lymphatic and capillary walls. Function: facilitates diffusion and osmosis.
2. Simple cuboidal epithelium: single layer of cube-shaped cells; located in certain endocrine glands such as thyroid and ovaries. Function: secretion.
3. Simple columnar epithelium: tall, columnar cells; located in lining of small intestine. Functions: absorption and secretion.
4. Ciliated columnar epithelium: columnar cells with cilia extending from them; located in lining of respiratory tracts and uterine tubes. Function: protect deeper tissues by trapping and removing foreign material.
5. Stratified squamous epithelium: several layers of epithelial cells; keratinized and non-keratinized; located in lining of mouth and epidermis of skin. Function: protection of deeper tissues.
6. Transitional: several strata of cells; located in wall of urinary bladder. Function: permits distension or stretching without rupturing of cells.
B. Connective (supporting) tissue: anatomic features are (1) richly supplied with blood vessel, (2) presence of intercellular material (matrix).
1. Adipose tissue: nucleus pushed to one side; stores fat molecules; located under skin, around all organs. Functions: primary reserve of food supply; heat insulator.
2. Blood (hemopoietic) tissue: liquid intercellular material with cells floating in it; found in blood vessels. Function: connects nutrient sources and excretory organs to all body cells.

3. Tendons and ligaments: jellylike intercellular material with many fibers; tendons attach muscles to bones; ligaments attach bones together.
4. Cartilage: elastic and pliable; surrounded by perichondrium.
   a. Hyaline: white and glassy; located at articulating surfaces of bones. Function: firm but flexible support.
   b. Elastic: yellow elastic fibers in matrix; located in external ear, epiglottis, and larynx. Function: allows some degree of stretch and change.
   c. Fibrous: composed of collagenic fibers; located in intervertebral disks and semilunar disks. Function: firm but flexible support.
5. Loose (areolar) connective: large number of fibers intermixed in a soft, jelly matrix; location beneath skin and epithelial tissues. Function: support and maintain position of structures.
6. Bones (osseous) tissue: rigid matrix; osteocytes in lacunae; located in all 206 bones. Function: support and protect all areas of body.

C. Muscle tissue
1. Visceral (smooth, involuntary): no striations; located in walls of stomach and intestines. Function: contracts involuntarily to move materials.
2. Skeletal (striated, voluntary): striations present in muscle tissue; attached to bones. Function: contracts voluntarily to move bones.
3. Cardiac: fibers have striations; contracts involuntarily; located in heart. Function: movement of blood through heart.

D. Nerve Tissue
Composed of neurons; located in all nerves, brain, and spinal cord. Function: coordinates activities of all organs and systems.

## Membranes

Combinations of two or more kinds of tissues; cover and line body surfaces; divide organs into sections.

A. Serous: secretes a thin watery serous fluid; fluid reduces friction when organs rub against each other; lines closed cavities (thoracic and abdominopelvic); composed of epithelial and connective.
B. Mucous: outer layer of epithelial and inner layer of connective tissue; line body cavities that open to outside of body (respiratory, digestive, and urinary).
C. Synovial: composed of connective tissue; secrete synovial fluid; line freely movable joints; function is to reduce friction between bones.
D. Fascial: composed of connective tissues; do not secrete a fluid; act to retain and support structures.
E. Miscellaneous fibrous membranes
1. Periosteum: covers surfaces of bones; point of attachment for ligaments, arteries, and veins.
2. Sclera: outer white layer of eye; protects deeper, sensitive layers of eyes.
3. Dura mater: outer covering of brain and spinal cord.

## Diseases and Their Relationship to Membranes

Membranes are prime sites for infections; examples are common cold (rhinitis), peritonitis, and gonorrhea.

## Introduction to Anatomy–Physiology of the Body

### Matching

1. The nose is _____ to the mouth.    **A.** lateral
2. The hand is _____ to the upper arm.    **B.** medial
3. The ears are _____ to the nose.    **C.** superior
4. The heart is _____ to the lungs.    **D.** distal
5. The breasts are _____ to the head.    **E.** inferior
6. The two major body cavities are dorsal and thoracic.    True (A) or False (B)

### Matching

7. mitochondria    **A.** synthesize proteins
8. endoplasmic reticulum    **B.** store and release digestive enzymes
9. ribosomes    **C.** release ATP
10. lysosomes    **D.** packaging of proteins and carbohydrates
11. Golgi complex    **E.** transport materials
12. Which of the following is defined incorrectly?
    (a) Osmosis: movement of water from a low solute to a high solute concentration through a membrane permeable to water only.
    (b) Filtration: pushing of water from a high pressure to a low pressure through a membrane.
    (c) Active transport: movement of substances through a membrane from a high to low concentration.

The following statement refers to questions 13 to 18. The first item in each pair of items names a structure or a location or a process. If the second item is located in or is in some way part of the first item, circle A. If not, circle B.

A  B    **13.** Simple squamous epithelium
              Single layer of columnar cells

A  B    **14.** Connective tissue
              Blood vessels and matrix

A  B    **15.** Metaphase
              Movement of chromatids toward centrioles

A  B    **16.** Transcription
              Attachment of t-RNA to m-RNA

A  B    **17.** Secretion of thin watery fluid
              Serous membrane

A  B    **18.** Hyperosmolar fluid
              2% NaCl and 10% glucose (dextrose)

# Chapter 5

# NERVOUS SYSTEM

After reading and studying this chapter, a student should be able to:

1. Describe a homeostatic mechanism as to its three parts and four characteristics.
2. Describe the anatomy of the different types of neurons and a synapse.
3. Describe the events that lead to nerve impulse conduction.
4. Recognize a description of the internal anatomy of the spinal cord and the meninges that cover it and the brain.
5. Write the names of the four spinal plexuses and a major nerve that exits from each.
6. Give the components and function of a stretch, flexor, and cross-extensor reflex.
7. Describe the parts and functions of the hindbrain and midbrain.
8. Describe the lobes of the cerebral cortex as to location, functions, and association areas.
9. Write a description of sensory and motor nerve pathways.
10. Compare short- and long-term memory.
11. Recognize a description of the pathway that CSF follows from where it is secreted until absorbed into venous sinuses.
12. Give the name, number, and function of each of the 12 cranial nerves.
13. Describe the location and function of the sympathetic and parasympathetic divisions of the autonomic nervous system.

*In Chapter 2 we described homeostasis (steady state) as a dynamic state of equilibrium of bodily processes. In this chapter we will study how the nervous system coordinates the activities of other organ systems and thereby maintains homeostasis.*

# 1 HOMEOSTATIC MECHANISMS

Homeostasis is defined as a dynamic equilibrium of a physiological activity. When physiological activities are in homeostasis, a person is in a normal state of health. When they are not, a person is ill. To maintain homeostasis, each organ system utilizes homeostatic mechanisms. Each mechanism consists of three parts (Figure 5–1):

- A **sensory receptor** that is stimulated by any change in the internal or external environment of the body.

- A **nerve circuit** that transmits a sensory nerve impulse to the central nervous system and then transmits a motor impulse to an effector organ.

- An **effector organ** that responds to the motor impulse and restores homeostasis (Figure 5–1).

Four characteristics describe each homeostatic mechanism:

- Self-regulating: Each mechanism is activated automatically in a healthy person. However, in an ill person one or more of the three parts malfunctions so that self-regulation is not possible.

- Compensatory: The response by a mechanism is a compensatory one to counteract the abnormal condition.

- Negative feedback: This feedback involves transmission of motor impulses to the effector organ(s) that result in physiological responses being directed or adjusted back to normal.

- More than one negative feedback system may be involved. Most examples of where homeostasis is restored involve negative feedback of more than one system. See the example in Figure 5–1.

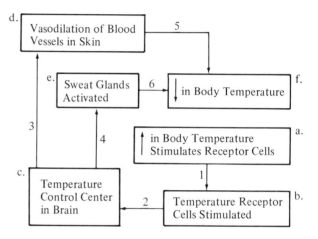

**Figure 5-1.** The three parts of a homeostatic mechanism are receptor, (b); nerve circuit, 1 to 6; effector organ, (d) and (e). The four characteristics of a mechanism are: self-regulating, 1 and 2; compensatory, (f); negative feedback, 5 and 6; more than one negative feedback system involved, (d) and (e).

# 2 ORGANIZATION OF THE NERVOUS SYSTEM

The nervous system is the most complex and highly organized system of the body. It is made up of several subdivisions, all of which function as a whole. To study this system, we must divide it into its subdivisions. The subdivisions are described in Table 5–1.

## NEURON: BUILDING BLOCK OF NERVOUS TISSUE

The basic cell making up nerve tissue is the **neuron** or nerve cell. A neuron exhibits the characteristic of "structure determines function," and vice versa, very

### TABLE 5-1. The Nervous System

| | ANATOMIC CHARACTERISTICS | PHYSIOLOGIC CHARACTERISTICS |
|---|---|---|
| Central nervous system (CNS) | Nerve tissue within the brain and spinal cord | Voluntary nerve impulses are carried to skeletal muscles and the skin; carries involuntary impulses to smooth muscles, cardiac muscles, and glands |
| Peripheral nervous system | All nerves that connect to the brain and spinal cord, cranial and spinal nerves | Both voluntary and involuntary nerve impulses are carried by these nerves |
| Autonomic or involuntary system | Autonomic nerves connect the CNS with all internal organs | This system controls all the organs that cannot be voluntarily controlled; the organs operate without your conscious control, or automatically |

well. Most neurons are thin elongated structures. This structure enables them to transmit nerve impulses rapidly. Some neurons may be quite long, 3 to 4 feet in some areas, and others may be only a fraction of an inch long.

### Anatomy of Neurons

All neurons (Figure 5-2) exhibit the same basic anatomic structures.

**CELL BODY.** This rounded area contains the nucleus of the neuron. The nucleus of this cell, as well as the nucleus of any nucleated cell, is vital. If the cell body is damaged, the neuron will die; therefore, it is always in a fairly well protected area. Cell bodies are found only in the gray matter of the spinal cord and brain, and ganglia (round masses of nerve tissue near the spinal cord).

**AXON AND DENDRITE.** The cytoplasm of the cell is extended out into two types of processes that attach to the cell body. The **dendrite** (looks like roots of a tree) receives impulses and carries them to the cell body (Figure 5-2). The **axon** carries impulses away from the cell body to the next neuron or muscle cell. The dendrite is the input part of the cell and the axon is the output part of the cell. There can be many dendrites to a neuron, but only one axon.

**NERVE COVERINGS (SHEATHS).** Some neurons are enveloped by sheaths and some others are not. The two types of sheaths are **myelin** and **neurilemma.** Myelin is composed of lipids and proteins and has a whitish color. The myelin sheath is not continuous, as is seen in Figure 5-1. There are many constrictions along the myelin sheath, called the **nodes of Ranvier.** The nodes are points at which the myelin is absent. Neurons that have the myelin sheath present are called myelinated neurons and when grouped together they are called **white matter.** Neurons lacking the myelin sheath are unmyelinated neurons, and when grouped together they are called **gray matter.** In the central nervous system (CNS) the gray matter consists of unmyelinated neurons and white matter consists of myelinated neurons.

The neurilemma sheath (Figure 5-2), if present, is outside the myelin sheath or in direct contact with the axis cylinder. It is found on peripheral neurons only and not in the CNS.

**FUNCTIONS OF NEURON SHEATHS.** Myelin insulates a neuron against $Na^+$ and $K^+$ ions. The nodes of Ranvier are the only points at which $Na^+$ and $K^+$ can enter and leave a neuron. This is significant in conduction of nerve impulses, as will be discussed shortly.

---

**Multiple sclerosis** is a disease characterized by degeneration of the myelin sheath on CNS nerves. The cause is unknown, and it is incurable.

---

The neurilemma acts to regenerate the neurons. If a peripheral neuron is damaged, it can regenerate itself by action of the neurilemma sheath. The neurilemma sheath is absent from CNS nerves and, therefore, they cannot regenerate themselves if damaged.

### Types of Neurons

We will discuss the different types of neurons according to which direction they transmit nerve impulses.

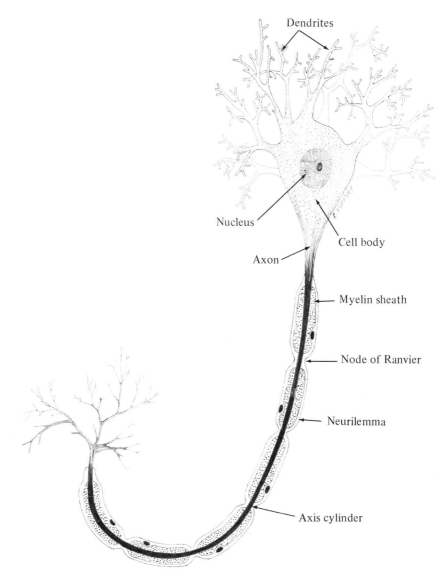

**Figure 5-2.** Anatomy of a myelinated neuron. A neuron contains a nucleus in the cell body. The cytoplasm of a neuron extends into two processes, axon and dendrite. Some neurons are enveloped by a myelin and neurilemma sheath, whereas others are not.

**AFFERENT (SENSORY) NEURONS. Afferent neurons** transmit sensory stimuli from the peripheral nervous system to the CNS. These neurons initially receive sensory stimuli by specialized sensory receptors (at distal ends of dendrites). The dendrite carries the impulse to the cell body in ganglia next to the spinal cord. The axon carries the impulse from the cell body into the CNS (either the spinal cord or the brain). These **sensory receptors** are specialized so that they are able to receive only a single type of stimulus (Figure 5-3). The receptors for pain, temperature, touch, and pressure are located in the skin and skeletal and visceral muscles. In addition, sensory receptors are located in the eyes (vision), tongue (taste), ear (hearing and equilibrium), and nose (olfactory or smell).

Sensory (afferent) neurons ultimately carry information about changes in the internal environment and external environment of the body to specific sites in the brain.

**EFFERENT (MOTOR) NEURONS. Efferent neurons** (Figure 5-3) transmit motor impulses from the

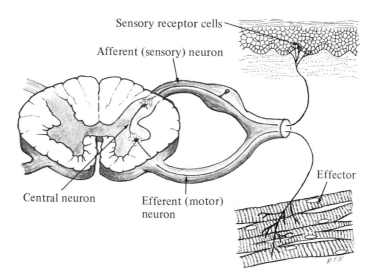

Figure 5-3. Types of neurons.

CNS to **effectors** (muscles and glands that carry out the command from the CNS). These neurons can arise in various areas of the brain and the spinal cord.

**INTERNUNCIAL (CENTRAL, ASSOCIATION, AND INTERMEDIATE) NEURONS. Internuncial neurons** primarily connect afferent to efferent neurons, but they also may connect various areas of the brain to each other. They are found only within the brain and spinal cord in the gray matter.

### Nerve Fibers, Nerves, and Tracts

A single neuron also is called a **nerve fiber** because it is long, thin, and fibrous in appearance. A **nerve** is composed of many, many bundles of nerve fibers, which may consist of thousands of nerve fibers. A peripheral nerve is composed of both afferent (sensory) fibers and efferent (motor) fibers (Figure 5–4). This means that a peripheral nerve has fibers carrying both input (sensory) information and fibers carrying output (motor or com-

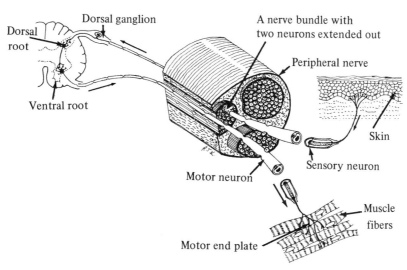

Figure 5-4. Component parts of a nerve. A peripheral nerve with three nerve bundles is shown. Each bundle is composed of many motor and sensory neurons, two of which are shown.

mand) stimuli. A **nerve tract** is bundles of nerve fibers in the CNS. All nerve tracts and fibers in the CNS are myelinated; therefore, they are white matter.

## SYNAPSE

A **synapse** is a junction between the axon end of one neuron and the dendrite or cell body of another neuron. Each neuron is a separate structure from the next neuron. In other words the cytoplasm and axis-cylinder of one neuron are not continuous with the next one. However, the axon of a neuron comes in close contact with the dendrites or cell bodies of another neuron or forms a synapse. Actually, the dendrites and axons of neurons do not come in direct contact. There is a slight gap between the dendrites and axons that is called a **synaptic cleft** (Figure 5–5). The neuron that conducts an impulse to a synapse is called a **presynaptic neuron,** and a neuron that conducts an impulse away from a synapse is a **postsynaptic neuron.** A nerve impulse

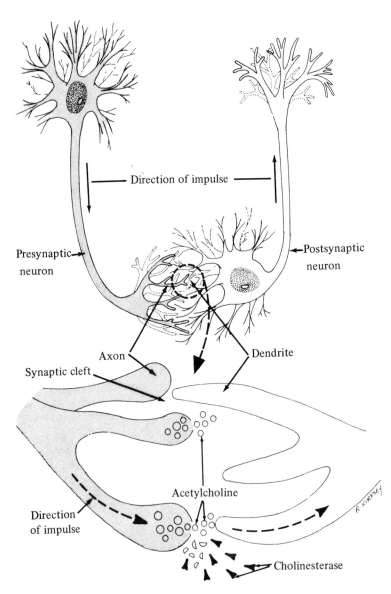

**Figure 5-5.**   A synapse between a presynaptic and postsynaptic neuron, along with a transmitter chemical (acetylcholine) and an inhibitor (cholinesterase).

must cross this synaptic cleft, and it does so by means of a chemical transmitter. This process will be discussed in detail shortly.

# 3 NERVE IMPULSE CONDUCTION

Understanding how a nerve impulse moves along a nerve fiber involves the following concepts and information:

1. Na⁺ is primarily an extracellular ion (outside neurons); K⁺ is primarily an intracellular ion (inside neurons). Cl⁻ is equally distributed between the inside and outside of neurons. Proteins inside neurons exist in an ionized state.

2. Active transport is involved with Na⁺ and K⁺.

3. Ions with like charges (+ and +; − and −) repel each other. Ions with unlike charges (+ and −) attract each other.

4. A nerve impulse is in reality a self-propagating wave of action potentials.

5. The neuron cell membrane normally is impermeable to Na⁺ ions entering and K⁺ ions leaving.

## *CELL MEMBRANE POTENTIAL*

Figure 5-6 shows that the outside of a neuron is positively charged and the inside negatively charged. This unequal distribution of + and − ions is a **polarized state.** The difference in electrical charge between the inside and outside of the membrane is about 85 millivolts and is called the **resting potential.**

**ACTIVE TRANSPORT AND MAINTENANCE OF RESTING POTENTIAL.** A resting neuron maintains a polarized state by actively transporting sodium ions and potassium ions back to their normal locations. This process is required because Na⁺ diffuse inward slowly and K⁺ outward.

## *THE NERVE IMPULSE*

The conduction of a nerve impulse involves several events, which are listed in Table 5-2 and illustrated in Figure 5-6. A neuron can be stimulated by changes in

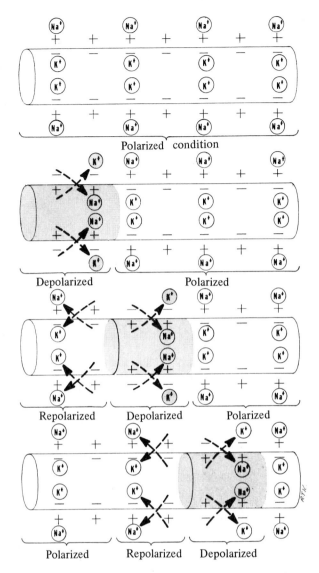

**Figure 5-6.** Nerve impulse conduction. A resting neuron is polarized. A nerve impulse is conducted along a neuron when a depolarized region is adjacent to a polarized region. A neuron must be repolarized before it can conduct another impulse.

the environment that are of **threshold strength** intensity. A threshold stimulus is one that disturbs the resting or polarized state of the neuron. Examples of stimuli that can stimulate a neuron are changes in temperature, pressure, chemical concentration, or electrical change.

## *Action Potential*

Conduction of a nerve impulse is possible once an **action potential** is initiated. An action potential is a sequence of electrical changes that occurs when a nerve

### TABLE 5–2. *Sequence of Events That Initiate a Nerve Impulse on a Neuron*

1. Establishment of resting potential or polarized state on membrane.
2. Reception of threshold strength stimulus.
3. Change in membrane permeability.
4. Sodium channels in membrane open and sodium ions rush in.
5. Potassium channels in membrane open and potassium ions rush out.
6. Membrane becomes less permeable to sodium and potassium as the channels close.
7. Depolarized state of neuron.
8. Action potential established.
9. Transmission of action potentials as a nerve impulse.
10. Repolarization and reestablishment of a resting potential by active transport.

cell membrane is exposed to a threshold strength stimulus. The following discussion explains the electrical changes of an action potential. Again, they are listed in Table 5–2 and shown in Figure 5–6.

**CHANGE IN MEMBRANE PERMEABILITY.** A threshold-strength stimulus causes a sudden change in membrane permeability. Channels for sodium ions open up and they rush inward in large numbers (Figure 5–6). Almost simultaneously, channels open up that allow potassium ions to rush out of the neuron. The channels close quickly after opening.

**DEPOLARIZATION.** The inward movement of sodium ions results in the membrane losing its electrical charge, or it is **depolarized.** The inside of the neuron in the depolarized region becomes positively charged (Figure 5–6). This sequence of changes is an **action potential,** and it stimulates an action potential in the adjacent portions of the neuron membrane. These in turn stimulate other areas or they are self-propagating. The transmission of action potentials along a neuron constitutes a nerve impulse.

**REPOLARIZATION.** Following depolarization, the cell membrane actively transports sodium ions out and potassium ions into the neuron. This event reestablishes the polarized condition or the resting potential.

## MOVEMENT OF NERVE IMPULSE ACROSS SYNAPSE

### Neurotransmitters

When a nerve impulse reaches the axon endings (Figure 5–4), a neurotransmitter substance is released; it diffuses from the axon to dendrites or the cell body of the

next neuron. In other words, the neurotransmitter substance diffuses across the synapse between neurons. It changes the membrane permeability (Figure 5–5) of the next neuron, so depolarization occurs and a new impulse is started.

Two common neurotransmitters are **acetylcholine** and **norepinephrine.** If these compounds were to remain in the synapse for any length of time, a neuron could not repolarize and receive new stimuli. **Cholinesterase** is an enzyme that breaks down acetylcholine. It acts quickly to break down acetylcholine and allow a neuron to repolarize.

The myoneural junction is a junction point at which a nerve impulse is transmitted from a motor (efferent) nerve to muscle tissue (Figure 5–7) by a neurotransmitter substance.

## RATE OF NERVE IMPULSE CONDUCTION

The myelinated nerves transmit impulses much more rapidly than do the unmyelinated nerves. Previously we said that the myelin sheath functions as an insulator. It insulates the nerve against passage of $Na^+$ and $K^+$ ions, except at the nodes of Ranvier. A nerve impulse, then, does not pass along the entire length of a myelinated nerve, but rather jumps from node of Ranvier to node of Ranvier. This process is called **saltatory conduction.** This jumping process enables a nerve impulse to pass along a myelinated neuron much faster than along an unmyelinated one. In the CNS the myelinated nerves compose white matter and conduct impulses from one point to another.

The diameter of neurons also affects the rate of impulse conduction. The larger the diameter, the faster a neuron conducts an impulse.

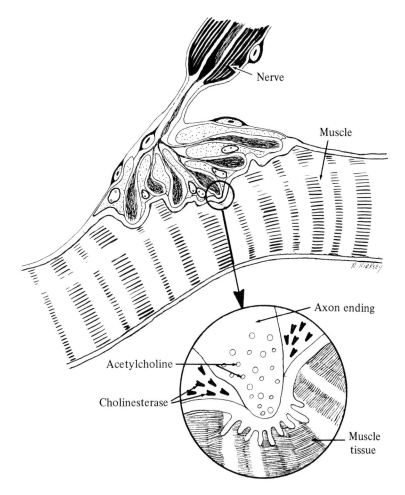

**Figure 5-7.** Myoneural junction. A nerve impulse is transmitted from neurons to muscle tissue by neurotransmitters, such as acetylcholine. Acetylcholine acts to depolarize the muscle tissue and thereby initiate a nerve impulse.

# 4  SPINAL CORD AND SPINAL NERVES

The spinal cord is like a major freeway in that afferent (sensory) nerves continue from the peripheral area into the spinal cord and up to the brain. The **efferent (motor)** nerves move down the spinal cord from the brain and exit to the various effectors.

## ANATOMY AND LOCATION OF SPINAL CORD

The spinal cord is oval shaped and is about 40 to 45 centimeters in length (Figure 5-8). The cord has two slight bulges in the cervical and lumbar regions. The anterior surface of the cord is distinguishable by a wide, deep fissure, the **anterior median fissure.** The cord extends downward from the **foramen magnum** (opening into the base of the skull) to the level of the first or second lumbar vertebra (L-1 or L-2). It is located in the spinal (vertebral) cavity but does not extend the full length of the cavity. The spinal cord coverings do continue the length of the cavity, which is to the bottom of the vertebral column (Figure 5-9).

### Meninges (Coverings) of the Spinal Cord

Three **meninges** surround the spinal cord: dura mater, arachnoid, and pia mater. These meninges continue up and surround the brain also.

**Dura mater** is the outer meninge, and it is the toughest and thickest of the three. It is composed of connec-

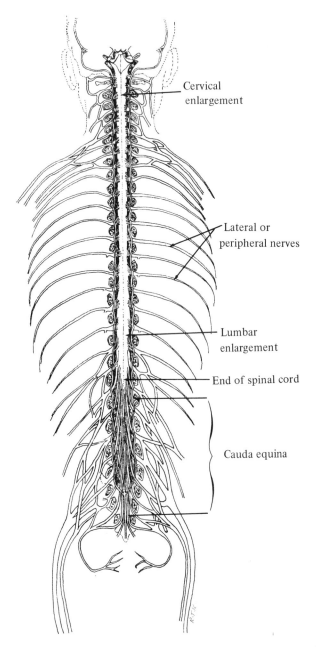

Cervical
enlargement

Lateral or
peripheral nerves

Lumbar
enlargement

End of spinal cord

Cauda equina

**Figure 5-8.** Posterior view of spinal cord. The spinal cord extends from the foramen magnum to the level of L-1 or L-2 vertebra. Nerves that descend downward from the spinal cord form the cauda equina (horse's tail). The spinal cord exhibits two enlargements, cervical and lumbar.

tive tissue and continues below the L-2 level down to the second sacral vertebra (S-2), where it ends as a sac (Figure 5-10).

Between the surface of the dura mater and the walls of the vertebral cavity is a space called **epidural space** (Figure 5-11). This space is filled with fluid, blood vessels, adipose and areolar connective tissue. Anesthetics can be injected into this space, below the level of the spinal cord, to produce **caudal anesthesia.** This type of anesthesia can be used during childbirth to reduce pain. The anesthetic acts to block transmission of sensory nerve impulses that originate in the uterus from reaching the brain. However, motor impulses to the uterus are not blocked; therefore, the woman feels no pain from the uterus but it will contract during labor.

**Arachnoid** is the second meninge. The name refers to the fact that it resembles a spider web. It is composed of connective tissue and continues to the end of the spinal cavity (Figure 5-10).

The **arachnoid** is attached loosely to the inner meninge by fibers, so that there is a space between the arachnoid and the inner meninge, pia mater. The space is referred to as the **subarachnoid space** (Figure 5-25) and is important, since cerebrospinal fluid (CSF) circulates around the brain and spinal cord through it. A spinal tap or lumbar puncture is performed by the insertion of a long needle into the subarachnoid space, between L-1 and L-5. CSF fluid is withdrawn and analyzed for diagnostic purposes.

Immediately below the spinal cord is a cavity called the **lumbar cistern,** which is located at about L-2 to L-5. CSF circulates from the skull all the way to the end of the subarachnoid space, which is this **lumbar cistern.** Actually, CSF that is withdrawn for diagnostic purposes is withdrawn from this cavity. An anesthetic can be injected into this lumbar cistern to produce **spinal anesthesia** for surgical operations in the lower abdomen, pelvis, and lower extremities.

The epidural space lies outside the lumbar cistern and continues below it.

**Pia mater** is the innermost meninge and is attached directly to the nerve tissue of the brain and spinal cord. It is composed of connective tissue, but is very delicate compared to the other two. The blood supply to the nerve tissue of the brain and spinal cord courses through the pia mater.

**Meningitis** (*mening*—membrane; *itis*—inflammation) is inflammation of the meninges, and can be caused by bacteria, viruses, and fungi. It can be present in one or all of the meninges of the brain and spinal cord. The most common form of meningitis is caused by the diplococcus *Neisseria meningitidis.* Pneumococci, streptococci, and staphylococci are other cocci that can cause meningitis. These organisms spread to the meninges from the upper respiratory tract.

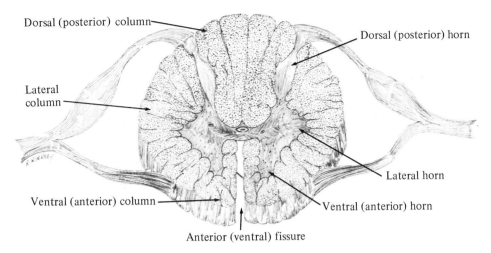

**Figure 5-9.** Internal anatomy of the spinal cord. The gray matter of the spinal cord is shaped like a flying H. Gray matter is composed of unmyelinated nerves. White matter surrounds the gray matter and it is composed of myelinated nerves.

Meningocele (*mening*—membrane; *ocele*—hernia) is a hernia of the meninges, which protrudes through an opening in the skull or spinal column.

| cervical | 8 pairs | C-1 to C-8 |
|----------|---------|------------|
| thoracic | 12 pairs | T-1 to T-12 |
| lumbar | 5 pairs | L-1 to L-5 |
| sacral | 5 pairs | |
| coccygeal | 1 pair | |

## *Internal Anatomy of the Spinal Cord*

A cross section of the spinal cord shows a gray matter area shaped like a flying H. This area is composed of gray matter (unmyelinated nerves). The gray matter is surrounded by white matter (myelinated nerves). The white and gray matter areas are composed of anterior and posterior columns and horns (Figure 5–9 and 5–10).

The white matter is composed of myelinated nerves, which conduct ascending and descending impulses. The ascending nerves carry sensory (afferent) information up to specific areas of the brain. The descending nerves carry motor (efferent) impulses down the cord to the proper level, where they exit to the effectors.

## THE SPINAL NERVES

### *Designations of Spinal Nerves*

There are 31 pairs of spinal nerves (Figure 5–10) attached to the spinal cord. They are numbered according to the spinal cord segment from which they originate. The segments and the number of nerves in each are:

## *Roots of Spinal Nerves*

Each spinal nerve is formed by two roots, the dorsal (posterior) and the ventral (anterior) (Figure 5–10).

The **dorsal (posterior) root** contains afferent (sensory) nerves only; therefore, it is called the **sensory root.** An enlarged area of the root is called the dorsal root ganglion. It contains the cell bodies of afferent neurons (remember that the cell bodies of neurons have to be in protected positions).

The **ventral (anterior) root** contains efferent (motor) nerves only; therefore, it is called the **motor root.**

Notice that in Figure 5–11 the two roots join together to finally form a spinal nerve. All this area is protected by the bony vertebrae. A short distance after the two roots join, the spinal nerve gives off into two branches, anterior (ventral) ramus and posterior (dorsal) ramus or anterior and posterior branches (Figure 5–11). The posterior rami pass posteriorly or dorsally and consist of sensory and motor fibers that supply the skin and back muscles. The anterior rami are larger, and they contain motor and sensory fibers that supply the extremities and the anterior and lateral tissues of the trunk. The anterior (ventral) rami that come off the cer-

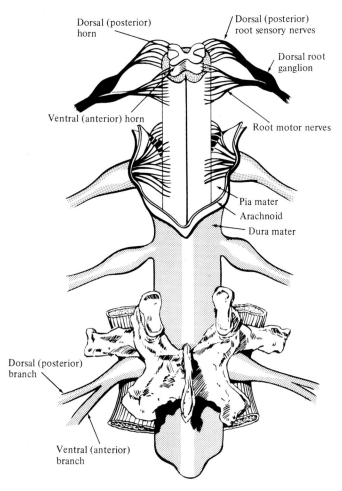

Dorsal (posterior) horn

Dorsal (posterior) root sensory nerves

Dorsal root ganglion

Ventral (anterior) horn

Root motor nerves

Pia mater
Arachnoid
Dura mater

Dorsal (posterior) branch

Ventral (anterior) branch

**Figure 5-10.** Spinal nerves and anatomy of spinal cord. Each spinal nerve is composed of dorsal and ventral roots. The dorsal root carries sensory impulses into the dorsal column of gray matter. The ventral root carries motor impulses away from the ventral column of gray matter. The three meninges are also shown.

vical, lumbar, and sacral regions first combine to form complicated networks of nerves called **plexuses.**

## SPINAL PLEXUSES

There are four major regions along the spinal cord where the anterior (ventral) rami form a complicated network of nerves called plexuses. These plexuses are called cervical, brachial (cervical and thoracic rami), lumbar, and sacral (Figures 5-12 and 5-13).* Nerves leave each of these plexuses and supply various regions.

* Some sources combine lumbar and sacral together as one plexus called the lumbosacral plexus.

The names of the nerves depend upon the regions and structures they supply. Table 5-3 presents a summary of all four plexuses.

### Cervical Plexus

The anterior rami of the first four cervical nerves, C-1 to C-4, combine to form the cervical plexus (Figure 5-12). The nerves that leave the plexus are the lesser occipital, the great auricular, the transverse, the supraclavicular, and the phrenic. All these nerves, except the phrenic, supply the muscles and tissues of the back of the skull and neck. The phrenic is the most vital nerve of the five since it supplies motor fibers to the muscular diaphragm. This muscle is the primary respiratory muscle. Severing or crushing of the spinal cord above C-4 will result in paralysis of the diaphragm since the phrenic nerve is also cut. This will result in death since the person will not be able to breathe.

### Brachial Plexus

The anterior rami of C-5 through C-8 and T-1 form the brachial plexus (Figures 5-12 and 5-13). As the name indicates, the nerves supply muscles in the brachial region as well as the entire upper extremity, neck, and shoulder. The major nerves that emerge from the plexus and areas they supply are as follows:

**RADIAL.** This is the largest branch, and it supplies motor and sensory fibers to the upper arm, lower arm (forearm), and hand (Figure 5-13).

**ULNAR.** The **ulnar** supplies motor fibers to the flexor muscles in the lower arm (forearm) and hand that are located anterior and medial.

**MEDIAN.** The **median** supplies motor fibers to the flexor muscles of the lower arm (forearm) and hand that are located anteriorly and laterally.

Injuries to the brachial plexus are common. People that improperly use crutches can cause a temporary paralysis of the radial nerve. Also injections given slightly inferior to the deltoid muscle can cause temporary paralysis of the radial nerve. Injury to the nerve is characterized by inability to extend the hand at the wrist.

### Lumbar Plexus

Anterior rami of the L-1 through L-4 nerves combine to form the lumbar plexus (Figure 5-12). Nerves from this plexus supply motor and sensory fibers to the muscles

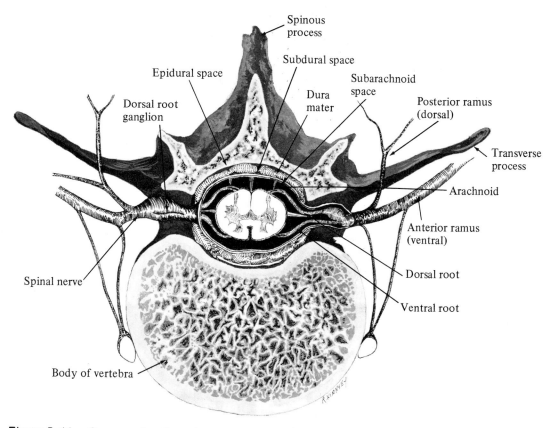

**Figure 5-11.** Cross section through spinal vertebra and spinal cord showing protection of spinal nerves and spinal cord by vertebra.

and skin of lower body wall, gluteal region, and anterio-medial region of the thigh. The femoral and obturator nerves are the main ones that emerge from this plexus. The femoral nerve carries motor impulses to the iliop-

soas muscle, which flexes the thigh. It also innervates the quadriceps femoris muscle, which extends the tibia or lower leg. The obturator nerve carries motor impulses to the adductor muscles of the thigh (adductor

TABLE 5-3.  *Summary of Spinal Plexuses*

| Plexus | Nerves Composing Plexus | Nerves Exiting Plexus | Areas Supplied |
|---|---|---|---|
| 1. Cervical | C-1 to C-4 | Occipital, great auricular, transverse supraclavicular, and phrenic (most vital) | Tissues at back of skull and neck; diaphragm |
| 2. Brachial | C-5 to C-8 and T-1 | Radial, ulnar, and median | Brachial region; upper extremity; neck and shoulder |
| 3. Lumbar | L-1 through L-4 | Femoral; obturator | Lower body wall, gluteal region, and anteriomedial region of thigh |
| 4. Sacral | L-4 and L-5 combine with S-1 to S-4 | Sciatic | Posterior leg muscles |

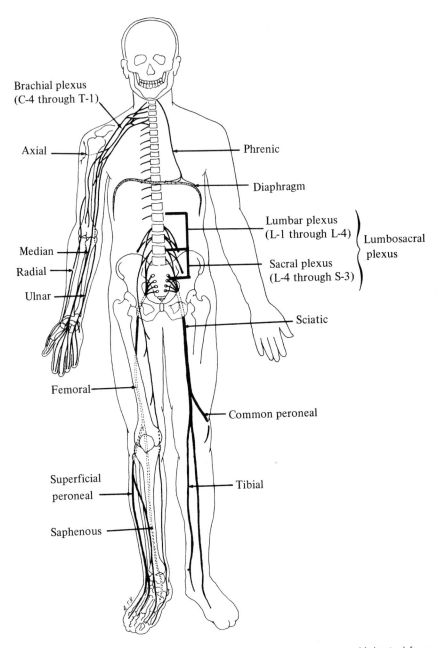

**Figure 5-12.** Anterior view of peripheral nerves and plexuses. [Adapted from Ellen E. Chaffee and Esther M. Greisheimer, *Basic Physiology and Anatomy*, 3rd edition (Philadelphia: J. B. Lippincott, 1974)]

brevis, longus, and magnus), which results in adduction of the thighs as when grasping a saddle while riding a horse.

Fractures of the hipbone (pelvis) and thigh (femur) can result in an inability to extend the lower leg and flex the thigh.

### Sacral Plexus

Anterior rami of L-4 and L-5 combine with rami from S-1 through S-4 to form the sacral plexus. The major nerve coming from this plexus is the sciatic nerve, which is the largest and longest nerve in the body. The

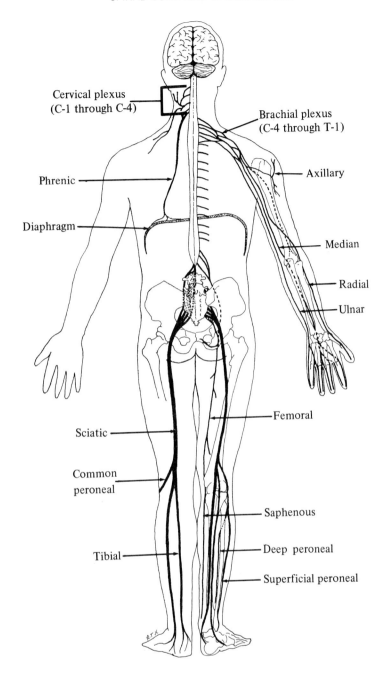

**Figure 5-13.** Posterior view of peripheral nerves and cervical plexus. [Adapted from Ellen E. Chaffee and Esther M. Greisheimer, *Basic Physiology and Anatomy,* 3rd edition (Philadelphia: J. B. Lippincott, 1974)]

sciatic nerve courses through the thigh, giving off branches to the posterior muscles (Figure 5-13), and continues into the lower leg, where it divides into the tibial and common peroneal nerves.

The gluteus maximus muscle covers the origin of the sciatic nerve. This muscle is a common site for intramuscular injections and if the needle is not inserted properly, the sciatic nerve can be injured. This injury results in an inability to contract various muscles of the thigh and lower leg.

## SPINAL CORD REFLEXES

**A reflex is an automatic act that does not require any conscious help on our part.** Reflexes are described as the functional units of the nervous system since reflexes constitute a large part of the nervous system's activity. In humans some complicated reflexes involve the brain in addition to the spinal cord.

Reflexes that involve synapses in the spinal cord are called spinal reflexes. There are three types of spinal reflexes: stretch, flexor, and cross-extensor. Figures 5–14, 5–15, and 5–16 show the component parts of these reflexes.

### Stretch (Extensor) Reflexes

This reflex involves two neurons (Figure 5–14). The simple knee jerk is initiated when the patellar tendon, slightly inferior to the patella, is tapped lightly. Nerve impulses are carried by afferent dendrites to the dorsal root ganglion and then by axons through the dorsal horns of gray matter. The impulse does not travel through a central neuron, but rather synapses with an efferent neuron in the ventral horn of gray matter. The efferent neuron carries the impulse through the ventral spinal root to the quadriceps femoris, which contracts and causes extension of the lower leg.

These reflexes are initiated when stretch receptor cells are stimulated, and they result in contraction of extensor muscles. The importance of stretch reflexes is that contraction of extensor muscles (quadriceps

femoris and gluteus maximus) enables one to remain in an upright position.

### Flexor Reflexes

This reflex involves three neurons (Figure 5–15). A flexor reflex is initiated whenever pain receptor cells in

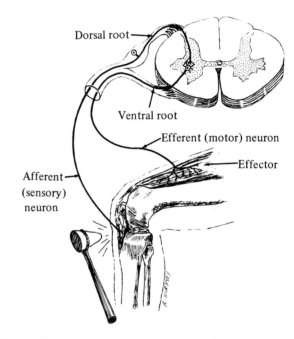

**Figure 5–14.** Simple reflex arc. A simple reflex involves a synapse between an afferent and an efferent neuron. A reflex is an involuntary response to a stimulus.

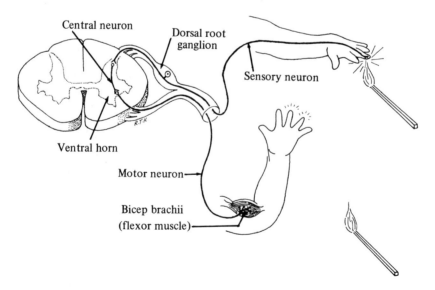

**Figure 5–15.** Flexor reflex or three-neuron reflex.

the extremities are stimulated. The sensory neurons synapse with inter neurons, and then efferent neurons carry motor impulses to flexor muscles and inhibitory impulses to antagonistic muscles. Inhibition of the antagonistic muscles allows a stronger flexor contraction. Flexor reflexes are protective in that they allow a person to withdraw an extremity from a painful stimulus (Figure 5-15).

### Cross-Extensor Reflexes

This reflex occurs simultaneously with a flexor reflex. At the same time that a limb is flexing away from a stimulus, the other limb is extending (Figure 5-16). This process involves an inter neuron carrying the sensory impulse across the cord to an efferent neuron, which stimulates contraction of an extensor muscle on the opposite side of the body. The purpose of this extensor contraction is that it supports and pushes the body away from the painful stimulus. Figure 5-16 shows the importance of this reflex. The extension of muscles in the leg, opposite to the one that flexed, allows the person to support his weight as the other leg flexes away from the painful stimulus.

## WHITE MATTER TRACTS IN THE SPINAL CORD

The white matter (myelinated neurons) in the spinal cord conducts impulses up and down the spinal cord. The neurons are grouped together into nerve tracts. Sensory impulses are carried by ascending tracts up to the brain, and motor impulses are carried by descending tracts down to certain levels of the spinal cord.

### Ascending Tracts

The ascending tracts are mainly three (Figure 5-17): the **dorsal (posterior) columns** (conscious muscle sense, discriminate touch and pressure), the **ventral (anterior) spinothalamic tract** (light touch), and the **lateral spinothalamic tracts** (pain and temperature).

**DORSAL (POSTERIOR) COLUMNS.** Sensory neurons concerned with conscious muscle movement and precise touch ascend to the cerebral cortex in the fasciculus gracilis tract (Figure 5-17).

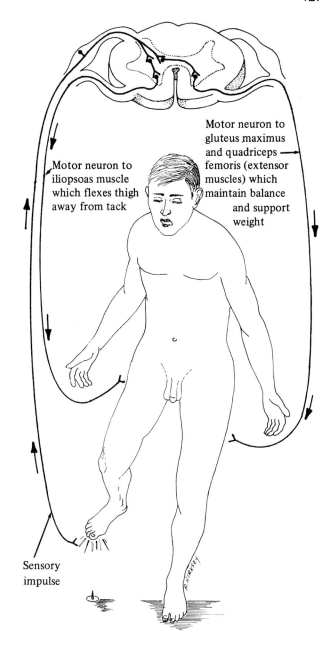

Figure 5-16. Nerve pathway for flexor–cross extensor reflex.

**VENTRAL (ANTERIOR) SPINOTHALAMIC TRACT.** Any sensory impulses that involve light touch are carried by sensory neurons up the spinal cord, in the **ventral (anterior) spinothalamic tract** (Figure 5-17), to the cerebral cortex.

**LATERAL SPINOTHALAMIC TRACT.** Pain and temperature stimuli ascend the cord in this tract (Figure 5-17) to the parietal lobe.

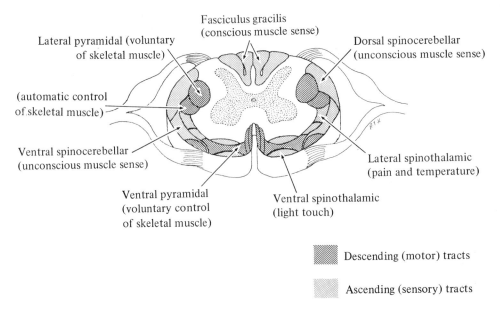

**Figure 5-17.**  Main nerve tracts that ascend and descend through the spinal cord. The primary type of nerve impulses carried by each tract is given.

---

**Injuries to the Ascending Tracts.**   Fractures of the vertebral column, diseases of the spinal cord, and tumors that damage the ascending tracts result in loss of sensations related to touch, pressure, pain, temperature, and muscle sensations. As a result, the person lacks coordinated muscle movement, muscle tone, and touch discrimination.

---

### Descending Tracts

The descending tracts carry impulses from the brain down the spinal cord to certain levels where they then leave and go to effectors. There are two groups of descending tracts: pyramidal and extrapyramidal (Figure 5–17).

**PYRAMIDAL OR CORTICOSPINAL TRACTS.** The neurons in this tract originate in the motor lobe along the precentral gyrus. The term pyramid is derived from the way in which the neurons are arranged. The motor neurons descend through the internal capsule to the medulla, where 80 to 90 percent **decussate** (cross over to the opposite side of the cord). The neurons that cross continue down the cord in the lateral pyramidal (crossed pyramidal) tract (Figure 5–17). The neurons that do not cross over in the medulla continue down the

cord in the uncrossed pyramidal (anterior corticospinal) tract. The pyramidal tract carries impulses that are concerned with voluntary movements of muscles in the hands and fingers. These impulses allow one to accomplish skilled movements such as playing a guitar.

**EXTRAPYRAMIDAL TRACTS.** The descending motor neurons in this tract do not descend directly down the cord; but, rather, they interconnect with regions of the brain below the cortex prior to descending through white matter of the cord (Figure 5–17). For example, motor neurons from the precentral cortex may interconnect with the thalamus and hypothalamus prior to descending through the cord. The neurons in this tract carry impulses that affect postural adjustments and maintenance of muscle tone.

**INJURIES TO DESCENDING TRACTS.** Two motor neurons are involved in the movement of motor impulses from the brain to an effector (Figure 5–25). The first neuron is called an upper motor neuron and carries the impulse from the motor cortex down the cord to a second motor neuron. The second motor neuron is also called a lower motor neuron. Injuries to upper motor neurons result in spastic skeletal muscle contractions. The muscles still are able to contract since some motor impulses are carried by the lower motor neurons to the muscles. Injuries to the lower motor neurons prevent impulses from reaching the muscles; the muscles are paralyzed and gradually they atrophy.

**Poliomyelitis** is a viral disease that usually spreads from the nose and throat to the ventral roots of the spinal nerves. It tends to destroy the cell bodies of the motor neurons. A person cannot conduct motor impulses out to the effectors; therefore, the individual is paralyzed. Afferent sensory neurons are not affected.

# 5   THE BRAIN

The brain is the final destination of most afferent (sensory) impulses. The impulses go to specific sensory areas where they are registered. Efferent (motor) impulses originate in the brain at various specific points before they are carried to the effectors. The brain (Figures 5–18 and 5–19) is a large organ weighing about 2 to 3 pounds. It is quite complex and has three primary subdivisions: forebrain, midbrain, and hindbrain. We will start our discussions with the base of the brain (hindbrain), which is where afferent impulses first enter the brain from the spinal cord.

## HINDBRAIN

The hindbrain has three parts: medulla oblongata, pons, and cerebellum.

### Medulla Oblongata

The **medulla** is an enlarged bulb-shaped area. It is the first part of the brain after the spinal cord goes through the large skull opening called foramen magnum. The medulla is composed mainly of white matter, but there are round nuclei of gray matter located deep within it. These nuclei are called the **vital reflex centers.** These centers coordinate vital reflex activities of the body. The vital reflex centers located in the medulla and their functions are discussed next.

**CARDIAC CENTER.**  This center controls the rate of heart contractions. In stress situations the heart rate needs to be speeded up. Following the stress, the rate is slowed to its normal pace. Sensory nerves transmit impulses about changes in heart rate to the cardiac center. The information is integrated by the center and a motor

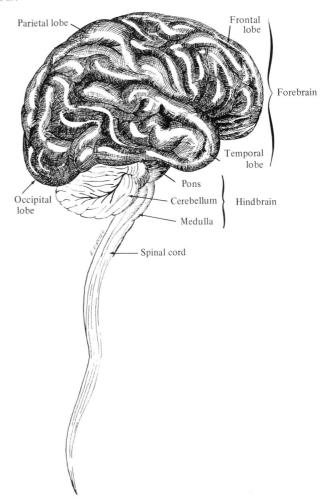

Figure 5-18.   Lateral view of the brain. The brain is a large organ that is subdivided into the forebrain, midbrain, and hindbrain. The midbrain is not shown.

impulse is transmitted back to the heart, which regulates its rate.

**VASOMOTOR CENTER.**  Sensory impulses concerning blood pressure are transmitted to the vasomotor center. If the pressure is too high, vasodilation impulses are transmitted to blood vessels, resulting in a decrease in blood pressure. If pressure is too low, vasoconstriction impulses are sent to blood vessels, resulting in an increase in blood pressure.

**RESPIRATORY CENTER.**  This center increases or decreases the respiratory rate. As an example, if the oxygen ($O_2$) level of the blood is low, the center receives this information via a sensory impulse. A compensatory motor impulse is transmitted to the respiratory muscles, thereby increasing the rate of respiration and oxygen consumption.

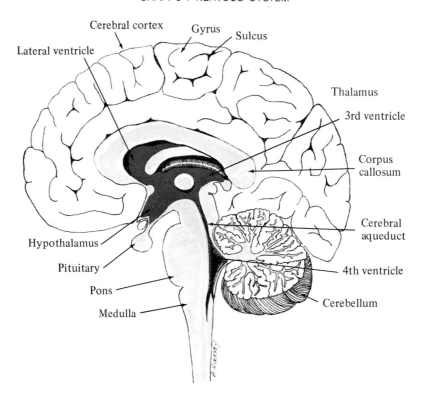

**Figure 5-19.**   Sagittal view of brain.

## Pons (Bridge)

The **pons** essentially is a link or conduction pathway between the hindbrain and midbrain. It is made up of both longitudinal and transverse white fibers. The transverse fibers conduct impulses between the right and left halves of the cerebellum. Also, the pons contains a respiratory nucleus, the **pneumotaxic center.** This respiratory center, and the one in the medulla, work together to regulate respiratory rate. Cranial nerves 5, 6, 7, and 8 have nuclei here.

## Cerebellum (Little Brain)

The **cerebellum** is the second largest part of the brain. It is dorsal to the pons and medulla. It is composed of two hemispheres and a central connecting area. The outer surface is gray matter and is called the **cerebellar cortex.** The cerebellum carries out the following functions:

**COORDINATION OF VOLUNTARY MUSCLE MOVEMENT.** All voluntary muscle movement impulses occur in the **forebrain (cerebrum).** As the impulses course downward, they are modified by impulses from the cerebellum. The cerebellum refines or makes muscle movements smoother and more coordinated. Without modification and refinement from the cerebellum, skeletal muscle movement tends to be jerky and uncoordinated.

**MAINTENANCE OF BALANCE, EQUILIBRIUM, AND ORIENTATION.** The semicircular canals of the inner ear contain equilibrium and orientation sensory cells. Sensory impulses concerning equilibrium and orientation enter the cerebellum where they are integrated. The cerebellum sends out motor (efferent) impulses to the proper skeletal muscles to restore or maintain equilibrium.

**MAINTENANCE OF MUSCLE TONE AND POSTURE.** Various muscles are involved in maintaining posture, and the cerebellum helps maintain these. Muscle tone involves contraction of a certain number of muscle fibers within a muscle. It enables muscles to respond quickly to stimuli.

Diseases, injuries, and other types of damage to the cerebellum usually result in muscle incoordination, lack of muscle tone, tremors, and disturbances of gait and equilibrium.

## MIDBRAIN

The **midbrain** is a small, short segment that lies superior to the pons and inferior to the cerebrum (forebrain). It connects the hindbrain to the forebrain. A canal called the **cerebral aqueduct** passes lengthwise through it and connects the third ventricle (fluid-filled cavity) of the forebrain to the fourth ventricle. The dorsal portion of the midbrain contains four small rounded bodies, **corpora quadrigemina** (*corpora*—bodies; *quadri*—four; *gemina*—round). These four rounded bodies are involved with visual reflexes, in which two of the bodies regulate movement of the eyes in accordance with the position of the head, and auditory reflexes, in which two of the bodies regulate the movement of the head to hear sounds that originate to the side of a person. Two bundles of white nerve fibers compose the ventral portion of the midbrain. These bundles are called **cerebral peduncles,** and they conduct sensory and motor impulses between the forebrain and the hindbrain.

In summary, the midbrain is a major conduction pathway for both sensory and motor impulses, through the cerebral peduncles, between the forebrain and hindbrain. Also, it coordinates visual and auditory reflexes.

## FOREBRAIN

The upper part of the brain is divided into two main parts, the **diencephalon** and the **telencephalon** (cerebral hemispheres).

### Diencephalon

The diencephalon region is superior to the midbrain and is covered completely by the cerebral hemispheres. It is composed of two parts, the **thalamus,** in the dorsal region, and the **hypothalamus,** in the ventral region.

**HYPOTHALAMUS.** The **hypothalamus,** as the name indicates, is inferior to the thalamus. It makes up the floor and lateral walls of the third ventricle. Reflex centers located deep within the hypothalamus control the activities of the visceral organs in the thoracic and abdominopelvic cavities. Some of these reflexes are vital and are the same as the ones that the medulla regulates. The hypothalamus is similar to a higher executive, compared to the medulla. This means that some sensory stimuli that come to the medulla oblongata re-

quire coordination from the next highest area of the brain, the hypothalamus (see Figure 5–19). The functions of the hypothalamus are as follows:

1. *Cardiac center.* The hypothalamus and the medulla interact to speed or slow the rate of heart contractions. The nerves that carry impulses to the heart from these areas will be discussed in more detail later.

2. *Vasomotor center.* The vasodilation and vasoconstriction of the blood vessels can be controlled by the hypothalamus as well as the medulla. Controlling the size of the blood vessels actually helps to regulate the body temperature. If the vessels dilate, more heat is given off; if they constrict, less heat is given off. These activities will be discussed in more detail.

3. *Respiratory center.* Reflex changes in the rate and depth of respiration are coordinated by the hypothalamus as well as the medulla.

4. *Regulation of water balance.* A hormone called ADH (antidiuretic hormone) is produced by the hypothalamus and stored in the pituitary gland. ADH is carried by the blood from the pituitary to the kidneys. It regulates the amount of water the body retains or excretes. A deficiency of ADH results in a person passing large quantities of urine; this is called **diabetes insipidus.**

5. *Regulation of appetite control.* Experiments indicate that the hypothalamus is able to control appetite and, therefore, the amount of food intake. People with tumors in this area eat tremendous amounts of food and gain large amounts of weight.

**THALAMUS.** The thalamus is composed of right and left parts, which are elongated masses of gray matter. They are located superior to the hypothalamus and make up the lateral walls of the third ventricle. The thalamus has extensive connections with the cerebral cortex, hypothalamus, and medulla. The functions of the thalamus (Figure 5–19) are as follows:

1. *Crude recognition of sensory stimuli.* Myelinated nerves bring sensory stimuli into the thalamus where they synapse with other neurons in gray matter. The thalamus is able to distinguish crudely between different sensory stimuli. For example, it can distinguish between pain and temperature impulses.

2. *Relay of sensory impulses to cerebral cortex.* The sensory neurons from the lower parts of the body synapse with appropriate sensory neurons that carry impulses to the proper areas of the cerebral cortex.

In other words, pain and temperature impulses that enter simultaneously are distinguished from each other and are relayed to the proper areas of the cerebral cortex.

## The Reticular Activating System

The reticular system is composed of many nuclei of gray matter with interconnecting white fibers (Figure 5-20). The system extends from the medulla up through the center of the brain stem, through the midbrain, and into the hypothalamus. It receives branches from sensory neurons as they course upward through this region. The reticular system gives off many branches into the cerebral cortex, as well as to lower areas of the brain.

The name **reticular activating system** is appropriate since the system activates all the regions of the brain for incoming sensory impulses. As the sensory impulses course upward, the reticular system is stimulated. Likewise, the reticular system stimulates the upper areas of the brain so that they are ready to receive the sensory impulses. Actually, the brain is alerted and stimulated into consciousness. A person is conscious only when the reticular activating system is functioning.

Unconsciousness results whenever conduction by the reticular activating system is blocked. This can be done voluntarily with general anesthetics and hypnotic drugs. These compounds produce a state of uncon-sciousness, which is desirable for operations as well as other situations. Also, tumors and hemorrhages in this area can result in unconsciousness. Severe damage to this system can result in coma from which the victim cannot regain consciousness. Amphetamines, epinephrine, and other compounds stimulate the reticular activating system and cause the brain to be hyperalert.

## Telencephalon

The **telencephalon** is composed entirely of two cerebral hemispheres. The right and left hemispheres are identical to each other in size and shape. The cerebral hemispheres are the final destination for most afferent (sensory) impulses and the origin for most efferent (motor) impulses (Figure 5-19).

The **cerebral cortex** is the site of intelligence, memory, personality, and character. This is the largest area of the human brain, which would lead one to think that humans have a great potential for intelligence, memory, and personality. There are other animals on earth that have brains as large as humans; however, they are not as intelligent because their cerebral cortex is not as large and as well developed as humans.

The cerebral hemispheres are connected near their inferior surface. Each hemisphere is divided into four regions called **lobes (frontal, parietal, occipital and temporal)** (Figure 5-21). Each cerebral hemisphere is

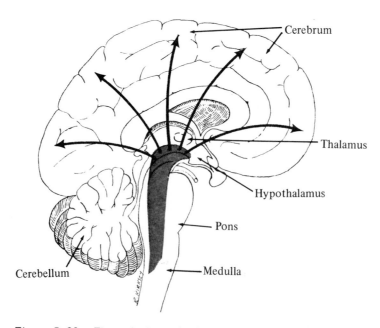

**Figure 5-20.**   The reticular activating system is shown sending impulses to the various areas of the brain.

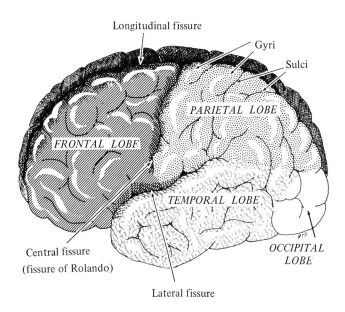

Longitudinal fissure

Gyri

Sulci

*PARIETAL LOBE*

*FRONTAL LOBE*

*TEMPORAL LOBE*

*OCCIPITAL LOBE*

Central fissure
(fissure of Rolando)

Lateral fissure

**Figure 5–21.** Lateral view of cerebral hemispheres. Each hemisphere is subdivided into four lobes by fissures. The surface is characterized by convolutions or gyri and grooves or sulci.

subdivided into (1) cerebral cortex, (2) white matter, (3) lobes of cerebral cortex, and (4) basal ganglia.

**CEREBRAL CORTEX.** Cortex always refers to the outer region of whatever structure one is studying. The cerebral cortex is composed of gray matter (unmyelinated nerves and cell bodies). This is the area in which sensory impulses are finally received, perceived, and integrated. Motor impulses also originate here. The amount of gray matter is somewhat indicative of potential intelligence. The surface is arranged in folds called **gyri (convolutions)**, which are separated from each other by grooves called **sulci** (Figure 5–21). **Fissures** are deep grooves that separate the various areas of the brain. Three fissures are important:

- *Longitudinal fissure.* The cerebral hemispheres are separated from each other by this fissue. The fissure extends down to the **corpus callosum**, which is a band of white fibers that connects the two hemispheres.
- *Central fissure.* The **central fissure (fissure of Rolando)** extends laterally from the longitudinal fissure down the side of the brain, to the lateral fissure. It separates the frontal lobe from the parietal lobe.
- *Lateral fissure.* The **lateral fissure (fissure of Sylvius)** extends along the lateral surface of the brain and

separates the temporal lobe from the parietal and frontal lobes.

**WHITE MATTER.** Below the cerebral cortex is **white matter**. The white matter is organized into three tracts that transmit impulses to various areas of the brain (Figure 5–22). These three tracts are association fibers, projection fibers, and commissural fibers.

- *Association fibers.* These fibers transmit impulses from one part of the cerebral cortex to another (Figure 5–22). However, they do not transmit impulses from one hemisphere to the other.
- *Projection Fibers.* **Projection fibers** transmit impulses between the different levels of the central nervous system (CNS) (Figure 5–22). For example, they transmit impulses back and forth between the cerebral cortex, midbrain, and hindbrain. The **internal capsule** is a region through which all the projection fibers pass as they course between the cerebral cortex and the hindbrain.
- *Commissural fibers.* The two hemispheres transmit impulses back and forth between themselves. The majority of these fibers pass through the corpus callosum (Figure 5–22).

Each hemisphere is divided into lobes that have specific functions; however, each is linked to the others and to lower areas of the brain by the white matter tracts. These tracts allow information to be shared between the hemispheres and areas of the brain. This means that each sensory impulse is transmitted among the different brain areas and that several areas of the cortex are involved in the final integration and coordination of the sensory impulse.

**LOBES OF THE CEREBRAL CORTEX.** The three fissures separate the cerebral hemispheres into lobes that have specific functions. These lobes are frontal, parietal, temporal, and occipital.

- *Frontal lobe.* The central fissure separates the frontal and parietal lobes (Figure 5–23). All the cortex anterior to the central fissure and dorsal to the lateral fissure makes up the **frontal lobe**. This area could be called the **motor cortex**, since voluntary movement impulses originate here. The frontal lobe of each cerebral hemisphere is independent of the other.

  The frontal lobe receives sensory impulses after they have been to the other lobes and sends out motor impulses to the voluntary effectors of the body.

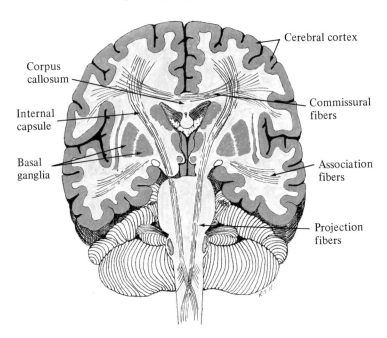

**Figure 5-22.** The cerebral cortex is composed by gray matter. White matter, below the cerebral cortex, is organized into three tracts: association, projection, and commissural fibers.

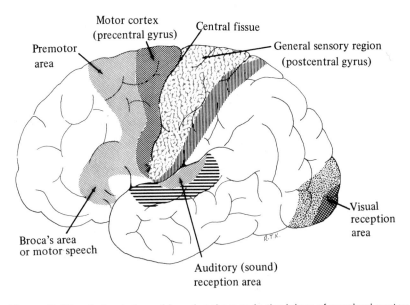

**Figure 5-23.** Lateral view of functional areas in the lobes of cerebral cortex.

One would assume that the right frontal lobe controls movements of the right side of the body, and the left controls the left side of the body, but that is not true. The left frontal lobe controls activities of voluntary muscles on the right side of the body, and the right frontal lobe controls voluntary activities on the left side of the body. This results from the fact that most sensory (afferent) impulses cross the cord, prior to being registered in the cerebral cortex. Sensory impulses that originate on the left side of the body are registered in the right cerebral cortex, and vice versa. The efferent (motor) impulses that are sent out as a response to a stimulus that originates on the left side of the body originate in the right cerebral cortex and then **decussate** (cross over) in the medulla to the left side.

- *Parietal lobe.* The **parietal lobe** extends posteriorly from the central fissure to the **occipital lobe** (Figure 5–23). This is the cutaneous lobe in that touch, pain, temperature, and pressure impulses are received from the skin. Sensory impulses from specific areas of the skin are received at specific points in the parietal lobe (postcentral gyrus) along the central fissure.

- *Temporal lobe.* The **temporal lobe** is inferior to the lateral fissure and extends posteriorly to the occipital lobe (Figure 5–23). This lobe receives auditory (sound) impulses and olfactory (smell) impulses.

- *Occipital lobe.* The **occipital lobe** is the most posterior lobe (Figure 5–23), and it receives visual impulses from the eyes.

Each of the lobes has its own memory storage area or **association area**. These areas store information and give the brain a memory capacity. The brain is able to relate current sensory impulses with those received before. These different association areas transmit impulses between themselves by means of association fibers. This enables the different lobes to associate their information before a motor impulse is initiated.

Brain damage or diseases to the cerebral hemispheres have different effects, depending on the lobe and area damaged. For example, if a person suffers a stroke and is paralyzed, the frontal (motor) lobe is affected. If a car accident damages a person's occipital lobe, the ability to see is affected.

**BASAL GANGLIA.** The basal ganglia are four round masses (nuclei) of gray matter located deep inside the cerebrum. These nuclei help the motor lobe bring about orderly, smooth, and purposeful muscle contractions.

Table 5–4 presents a summary of the subdivisions, parts, and functions of the brain.

### TABLE 5–4.   *Brain Parts and Functions*

| Subdivision | Part | Function |
| --- | --- | --- |
| Hindbrain | Medulla oblongata | Controls heart rate, respiratory rate, and diameter of blood vessels |
|  | Pons | Conducts impulses between hindbrain and midbrain; helps control respiratory rate |
|  | Cerebellum | Coordination of muscle movement; maintenance of equilibrium and orientation; maintenance of muscle tone |
| Midbrain | Corpora quadrigemina | Visual and auditory reflexes; conduction pathway between forebrain and hindbrain |
| Forebrain | Hypothalamus | Controls heart rate, respiratory rate; regulates water balance and appetite; controls secretions and contractions of digestive organs |
|  | Thalamus | Crude recognition of sensory stimuli; relay of sensory stimuli; relay of sensory impulses to cerebral cortex |
|  | Cerebral hemispheres:<br>1. Cerebral cortex | 1. Receives sensory impulses; originates voluntary muscle impulses |
|  | 2. White matter | 2. Transmits impulses within hemispheres and between them |
|  | 3. Lobes of cerebral cortex<br>  a. Frontal<br>  b. Parietal<br>  c. Temporal<br>  d. Occipital | a. Originates voluntary motor movements<br>b. Receives cutaneous sensory impulses<br>c. Receives auditory and olfactory impulses<br>d. Receives visual impulses |

## PATHWAYS FOR SENSORY AND MOTOR IMPULSES

In this area we will discuss the total pathway that sensory and motor impulses follow as they ascend to and descend from the brain. Concerning the pathway of sensory impulses that originate below the brain, sensory impulses travel over three neurons, through the ascending tract of the spinal cord, to reach the brain. These neurons will be designated as sensory neurons 1, 2, and 3.

Sensory neuron 1 (Figure 5–24) conducts impulses from the receptor cell through the **dorsal (afferent or sensory)** spinal root into the gray matter of the spinal cord. It synapses with sensory neuron 2 in the gray matter.

Sensory neuron 2 (Figure 5–24) crosses to the other side of the cord into white matter and continues upward to the thalamus. In the thalamus it synapses with sensory neuron 3.

The thalamus has crude recognition ability. It can detect the type of sensation and whether it is a pleasant or an undesirable sensation. After this recognition has occurred, the second neuron synapses with the proper third sensory neuron (Figure 5–24). The third sensory neuron travels through **projection fibers (internal capsule)** to the proper area of the cerebral cortex.

General sensory impulses finally synapse in the **cerebral cortex (gray matter)** of the **parietal lobe.** Projection, association, and commissural fibers now carry the impulse to various areas of the two cerebral hemispheres and to lower levels of the brain. The current sensory impulse will be integrated in the association areas with previously received impulses. The sensory impulse ultimately will go to the **frontal lobe (motor lobe).**

Voluntary motor impulses originate in the frontal lobe and are transmitted by a total of two motor neurons, through pyramidal tracts, to the skeletal muscles (effectors) (Figure 5–25). The impulse crosses to the opposite side of the brain from which it originates.

The transmission of a voluntary motor impulse originates with motor neuron 1 on one side of the brain descending on the same side through the internal capsule and into the hindbrain. As the motor impulse passes the cerebellum, it is modified into a smoother, more coordinated impulse. In the medulla, motor neuron 1 crosses to the other side of the brain. It then traverses downward through the spinal cord until it reaches a certain level of the cord where it synapses in gray matter with motor neuron 2. The second motor neuron leaves the cord through the **ventral root (motor or efferent root)** and transmits the motor impulses to the skeletal muscles that carry out the impulse.

## SHORT- AND LONG–TERM MEMORY

One outstanding feature of the human cerebral cortex is the ability to store and recall information. The storage and recall of information is called **memory** and is the basis of learning and intelligence. Previously we said that there were association areas for each of the sensory input regions in the cerebral cortex. As a person receives current sensory stimuli, they will be associated with stored material in the memory banks.

There are two types of memory: long term and short term. **Short-term** memory enables a person to store information for a few minutes to a few hours. For example, at a party where you are introduced to several new people, you probably will be able to remember their names during the party; however, several days later you probably will not be able to recall their names. The names of these people could be converted to **long-term** memory if you had repeated their names to yourself many times. To convert current information to long-term memory requires repetition or rehearsal of the information. Once a person has been able to convert information to long-term memory, the information has been learned. He should be able to recall the information from the memory association banks when called upon to do so.

Recent research indicates that long-term memory involves production of RNA and subsequent synthesis of proteins in the cerebral cortex. When a specific group of neurons in regions of the brain is stimulated over and over by the same information or stimuli, changes occur with the production of RNA. The RNA molecules stimulate synthesis of specific proteins that possibly act to strengthen the synapses of these specific neurons. The proteins also seem to stimulate new interconnections and synapses within the group of neurons. The production of proteins and the results they produce appear to be essential for long-term memory and, therefore, learning.

The mechanism involved in recalling or retrieval of learned information is not known. The more association areas in which specific information has been stored on a long-term memory basis, the greater are the chances that a person probably will recall some specific information. For example, if a student has some specific information to learn, but only reads the material

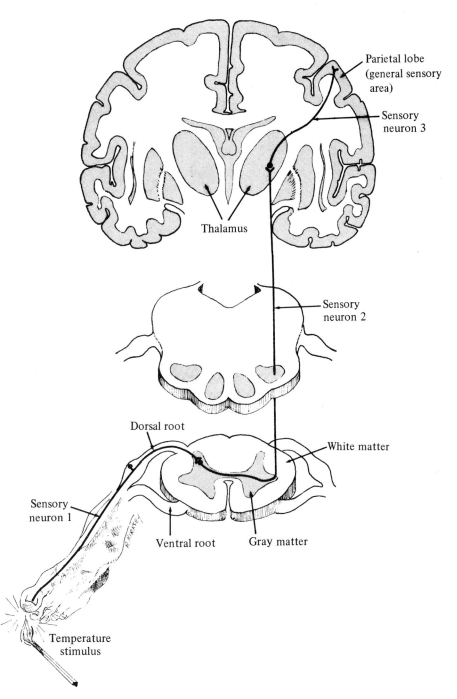

**Figure 5-24.** Sensory impulse pathway. Sensory impulses cross over to the opposite side of the cord from which they originate. They travel over three neurons to the sensory area of the cerebral cortex.

repetitively, he or she is storing the information in only the visual association area of the brain. On a test the person has only the visual association area from which to retrieve or recall the information. However, if the person repetitively reads, writes, and says aloud the in-

formation, he or she stores the information in the visual, touch, and sound association regions of the cortex. These areas all are interconnected by association fibers. On a test the student then has three association areas from which to recall or retrieve the information.

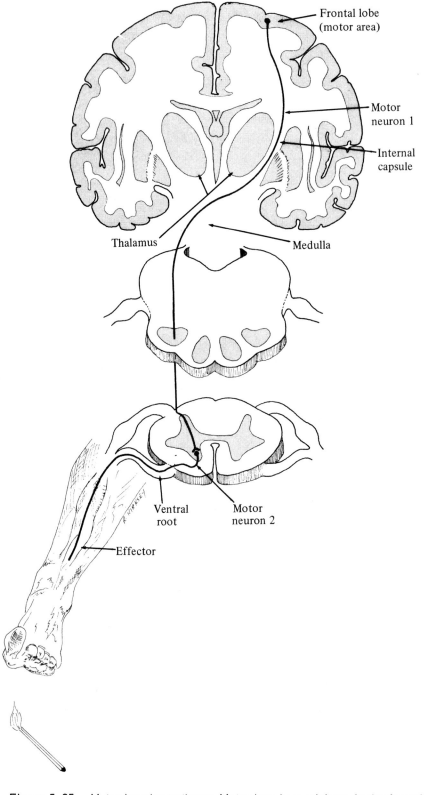

**Figure 5-25.** Motor impulse pathway. Motor impulses originate in the frontal lobe with motor neuron 1. Three-fourths of the impulses decussate or cross over to the opposite side of the spinal cord in the medulla. Motor neuron 2 leaves the spinal cord through the ventral root and goes to an effector.

## CRANIAL MENINGES AND CEREBROSPINAL FLUID

The brain is protected by membranes (meninges), cerebrospinal fluid, and cranial bones. The cranial bones will be discussed in Chapter 10. The meninges that cover the brain are continuations of those that cover the spinal cord: dura mater, arachnoid, and pia mater.

### Cranial Meninges

The **dura mater** in the brain (Figure 5-26) is composed of two layers. One layer lines the interior of the skull, and the other covers the brain. In some places these two layers are separated from each other, forming spaces called **cranial venous sinuses.** These sinuses are filled with blood that flows from the brain to the heart. Cerebrospinal fluid circulates around the brain and spinal cord and is finally absorbed into the *venous sinuses.*

The **arachnoid** is the next meninge. It is attached loosely (Figure 5-26) to the inner meninge (pia mater) by fibers, so that a space is created between the arachnoid and pia mater. This space is the **subarach-** noid space, and cerebrospinal fluid circulates through it. The arachnoid also sends tuftlike extensions up through the inner layer of the dura mater into the venous sinuses. These extensions are called **arachnoid villi,** and they aid in the return of cerebrospinal fluid to the blood.

The **pia mater** is the innermost meninge and is attached directly to the surface of the brain. It is composed of delicate connective tissue in which many blood vessels are found.

### Ventricles and Cerebrospinal Fluid (CSF)

**VENTRICLES OF THE BRAIN.** There are four elongated fluid-filled cavities in the brain, called **ventricles** (Figure 5-27). The first and second ventricles are located in the lateral hemispheres, and each contains a choroid plexus (a network of blood capillaries). The third ventricle, located between the right and left thalami, is a slitlike cavity. The first and second ventricles open into it by means of the **interventricular foramen** (foramen of Monro). The fourth ventricle is located between the medulla and pons and is connected to the third ventricle by the cerebral aqueduct. The fourth ventricle has three openings into the subarachnoid space.

**PRODUCTION, QUANTITY, AND CHARACTERISTICS OF CSF.** CSF, along with other body fluids, originates in the blood. The choroid plexuses in the

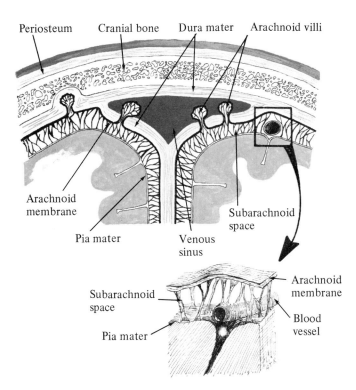

Figure 5-26. Cranial meninges and venous sinuses. The separation of the two layers of dura mater and blood in the venous sinus is shown. The arachnoid, pia mater, and subarachnoid space are also shown.

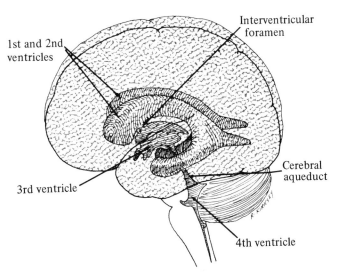

Figure 5-27. The four ventricles are shown from a lateral view. The interventricular foramen is shown connecting the first and second ventricles to the third ventricle. The cerebral aqueduct connects the third ventricle to the fourth ventricle.

first, second, and third ventricles are the sites of CSF production (Figure 5-28). The blood pressure in the plexuses is great enough to cause filtration or the pushing of fluids out of the blood. CSF is similar to blood in its contents of $H_2O$, NaCl, $K^+$, and glucose. The specific gravity of CSF is 1.004 to 1.008. The average quantity of CSF in an adult at any one time is 100 to 200 cc; however, the body actually produces approximately 550 cc during a 24-hour period. To maintain this 100 to 200 cc, CSF constantly osmoses through arachnoid villi into blood in the venous sinuses. Before CSF moves into the venous sinuses, it circulates through the ventricles and around the brain and spinal cord in the subarachnoid space. The passageway that CSF follows as it moves downward into the subarachnoid space can be important clinically; therefore, we will discuss this passageway (Figure 5-28).

CSF is produced by the **choroid plexus** in the first and second ventricles and flows through the interventricular foramen into the third ventricle. More CSF is produced in the third ventricle, and all of it flows through the **cerebral aqueduct** into the fourth ventricle. From the fourth ventricle, there are three openings into the subarachnoid space. The fluid, now in the subarachnoid space, flows around the brain and spinal cord.

The majority of CSF passes through the arachnoid villi into blood in the venous sinuses (Figure 5-28). It is

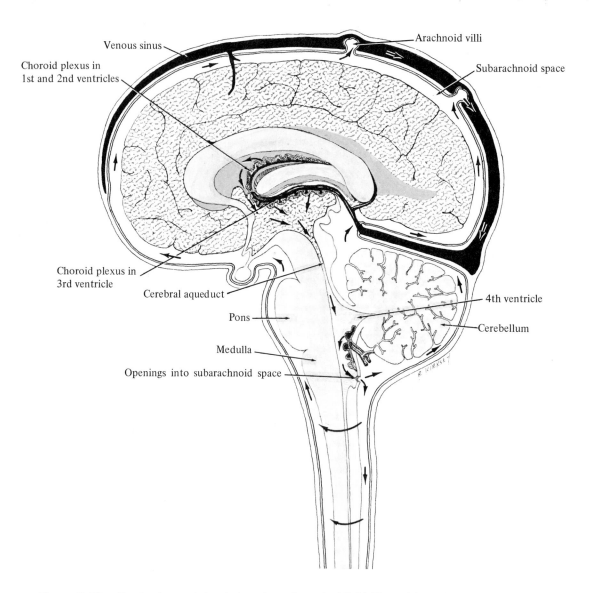

**Figure 5-28.** Production and circulation of cerebrospinal fluid. The origin and circulation of CSF is shown by arrows. CSF finally passes through arachnoid villi into venous sinuses by means of osmotic pressure.

thought that CSF passes into the venous sinuses by osmosis. The blood in these sinuses has a low blood pressure and a high osmotic pressure (pulling pressure). The high osmotic pressure is caused by the concentration of blood proteins. This high "osmotic pulling pressure" causes CSF to osmose into the venous blood.

**INTERNAL HYDROCEPHALUS (HYDRO—WATER; CEPHALUS—BRAIN).** If anything interferes with the passage of CSF, the rate of absorption into venous blood is reduced. This interference, however, does not reduce the rate of production. This unequal production and absorption increase the quantity of CSF and result in internal hydrocephalus. Tumors in the midbrain can cause constriction of the cerebral aqueduct so that CSF cannot pass this point; it continues to be produced but cannot circulate past the constriction and cannot be absorbed. The resulting accumulation of CSF in the first and second ventricles can cause swelling of the brain and an increase in cranial pressure.

**SPINAL PUNCTURE AND EXAMINATION OF CSF.** A spinal puncture is a process by which a long needle is inserted into the subarachnoid space between L-1 and L-5, and CSF is withdrawn or anesthetics are introduced. CSF is withdrawn for diagnostic purposes. The CSF is checked for the presence of white blood cells and blood; glucose and protein concentration is determined, and bacterial cultures are set up. Diseases such as meningitis, syphilis, and tuberculosis can be detected and identified by the type of bacteria present. Anesthetics are introduced into this space prior to surgery.

**FUNCTIONS OF CEREBROSPINAL FLUID (CSF).** CSF primarily acts as a water shock absorber. It totally surrounds the brain and spinal cord; therefore, any blows to the head or spinal cord region are absorbed by the CSF. It also acts as a carrier of nutrient and waste materials between the blood and central nervous system.

## CRANIAL NERVES

So far we have discussed spinal and peripheral nerves that are located inferior to the brain. Nerves that attach directly to the brain are called cranial nerves (Figure 5-29). Twelve pairs of cranial nerves are attached to the inferior surface of the brain. They pass through small skull openings (foramina) to reach their destination. The nerves are numbered, by Roman numerals, according to their position on the brain from anterior to posterior. Their names indicate their function or destination. Five of the nerves carry only motor impulses to effectors; three nerves carry only sensory impulses; four nerves carry both motor and sensory impulses. Table 5-5 lists the cranial nerves and their functions and whether they are sensory, motor, or both. The table also gives two mnemonics (device to help one memorize something). These two mnemonics can be used to learn the names of the nerves and the type of impulses (sensory, motor, or both) they carry. After the mnemonic for the names is memorized, the first letter of each cranial nerve corresponds to the first letter of each word in the mnemonic. The same procedure applies to the mnemonic for the type of nerve impulses (sensory, motor, or both).

Most of the cranial nerves carry motor impulses to skeletal muscles or they carry somatic impulses; however, cranial nerves III, VII, IX, and X carry both somatic and visceral impulses.

### Location and Function of Cranial Nerves*

I. The **olfactory nerves** originate in the superior region of the corresponding nasal cavity. The nerve transmits smell impulses to the olfactory region in the temporal lobe. Current smell impulses will be associated with past smell impulses.

II. The fibers of each **optic nerve** originate in the retinal layer of the corresponding eye. The optic nerves transmit visual sensory impulses to the occipital lobe of the brain; current visual impulses are associated with past visual impulses in the visual association area.

III. The **oculomotor nerves** transmit somatic motor impulses to four of six extrinsic muscles attached to the eye (Figure 5-29). These skeletal muscles are responsible for moving the eye, and only the **superior oblique** and **lateral rectus** muscles are not supplied by the oculomotor nerve. Somatic fibers also innervate the **levator palpebrae superioris** muscle, which raises the upper eyelid.

Visceral impulses are transmitted by this nerve to constrictor muscles of the iris and muscles that change the shape of the lens in the eye (Figure 5-29). The iris (colored part of the eye) is composed of smooth muscles that constrict and dilate the size of the pupil (opening in the iris), thereby regulating the entrance of light into the eye.

---

*Roman numerals are used to number cranial nerves since they are recognized the same internationally, whereas Arabic numerals are not.

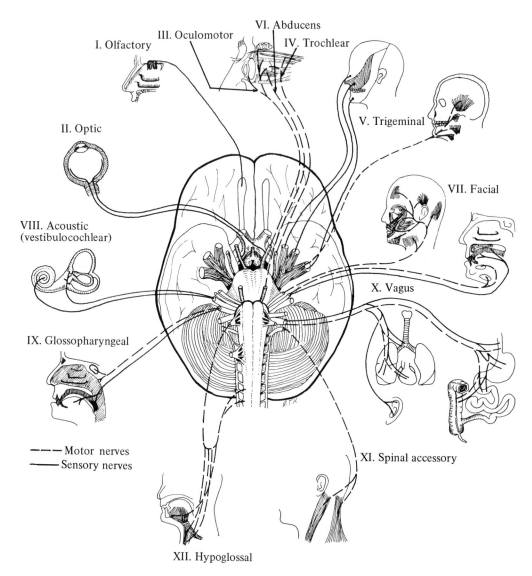

**Figure 5–29.** The twelve cranial nerves and the structures that their motor and sensory fibers innervate are shown.

IV. The **trochlear nerves** carry both sensory and motor fibers to and from the superior oblique muscles (Figure 5–29) attached to the eye.

V. The **trigeminal nerves** are the largest of the cranial nerves and are composed of three branches: opthalmic, maxillary, and mandibular branches.

The nerve transmits both sensory and motor fibers. The ophthalmic branch transmits sensory impulses from the orbits and head. The maxillary branch transmits sensory impulses from the face superior to the lower jaw. The mandibular branch transmits sensory impulses from the lower jaw (mandible) region. These sensory impulses are transmitted to the postcentral gyrus (general sensory region) of the parietal lobe.

Motor impulses are transmitted by the mandibular branch to the muscles of mastication (chewing).

VI. The **abducens nerves** transmit motor and sensory fibers to and from the lateral rectus muscle of the eye. The (III) oculomotor, (IV) trochlear, and (VI) abducens nerves all innervate extrinsic muscles of the eyes. Motor impulses to these muscles are responsible for movement of the eyes. The oculomotor, in addition, is responsible for constricting (decreasing the size of) the pupil and changing the shape of the lens. The importance

### TABLE 5-5.   Cranial Nerves and Their Functions

| Nerve | Function | Mnemonic for Name | Mnemonic for Motor, Sensory, or Both |
|-------|----------|-------------------|--------------------------------------|
| I. Olfactory | Sensory: smell impulses to brain | On | Some |
| II. Optic | Sensory: visual impulses to brain | Old | Say |
| III. Oculomotor | Motor: movements of eye; regulates size of pupil and amount of light entering eye | Olympus | Marry |
| IV. Trochlear | Motor: causes rotation of eyes | Towering | Money |
| V. Trigeminal | Both: has three branches; sensory fibers from skin of head and face; motor fibers to chewing muscles | Tops | But |
| IV. Abducens | Motor: lateral movement of eyes | A | My |
| VII. Facial | Both: sensory impulses for taste; motor impulses for muscles of facial expression | Finn | Brother |
| VIII. Acoustic (vestibulocochlear) | Sensory: impulses for hearing and balance | And | Says |
| IX. Glossopharyngeal | Both: sensory impulses for taste; motor impulses for swallowing | German | Bad |
| X. Vagus | Both: motor fibers to most organs in thoracic and abdomino-pelvic cavities. Sensory impulses from pharynx, larynx, and trachea. | Viewed | Business |
| XI. Spinal accessory | Motor: allows movement of head by causing contraction of trapezius and sternocleidomastoid muscles | Some | (to) Marry |
| XII. Hypoglossal | Motor: tongue movements | Hops | Money |

of these two actions in forming visual images will be discussed later.

VII. The **facial nerves** transmit both motor and sensory fibers to and from muscles and glands of the face and scalp. Afferent (sensory) fibers concerning taste are carried from the anterior two-thirds of the tongue to the taste association area in the temporal lobe (Figure 5-29). Somatic efferent (motor) impulses are transmitted to the muscles involved with facial expressions. Visceral efferent fibers stimulate the secretion of saliva in the sublingual and submaxillary salivary glands.

VIII. The **acoustic nerves** (vestibulocochlear nerves) are composed of vestibular and cochlear branches. The vestibular branch transmits sensory impulses concerning equilibrium from the semicircular canals of the inner ear to the cerebellum. The cochlear branch transmits sound impulses from the cochlea of the inner ear to the sound association area in the temporal lobe.

IX. The **glossopharyngeal nerves** transmit motor and sensory impulses to and from the tongue and pharynx (throat) muscles. They transmit taste sensory impulses from the posterior one-third of the tongue to the taste association area in the temporal lobe. Sensory impulses are transmitted from the lining of the pharynx to the swallowing reflex center in the medulla oblongata. Sensory impulses concerning blood pressure and oxygen level are transmitted from the carotid artery to the vasomotor and cardiac reflex centers in the medulla oblongata. Somatic motor impulses are transmitted to muscles of the tongue and constrictor muscles in the pharynx, which are responsible for swallowing. Visceral motor impulses are transmitted to the parotid salivary gland, stimulating it to secrete saliva.

X. The **vagus nerves** (wandering nerves) transmit motor and sensory impulses to many organs inferior to the head and neck. Sensory impulses are transmitted from mucous membranes of the pharynx (throat), larynx, and trachea. Somatic motor impulses are transmitted to the muscles of the mouth and throat, which help one to swallow; also, motor impulses are transmitted to the larynx, which help one to speak.

The majority of impulses transmitted by the vagus are visceral efferent impulses to smooth muscles in the pharynx, larynx, heart, and digestive system. These impulses play important roles in maintaining and restoring homeostasis in the thoracic and abdominopelvic cavities.

XI. The **spinal accessory nerves** primarily transmit somatic motor impulses to the trapezius and sternocleidomastoid muscles. Contraction of these muscles allows one to raise the shoulders and rotate the head.

XII. The **hypoglossal nerves** transmit motor impulses to deep muscles of the tongue.

---

The disorders of the following six cranial nerves probably are the most important disorders involving the cranial nerves.

**Loss of Smell.** Damage to the olfactory (I) nerve often results in impairment or loss of smell.

**Blindness.** Damage to the optic (II) nerve by syphilis organisms and excessive eye pressure are disorders that can result in blindness.

**Neuralgia.** Injury to or abnormal pressure on the trigeminal (V) nerve can result in severe pain in the face. This condition is called *tic douloureux*.

**Bell's Palsy.** Damage to the facial (VII) nerve results in paralysis of facial muscles. The paralysis typically occurs on one side of the face only, with a distorted appearance resulting.

**Deafness and Loss of Equilibrium.** Injury to the acoustic (vestibulocochlear) (VIII) nerve can result in deafness and loss of equilibrium.

**Reduction of Nerve Impulses to Various Visceral Organs.** Various branches of the vagus (X) nerve can be cut to reduce the flow of nerve impulses to certain visceral organs. For example, stomach ulcers can be helped by cutting the branch of the vagus that goes to the stomach. Stomach ulcers result from an excessive amount of hydrochloric acid (HCl). The vagus nerve stimulates glands in the stomach to release HCl. A large number of impulses carried by the vagus nerve can cause the stomach to release excessive quantities of HCl.

# 6 THE AUTONOMIC NERVOUS SYSTEM

So far our discussions concerning the nervous system and brain primarily have been about the voluntary (somatic) nervous system. This system voluntarily controls the contraction of skeletal muscles. The autonomic nervous system controls the activities of all smooth and cardiac muscles. Since all the visceral organs are composed of smooth muscle except the car-diac muscle in the heart, the autonomic nervous system controls the activities of the visceral organs. The activities of the visceral organs cannot be controlled voluntarily, and they function without our being aware of their activities.

## PARTS OF THE AUTONOMIC SYSTEM

The autonomic system is divided into the **sympathetic** and **parasympathetic** divisions. Both divisions innervate most visceral organs.

### Sympathetic or Thoracolumbar Division

The sympathetic division is responsible for preparing the body to respond to emergency situations and cases of fear, anger, worry, and strenuous activity (Figure 5–30). In other words, it is primarily concerned with processes involving the expenditure of energy. Sympathetic impulses exit the spinal cord from the thorax and lumbar regions of the spinal cord.

### Parasympathetic or Craniosacral Division

The parasympathetic division (Figure 5–30) controls activities of the organs under normal circumstances. The motor (efferent) nerves leave the spinal cord from the cranial and sacral regions, therefore, the name craniosacral region.

These two divisions tend to be antagonistic in that the sympathetic division activates the body to meet emergency situations. When the emergency situation has passed, the parasympathetic division deactivates the body back to a normal state. In other words, it is primarily concerned with activities that restore and conserve body energy.

### Autonomic Chemical Transmitters

Previously we said that nerve impulses were transmitted across a synapse by acetylcholine. In the sympathetic and parasympathetic ganglia, acetylcholine carries impulses from preganglionic to postganglionic fibers (Figure 5–31). Most of the sympathetic postganglionic fibers release **norepinephrine** at the **neuroeffector junction** (junction between muscle and nerve).

Autonomic fibers that release acetylcholine are referred to as **cholinergic fibers.** Fibers that release norepinephrine (adrenalin) are referred to as **adrenergic fibers.** The effects of cholinergic fibers are short-lived

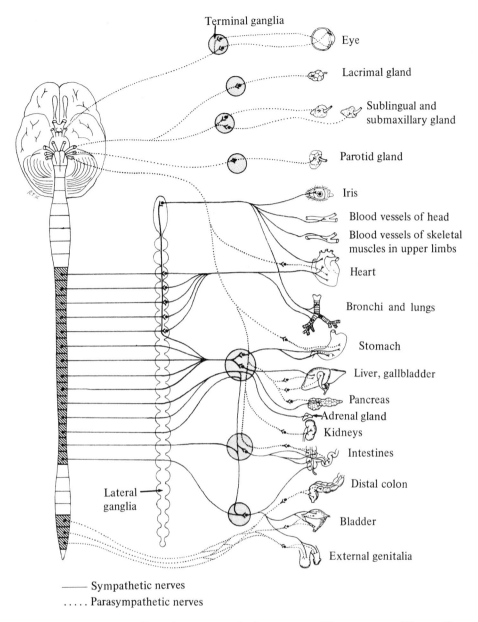

**Figure 5-30.** Sympathetic and parasympathetic nerves and the organs and tissues they innervate.

_____ Sympathetic nerves
. . . . . Parasympathetic nerves

and local; those of adrenergic fibers are longer lasting and more widespread.

## FUNCTIONS OF THE AUTONOMIC SYSTEM

The sympathetic and parasympathetic divisions together function to maintain homeostasis. However, it is especially important during times of stress for the sympathetic division to accelerate body activities, so

that the body can respond properly to the stress condition. Following a time of stress, the parasympathetic tends to slow down body activities or bring them back to their normal state. A specific example of how these two divisions work might make this clearer. Assume you are walking down a street at night, when suddenly a robber jumps out from an alley and sticks a gun in your face. Let's look at some of the body changes that occur as a result of the actions of the sympathetic system, and what changes the parasympathetic system brings about to restore normal body activities.

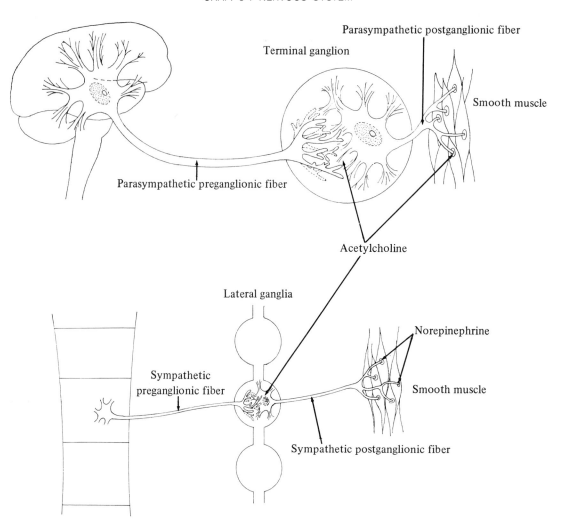

**Figure 5-31.** Chemical transmitters released by sympathetic and parasympathetic neurons. Notice that acetylcholine is released by preganglionic neurons of the parasympathetic and sympathetic systems as well as the post ganglionic neurons of the parasympathetic system. The postganglionic neurons of the sympathetic system release norepinephrine.

- The pupils in the eyes dilate allowing more light to enter to better see the robber and gun.
- The heart rate increases, and the force of the contractions increases. Blood has to be moved faster to the effectors.
- The respiratory rate increases. More $O_2$ is needed by the tissues, and the $CO_2$ must be removed.
- The bronchi (air tubes) dilate to carry air into the lungs.
- Elevated blood pressure occurs because of increased capillary bed constrictions and more rapid heart contractions.

- The rate of digestion is inhibited. The energy needed for this process is diverted to help speed up other activities.
- Sweat glands are stimulated to produce more sweat. Increasing activities of the body increase body temperature; therefore, the process of sweating helps to maintain normal body temperature.

Whether you decide to fight the robber or flee, the skeletal muscles would be strongly stimulated. Notice that all the body activities are speeded up except for digestion. During a time of stress, only body activities that are vital to overcoming the situation are speeded up.

Body activities not vital to overcoming the situation (digestion and urination) are inhibited.

After this condition is passed, all the activities that were accelerated or inhibited are restored to normal by a cessation of sympathetic nerve impulses.

Sympathetic and parasympathetic divisions of the autonomic system are very important. We will refer to them and the reactions they initiate as we discuss each system of the body. A summary of some of the more important reactions they cause is listed in Table 5–6.

### TABLE 5–6. *Autonomic Functions*

| STRUCTURE AND ACTIVITY | EFFECTS DUE TO PARASYMPATHETIC IMPULSES | EFFECTS DUE TO SYMPATHETIC IMPULSES |
|---|---|---|
| Heart | | |
| Rate of contractions | Decrease (−) | Increase (+) |
| Heart capillaries | Constriction | Dilation |
| Blood vessels | | |
| Abdomen | No effect | Vasoconstriction increases blood pressure |
| Skin | No effect | Vasoconstriction increases blood pressure |
| Skeletal muscles | No effect | Vasodilation decreases blood pressure and more blood flows into muscles |
| Respiratory system | | |
| Rate of breathing | Decrease (−) | Increase (+) |
| Bronchioles (air tubes) | Constriction decreases amount of air flowing into lungs to normal | Dilation increases amount of air flowing into lungs |
| Digestive system | | |
| Digestive movements | Increase | Decrease; energy for movements is used to meet emergency |
| Digestive secretions | Increase | Decrease |
| Muscular sphincter valve | Relaxes | Contracts |
| Conversion of blood glycogen to glucose | No effect | Increase |
| Pupil of the eye | Constriction | Dilation |

# SUMMARY

### Homeostatic Mechanisms
A. A mechanism consists of three parts: sensory receptor, nerve circuit, and effector organ.
B. Four characteristics of each homeostatic mechanism:
(1) self-regulating, (2) compensatory, (3) negative feedback, (4) more than one negative feedback system may be involved.

### Organization of the Nervous System
A. Neuron: structural and functional unit of nervous tissue
1. Anatomy: cell body, axon and dendrite, nerve coverings (myelin and neurilemma).
2. Types of neurons: afferent (sensory), transmit sensory stimuli from PNS to CNS; ef-

ferent (motor), transmit motor impulses to effectors; internuncial (central, association, and intermediate), primarily connects afferent to efferent neurons.

3. Nerve fibers, nerves, and tracts: nerve fiber, a single neuron; nerve, composed of many nerve fibers; nerve tract, bundles of nerve fibers in CNS.

B. Synapse

A contact point between a presynaptic and a postsynaptic neuron.

## Nerve Impulse Conduction

A. Resting potential and action potential

1. Resting potential: difference in electrical charge between the inside and outside of a nerve membrane; membrane in a polarized state.
2. Action potential: sequence of electrical changes in a nerve cell membrane when exposed to a threshold stimulus.

B. Polarization, depolarization, and repolarization: polarization, a separation of + charges (on outside of neuron) from − charges (on inside of neuron); depolarization, movement of $Na^+$ inside and $K^+$ outside neuron and starts an action potential; repolarization, reestablishment of polarized condition by active transport of $Na^+$ and $K^+$ back to their original positions.

C. Movement of nerve impulse across synapse

1. Neurotransmitters: a neurotransmitter is released from a presynaptic neuron; diffuses across a synaptic cleft and initiates an action potential at a postsynaptic neuron; two examples are acetylcholine and norepinephrine; cholinesterase breaks down acetylcholine.
2. Rate of nerve impulse conduction: myelinated nerves transmit impulses more rapidly than unmyelinated as a result of saltatory conduction (impulse jumping from node to node).

## Spinal Cord and Spinal Nerves

A. Anatomy and location of spinal cord: 40 to 45 cm in length; enlargements in cervical and lumbar regions; anterior median fissure on anterior surface; extends downward from foramen magnum to L-1 or L-2 vertebra.

1. Meninges (coverings) of spinal cord:
   a. Dura mater: outer meninge; tough fibrous connective tissue; protects spinal cord.
   b. Arachnoid: resembles a spider web; subarachnoid space is site where CSF circulates around brain and spinal cord.
   c. Pia mater: innermost meninge attached to nerve tissue; very vascular.

B. Internal Anatomy: cross section of cord reveals gray matter in an H shape; white matter surrounds gray matter and transmits sensory and motor impulses.

C. Spinal nerves

1. Designation: 31 pairs named according to the spinal segment from which they originate.
2. Roots: each spinal nerve formed by union of dorsal (posterior) and ventral (anterior) roots.

D. Spinal plexuses

1. Four major plexuses (a complicated network of nerves):
   a. Cervical: C-1 to C-4 nerves; phrenic nerve exits plexus and innervates diaphragm.
   b. Brachial: C-5 through T-1; nerves supply brachial region, upper extremities, neck and shoulder.
   c. Lumbar: L-1 through L-4 nerves; femoral and obturator nerves are main nerves supplying impulses to lower body wall, gluteal region, and thigh.
   d. Sacral: L-4 through S-5; sciatic is major nerve, which supplies impulses to thigh and lower leg muscles.

E. Spinal cord reflexes

Reflex is an automatic act that does not require conscious help.

1. Stretch (extensor) reflex: two neurons, sensory and motor.

*Ex.*: reflex contraction of quadriceps femoris and gluteus maximus enable one to remain upright.

2. Flexor: three neurons, sensory, motor, and central; protective reflex that flexes body parts away from painful stimulus.

3. Cross-extensor reflexes: one limb reflexly extends while the other flexes; extension is for purpose of supporting one side of body while the other side is flexed away from stimulus.

F. White matter tracts in spinal cord

Myelinated neurons are grouped together into nerve tracts; ascending tracts transmit sensory impulses up cord to brain; descending tracts transmit motor impulses down cord.

## The Brain

A. Hindbrain

1. Medulla oblongata: first part of brain after spinal cord enters skull. Functions: cardiac center, regulates heart rate; vasomotor center, regulates dilation and constriction of blood vessels, thereby lowering or raising blood pressure, respectively; respiratory center, increases or decreases respiratory rate depending upon $O_2$ and $CO_2$ level of blood.

2. Pons: link between hindbrain and midbrain; contains pneumotaxic center that works with medulla to regulate respiration.

3. Cerebellum: dorsal to pons and medulla; composed of two hemispheres; outer surface is cerebellar cortex. Functions: (1) coordination of muscle movement, (2) maintenance of balance, equilibrium, and orientation, (3) maintenance of muscle tone and posture.

B. Midbrain

1. Location: superior to pons and inferior to cerebrum.

2. Function: coordinates visual and auditory reflexes; major conduction pathway for both sensory and motor impulses.

C. Forebrain

1. Diencephalon

a. Hypothalamus: inferior to thalamus and composes floor and lateral walls of third ventricle. Functions: (1) cardiac, regulates heart rate, (2) vasomotor, regulates vasodilation and vasoconstriction of blood vessels, (3) respiratory, regulates rate of respiration, (4) regulation of water balance, (5) regulation of appetite control.

b. Thalamus: superior to hypothalamus; composes lateral walls of third ventricle. Functions: (1) crude recognition of sensory stimuli, (2) relay of sensory impulses to cerebral cortex.

D. Telencephalon

1. Anatomy: composed of two cerebral hemispheres; each hemisphere is divided into (1) cerebral cortex, (2) white matter, (3) lobes of cerebral cortex, and (4) basal ganglia.

2. Lobes of cerebral cortex: (a) frontal lobe, initiates motor impulses to tissues; left lobe controls motor movements of right side of body, and vice versa for right lobe; (b) Parietal lobe, general sensory lobe; receives and interprets pain, temperature, touch, and pressure impulses from all parts of body; (c) temporal lobe, receives auditory and olfactory impulses; (d) occipital, receives visual impulses.

3. Association areas: each lobe has a memory storage or association area; allows brain to relate current sensory impulses with those stored in association area.

E. Pathways for sensory and motor impulses

1. Three neurons compose pathway for sensory impulses from receptor cells to cerebral cortex; second neuron frequently decussates (crosses over) to opposite side of cord.

2. Two neurons compose pathway of motor impulses from frontal lobe to tissues; motor neuron 1 frequently decussates in medulla.

F. Short- and long-term memory

1. Short term: storage of information in memory areas for only a short time (few hours).

    2. Long term: repeated repetition of information results in synthesis of RNA and protein, which are stored and can be recalled for a long term.

G. Cranial meninges and cerebrospinal fluid
    1. Three meninges (membranes) protect brain: (1) dura mater, outer meninge; (2) arachnoid, attached loosely to pia mater by fibers so that a subarachnoid space is created; (3) pia mater, innermost meninge and attached directly to brain; very vascular.
    2. Ventricles and cerebrospinal fluid (CSF). Four ventricles (cavities) are located in brain; choroid plexus in each secretes cerebrospinal fluid (CSF), which circulates through each ventricle until it enters subarachnoid space at fourth ventricle; CSF is absorbed into blood in venous sinuses. Function of CSF: shock absorber.

H. Cranial nerves: 12 pairs of nerves originate on inferior surface of brain; numbered by Roman numerals according to their position on brain from anterior to posterior; five nerves are motor in function, three are sensory, and four are both motor and sensory.

## The Autonomic Nervous System

A. Sympathetic (thoracolumbar): prepares body to respond to emergency situations, fear, anger, and worry; primarily concerned with processes involving expenditure of energy; sympathetic nerves exit the spinal cord from the thorax and lumbar regions.

B. Parasympathethic (craniosacral): controls activities of internal organs under normal circumstances; primarily concerned with processes that conserve energy; parasympathetic nerves exit from the cranial (brain) and sacral region of spinal cord.

C. Autonomic chemical transmitters: sympathetic and parasympathetic neurons release acetylcholine at synapses in ganglia; parasympathetic nerves release acetylcholine at neuromuscular junction; sympathetic neurons release norepinephrine at neuromuscular junctions.

D. Functions of the autonomic system: sympathetic division tends to activate most organs in order to meet stress; parasympathetic tends to restore homeostasis, after stress, by slowing organ activity; specific functions of each division are presented in Table 5–6.

## Nervous System

1. Afferent neurons are to transmission of sensory stimuli as efferent neurons are to (a) transmission of motor impulses, (b) synapse between sensory and motor, (c) transmission of impulses from CNS to effectors, (d) a and c, (E) b and c.

2. A stretch reflex involves two neurons and is important in enabling one to remain in an upright position. True or false?
   The following statement refers to Questions 3 to 6. The first item in each pair of items names a structure, a location, or a process. If the second item is located in or is in some way part of the first item, underline A. If not, underline B.

3. A  B  Cerebellum
      Coordinates visual and auditory reflexes

4. A  B  Parietal lobe
      Reception of pain impulses from skin.

5. A  B  Telencephalon
      Cerebral hemispheres

6. A  B  Left frontal lobe
      Controls motor movements of left side of body

7. CSF functions as a shock absorber. True or False?

8. Which of the following are incorrectly paired?
   (a) oculomotor—transmit visual impulses; (b) glossopharyngeal—swallowing; (c) VI—facial nerve; (d) none of these; (e) a and c

Matching. Questions 9 to 13.

9. sympathetic division

10. parasympathetic division

11. secretion of CSF

12. adrenergic fibers

13. sympathetic impulses

A. choroid plexus

B. prepare body for stress

C. thoracolumbar

D. norepinephrine as neurotransmitter

E. craniosacral

# Chapter 6

# ENDOCRINE  SYSTEM

After reading and studying this chapter, a student should be able to:
1. Define a hormone.
2. Describe how blood chemicals and the autonomic nervous system regulate secretions of hormones.
3. Recognize an anatomical description of the anterior and posterior lobes of the pituitary gland.
4. Give the names of the hormones secreted by the anterior and posterior pituitary, as well as their target organs and functions.
5. Name the hormones secreted by the thyroid gland, their functions, and symptoms of hyper- and hyposecretions.
6. Describe functions of hormones secreted by parathyroid glands, as well as symptoms of hypo- and hypersecretions of each.
7. Recognize the names of hormones secreted by adrenal cortex and medulla and their functions, plus symptoms associated with hypo- and hypersecretions.
8. Name the hormones secreted by the pancreas and their functions, as well as symptoms of hypo- and hypersecretions of each.

*Various physiologic activities occur very slowly and over a prolonged period of time. Body growth, sexual maturation and metabolic functions are examples. The organs responsible for these activities require constant and long-lived coordination. The nervous system, acting alone, cannot coordinate these activities. The endocrine and nervous systems interact to control these activities, as well as others.*

# 1 CHARACTERISTICS OF THE ENDOCRINE SYSTEM

The endocrine system is composed of glands called "ductless glands" since they do not have ducts. Each gland secretes chemical compounds called hormones directly into the blood. A **hormone** is defined as a chemical messenger secreted into the blood. It coordinates the physiologic activities of effectors distant from the point of secretion. The amount of time it takes for a hormone to be secreted and to be moved to the effectors is much slower than that for a nerve impulse.

# 2 REGULATION OF HORMONE SECRETION

Small quantities of hormones are quite effective; therefore, the amounts being secreted have to be regulated to maintain homeostasis. The secretions of hormones are controlled by the following.

## BLOOD CHEMICALS

The concentrations of certain blood chemicals stimulate or inhibit secretion of hormones. For example, if the concentration of blood glucose rises, the pancreas is stimulated to secrete more insulin. As the concentration of glucose drops, the secretion of insulin decreases.

Other blood chemicals and the corresponding hormones, whose secretions are stimulated and inhibited, will be discussed later.

## NERVOUS SYSTEM (AUTONOMIC)

The autonomic system stimulates the medulla region of the adrenal gland to release epinephrine and norepinephrine. These hormones are utilized by both the endocrine and nervous systems.

### Negative Feedback Mechanism

Several glands are regulated by negative feedback (which is always an inverse relationship) of another hormone. An example is secretion of thyroid-stimulating hormone (TSH). Whenever the thyroxine hormone level drops, this concentration feeds back to the pituitary gland, causing it to release more TSH. The increased level of TSH stimulates the thyroid gland to release more thyroxin, thereby restoring the normal range. A word equation that expresses this inverse negative feedback mechanism is

↓ Thyroxin = ↑ stimulation of = ↑ secretion = pituitary gland of TSH

↑ stimulation of = ↑ thyroxin thyroid gland

## 3    ENDOCRINE GLANDS: THEIR HORMONES AND TARGET ORGANS

Figure 6–1 shows the various endocrine glands. Each endocrine gland releases a hormone or hormones that stimulate changes in the cells of an organ or group of organs. These are called the **target organs.** In the discussion that follows each gland and the hormones that it secretes will be discussed along with the effects of the hormones on the **target organs.**

## PITUITARY GLAND (HYPOPHYSEAL)

This gland is about the size of a pea and is located at the base of the brain, inferior to the hypothalamus (Figure 6–2). The pituitary is protected by the sphenoid bone and is attached to the hypothalamus by means of hypophyseal stalk.

**ANATOMY OF THE PITUITARY GLAND.** The pituitary is composed of two lobes, anterior and posterior. The anterior lobe is glandular in makeup; therefore, it is called **adenohypophysis** (*adeno*—gland; *hypo*—under). Seven different types of secretory cells are found in the

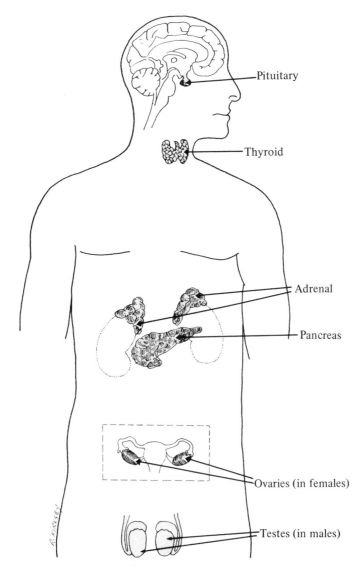

Figure 6–1.    Endocrine glands.

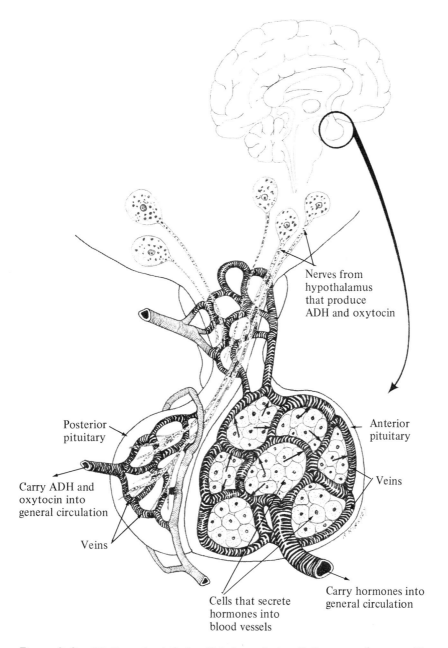

Nerves from
hypothalamus
that produce
ADH and oxytocin

Posterior
pituitary

Anterior
pituitary

Carry ADH and
oxytocin into
general circulation

Veins

Veins

Carry hormones into
general circulation

Cells that secrete
hormones into
blood vessels

**Figure 6-2.**   Pituitary gland. Cells within the anterior pituitary secrete seven different hormones into the bloodstream. ADH and oxytocin are produced by nerve tissue in the hypothalamus and are sent to the posterior pituitary. [Adapted from Ellen E. Chaffee and Esther M. Greisheimer, *Basic Physiology,* 3rd edition (Philadelphia: J.B. Lippincott, 1974)]

adenohypophysis, each one thought responsible for synthesis and secretion of one of the seven anterior pituitary hormones. The anterior pituitary does not receive an arterial blood supply like other tissues. Veins from the hypothalamus bring blood to the anterior pituitary.

The posterior lobe originates from the hypothalamus and also can be called **neurohypophysis** (*neuro*—nervous; *hypo*—under). It is composed of thousands of axons that descend into it from the hypothalamus (Figure 6-2). The posterior pituitary has the normal arterial and venous capillary blood supply to it.

**PITUITARY PORTAL SYSTEM AND HYPOTHA-
LAMIC CONTROL OF THE ANTERIOR LOBE.**
Small branches from the internal carotid arteries go to
the proximal portion of the **hypophyseal stalk** (Figure
6–2). Veins then carry blood into the anterior pituitary.
This arrangement of blood vessels is called the **pituitary
portal system.** Special neurons course down from the
hypothalamus to the pituitary portal system in the hypophyseal stalk.

Specialized nerve cells in the base of the hypothalamus secrete hormones called **neurosecretory substances** or **releasing factors (RF),** which are carried by
neurons to and stored in neurons in the capillary region

of the hypophyseal stalk. When certain stimuli reach
the base of the hypothalamus, they are relayed to where
the releasing factors are stored. The releasing factors
are carried by the pituitary portal system to the anterior
pituitary where they stimulate the secretion of one or
more of the anterior pituitary hormones.

**HORMONES OF THE ANTERIOR PITUITARY
(ADENOHYPOPHYSIS).** The anterior pituitary secretes seven hormones. Six of these are trophic; that is,
they regulate the growth and secretions of other endocrine glands (Figure 6–3).

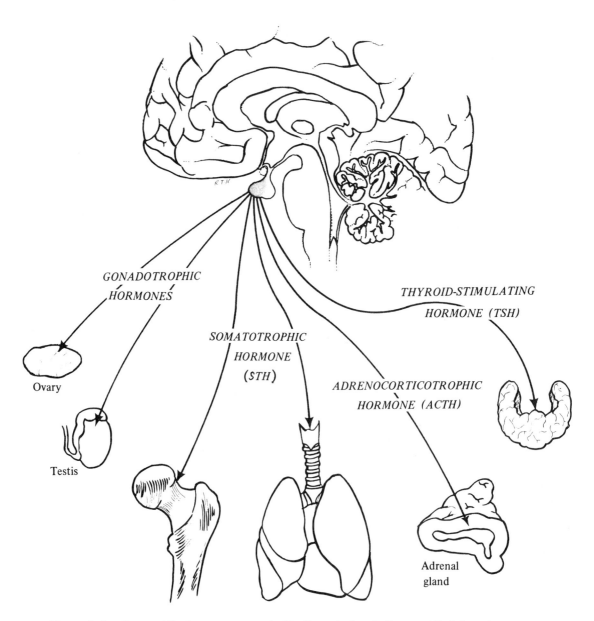

**Figure 6–3.** Some of the hormones secreted by the anterior pituitary and their target organs.

1. *Somatotrophic hormone (STH): growth hormone.* This hormone promotes growth of bones, muscles, and other organs of the body (Figure 6–3). It accomplishes this by increasing the metabolism of proteins, fats, and carbohydrates. If a lower-than-normal amount of growth hormone is secreted (hyposecretion) during the growing years, **dwarfism** results. A decreased production of somatotrophic hormone results in a decreased production of cells by the epiphyseal cartilage in long bones.

   If an overabundance of growth hormone is secreted (hypersecretion) during the growing years, **gigantism** occurs. This condition results in an increase in the production of cells by the epiphyseal cartilage of long bones. If hypersecretion occurs in adult years, it results in **acromegaly**. This condition is characterized by a protruding jaw, prominent cheek bones, and large hands.

2. *Gonadotrophic hormones.* Three hormones control the growth, development, and secretion of the gonads (testes and ovaries) (Figure 6–3). The three hormones are the **follicle-stimulating hormone (FSH)**, **luteinizing hormone (LH)**, and **lactogenic hormone (LTH)**. The details concerning the functions of these hormones will be discussed in Chapter 21.

3. *Thyroid-stimulating Hormone (TSH).* This hormone coordinates the growth, development, and secretion of the thyroid gland (Figure 6–3).

4. *Adrenocorticotrophic hormone (ACTH).* ACTH stimulates the growth and secretion of the cortex region of the adrenal gland (Figure 6–3).

Table 6–1 summarizes the anterior pituitary hormones and their effects.

**HYPOTHALAMIC CONTROL OF THE POSTERIOR LOBE.** Figure 6–2 shows some of the nerves that descend into the posterior lobe from specialized nerve cell bodies in the hypothalamus. The hypothalamic cell bodies produce **antidiuretic hormone (ADH)** and **oxytocin,** which slowly move down and are stored at the ends of the nerves in the posterior lobe. When the blood circulating through the hypothalamus brings certain messages to it, impulses are sent from the hypothalamus down nerves to the posterior lobe, which releases the appropriate hormone into the venous blood.

**HORMONES OF THE POSTERIOR PITUITARY (NEUROHYPOPHYSIS).** Two hormones are released from the posterior pituitary, **oxytocin** and **antidiuretic hormone (ADH)** (Figure 6–4). Oxytocin (pitocin) stimulates the smooth muscles of the uterus during pregnancy to contract forcefully and aid in the birth of the child (Figure 6–4). **ADH** increases the water-absorbing ability of the blood vessels in the kidney nephrons (Figure 6–4). ADH is also called **vasopressin** because it stimulates the contraction of arteries and arterioles, thereby increasing blood pressure.

## THYROID GLAND HORMONES

The thyroid gland is located inferior to the larynx (voice box). It is composed of two lobes connected to each other by a narrow strip of tissue (Figure 6–5). The secretory portion of the thyroid is composed of follicles that secrete the thyroid hormones **thyroxin, triiodothyronine,** and **calcitonin.** Thyroid-stimulating hormone (TSH) controls the growth, development, and secretion of the thyroid follicles.

**Thyroxin** and **triiodothyronine** are compounds composed of iodine and amino acids. The follicles remove iodine and amino acids from the blood to make

*TABLE 6–1. Summary of Anterior Pituitary Hormones*

| Hormone | Function | Effects of Hyposecretion | Effects of Hypersecretion |
|---|---|---|---|
| Somatotrophic | Promotes growth of body tissues | Dwarfism (growing years) | Gigantism (growing years) Acromegaly (adult years) |
| Follicle-stimulating hormone Luteinizing hormone (LH) Lactogenic hormone (LTH) | Details will be discussed in Chapter 21. | | |
| Thyroid-stimulating hormone | Coordinates growth, development, and secretion of thyroid gland | See Table 6–2. | See Table 6–2. |
| Adrenocorticotrophic hormone (ACTH) | Stimulates growth and secretion of cortex region of adrenal gland | See Table 6–3. | See Table 6–3. |

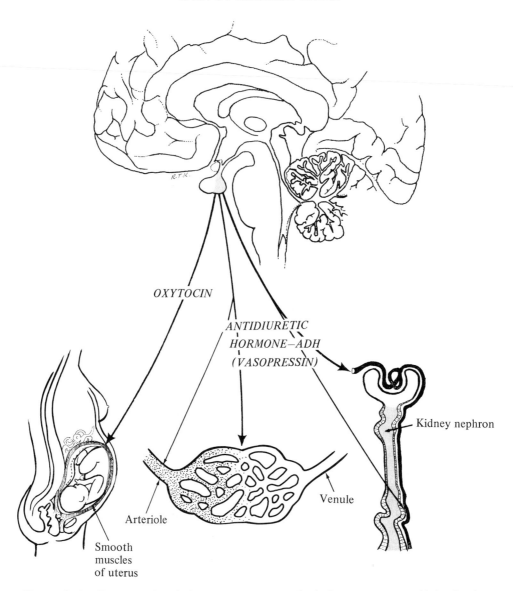

**Figure 6-4.** The posterior pituitary secretes oxytocin during pregnancy, which stimulates the muscles of the uterus. It also secretes ADH or vasopressin, which increases absorption of water out of kidney nephrons and contraction of arterioles, which increases blood pressure.

these two hormones. Iodine is combined with amino acids to form thyroxin ($T_4$, composed of four iodines) and triiodothyronine ($T_3$, composed of three iodines).

TSH stimulates the thyroid follicles to secrete thyroxin ($T_4$) and triiodothyronine ($T_3$) into the blood where they combine with plasma proteins. These hormones, bound to proteins, are called protein bound iodine (PBI) and are carried throughout the body.

**FUNCTIONS OF THYROXIN, TRIIODOTHYRO-NINE, AND CALCITONIN.** Thyroxin ($T_4$) and triiodothyronine ($T_3$) primarily act to regulate the production of heat and energy in the body tissues or regulate body metabolism. Their site of action appears to be the mitochondria. They tend to regulate the catabolism reactions or the reactions responsible for producing heat and energy in the body. Also, these two hormones are important in growth and mental development.

**Calcitonin** functions to lower the level of blood calcium. It does this by stimulating the bones to take up more calcium. Its secretion is regulated by the level of blood calcium. When the level of blood calcium is high, the thyroid is stimulated to release calcitonin, which causes bones to take up and store calcium. Once the

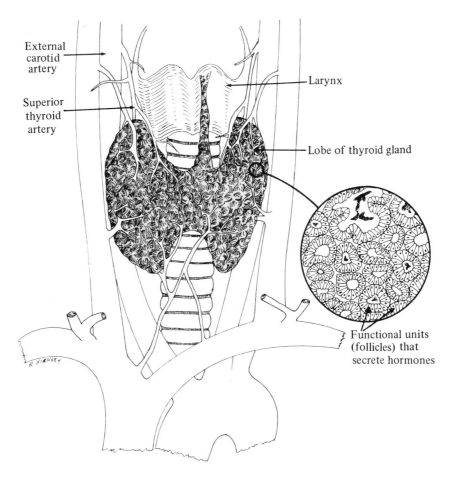

External
carotid
artery

Superior
thyroid
artery

Larynx

Lobe of thyroid gland

Functional units
(follicles) that
secrete hormones

**Figure 6-5.** Thyroid gland. The two lobes of the thyroid gland and the narrow connecting strip are shown. Also shown are the follicles that secrete thyroxin, triiodothyronine, and calcitonin into the blood.

level of blood calcium is within the normal range, the thyroid gland in inhibited from releasing calcitonin.

**HYPOSECRETION AND HYPERSECRETION OF THYROID HORMONES.** Various conditions (such as dietary deficiency of iodine) may cause an undersecretion (hyposecretion) of the thyroid gland. Hyposecretion of these hormones will lower the overall ability of body cells to produce energy, grow, and develop.

Cretinism is caused by hyposecretion of the thyroid gland at birth. It can result from the absence of a thyroid gland or insufficient iodine in the mother's diet during pregnancy. A child with this disorder is called a cretin. He or she does not mature physically or mentally, resulting in a dwarf who is mentally retarded. Skeletal growth can be helped if thyroxin is supplied to the child; however, mental retardation will be permanent unless treatment is started a few months after birth.

Hyposecretion of the thyroid gland in the adult causes myxedema. The term **myxedema** implies that the disorder has something to do with edema. Thyroxin tends to function like a diuretic and, therefore, aid in elimination of water. If a hyposecretion of thyroxin occurs, such as in myxedema, then the individual tends to retain water. This is evidenced by edema in the facial tissues causing them to be quite puffy. The increased water level in the body results in elevated blood volume (**hypervolemia**), which results directly in increased blood pressure. Other problems that accompany myxedema are slow heart rate, low body temperature, and weight gain. Females suffer from myxedema eight times more frequently than do males.

Oversecretion or hypersecretion of the thyroid causes an elevation of the basal metabolic rate (BMR). An increased BMR results in rapid respiration, weight loss, increased sweating, protrusion of eyeballs (or **exophthalmos**), and increased nervousness.

Often hyperthyroidism or Grave's disease causes an enlargement of the thyroid gland or an **exophthalmic goiter.** This often is visible as an enlargement on the lateral surface of the neck. Exophthalmos or protrusion of eyeballs and exophthalmic goiter both can be present at the same time.

Table 6-2 summarizes the effects of thyroid hormones.

**LAB TESTS FOR THYROID FUNCTION.** Lab tests are performed to determine how the thyroid gland is functioning. Two important tests are based on the concentration and uptake of iodine.

1. *Protein-bound iodine (PBI) test.* This test consists of measuring the concentration of protein-bound iodine. The concentration is measured in terms of micrograms ($\mu$g) per 100 ml of plasma.
2. *Radioactive iodine uptake.* $^{131}I$ is administered orally in distilled water. Twenty-four to forty-eight hours later the amount of radioactive iodine ($^{131}I$) uptake is measured by means of a radiant energy counter.

## PARATHYROID GLANDS AND HORMONES

The **parathyroid glands** are small roundish bodies located close to the posterior surface of the thyroid gland (Figure 6-6). There are two parathyroid glands in each lobe of the thyroid gland, and they may be embedded in the thyroid tissue.

**PARATHYROID HORMONE (PTH).** PTH plays an important role in increasing the level of calcium ions ($Ca^{2+}$) in the blood. Calcium ions play an important role in muscle contractions and nerve impulse conduction;

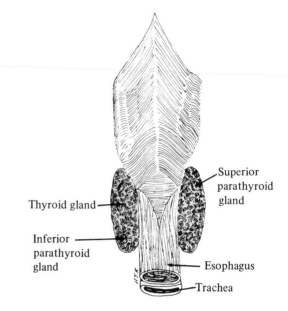

**Figure 6-6.** Two parathyroid glands are attached to the posterior surface of each lobe of the thyroid gland.

therefore, a normal level of blood calcium is important. PTH acts on three tissues to increase the concentration of $Ca^{2+}$ in the blood. It acts on bone tissue to release $Ca^{2+}$ into the blood. PTH stimulates the kidneys to resorb more $Ca^{2+}$ into the blood as they form urine. The third tissue acted on by PTH is the small intestine. PTH increases the rate of $Ca^{2+}$ absorption through the small intestine into the blood.

**HYPERPARATHYROIDISM.** The overproduction of PTH from the parathyroid gland is called hyperparathyroidism and is characterized by a large amount of calcium being released from bones into the blood. This condition is called hypercalcemia, and it causes the bones to weaken and fracture easily. Another problem with this condition is the formation of kidney stones be-

## TABLE 6-2.  *Summary of Thyroid Gland Hormones*

| HORMONE | FUNCTION | EFFECTS OF HYPOSECRETION | EFFECTS OF HYPERSECRETION |
|---|---|---|---|
| Thyroxin ($T_4$) and triiodothyronine ($T_3$) | Regulate body metabolism<br>Important in growth and mental development | Cretinism (infant)<br>  Dwarf size<br>  Mentally retarded<br>Myxedema (adult)<br>  Retention of water<br>  Slow heart rate<br>  Low body temperature | Grave's disease<br>  Enlargement of thyroid gland<br>  Rapid respirations<br>  Weight loss<br>  Protrusion of eyeballs (exophthalmos) |
| Calcitonin | Decrease blood calcium level by increasing absorption of Ca into bone tissue | Increase in blood calcium above normal, or hypercalcemia | Decrease in blood calcium below normal, or hypocalcemia |

cause of the increased concentration of calcium ions in the blood. Kidney stones can cause considerable damage to kidney tissue.

**HYPOPARATHYROIDISM.** This condition accompanies an undersecretion of PTH, and the symptoms are caused by a low blood calcium level. The most obvious symptom is increased excitability of the nervous system, leading to **tetany,** which is characterized by intermittent muscular contractions, tremors, and muscular pain. This condition often is evidenced by a sharp flexion (inward movement) of the hands and feet. It can lead to respiratory paralysis, if the respiratory muscles quit functioning properly.

**REGULATION OF PTH AND CALCITONIN SECRETION.** Previously, we stated that regulation of hormone secretion was controlled in three ways. The level of calcium in the blood that feeds back to the parathyroids regulates the amount of PTH secretion. The normal range of blood calcium is 4.5 to 5.8 mEq/liter. Figure 6-7 shows that when blood $Ca^{2+}$ drops below the normal range the parathyroid gland releases parathormone. Parathormone acts on bones, kidneys and intestines, and the end result is an increase in blood $Ca^{2+}$ back into the normal range. Figure 6-7 also shows that when the upper limit of $Ca^{2+}$ is exceeded the thyroid is stimulated to release calcitonin. It inhibits the activities of the same tissues that parathormone stimulates. The end result is that blood $Ca^{2+}$ is lowered into the normal range. Figure 6-8 shows how the **negative feedback** control mechanism is working to bring blood $Ca^{2+}$ back toward the normal range by calcitonin hormone. The

Normal Blood
Ca⁺⁺ Range

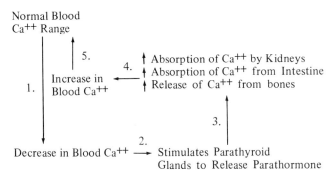

**Figure 6-7.** Increase in blood $Ca^{2+}$ by actions of parathormone: (1) A decrease in blood $Ca^{2+}$ results in (2) stimulation of parathyroid glands and release of PTH, which results in (3) increased activity of kidneys, intestines, and bones, which results in (4) increase in blood $Ca^{2+}$, which results in (5) normal blood $Ca^{2+}$ range being restored.

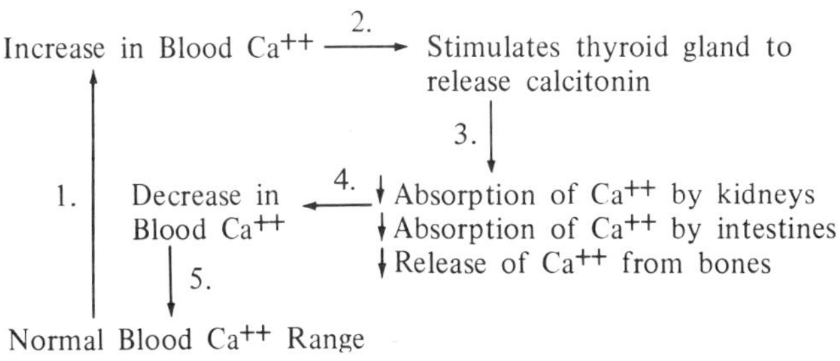

Increase in Blood Ca⁺⁺ —²·—→ Stimulates thyroid gland to
release calcitonin

3.

1. │ Decrease in —⁴·— ↓ Absorption of Ca⁺⁺ by kidneys
Blood Ca⁺⁺     ↓ Absorption of Ca⁺⁺ by intestines
5.            ↓ Release of Ca⁺⁺ from bones

Normal Blood Ca⁺⁺ Range

**Figure 6-8.** Decrease in blood $Ca^{2+}$ by actions of calcitonin: (1) a high level of blood $Ca^{2+}$ results in (2) stimulation of thyroid gland to release calcitonin, which results in (3) decreased activity of intestines, bones, and kidneys, which results in (4) decreased $Ca^{2+}$ level in blood, which results in (5) normal range of blood $Ca^{2+}$ being restored.

word equations for the relationships between $Ca^{2+}$, parathormone, and calcitonin are

$$\downarrow \text{Blood } Ca^{2+} = \uparrow \text{ release of } = \uparrow \text{ Blood } Ca^{2+}$$
$$\text{PTH}$$

$$\uparrow \text{Blood } Ca^{2+} = \uparrow \text{ release of } = \downarrow \text{ Blood } Ca^{2+}$$
$$\text{calcitonin}$$

## ADRENAL GLANDS (SUPRARENAL GLANDS)

The **adrenal glands** are two small glands, one of which is located on the superior surface of each of the kidneys (Figure 6-9). The outer portion of the adrenal gland is the cortex, and the inner region is the medulla. The two regions secrete their own hormones.

**ADRENAL CORTEX HORMONES.** The adrenal cortex is stimulated by **adrenocorticotrophic hormone (ACTH),** from the anterior pituitary, to release three groups of hormones, **mineralocorticoids, glucocorticoids,** and **sex hormones.** All the hormones belong to the organic group called **steroids.**

- *Mineralocorticoids.* The primary mineralocorticoid is **aldosterone,** and it stimulates the kidneys to absorb more sodium ($Na^+$) and water and excrete more potassium ($K^+$).

- *Glucocorticoids.* **Cortisone** is an example of a glucocorticoid. It acts to conserve the carbohydrate reserve by changing amino acids to simple sugars rather than to proteins. This conversion of amino acids to simple sugars helps to conserve carbohydrate reserves. This hormone is released in large quantities during times of stress, but the exact way it helps in stress situations

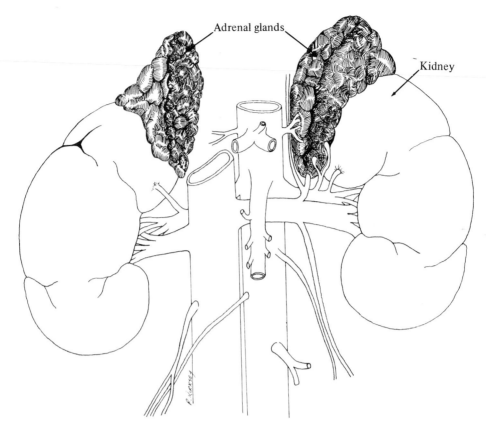

**Figure 6-9.** Each adrenal gland is located on the superior surface of each kidney.

is not clear. Cortisone and other glucocorticoids also are important since they act as antiinflammatory agents. They are useful in the treatment of inflammatory diseases such as arthritis, rheumatic fever, and acute kidney disease.

- *Sex hormones.* The sex hormones include both male and female hormones. The male sex hormone is testosterone, and the female sex hormones are estrogen and progesterone. These hormones and their functions will be discussed in more detail in Chapter 21.

**ADRENAL MEDULLA HORMONES.** The hormones of the adrenal medulla are **epinephrine** and **norepinephrine** (Figure 6-10). These hormones are similar in chemical structure, and their actions are similar but not identical. In general, their actions are the same as those of the sympathetic nervous system. They prepare the body to meet stress situations by stimulating certain systems and activities of the body and inhibiting others.

The secretion of these hormones is directly under the control of the sympathetic nervous system; the nervous and endocrine systems are dependent upon each other. The adrenal medulla and the hormones it secretes are good examples of this relationship. The sym-

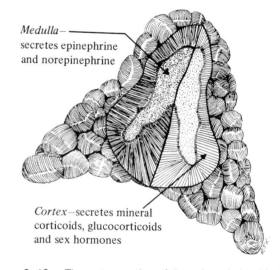

**Figure 6-10.** The outer portion of the adrenal gland is the cortex, and it secretes three groups of hormones. The inner portion is the medulla, and it secretes epinephrine and norepinephrine.

pathetic system stimulates the adrenal medulla to release epinephrine and norepinephrine; lack of sympathetic impulses inhibits the release of these hormones. These two hormones travel through the blood and coordinate activities of various effectors. **Norepinephrine** is the chemical transmitter released by the sympathetic postganglionic neurons. This means that norepinephrine is released by the adrenal medulla and sympathetic postganglionic neurons and serves to reinforce the actions of both the nervous and endocrine systems.

---

**HYPERSECRETION OF THE ADRENAL CORTEX.** *Cushing's disease* exhibits various symptoms that result from excessive amounts of glucocorticoids, mineralocorticoids, and sex hormones. The symptoms include an abnormal distribution of fat in the face (round moon face) and shoulders. The abdomen tends to enlarge considerably. The level of blood glucose increases considerably, probably because of the increased level of glucose production (glucocorticoids). This persistent high level of glucose can damage cells in the pancreas and lead to *diabetes mellitus.*

*Adrenogenital syndrome* results primarily from excessive amounts of sex hormones. The symptoms in a young male include early development of sexual organs (precocious puberty). In the female, the symptoms tend toward masculinization—excessive facial hair, atrophy of breast, enlargement of clitoris, and enlargement of skeletal muscles.

**HYPOSECRETION OF THE ADRENAL CORTEX.** *Addison's disease* results from tuberculosis organisms damaging the cortex of the adre-

---

nal glands. Some important signs and symptoms of this disease are increased blood potassium and decreased blood sodium (caused by lack of aldosterone), little resistance to infection, muscular weakness, fatigue, low blood pressure, and low blood sugar.

---

Table 6–3 summarizes the effects of the adrenal gland hormones.

## PANCREAS

The **pancreas** is a long, thin flattened organ. It is located inferior to the stomach and extends from the duodenum laterally to the spleen. The pancreas is both an endocrine and an exocrine gland. It secretes hormones (**endocrine function**) into the blood and digestive juices into the first part of the small intestine (**exocrine function**). The exocrine functions will be discussed in Chapter 19.

**HORMONES SECRETED BY PANCREAS.** Specialized cells scattered throughout the pancreas called **islands of Langerhans** (Figure 6–11) secrete hormones. Two types of cells, **alpha** and **beta,** each secrete a particular hormone.

*Insulin (beta cells).* **Insulin** is a very important hormone secreted by beta ($\beta$) cells (Figure 6–11). It functions in several ways:

**TABLE 6–3.** *Summary of Adrenal Gland Hormones*

| Region | Hormone | Function | Effects of Hyposecretion | Effects of Hypersecretion |
|---|---|---|---|---|
| Adrenal cortex | Aldosterone | Increases Na+ absorption<br>Decreases K+ absorption | Addison's disease<br>Increased Blood K+<br>Decreased Blood Na+ | Cushing's disease<br>Increased blood glucose<br>Enlarged abdomen<br>Abnormal deposition of fat in face and shoulders |
| | Cortisone | Changes amino acids to sugars (conserves carbohydrates)<br>Antiinflammatory | Muscular weakness<br>Fatigue<br>Low blood pressure<br>Low blood sugar | |
| | Male and female sex hormones | Influences secondary sexual characteristics | | Adrenogenital syndrome<br>Early development of sexual organs<br>Masculinization of features in females |
| Adrenal medulla | Epinephrine and nor-epinephrine | Prepares body to meet stress conditions | | |

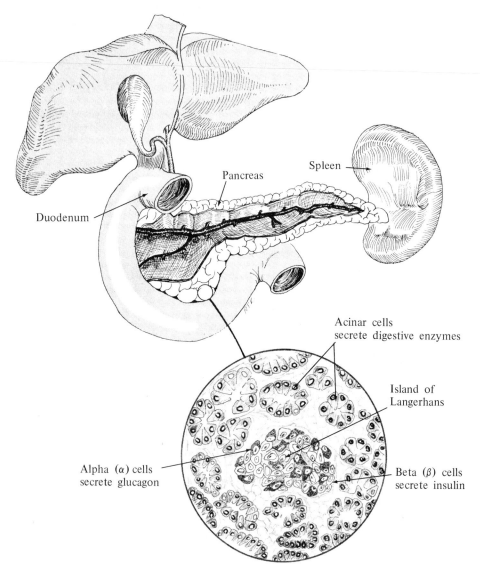

**Figure 6-11.** The structure and location of the pancreas are shown. Also shown is an Island of Langerhans with alpha (α) cells and beta (β) cells.

- **Aids entry of glucose into cells.** Glucose is the primary source of energy for cells, and insulin facilitates its passage into certain cells—liver, muscle, and fat. Other cells in the body do not require insulin to move glucose across their membranes.

- **Decreases blood glucose level.** Insulin helps to maintain a normal level of blood glucose by moving glucose from the blood into cells.

- **Inceases synthesis of glycogen in liver.** Insulin speeds up synthesis of glucose into glycogen in liver. Glycogen is composed of many glucose molecules and is the form in which glucose is stored until it is

needed. When glucose is needed, glycogen can be broken down to glucose molecules.

*Glucagon (alpha cells).* The **alpha cells** of the islands of Langerhans secrete the hormone, **glucagon.** Glucagon is carried by the blood to the liver where it accelerates the conversion of glycogen to glucose. Glucagon is released by the pancreas whenever the concentration of glucose drops to a certain level.

**REGULATION OF HORMONAL SECRETION FROM PANCREAS.** There are no hormones from the anterior pituitary that regulate the secretion of insulin and glucagon. Their secretion is regulated by the level of blood glucose that flows through the pancreas. When the level of blood glucose is high, the secretion of insulin is increased; glucagon secretion is increased when the level of glucose drops. These antagonistic hormones maintain a normal level of blood glucose. The word equations that express these relationships are

$$\downarrow \text{Blood glucose} = \uparrow \text{secretion of glucagon} = \uparrow \text{blood glucose}$$

$$\uparrow \text{Blood glucose} = \uparrow \text{secretion of insulin} = \downarrow \text{blood glucose}$$

**HYPOSECRETION OF INSULIN.** A lack of insulin means that less glucose can move into the cells; therefore, the blood glucose level will rise, causing hyperglycemia or diabetes mellitus. A diabetic must take daily injections of insulin to reduce the level of blood glucose.

**HYPERSECRETION OF INSULIN.** In some cases a tumor in the islands of Langerhans causes an overproduction of insulin. This means that more than the normal amount of glucose moves into the cells. This condition results in **hypoglycemia** (low blood sugar), which can lead to coma, convulsions, and death.

Table 6-4 summarizes the effects of pancreatic hormones.

## OVARIES AND TESTES

Earlier in the chapter we said that there were three hormones that controlled the growth, development, and secretion of the testes and ovaries (gonads); however, we did not discuss the gonads as endocrine glands. These glands and their hormones will be discussed in more detail in Chapter 21.

**TESTES.** The testes secrete the hormone **testosterone**. This hormone is responsible for the development of male secondary characteristics—deep voice, facial hair, pubic hair, and sex drive.

**OVARIES.** The ovaries produce **estrogen,** which is the female equivalent of testosterone. Estrogen stimulates the development of female secondary sex characteristics—enlargement of breast, widening of hips, pubic hair, lowering of voice, and beginning of menstruation.

**TABLE 6-4.** *Summary of Pancreas Hormones*

| HORMONE | FUNCTION | EFFECTS OF HYPOSECRETION | EFFECTS OF HYPERSECRETION |
|---|---|---|---|
| Insulin | Helps sugar enter cells (muscle, fat, and liver) Decreases blood glucose Increases glucose level in liver | Hyperglycemia or diabetes mellitus Increased urination High blood glucose Glucose in urine | Hypoglycemia Low blood glucose Weakness Easily fatigued Coma Convulsions |
| Glucagon | Increases level of blood glucose by breaking down glycogen | | |

# SUMMARY

**Characteristics of the Endocrine System**
Composed of ductless glands that secrete hormones; a hormone is a chemical messenger secreted into blood.

**Regulation of Hormone Secretion**
A. Blood chemicals: concentrations of certain chemicals stimulate or inhibit secretion of hormones.
   *Ex.*: drop in blood glucose results in increase in secretion of insulin by pancreas.

B. Nervous system (autonomic): release of epinephrine by adrenal gland is regulated by autonomic nervous system.
C. Negative feedback: secretion of hormones by several glands is inhibited or stimulated by level of another hormone.
    Ex.: level of thyroxin controlling amount of thyroid-stimulating hormone (TSH) released by anterior pituitary.

### Endocrine Glands: Their Hormones and Target Organs

A. Target organs: organ or group of organs stimulated by a hormone.
B. Pituitary gland: located at base of brain; composed of two lobes, anterior and posterior.
    1. Hormones of anterior pituitary
        a. Somatotrophic hormone (STH): promotes growth of tissues; hyposecretion results in dwarfism; hypersecretion results in giantism; hypersecretion in adult years, acromegaly.
        b. Gonadotrophic: FSH, LH, and LTH all affect growth, development, and secretion of gonads.
        c. Thyroid-stimulating hormone (TSH): growth, development, and secretion of thyroid gland.
        d. Adrenocorticotrophic hormone (ACTH): stimulates growth and development of cortex region of adrenal gland.
    2. Hormones of the posterior pituitary (neurohypophysis)
        a. Antidiuretic hormone (ADH): increases water absorption in kidneys.
        b. Oxytocin (pictocin): stimulates uterine muscles to contract forcefully to aid in birth of child.
C. Thyroid gland hormones
    1. Thyroxin ($T_4$) and Triiodothyronine ($T_3$) regulate release of heat and energy in body tissues or regulate body metabolism; hyposecretion results in cretinism of infant and myxedema in adult; hypersecretion results in increased BMR and exophthalmic goiter.
    2. Calcitonin: lowers blood calcium; stimulates absorption of calcium by bone tissue.
D. Parathyroid glands and hormones
    1. Four roundish bodies on posterior surface of thyroid gland.
        a. Parathyroid hormone (PTH). Stimulates bone tissue, kidneys, and small intestine in ways that raise blood calcium. Hyperparathyroidism results in large amount of calcium being released from bones, thereby weakening them; hypoparathyroidism, low blood calcium level results in muscle tetany.
E. Adrenal glands (suprarenal glands)
    1. Located on superior surface of kidneys.
    2. Adrenal cortex, stimulated by ACTH, secretes three groups of hormones: (a) mineralocorticoids: aldosterone stimulates kidneys to absorb $Na^+$ and excrete $K^+$; (b) glucocorticoids: cortisone conserves carbohydrates by changing amino acids to simple sugars; also functions as antiinflammatory agent; (c) sex hormones: testosterone.
        a. Hypersecretion of adrenal cortex
            (1) Cushing's disease, characterized by abnormal distribution of fat in face and shoulders; abdomen enlarges.
            (2) Adrenogenital syndrome: excessive levels of sex hormones; in males causes early development of sexual organs; in females causes development of masculine features (excessive facial hair and atrophy of breasts).
        b. Hyposecretion of adrenal cortex. Addison's disease: symptoms, increased blood potassium, decreased blood sodium, decreased resistance to infection, muscular weakness, fatigue, low blood pressure, and low blood sugar.
    3. Adrenal medulla: secretes epinephrine and norepinephrine; both prepare body to meet stress.

F. Pancreas

1. Long, thin flattened organ; inferior to stomach and extends from duodenum laterally to spleen.
2. Secretes insulin. Functions: (a) aids entry of glucose into cells, (b) decreases blood glucose level, (c) increases synthesis of glycogen in liver.
3. Secretes glucagon. Function: accelerates conversion of glycogen to glucose or increases blood glucose.
4. Regulation of hormonal secretion from pancreas: no hormones regulate release of hormones from pancreas; release is regulated by level of blood glucose:

$\downarrow$ Blood glucose = $\uparrow$ secretion of glucagon = $\uparrow$ blood glucose

$\uparrow$ Blood glucose = $\uparrow$ secretion of insulin   = $\downarrow$ blood glucose

## Endocrine System

Matching. Questions 1 to 5.

| | | | |
|---|---|---|---|
| **1.** | thyroxin (T$_4$) | **A.** | aids entry of glucose into cells |
| **2.** | posterior pituitary | **B.** | hyposecretion of adrenal cortex |
| **3.** | cortisone | **C.** | changes amino acids to glucose |
| **4.** | Addison's disease | **D.** | ADH and oxytocin |
| **5.** | insulin | **E.** | regulates body metabolism |

True (A) or false (B). Questions 6 to 10.

**6.** An increase in TSH results in an increased release of thyroxin.

**7.** The level of hormones is regulated by blood chemicals, autonomic nervous system, and positive feedback.

**8.** ACTH stimulates the release of norepinephrine from the adrenal medulla region.

**9.** PTH raises blood calcium and calcitonin lowers it.

**10.** Hormones secreted by the pancreas are regulated by the level of blood glucose.

In questions 11 to 14, circle the letter preceding the hormone that produces the given effect or condition.

**11.** High basal metabolic rate (BMR)

   (a). thyroxin
   (b). calcitonin

**12.** Low level of blood calcium

   (a). calcitonin
   (b). parathormone

**13.** Cushing's disease

   (a). mineralcorticoids
   (b). norepinephrine

**14.** Decrease in blood glucose level

   (a). glucagon
   (b). insulin

# Chapter 7

# THE BLOOD

After reading and studying this chapter, a student should be able to:

1. Name and give the function of each plasma protein.
2. Describe RBCs as to structure, number, and functions.
3. Describe the structure of hemoglobin molecules.
4. Give the name of each granular leukocyte along with its percent of all WBCs and function.
5. Name the nongranular leukocytes and give the percent and function of each.
6. Write a description of the three steps involved in blood clotting.
7. Describe each blood type as to which antigen (agglutinogen) and antibody (agglutinin) characterize it.
8. Describe the erythroblastosis fetalis condition as to the blood type of the fetus and mother; also discuss problems associated with an increase in Rh antibody titer.
9. Give the blood type that is known as the universal blood donor and universal recipient and discuss why they are designated as such.

# 1 GENERAL PROPERTIES OF BLOOD

**Blood** is classified as a connective tissue. It is composed of a liquid matrix called **plasma** and **cells** suspended in the plasma that are called **formed elements.** Blood also is classified as a chemical mixture. It is composed of many chemical compounds that are not chemically combined, and these compounds can be separated by physical and chemical means. Blood tests are based on the fact that the components can be separated.

The types of cells are red blood corpuscles (RBC), white blood cells (WBC), and platelets (thrombocytes). The plasma composes 55 percent of the blood and the formed elements 45 percent.

The **quantity** of blood circulating in the body is approximately 4 to 5 liters or about 7 percent of the body weight.

The **pH** of blood is between 7.35 and 7.45. The **specific gravity** of blood refers to the weight of a certain volume of blood compared to the weight of the same volume of water. The specific gravity of water is 1.000. The normal specific gravity of whole blood is between 1.055 and 1.065. Whole blood is heavier than water because of the formed elements and the chemical compounds dissolved in plasma.

The **hematocrit** is the percentage of formed elements in the blood. A hematocrit is measured by centrifuging a quantity of whole blood and measuring the percentage of formed elements (Figure 7–1). For example, a tube containing 10 cc of blood is centrifuged and the formed elements, in the bottom of the tube, make up 4.0 cc of the entire 10 cc of blood. The hematocrit of this person is 40 percent. The clear fluid above the formed elements is called plasma.

A normal hematocrit indicates that a person has the

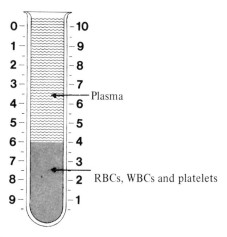

**Figure 7–1.** Hematocrit. The percentage of formed elements in a tube represents 40% formed elements and, therefore, the hematocrit is 40.

proper amount of cells, especially red blood cells. An abnormally low hematocrit indicates a lower number of cells, and this is called an **anemic** condition. The normal hematocrit values are, female, 38 to 45 percent; male, 42 to 50 percent. Values lower than these indicate a person is anemic or has a lower than normal number of formed elements.

# 2 CHEMICAL COMPONENTS OF PLASMA

Plasma contains many chemicals, some of which are vital for its protective functions. Ninety percent of plasma is water. The other 10 percent is composed of proteins, nutritive materials, electrolytes, gases, waste products, hormones, antibodies, and enzymes.

## PLASMA PROTEINS

Four important proteins are found in plasma. The liver is the primary source of all of them. These proteins carry out their functions only in the plasma and do not move into the tissue cells.

**Fibrinogen** is produced by the liver and circulates in a liquid form. It plays an important role in the clotting of blood, when it is changed into an insoluble form.

**Prothrombin** is produced by the liver, if an adequate amount of vitamin K is available. This protein also is important in the clotting process.

**Albumin** is the third of the four proteins produced by the liver. This is the most prevalent protein in blood plasma. It is the primary colloid in determining **colloidal osmotic pressure.** This is the "pulling force" that acts to pull fluids and materials from the interstitial compartment into the plasma compartment through the venous end of capillaries. This protein primarily functions to maintain a constant level of fluid in the plasma compartment. It may be administered intravenously, following a hemorrhage, to increase the colloidal osmotic pressure, thereby increasing the blood volume as more fluid is pulled into the plasma compartment.

The last plasma protein, **globulin,** circulates in the plasma in three forms—alpha, beta, and gamma. Gamma globulin is the only form not produced by the liver. It is formed by plasma cells that make up the **reticuloendothelial system (RES).** Gamma globulin functions as an antibody combining with and inactivating antigens that invade the body. The alpha and beta forms do not function in protective roles.

## NUTRITIVE MATERIALS

The nutritive materials include the basic chemical building blocks of proteins (amino acids), lipids (fatty acids and glycerol), and carbohydrates (glucose, fructose, and galactose). These materials move from the plasma compartment into the cells.

## ELECTROLYTES OR IONS

Cations and anions are transported by plasma. These ions are involved in a multitude of activities such as muscle contractions, transmission of nerve impulses, and acid–base buffer reactions. The concentration of these electrolytes makes up the electrolyte balance, which is vital for maintenance of homeostasis.

## GASES

Three gases dissolve in and are transported by the plasma. A small amount of oxygen gas and a large amount of carbon dioxide, in the form of bicarbonate ($HCO_3^-$) ions and sodium and potassium bicarbonate compounds ($Na^+HCO_3^-$ and $K^+HCO_3^-$), are carried in the plasma. Nitrogen gas is transported in the plasma but has no physiologic role in the body.

## WASTE PRODUCTS

Various waste products that result from chemical reactions are transported to the kidneys for excretion. Some examples of waste products are uric acid, urea, and lactic acid. Plasma carries these compounds to the glomeruli in the Bowman's capsules, where the waste materials are removed from the blood by filtration.

## HORMONES

The numerous hormones produced by the endocrine glands are transported by plasma to the target organs. Plasma also transports hormones to the liver, where they are broken down after they have stimulated the various target organs.

## ANTIBODIES

The plasma cells of the reticuloendothelial system manufacture antibodies in the form of immunoglobulin (Ig) proteins.

## ENZYMES

Plasma carries enzymes to many different areas of the body where they function to speed up the rate of chemical reactions.

# 3  FORMED ELEMENTS: THE BLOOD CELLS

## *RED BLOOD CORPUSCLES (RBCs) OR ERYTHROCYTES*

Red blood corpuscles (RBCs) are small biconcave discs (Figure 7–2) that are very flexible. They also are referred to as erythrocytes and red blood cells. The term red corpuscle means "red body." This term scientifically is more accurate than red blood cell, since the mature red blood corpuscles lack a nucleus.

Erythrocytes number 4.5 to 5.5 million per cubic millimeter of blood, and there are approximately 5000 ml of blood in a person. This means that there is a total of approximately 25 trillion RBCs in the blood at any one time. Millions of the RBCs are being destroyed every second of each day; however, millions constantly are being formed to replace them. Mature RBCs lack a nucleus; therefore, they cannot reproduce themselves.

**PRODUCTION OF RED BLOOD CORPUSCLES: ERYTHROPOIESIS.**  In the developing fetus, RBCs are produced by the liver, spleen, and bone marrow; however, when a child is born, RBC production is limited only to red bone marrow. Almost every bone has functional red bone marrow until a person becomes an adult. At this point red bone marrow, in long bones, is limited to the **proximal epiphyses** (Figure 7–3) of the femur and humerus. In addition, functional red bone marrow and production of RBCs occur in the sternum, os coxae, ribs, cranial bones, clavicles, and vertebrae.

**FACTORS THAT REGULATE RBC PRODUCTION.**  The oxygen need of the tissues is a primary fac-

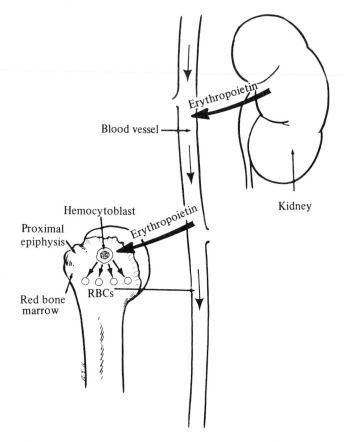

**Figure 7–3.**  Influence of erythropoietin on RBC production.

tor that stimulates the production of RBCs. As the level of oxygen in the body drops or as the body needs more oxygen, a compound called **erythropoietin** is released from the kidneys (Figure 7–3) into the blood. It is carried to bone marrow where it stimulates RBC development from **hemocytoblasts.** The production and maturation of RBCs also is called **erythropoiesis.** The increased production of RBCs increases the oxygen-carrying capacity of the blood to satisfy the needs of the tissues.

Vitamin $B_{12}$ is important for the proper maturation of RBCs from hemocytoblasts. Vitamin $B_{12}$ is ingested in the food we eat and is synthesized by bacteria in the large intestine. It is stored in the liver until needed by the bone marrow.

**DESTRUCTION OF RBCs.**  The life span of RBCs is approximately 90 to 120 days. They are subjected to much wear and tear as they pass through narrow capillaries in single file fashion, as well as through the heart, arteries, and veins. The RBC membrane finally wears out, at which time either it ruptures or the entire

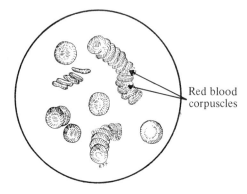

**Figure 7–2.**  Red blood corpuscles, showing the biconcave disc shape.

RBC is digested. Most of the RBC destruction occurs in the spleen, liver, and bone marrow by **reticuloendothelial cells.** The iron in the hemoglobin molecules is not broken apart and is sent to the red bone marrow for future RBC production. The remainder of the hemoglobin is converted to **bilirubin,** which is excreted by the liver in bile. If the liver does not excrete bilirubin properly, the quantity builds up and spills over into the bloodstream. This causes the skin to become yellowish and the condition is called **jaundice.**

**HEMOGLOBIN.** About one-third of the weight of every RBC is hemoglobin. Hemoglobin is a complex protein molecule that is composed of four subunits (Figure 7–4). Each subunit is composed of a simple protein, **globin,** which is attached to a pigment called **heme,** which contains iron ($Fe^{2+}$). It is the iron portion of each subunit that combines with the one oxygen molecule to form **oxyhemoglobin.** Since each hemoglobin molecule contains four iron ($Fe^{2+}$) atoms, each hemoglobin can combine with four oxygen molecules. A single RBC contains 200 to 300 million hemoglobin molecules, and each molecule can transport four molecules of oxygen. In other words, each RBC has a tremendous oxygen-carrying capacity.

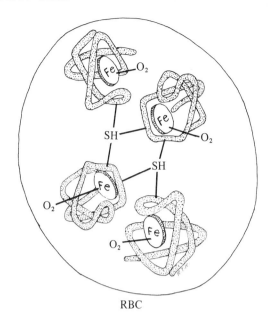

RBC

**Figure 7–4.** Hemoglobin molecule. Hemoglobin is a protein that is composed of four subunits, each containing $Fe^{2+}$. $O_2$ molecules bind with the $Fe^{2+}$ of each subunit.

and loosely combines with the iron ($Fe^{2+}$) of hemoglobin. Oxygen also is transported in a dissolved form in the plasma. Chemical reactions and details concerning the reactions of $O_2$ with hemoglobin and buffers will be discussed in Chapter 16.

Second, the RBCs function in carbon dioxide transport. Carbon dioxide diffuses into RBCs and is transported in two ways. Most of it dissolves and is transported as sodium bicarbonate ($NaHCO_3$) and potassium bicarbonate ($KHCO_3$). Some of the carbon dioxide combines with hemoglobin to form **carboxyhemoglobin.** Details of these chemical reactions will be discussed in Chapter 16.

---

Anemia is a condition in which the number of RBCs or hemoglobin is below normal. Three common types of anemia are pernicious, iron deficiency, and sickle-cell anemia.

Pernicious anemia is a reduction in RBC production as a result of a decrease in vitamin $B_{12}$. The decrease results from the stomach not secreting an intrinsic factor, which is responsible for the absorption of vitamin $B_{12}$ into the blood.

Iron deficiency anemia is a decrease in hemoglobin production as a result of an inadequate amount of iron for RBC synthesis. The deficiency of iron in the blood frequently results from an inadequate amount in the diet, bleeding ulcers, and infants fed milk formulas without iron supplements.

Sickle-cell anemia is a hereditary disease characterized by the affected RBCs having a sickle or half-moon shape. This shape causes the RBCs to clump and rupture more easily than normal RBCs, resulting in anemia.

---

**FUNCTIONS OF RED BLOOD CORPUSCLES.** First, RBCs are involved in oxygen transport. Most of the oxygen that diffuses into blood moves into RBCs

## WHITE BLOOD CELLS: LEUKOCYTES

WBCs are larger than RBCs, and they contain a nucleus. They lack hemoglobin; therefore, they are not able to transport oxygen and carbon dioxide. WBCs number from 5000 to 10,000 per cubic millimeter of blood. Some are capable of moving out of capillaries (**diapedesis**) into tissues to attack microbes, and thereby help protect the body against disease.

There are two groups of WBCs, and they are distinguished from each other by the presence or absence of granules in the cytoplasm. The two groups are granular and nongranular leukocytes (Figure 7–5).

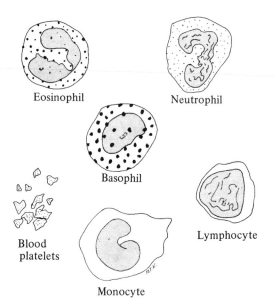

Figure 7-5. Leukocytes and platelets. The characteristic shapes of the three granular leukocytes (above) and non-granular leukocytes (below) are shown. The irregularly shaped blood platelets are also shown.

## Granular Leukocytes (Granulocytes)

This group contains granules in the cytoplasm of the cells, and their nuclei are lobed or branched. All the granular leukocytes are produced in the red bone marrow. The different types of granular leukocytes (granulocytes) are distinguished from each other by the type of stain that reacts with their granular cytoplasm.

- **Neutrophils** react with a neutral pH stain. The nucleus usually has three to four lobes. Approximately 60 to 70 percent of all WBCs are neutrophils. They easily move through the pores in capillary membranes by **diapedesis** into the tissues, where they attack foreign matter. Neutrophils are an important WBC in that they are ferocious phagocytes.

- **Eosinophils** react with an acid dye called **eosin.** They have a two-lobed nucleus with coarser granules than neutrophils. They form only 1 to 3 percent of all the WBCs. Eosinophils apparently act like antibodies to neutralize foreign **antigens** (proteins) that enter the blood. Evidence indicates that they may play a role in alleviating an allergic condition. Their role is not clear, but one theory is that an allergic condition causes the release of toxic materials, and possibly the eosinophils act to neutralize the toxins.

- **Basophils** react with basic dyes. Their nucleus is S-shaped and they constitute only 0.5 to 1.0 percent of all the WBCs. Their main function is the secretion of **heparin,** which is a compound that prevents blood from clotting.

## Nongranular Leukocytes (Agranulocytes)

This group lacks granules in the cytoplasm, and their nuclei are not branched. Nongranular leukocytes are formed in the lymph nodes and spleen.

- **Lymphocytes** are smaller than the other WBCs. Their nucleus occupies almost the entire volume of the cell, with only a thin layer of cytoplasm visible. Lymphocytes comprise 20 to 35 percent of the total number of WBCs. Lymphocytes primarily function as plasma cells to secrete antibodies. They also have an unusual ability to convert themselves into other cells, such as **monocytes** and **hemocytoblasts.**

- **Monocytes** are the largest of all the blood cells. Their nucleus may be round to kidney shaped. Monocytes constitute only 3 to 8 percent of the total number of WBCs. Monocytes function as phagocytes, exactly like neutrophils. However, monocytes are produced in the lymph nodes and spleen. After monocytes are formed, they rapidly move by diapedesis into tissue spaces to attack microbes and foreign materials. They are present in smaller numbers than neutrophils, but each monocyte can engulf and phagocytize as many as 100 microbes.

> Leukemia is a cancerous condition of the bone marrow. The cancerous cells cause a large production of white blood cells. Since only a certain number of blood cells can be circulated in blood plasma, the large number of WBCs reduces the number of circulating RBCs, thereby resulting in anemia.

The method by which neutrophils and monocytes move through capillary membranes is called **diapedesis.** This process involves the neutrophil and monocyte cells squeezing through pores of the endothelial lining of the capillaries (Figure 7-6). They move through the pores and into the tissues in an amoeboidlike movement. Some degree of diapedesis goes on all the time, but it increases considerably in the

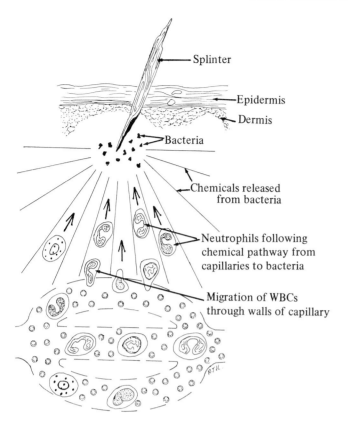

**Figure 7-6.** Diapedesis and chemotaxis. White blood cells are shown moving out of the capillaries and following a chemical pathway back to bacteria.

presence of an infection or when an injury occurs. Research indicates that these phagocytes are attracted to bacteria and pathogens by chemicals released from damaged cells. This type of attraction is called **chemotaxis.** The chemicals serve as a chemical trail, and the neutrophils and monocytes follow the trail to the bacteria or pathogens and destroy them by phagocytosis.

## BLOOD PLATELETS (THROMBOCYTES)

**Platelets** or **thrombocytes** are the third type of formed element found in the blood. Blood platelets are fragments of cells that do not have a definite shape (Figure 7-5). They lack a nucleus and color. Platelets contain a substance that functions to initiate clotting of blood. Their role in clotting will be discussed shortly. The number of platelets in the body varies from 200,000 to 400,000 per cubic millimeter. They are formed in red bone marrow from **megakaryocytes,** and have a life span of five to nine days. At the end of their life span they are destroyed by the reticuloendothelial system, especially in the spleen.

Table 7-1 summarizes information about blood cells.

## TABLE 7-1.  Blood Cells

| Name of Cell | Number in Plasma | Where Produced | Function |
|---|---|---|---|
| RBC (erythrocyte) | 4.5 to 5.5 million/mm³ | Red bone marrow | Oxygen transport Carbon dioxide transport Buffer action |
| White Blood Cells (leukocytes) | 5000 to 10,000/mm³ | | |
| A.  Granular | | | |
| 1. Neutrophils | 60% to 70% of all WBCs | Red bone marrow | Phagocytosis |
| 2. Eosinophils | 1% to 3% of all WBCs | Red bone marrow | Help alleviate allergic conditions |
| 3. Basophils | 0.5% to 1.0% of all WBCs. | Red bone marrow | Secrete heparin |
| B.  Nongranular | | | |
| 1. Lymphocytes | 20% to 35% of all WBCs | Lymph nodes | Secrete antibodies |
| 2. Monocytes | 3% to 8% of all WBCs | Lymph nodes and spleen | Phagocytosis |

# 4 BLOOD CLOTTING

The formation of a blood clot inhibits the normal flow of blood. Normally, blood does not clot in blood vessels due to the anticlotting compound, heparin, which is produced by the liver and also released from basophils. Blood clotting does protect against blood loss when vessels have been cut or ruptured. When hemorrhaging begins, several chemical compounds interact to form a clot in about 3 to 7 minutes. The clot acts to plug up the opening and prevent further blood loss.

## Steps in the Blood-Clotting Process

The steps in the blood-clotting process essentially involve the conversion of the proteins **prothrombin** and **fibrinogen** into an insoluble compound, *fibrin*.

**Step 1** is the formation and release of **thromboplastin**. To explain how it is formed, let us assume that you have received a jagged cut on the upper arm (Figure 7-7). As the platelets (thrombocytes) come in contact with the rough edges of the blood vessels and skin, they disintegrate and release the "blood platelet factor." Calcium ions and the antihemophilic factor react with the blood factor to form thromboplastin. Thromboplastin also is released by damaged tissue cells.

**Step 2** involves **thromboplastin** interacting with **prothrombin** to form **thrombin**. Calcium ions and other factors are necessary to speed up this reaction. Thromboplastin acts as a catalyst to convert prothrombin into thrombin.

**Step 3** is the interaction of **thrombin** with the soluble **fibrinogen** protein to form **fibrin** threads. Thrombin acts as a catalyst to convert fibrinogen into fibrin. These fibrous threads become entangled at the point of injury and actually form the clot. Red blood corpuscles become trapped in this clot and the flow of blood stops.

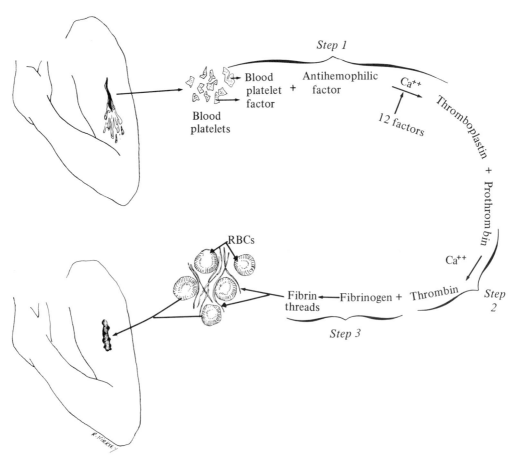

**Figure 7-7.** The three steps involved in the blood-clotting process as soluble proteins are converted into the insoluble protein fibrin.

*Important Point About Clotting*

The process of blood clotting involves the conversion of two plasma proteins, prothrombin and fibrinogen, into solid fibrous threads. Prothrombin and fibrinogen are produced by the liver. The formation of thromboplastin and thrombin, in addition to calcium ions and plasma factors, is vital for the conversion of prothrombin and fibrinogen, since they function as catalysts.

# 5  NORMAL PREVENTION OF CLOTTING

All the components for clotting circulate in the blood at all times and one might ask why the blood does not clot constantly. There are two reasons why the blood normally does not clot in blood vessels. The first reason is that the inner surface of blood vessels is smooth and wet. Platelets do not stick to it, and, therefore, they do not rupture and release their clot-initiating substance (blood platelet factor). The second reason is the presence of two anticlotting substances, **heparin** and **antithrombin. Heparin** is produced by the liver and other organs. It inhibits clotting in two ways: (1) It prevents **thrombin** from converting **fibrinogen** to **fibrin** (Figure 7–7). (2) It inhibits the conversion of **prothrombin** to **thrombin.**

# 6  ARTIFICIAL ANTICLOTTING CHEMICALS

Blood can still clot after it has been removed from the body. Various compounds are used to prevent clotting outside the body. Oxalate and citrate salts prevent clotting of blood by precipitating out calcium in the form of **calcium oxalate** and **calcium citrate.** Calcium ions play a vital role in the clotting process, and with them absent, clotting is inhibited.

Artificial preparations of heparin are administered to patients to reduce the formation of blood clots. The action of heparin is immediate but short-lived. **Dicumarol** is another artificial drug that can be administered to reduce clotting. Vitamin K is needed by the liver to produce the clotting protein prothrombin. Dicumarol interferes with vitamin K, thereby preventing synthesis of prothrombin. In contrast to **heparin,** dicumarol does not take effect for 48 hours.

# 7  BLOOD TRANSFUSIONS AND BLOOD GROUPS

A person who has lost a considerable amount of blood must receive a transfusion to maintain the normal level of blood. The person either can receive plasma or whole blood. Plasma can be transfused immediately, but it is not as desirable as whole blood since it does not contain any blood cells. If whole blood is transfused then the blood of the **donor** (person from whom the blood is removed) and **recipient** (person receiving the whole blood) must be crossmatched to make sure their bloods are compatible. The term **compatible bloods** means that the blood types of the donor and recipient are such that clumping will not occur when their bloods are mixed.

What makes bloods incompatible is the interaction of antigens and antibodies. Specific proteins are attached to the membranes (Figure 7–8) of red blood corpuscles (RBCs), and they are called **antigens** or **agglutinogens.** The most important antigens are designated as A, B, and Rh. In the blood plasma are found **antibodies** or **agglutinins** whose names correspond to the antigens. The antibodies are designated as *a* and *b*.

## BLOOD GROUPS

Blood groups are named according to the antigens that are attached to the RBCs. There are four different blood types: A, B, O, and AB.

A blood type is always designated with a capital letter according to the antigen or antigens that are present. Blood type O can be thought of as blood type "zero" since it contains no antigens; however, it does contain both antibodies, a and b.

Blood type AB contains both A and B antigens but no antibodies. Notice in Table 7–2 that each blood type contains the opposite antibody compared to the antigen that is present. This is vital, because if compatible antigens and antibodies come in contact, clumping of blood occurs. For example, if blood type A is mixed with blood type B, the A antigens combine with a antibodies. Also the B antigens combine with b antibodies. Figure 7–8 shows that antigens protrude from RBCs, and when compatible antigens and antibodies combine, protruding structures are formed. These structures prevent RBCs from flowing past each other and, as a result, the RBCs begin to aggregate or clump together.

Previously, we mentioned that prior to a blood trans-

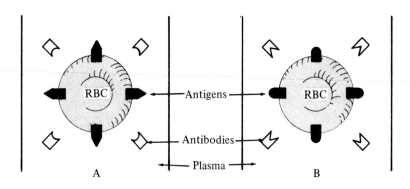

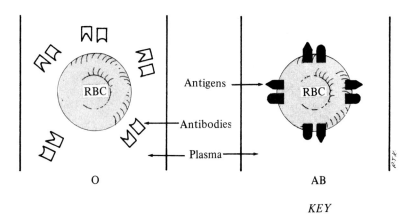

KEY

Antigen or                    Antibody or
agglutinogen                  agglutinin

◗ A          Σ a

◖ B          ⊐ b

**Figure 7-8.** The four ABO blood types along with their corresponding anti-bodies. A person's blood type is determined by which antigens are present on the RBCs.

### TABLE 7-2. Blood Types

| Type | Percentage of Occurrence | Agglutinogen (Antigen) | Agglutinin (Antibody) |
|---|---|---|---|
| A | 41 | A | b |
| B | 10 | B | a |
| O | 45 | None | a and b |
| (Type O is the universal donor) | 4 | A and B | None |
| AB | | | |
| (Type AB is the universal recipient) | | | |
| RH⁺ | 85 | Rh | None |
| Rh⁻ | 15 | None | None |

fusion the donor's and recipient's blood must be crossmatched to be sure that the bloods are compatible. The bloods are compatible if they do not contain complementary antigens and antibodies. For example, blood type A can be transfused with blood type A because they do not contain complementary antigens and antibodies; however, if blood types A and B were mixed (Figure 7–9), complementary antigens and antibodies would combine and clumping would result. Clumping of blood cells can be fatal, since the transport of oxygen and carbon dioxide by RBCs cannot take place.

The other protein that may be attached to RBCs is the Rh antigen. If the antigen is present, a person is said to be Rh⁺; and if it is not, a person is said to be Rh⁻. When crossmatching of bloods is done, the presence or absence of the Rh antigen has to be determined, in addition to that of the A and B antigen. For example, if the donor had A⁺ blood and the recipient A⁻, the donor's blood contains the Rh antigen, and the recipient's blood does not contain Rh antigens. In this case the recipient's blood would form antibodies that would react with the antigens from the donor's blood. However, if the donor were A⁻ and the recipient A⁺, there would be no reaction because the donor's blood contains no Rh antigens, and the recipient's blood already has Rh antigens present.

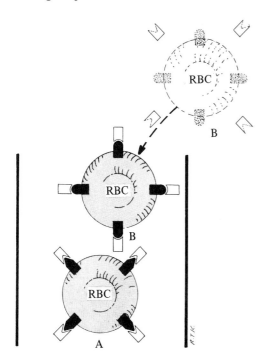

**Figure 7–9.** Transfusion of incompatible bloods. The reactions of antigens and antibodies between two incompatible bloods, types A and B, are shown when they are transfused. The protruding structures from the RBCs cause them to interact and clump.

There are two ways that an Rh⁻ person's blood can become sensitized to Rh⁺ antigens and thereby produce antibodies that will react with the antigens. One way is that an Rh⁻ person receives a transfusion of Rh⁺ blood. This is highly unlikely since the bloods will be crossmatched before transfusion. The second way is when the blood of a developing embryo which is Rh⁺ mixes with the blood of a mother who is Rh⁻. During the development of the child, the Rh antigen can diffuse from the child's blood into the mother's blood. The mother's blood then will become sensitized and will produce Rh antibodies to combat the Rh antigens. The antibodies can diffuse into the child's blood and react with the antigens, thereby destroying the RBCs. The destruction of the child's RBCs probably will not occur with the first child because the concentration of Rh antibodies produced by the mother usually is too low; however, the concentration of antibodies can increase to dangerous levels with the second and third Rh⁺ children. A reaction between the Rh antibodies of the mother and RBCs of the child is called **erythroblastosis fetalis.** The reaction causes clumping and rupturing of the RBCs in the developing embryo. The oxygen-carrying capacity of the blood is lowered considerably, and the hemoglobin that is released is transformed into the yellow pigment, bilirubin. These reactions often are fatal, and the child is born dead. If a wife is Rh⁻ and her husband is Rh⁺, there is a possibility that an embryo will inherit the Rh⁺ trait from the father, thereby possibly creating an erythroblastosis fetalis condition. If this does occur, it is now possible to prevent the buildup of Rh antibodies in the mother's blood by early drug treatments.

## 8 UNIVERSAL DONOR AND UNIVERSAL RECIPIENT BLOOD GROUPS

Blood type O negative (O⁻) is the universal blood donor type. This means it can be transfused into anyone's blood without agglutination occurring. This universal donor contains no A and B antigens or Rh antigens. It cannot react with a or b antibodies or cause production of Rh antibodies.

Blood type AB positive (AB⁺) is the universal blood recipient. It does contain all three types of antigens, A, B, and Rh; but it contains no a and b antibodies to react with the RBCs of the donor. The AB positive blood already contains Rh antigens; therefore, it will not produce Rh antibodies if Rh positive blood is introduced.

# SUMMARY

### General Properties
Classified as connective tissue; liquid matrix called plasma; cells called formed elements; quantity, 4 to 5 liters; pH = 7.35 to 7.45; hematocrit is percentage of formed elements in blood.

### Chemical Components of Plasma
A. Plasma proteins: (1) fibrinogen, important for clotting; (2) prothrombin, important for clotting; (3) albumin, most common protein and determines colloidal osmotic pressure; (4) globulin, functions as antibody in providing immunity.
B. Nutritive materials: amino acids, fatty acids and glycerol, and carbohydrates.
C. Electrolytes or ions: involved in muscle contractions, transmission of nerve impulses, and acid–base buffer reactions.
D. Gases: oxygen, carbon dioxide, and nitrogen are transported through blood.
E. Waste products: urea, uric acid, and lactic acid are transported by blood to excretory organs.
F. Hormones: all hormones are transported to target organs by blood.
G. Antibodies: immunoglobulin (Ig) proteins carried throughout body by blood.
H. Enzymes: many enzymes are found in blood.

### Formed Elements: The Blood Cells
A. RBCs or erythrocytes. Biconcave discs; 4.5 to 5.5 million/mm$^3$ of blood.
   1. Erythropoiesis: RBCs produced by liver, spleen, and bone marrow in fetus; in adults only the proximal epiphysis of some long bones.
      a. Factors that regulate erythropoiesis: decrease in oxygen stimulates release of erythropoietin, which increases erythropoiesis.
      b. Destruction of RBCs; life span of RBCs is 90 to 120 days; occurs in spleen, liver, and bone marrow; iron is recovered and reused, whereas remainder of hemoglobin is converted to bilirubin and excreted in bile.
      c. Hemoglobin: about one-third of the weight of RBC is hemoglobin; composed of four subunits, each composed of globin protein and pigment heme, which contains iron.
      d. Functions of RBCs: (1) transport of $O_2$, (2) transport $CO_2$ in form of carboxyhemoglobin, (3) buffering action.
B. White blood cells: leukocytes. Larger than RBCs; contain nucleus; 5000 to 10,000/mm$^3$ of blood.
   1. Granular leukocytes. Cells contain granules in cytoplasm, their nuclei are branched or lobed; produced in red bone marrow.
      a. Neutrophils: nucleus has three to four lobes; compose 60 to 70 percent of all WBCs. Function: phagocytosis.
      b. Eosinophils: two-lobed nucleus; make up 1 to 3 percent of WBCs. Function: neutralize antigens and help alleviate allergic conditions.
      c. Basophils: S-shaped nucleus; compose 0.5 to 1.0 percent of WBCs. Function: secretion of heparin.
   2. Nongranular leukocytes: cells lack granules in cytoplasm; nuclei not branched; formed in lymph nodes and spleen.
      a. Lymphocytes: smallest of WBCs; comprise 20 to 35 percent of all WBCs. Function: secrete antibodies.
      b. Monocytes: largest WBC; constitute 3 to 8 percent of WBCs. Function: phagocytosis.
C. Blood platelets (thrombocytes): fragments of cells; 200,000 to 400,000/mm$^3$; formed in red bone marrow from megakaryocytes. Function: blood clotting.

## Blood Clotting

Steps in blood-clotting process: (1) blood platelet factor plus antihemophilic factor and $Ca^{2+}$ result in formation of thromboplastin; (2) thromboplastin plus prothrombin results in formation of thrombin; (3) thrombin plus fibrinogen results in formation of fibrin threads.

## Normal Prevention of Clotting

Blood normally does not clot for two reasons: (1) inner surface of blood vessels is smooth and wet, therefore, platelets do not rupture and initiate clotting; (2) heparin and antithrombin inhibit clotting.

## Artificial Anticlotting Chemicals

Oxalate, citrate salts, and dicumarol prevent clotting of blood once it has been removed from body.

## Blood Transfusions and Blood Groups

A. Transfusions can be either plasma or whole blood; if plasma transfused, it must be crossmatched to avoid clumping of donor and recipient bloods.
B. Clumping results from interaction of like antigens and antibodies.
C. Blood groups: blood groups or types are named according to the antigens (agglutinogens) A, B, and Rh that are attached to an RBC membrane; if like antibodies (found in plasma) combine with like antigens, clumping of blood occurs (e.g., antigen A and antibody a). If Rh antigen is present, person is said to have positive blood; if absent, the blood is designated as negative.
D. Erythroblastosis fetalis: condition where pregnant woman is $Rh^-$ and fetus is $Rh^+$. Mixing of the two bloods results in mother producing antibodies against fetus's RBCs, which have Rh antigen; the end result can be destruction of fetal RBCs by mother's antibodies; usually does not occur with first $Rh^+$ baby but rather with second and third $Rh^+$ child.

## Universal Donor and Universal Recipient Blood Groups

A. Blood type O negative ($O^-$) is the universal blood donor type; it can be added to any blood type that is either + or − without fear of clumping; AB positive ($AB^+$) is universal recipient since it contains no antibodies to react with RBCs of any donor.

## The Blood

Matching

1. RBCs      **A.** oxygen and $CO_2$ transport plus buffering action
2. WBCs     **B.** percentage of formed elements in blood
3. platelets   **C.** help initiate blood clotting
4. erythropoiesis   **D.** functions include phagocytosis, immunity, and alleviate allergic conditions
5. hematocrit   **E.** none of these

True (A) or false (B). Questions 6 to 10.

6. Blood types are named according to which agglutinogens are present on RBC membranes.

7. Agglutination or clumping of donor and recipient's blood occurs when A antigen and b antibody combine.

8. Blood type B $^+$ means that a person has B agglutinogens on the RBC membrane and a agglutinins in plasma, plus Rh antigens on membrane.

9. Blood clotting involves three steps and the conversion of soluble prothrombin and fibrinogen proteins into an insoluble fibrin protein clot.

10. Erythroblastosis fetalis involves a Rh $^+$ mother and Rh $^-$ fetus and production of Rh antibodies by the fetus.

11. Which of the following is(are) incorrectly paired?
    **(a)** Neutrophils   — phagocytosis
    **(b)** Eosinophils   — secretion of heparin
    **(c)** Basophils    — alleviate allergic conditions
    **(d)** (a), (c)
    **(e)** (b), (c)

# Chapter 8

# THE CARDIOVASCULAR SYSTEM

After reading and studying this chapter, a student should be able to:

1. Write a description of the layers of the heart, heart valves, atria, and ventricles.
2. Describe the cardiac cycle as to diastole and systole.
3. Trace the path a nerve impulse follows through the heart.
4. Describe the P, Q, R, S, and T waves in an ECG measurement.
5. State the function and describe the layers of an artery, vein, and capillary.
6. Recognize a description of systemic, hepatic portal, and pulmonary circulatory units.
7. Describe how precapillary sphincters regulate peripheral resistance and thereby blood pressure.
8. Name and describe the five factors involved in the maintenance of arterial blood pressure.
9. Describe what the arterial pulse indicates.
10. Name the two reflex centers and describe their functions.
11. Describe the rate of blood flow in arteries and capillaries.

*In Chapters 5 and 6 we discussed how the nervous and endocrine systems function to coordinate the other organ systems to maintain and restore homeostasis. The cardiovascular system aids the endocrine and nervous systems by transporting nutrients ($H_2O$, $O_2$, sugars, electrolytes, and others) to the cells of the various tissues. The nutrients are exchanged for wastes produced by the cells ($CO_2$, ammonia, and others). The wastes are transported to the appropriate organs where they are eliminated from the body. In the discussions of the systems that follow, the arteries that transport nutrients, and veins that carry wastes from each system will be discussed.*

# 1 THE CARDIOVASCULAR SYSTEM

The **cardiovascular system** is composed of organs that circulate fluids through the body. These organs and their functions are as follows:

- *Heart* (pump): This organ, composed of cardiac muscle tissue, pumps blood through the arteries, veins, and capillaries.
- *Artery* (tube): An artery is a muscular tube that carries blood away from the heart to the capillaries. This tube primarily carries nutrients to the capillaries.
- *Capillary* (tube): A capillary is a minute, thin-walled, branched tubular organ that connects arteries to veins. It is the functional unit of the cardiovascular system, since the exchange of nutrients and wastes occurs here. Blood flows from the arterial end to the venous end of a capillary, and the exchange of nutrients and wastes occurs through the walls of the capillary.
- *Vein* (tube): A vein is a muscular, tubular-shaped organ that carries blood from capillaries to the heart. Primarily, it drains blood, containing waste materials, toward the heart (pump). The heart pumps blood to various organs (lungs and kidneys) that excrete the waste material.

The cardiovascular system is a closed system. The contractions of the heart generate blood pressure, which is vital for the movement of blood and exchange of materials. The anatomy, physiology, diseases, and malfunctions of these organs will be discussed next.

## ANATOMY OF THE HEART

The heart is a four-chambered muscular organ that is somewhat larger than a clenched fist. It is located between the lungs in the mediastinum space of the thoracic cavity. It is cone shaped with the **apex** (pointed end) of the heart directed downward and the base directed upward (Figure 8–1).

### The Wall of the Heart

The wall of the heart is composed of three tissue layers: **epicardium, myocardium,** and **endocardium.**

**EPICARDIUM (VISCERAL PERICARDIUM).** As the prefix epi- (outer) indicates, this is the outermost membrane of the heart. It is composed of **serous tissue.** Also it is the inner layer of the **pericardial sac,** which encloses the heart. The pericardial sac is composed of this inner serous layer and an outer **fibrous layer.** The fibrous layer gives protection to the heart, and the inner layer secretes serous fluid (pericardial fluid), which reduces friction between the two layers when the heart contracts.

**FUNCTION OF EPICARDIUM.** The epicardium functions to protect the heart. Every time the heart contracts it hits the thoracic wall and therefore needs protection against friction. The pericardial sac, outer layer, accomplishes this. The serous layer (epicardium) helps to reduce friction between the pericardial sac and the wall of the heart.

**MYOCARDIUM.** The middle layer of tissue is the thickest of the three. It is composed primarily of cardiac

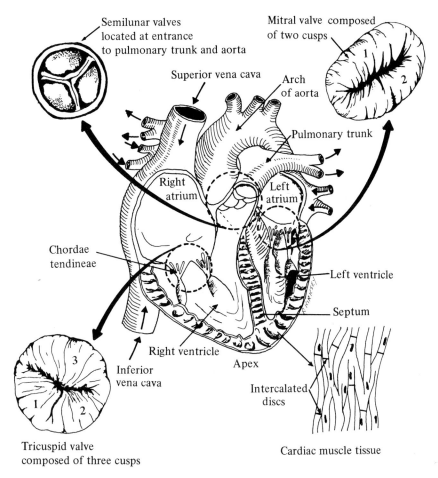

**Figure 8-1.** Internal parts of heart. The atria and ventricles of the heart are shown. The valves between the atria and ventricles as well as the valves at the entrance to the pulmonary trunk and arch of aorta are also shown.

muscle tissue. Cardiac muscle tissue is striated involuntary tissue. The anatomy of the **myocardium** is that of short, branched cells that interconnect with each other to form a muscular network. When one myocardium cell is stimulated by a nerve impulse, it contracts, but it also causes all the interconnected cells to contract. This type of contraction results in a network of cells contracting as a functional unit. The contraction of cells as a functional unit, in the heart, is absolutely essential to the effective movement of blood through the heart to the tissues. The ends of the cells are butted against each other in a manner that forms dark, thick-appearing areas called **intercalated discs** (Figure 8-1).

The myocardium varies from thin in the atria to thick in the ventricles. The myocardium is thinner in the atria (upper chambers) since they contract and pump blood against a low resistance and over a short distance—atria into ventricles. The myocardium layer is thicker in the ventricles (lower chambers) since they pump blood against a higher resistance and over a longer distance. The left ventricle is thickest since it pumps blood against the highest resistance and over the longest distance.

Since the myocardium contracts constantly everyday, it has to receive nutrients, to have its wastes removed, and to have its rate of contraction constantly altered to meet the body's needs. To accomplish this the myocardium is richly supplied with **coronary arteries** and **veins,** as well as sympathetic and parasympathetic nerves.

Normally, the cardiac muscle tissue contracts rapidly, continuously, and rhythmically about 72 times a minute without stopping. This rate of contraction can be increased or decreased by the sympathetic or parasympathetic nerves. **It should be emphasized here that these impulses simply increase or decrease the rate of the heart contractions, but they are not needed for contractions of the heart. Cardiac muscle tissue possesses inherent contractility. This means that if nerve impulses to the heart were stopped it would continue to contract due to its inherent contractility property.**

**FUNCTION OF MYOCARDIUM.** The myocardium is responsible for moving blood through and out of the heart to the tissues.

**ENDOCARDIUM (ENDOTHELIUM).** Endocardium is composed of simple squamous epithelium tissue (**endothelium**) with underlying connective tissue. This **endothelium** tissue also extends into the arteries and veins and constitutes, therefore, these arterie's and vein's linings. Endocardium lines all chambers of the heart and also covers the valves of the heart.

**FUNCTIONS OF ENDOCARDIUM.** The endocardium functions as an inner protective membrane to protect the myocardium from materials that may be in the blood.

### Atria and Ventricles

The heart is a four-chambered structure. A **septum** (divider) divides the heart into right and left halves (Figure 8–1). Each half consists of an upper chamber, the **atrium,** and a lower chamber, the **ventricle.** The atrium and ventricle on each side communicate with each other by a valve. The septum separates the right atrium and ventricle from the left atrium and ventricle. The heart can be described as a double pump. The right pump consists of the right atrium and ventricle. The left pump consists of the left atrium and ventricle. Each pump functions independently of the other, and blood is not mixed between the pumps.

*Function:* The atria receive blood from the body and pump it to the ventricles. The ventricles pump blood into the arteries, which carry blood to the capillaries.

### Heart Valves

Two types of valves are found in the heart, **atrioventricular** and **semilunar.** These valves are one-way valves since they allow blood to flow in only one direction.

Atrioventricular valves are located between atria and ventricles. The **tricuspid valve** (three cusps or flaps) (Figure 8–1) is located between the right atrium and the right ventricle. the **bicuspid** or **mitral valve** (two cusps or flaps) is located between the left atrium and the left ventricle. The mitral valve is much thicker than the tricuspid valve. The ventral surface of each valve flap is attached by connective tissue cords, **chordae tendineae,** to the ventricle walls. The cords prevent the valves from swinging into the atria when they close. The mitral and tricuspid valves open to allow blood to flow from the atria into the ventricles, but close to prevent backflow of blood into the atria.

**Semilunar valves** (half-moon shaped) are located at the entrance to the arteries leaving the ventricles. The aortic semilunar valve is located at the entrance to the aorta, which originates in the left ventricle. When the left ventricle contracts, the valve opens, allowing blood to flow into the aorta, and then closes to prevent backflow of blood into the left ventricle. The pulmonary semilunar valve is located at the entrance to the pulmonary trunk. When the right ventricle contracts, the pulmonary semilunar valve opens, allowing blood to flow into the pulmonary trunk, and then closes to prevent backflow of blood into the right ventricle.

#### Important Points

The heart is a double pump. The right atrium receives blood with a high concentration of $CO_2$ from the tissues. The right ventricle receives the blood from the atrium and pumps it to the lungs where $CO_2$ is exchanged for $O_2$. The left atrium receives oxygenated blood from the lungs. The left ventricle pumps the oxygenated blood into the aorta, which carries it to the capillaries. The only function of the right pump is to send unoxygenated blood to the lungs. The left pump sends oxygenated blood to the capillaries throughout the body.

The left pump works harder than the right pump. This means that the left ventricle must contract with greater force to generate a higher blood pressure than the right ventricle. Notice in Figure 8–1 that the walls of the left ventricle are much thicker than those of the right ventricle. This enables the left ventricle to contract with greater force.

## BLOOD SUPPLY TO THE HEART

Cardiac muscle tissue has to receive blood to carry out the same functions as other tissues. The arteries and blood supply to the cardiac muscles are called **coronary arteries** and **coronary blood supply.** The first arteries that branch off the aorta (the major blood vessel of the body; originates at the left ventricle) are the right and left coronary arteries (Figure 8–2).

The walls of the left ventricle receive the majority of coronary blood, which is reasonable since it works harder than the right ventricle. Oxygen and other nutrients are pushed by blood pressure through coronary capillaries into cardiac cells. Carbon dioxide plus other wastes move from the cardiac cells into the coronary capillaries. Coronary capillaries converge and enlarge to form **coronary veins** (Figure 8–2), which carry unoxygenated blood into the coronary sinus and then into the right atrium.

Blood clots often form in one part of the body and move through blood vessels to the small coronary arteries. They can plug the vessels and prevent an ade-

quate amount of blood from reaching the cardiac muscle cells. Death of heart tissue soon results from this condition. This dead area of the heart is called a **myocardial infarction.** An infarct area is weak compared to normal cardiac muscle tissue. This weak area causes tremendous pain and often is called a "heart attack" or a coronary.

## CARDIAC CYCLE AND REGULATION OF HEART CONTRACTIONS

Earlier we described the heart as being composed of the right and left pumps and traced the flow of blood through them. The manner in which these pumps con-

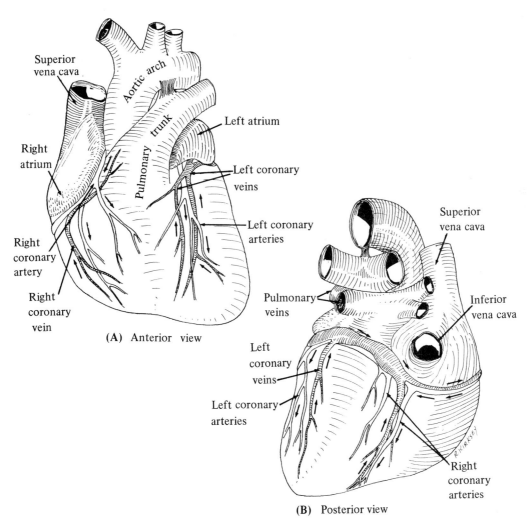

**Figure 8–2.** Cardiac muscle tissue receives blood from coronary arteries. Coronary veins drain blood from cardiac muscle tissue into the right atrium.

tract and relax determines how efficiently blood flows through the heart. If all four chambers contracted or relaxed simultaneously, heart contraction would be ineffectual; in other words, blood would not be effectively pumped out to the lungs and tissues.

The heart pumps quite efficiently by means of both the right and left atria relaxing and filling with blood simultaneously. They both contract simultaneously pumping blood into the two relaxed ventricles. The two ventricles both contract simultaneously and force blood into the pulmonary trunk and aorta. The interconnection of the cardiac muscle tissue is the reason the atria contract as a unit, and the ventricles also contract as a unit for the same reason.

The cardiac cycle is the heart's action that takes place during a single heartbeat. This cycle consists of the relaxation (diastole) and contraction (systole) of both atria, followed by the relaxation and contraction of the ventricles. The entire heart does not contract as a unit, but rather both atria relax simultaneously (atrial diastole) and contract simultaneously (atrial systole). Both ventricles likewise relax simultaneously (ventricular diastole) and contract simultaneously (ventricular systole).

To fully understand the cardiac cycle, we need to know what the atrioventricular and semilunar valves are doing during diastole and systole (we previously discussed their location and function). The atrioventricular valves must close to allow the atria to fill with blood during atrial diastole. During atrial systole, the valves open so that blood can be pumped into the ventricles. During ventricular systole, atrioventricular valves close to prevent a backflow of blood into the atria, but the pulmonary and aortic semilunar valves open to allow passage of blood into their respective arteries. The semilunar valves close during ventricular diastole to prevent backflow of blood into the ven-

tricles. The functions of the valves in relation to the atria and ventricles are summarized in Table 8-1.

### Heart Sounds

The opening and closing of these valves is vital for proper flow of blood through the heart. The opening and closing of the valves is important in another way: The actions of these valves create sounds that can be heard through a stethoscope placed on the chest over the heart. The first sound, **lub,** results from atrioventricular valves closing and ventricles contracting. A **lub** is lower and longer than the second sound, **dup.** A **dup** results from closing of semilunar valves.

Damaged valves cause abnormal sounds often known as **murmurs.** Murmurs can be caused by blood flowing rapidly in the usual direction through an abnormally narrowed valve, backflow through a damaged leaky valve, or flow between the two atria through a small hole in the septum. The resulting abnormal sounds are a valuable diagnostic tool to a physician.

## ABNORMALITIES OF THE HEART THAT AFFECT THE CARDIAC CYCLE

Various abnormalities in the heart and heart valves result from infections and diseases. **Rheumatic fever** is a streptococcal infection that originates in the connective tissues of joints. Approximately 60 percent of the time the streptococcal organisms spread to the heart. The organisms excrete poisonous compounds or toxins, which affect the endocardium of the heart, especially the mitral valve. The toxins cause **mitral stenosis,** "narrowing of the mitral valve." Mitral stenosis involves a

### TABLE 8-1.  Heart Valve Functions

|  | AV Valves | Reason | Semilunar Valves | Reason |
|---|---|---|---|---|
| Atrial diastole | Closed | Atria fill with blood | Open | Ventricles contracting |
| Atrial systole | Open | Pump blood into ventricles | Closed | Ventricles relaxed |
| Ventricular diastole | Open | Ventricles fill with blood | Closed | Prevent backflow of blood into ventricles |
| Ventricular systole | Closed | Prevent backflow of blood into atria | Open | Allow blood to flow into the arteries |

buildup of fibrous tissue on the flaps of the mitral valve. The flaps are changed into rigid, thickened structures, which reduce the opening between the left atrium and ventricle. These changes reduce the amount of blood that flows from the left atrium into the left ventricle. A buildup of blood occurs in the left atrium, and the cardiac cycle is altered as a result of this disease.

## REGULATION OF RHYTHMIC HEART CONTRACTIONS

The autonomic nervous system is responsible for regulating the rhythmic contractions of the heart. Specially modified cardiac muscle tissue transmits nerve impulses from the atria (Figure 8–3) to the ventricles. This specially modified tissue includes two nodes and two bundles of tissue. The nodes and bundles of tissue are the following:

1. The **sinoatrial node (SA node)** is a modified knot of cardiac tissue (Figure 8–3) in the right atrium. The SA node initiates the heartbeat and sets the rhythm of heart contraction; hence, it is called the pacemaker. It is well supplied with sympathetic and parasympathetic nerve fibers.

2. The **atrioventricular node (AV node)** is a second modified knot of tissue, and it is located at the junction of the right atrium and the right ventricle. The AV node (Figure 8–3) receives nerve impulses from the atria and conducts them to the ventricles through the **atrioventricular bundle (bundle of His).**

3. The **bundle of His (atrioventricular bundle)** is a group of modified muscle fibers (Figure 8–3) extending from the AV node through the ventricular septum. The fibers function to transmit nerve impulses from the AV node to the Purkinje fibers in the ventricles.

4. The **Purkinje fibers** branch off the bundle of His into the right and left walls of the ventricles (Figure 8–3). They conduct impulses to the walls of the ventricles, stimulating contractions in them.

Normally, the modified cardiac muscle tissue functions as follows: An electrical nerve impulse starts in the SA node (pacemaker) and spreads through the atria causing them to contract (Figure 8–4). When the impulse reaches the AV node, it is relayed through the bundle of His in the septum to the Purkinje fibers in the walls of the ventricles, where it causes them to contract. This anatomical organization facilitates nerve impulses moving from the atria through the AV node to the ventricles only. At the AV node the impulse is delayed for about 0.1 second.

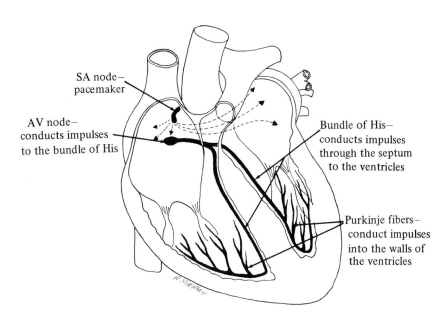

**Figure 8–3.**    The four parts of the nerve conduction system of the heart.

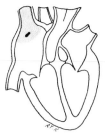 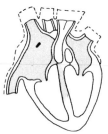 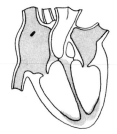 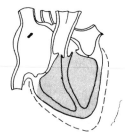

Gradual spread of nerve impulse from SA node through atria

Contraction of atria and spread of impulses through bundle of His

Gradual spread of impulses through bundle of His and purkinje fibers

Contraction of ventricles and relaxation of atria

**Figure 8-4.**  Spread of nerve impulses through the conduction system of the heart. The gray area indicates the spread of nerve impulses.

The orderly movement of impulses through the modified cardiac muscle tissue and the slight delay at the AV node cause rhythmical contractions of the atria, followed by contractions of the ventricles (Figure 8-4). These rhythmical contractions allow the atria and ventricles to completely fill and empty efficiently; therefore, blood is pumped through the heart to the various parts of the body.

The heart contractions are **intrinsic** (arise from inside the heart itself); and if all nerve connections are cut, the heart would continue to contract. Nerve impulses are necessary to regulate the rate of heart contractions as the body's needs vary. Without nerve impulses the heart possibly would contract less than 40 times per minute; whereas to maintain effective circulation, the heart contracts 70 to 90 times per minute.

## NERVOUS CONTROL OF HEART

The needs of the body often require that circulation be speeded up, which consequently increases the rate of heart contractions. The SA node is innervated by sympathetic (accelerator nerves) and parasympathetic (inhibitory nerves) fibers (Figure 8-5). These nerves serve to speed up and decrease the rate of the heart, respectively. For example, if you decide to run up some stairs rather than walk, the heart and circulatory rates are speeded up by impulses from the sympathetic (accelerator) nerves. When you reach the top of the stairs, the heart and circulatory rate are slowed by impulses from the parasympathetic (inhibitory) nerves.

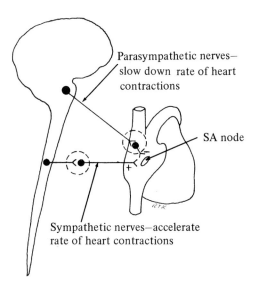

Parasympathetic nerves— slow down rate of heart contractions

SA node

Sympathetic nerves—accelerate rate of heart contractions

**Figure 8-5.**  Nervous control of heart rate. The effect of interaction of sympathetic and parasympathetic nerves on the rate of heart contractions is shown.

### Electrocardiogram

The transmission of electrical nerve impulses through the heart is accomplished by electrical changes in the cardiac tissue. These electrical changes are conducted from the heart through body fluids and tissues to the skin surface. Sensitive metal detectors conduct these impulses to an instrument, the electrocardiograph, that records these changes. These changes are valuable to physicians who are trying to diagnose heart disease and abnormalities.

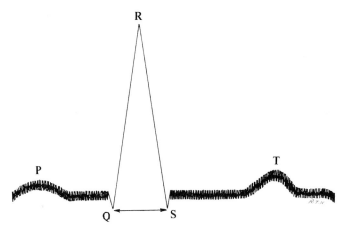

**Figure 8-6.** The movement of a nerve impulse through the atria and ventricles of the heart is shown by an electrocardiogram tracing.

Figure 8-6 illustrates a typical recording of these electrical changes. Each of the electrical deflections can be described:

1. **P wave:** This wave traces the spread of a nerve impulse from the sinoatrial (SA) node through the atria. The ascending part of the wave indicates the gradual spread of the impulse through the atria. When the wave is at its maximum height, the atria have contracted. The descending part of the wave indicates relaxation of the atria.

2. **Q, R, S waves:** The Q wave represents the origin of the impulse at the atrioventricular (AV) node. The ascending part of the R wave illustrates the spread of the impulse and gradual contraction of the ventricles. The height of the R wave illustrates total contraction of the ventricles. The relaxation of the ventricles is illustrated by the descent of the wave from R down to the S.

3. **T wave:** This wave represents the recovery phase of the ventricles. During the T wave the ventricle muscle tissue is preparing for the next impulse, or, in other words, repolarization is taking place. The muscle is incapable of another contraction during this wave.

4. **P–Q interval:** This measurement reflects the time it takes for the impulse to move through the atria to the AV node.

5. **P–R interval:** This measurement reflects the time it takes for the impulse to move through the atria to the ventricles. If this time is longer than normal, it in-dicates a possible block in the atrioventricular (AV) node and its branches.

6. **S–T interval:** This interval measures the time from the end of ventricle contraction to the beginning of the recovery phase. If this time is abnormally long, it could be an indicator of ventricular muscle injury.

*Important Points*

P, Q, R, S, and T measurements or the electrocardiogram are important because they indicate whether the heart is working properly and, if not, the source of the problem. One should keep in mind, however, that these measurements will not detect problems in the heart unless the pathology is severe enough to interfere with the heart's electrical activity.

## EFFECT OF IONS ON NERVOUS CONTROL OF HEART

In Chapter 2 we studied the concentrations of the various important electrolytes in the body and their various functions. Two of these electrolytes ($K^+$ and $Ca^{2+}$) are very important in the overall nervous regulation of the heart and therefore its ability to contract properly.

### Effects of Potassium Ions ($K^+$)

The normal range for plasma $K^+$ is 3.8 to 5.6 mEq/liter. As long as this normal range is maintained the heart contracts at its normal rate and rhythm. However, if a person's plasma $K^+$ level exceeds 5.6 mEq/l, the condition called **hyperkalemia** exists. This condition alters the normal polarized state of the cardiac muscle, thereby resulting in a decreased rate and force of heart contractions. **A seriously elevated plasma $K^+$ level constitutes a medical emergency, and cardiac arrest may be imminent.** If the plasma $K^+$ drops below the lower limit (approximately 3.8 mEq/l), a person is in a state of **hypokalemia.** This condition can result in abnormal cardiac rhythms (**arrhythmia**) and ultimately in cardiac arrest.

The main cause of **hyperkalemia** is renal failure; however, patients suffering from serious burns, crushing injuries, and infection possibly can develop this condition. Renal failure will be discussed in greater detail in Chapter 18.

## *Effects of Calcium Ions (Ca²⁺)*

The normal range for $Ca^{2+}$ is 4.7 to 5.5 mEq/l. If the upper limit is exceeded, a person is said to be in **hypercalcemia,** which usually results in a person's heart rate increasing. The major problem, though, is that the myocardium goes into a prolonged state of spastic contractions. The theory behind this problem is related to the fact that $Ca^{2+}$ helps initiate muscle contractions. This process will be discussed in detail in Chapter 13.

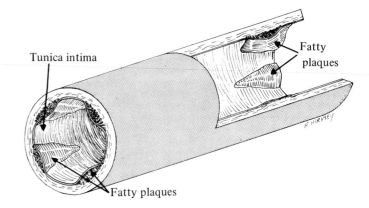

**Figure 8–7.**   Presence of plaques in arteries.

## VOLUME OF BLOOD PUMPED THROUGH THE HEART

If the ventricles are contracting normally, each will pump out about 70 ml of blood per contraction. The **stroke volume** is the amount of blood pumped out of a ventricle with each contraction (70 ml blood/contraction). Under normal conditions the heart contracts about 72 times each minute. One can see that

$$\text{Rate} \times \begin{pmatrix} \text{stroke volume of} \\ \text{a ventricle} \end{pmatrix} = \text{cardiac output}$$

$$72 \, \frac{\text{heart contractions}}{\text{min}} \times 70 \, \frac{\text{ml blood}}{\text{contraction}} = 5040 \, \frac{\text{ml}}{\text{min}}$$

That is, about 5040 ml of blood is pumped from each ventricle to all the tissues every minute. The **cardiac output** is the amount of blood pumped from a ventricle each minute: cardiac output = 5040 ml/min.

Under normal conditions the stroke volume and cardiac output will supply the needed nutrients and fluids to the tissues as well as carry away the waste products. If the activities of the body increase, tissue requirements for nutrients, fluids, and transport of waste products also increase. These increases are met by increasing the heart rate, thereby increasing the cardiac output of blood.

## ARTERIES

**Arteries** are vessels that transport blood away from the heart to the capillaries. They transport oxygenated blood (high concentration of $O_2$). A cross-sectional view of arteries compared to veins is illustrated in Figure 8–7. Arterial walls are composed of three tissue layers:

- **Tunica externa (adventitia)** is composed of white fibrous connective tissue. Some smooth muscle tissue is found in this layer also. This coat is relatively inelastic and tough. It limits the ability of the artery to stretch, and it also increases the strength of the artery.

- **Tunica media** is the middle layer and is composed of circular smooth muscle and elastic tissue. This layer, with the large amount of elastic tissue, allows an artery to dilate and then constrict. The tunica media also is responsible for alternately dilating and constricting an artery when it is cut. This causes blood to flow out in spurts.

- **Tunica interna** is the innermost layer and is composed of delicate simple squamous tissue (endothelium). Arterial injury or disease often damages this delicate layer. This is the only layer of tissue composing the walls of capillaries. The tunica externa and tunica media are absent from capillaries. The single layer of endothelium tissue is a continuation of the endothelium layer of the heart.

> Atherosclerosis is deposition of fatty plaques in the tunica intima of arteries (Fig. 8–7). The plaques reduce blood flow to tissues and can ultimately result in tissue death. Diabetics are more prone to develop plaques than nondiabetics.

Arteries possess two important properties as a result of their walls. First, they are elastic and when stimulated can stretch both in length and diameter. Second, the arteries can contract because of the presence of smooth muscle tissue in the walls. These two properties are important because they allow arteries to **vasodilate** (increase their diameter) and **vasoconstrict** (decrease their diameter). The movement of blood through arteries, arterial blood pressure, and the arterial pulse are influenced by vasodilation and vasoconstriction.

An aneurysm is a sac or bulged-out section of an artery or vein. The sac is at a weak region in a vessel. The aortic arch is a common site for an aneurysm. The main danger of an aneurysm is the possibility of rupture and death due to internal hemorrhaging and drop in blood pressure.

## VEINS

**Veins** transport blood away from capillary beds to the heart. With one exception, pulmonary veins, they transport blood low in $O_2$ but high in $CO_2$ toward the right atrium of the heart. The tissue layers composing the walls of veins are the same as for arteries but much thinner (Figure 8–8). The muscle and elastic tissues are less developed; therefore, veins are much less elastic than arteries.

Veins can adapt to the amount of blood passing through them; and many veins, especially ones in the limbs, possess one-way valves (Figure 8–9). Since the elasticity and contractility of the veins are reduced, the valves prevent blood from flowing back into the capillaries, but allow it to be pumped toward the heart. Veins collapse easily because of their lack of elasticity; and, if cut, they tend to remain wide open and allow blood to escape in a fairly steady flow. If an artery is cut, blood tends to flow out in an uneven stream or a spurt as a result of the alternate vasoconstriction and vasodilation, which result from the elastic and contractile properties of the artery.

Phlebitis is inflammation of veins and may be accompanied by edema and pain. Infection, varicose veins, pregnancy, and tumors can cause the condition. A major danger is the possibility of forming a blood clot or thrombophlebitis.

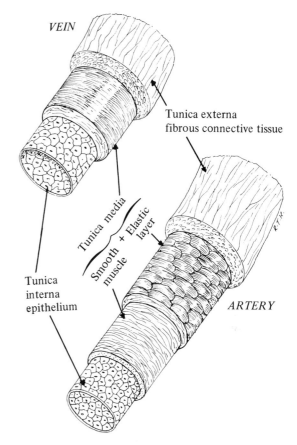

**Figure 8-8.** Tissue layers of arteries and veins. The elastic and smooth muscle tissue of the tunica media in veins is much thinner than that of arteries.

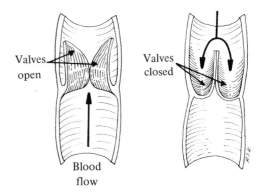

**Figure 8-9.** The opening and closing of valves in veins.

## CAPILLARIES

Capillaries are microscopic vessels consisting of a single layer of simple epithelium or endothelium tissue. Capillaries connect arteries to veins, or, more specifically, arterioles to venules. It is important to remember that arteries transport the necessary nutrients to the millions of cells throughout the body, but the actual exchange can occur only through the capillaries.

In Chapter 4, the simple squamous tissue was described as being important for passage of materials through it from the bloodstream to the tissues, and vice versa. The major function of capillaries is exchange of nutrients and wastes between the tissues and blood. For this reason many authorities refer to capillaries as the **functional unit** of the cardiovascular system. Details concerning how materials are exchanged across capillaries will be discussed in Chapter 16.

The structure of the capillary is not only important for allowing exchange of materials, but also it has elasticity that allows it to adapt to the amount and force of blood flowing into it.

### Size and Distribution of Capillaries

The diameter of capillaries varies from tissue to tissue. For example, in the lungs the **lumen** (the inner open space) is larger than it is in most of the capillaries throughout the rest of the body. The lumen in some capillaries is so small that only one red blood cell (RBC) can pass through it at a time; in others several RBCs can pass abreast through a capillary at the same time. The size of the lumen is regulated by **precapillary sphincter muscles** (Figure 8–17). These muscles will dilate or constrict the lumen depending on the amount of blood needed by the tissues surrounding the capillaries.

The distribution or numbers of capillaries within tissues varies according to the metabolic activity of the tissues. For example, muscle and nerve tissues are very metabolically active and need large quantities of oxygen, glucose, and other nutrients; therefore, they are well supplied with capillaries. In comparison, tissues such as hyaline cartilage, cornea, and epidermis of the skin are not very active and, therefore, are lacking in capillaries.

## 2　THE CIRCULATORY SYSTEM

Figures 8–10 and 8–12 show the major arteries and veins in the body. The circulatory system can be divided into three small units: systemic, hepatic portal, and pulmonary.

## SYSTEMIC UNIT

The **systemic unit** carries blood to and from all parts of the body, except the air sacs (alveoli) of the lungs.

### Major Arteries of the Systemic Circulation

The **aorta** is by far the largest artery in the body, and all major systemic arteries branch from the aorta. It leaves the left ventricle and curves posterior and inferior, anterior to the vertebral column. The aorta continues down through the body giving off many branches. Table 8–2 lists the regions of the aorta, branches, and areas supplied.

Other important systemic arteries are the **right** and **left subclavian arteries,** which branch off the aorta to the right and left upper arms. They then divide into the following branches:

subclavian arteries
→ axillary (armpit area)
　→ brachial (longest part of vessel in upper arm; at the elbow it gives off two branches)
　　→ radial (continues down thumb side of forearm and wrist into the hand)
　　→ ulnar (continues along medial or little finger side of arm into the hand)

The **brachial artery** is important since it is the artery in which blood pressure is measured. The **radial artery** is important for determining a patient's pulse.

The **circle of Willis** is a circle of arteries at the base of the brain. It is formed by the union of the right and left internal carotid arteries, anterior communicating, posterior communicating, and basilar arteries (Figure 8–11). The internal carotids and basilar arteries transport blood to the circle of Willis. The posterior communicating arteries connect the basilar artery to the internal carotids. The anterior communicating arteries connect the internal carotid arteries and thereby complete the circle of Willis. This group of vessels is quite important since they supply the brain cells with essential $O_2$ fluids, and nutrients.

The brain is very vulnerable when an interruption of blood flow occurs. The brain does not have any energy reserves such as lipids and glycogen. Almost all tissues such as cardiac and skeletal muscle tissues have these energy reserves; therefore, if a decreased blood flow oc-

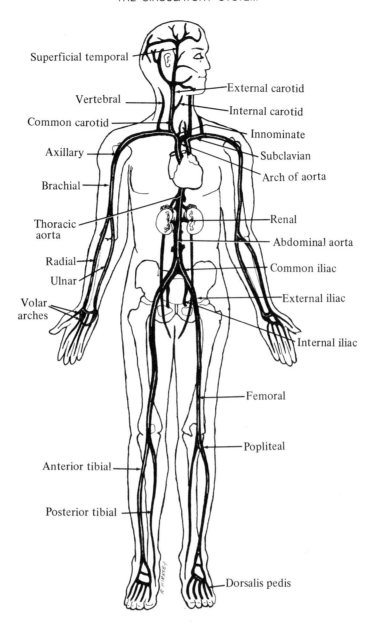

Figure 8-10. Major arteries of the body.

curs to them, they can rely upon these reserves to get their energy. However, a total interruption of blood flow to the brain for 4 minutes results in widespread and irreversible damage to the affected brain region. This occurs because the brain cells do not have the necessary nutrients to form ATP, the energy source that powers each nerve cell. This interruption of blood flow to the brain is called a **stroke.** This is by far the most common serious disease of the nervous system, and it actually results from a malfunction of the cardiovascular system. Seventy-eight percent of strokes are the result of an **occlusion** (an obstruction) of the arteries leading to or in the circle of Willis. The **occlusion** is either an **embolus** or **thrombus.** Details concerning these will be discussed later.

The various vessels of the circle of Willis (Figure 8-11) and the areas of the brain that each supplies arterial blood to are as follows:

Anterior cerebral artery → *Frontal lobe*
Middle cerebral artery → *Precentral gyrus*
Regulates voluntary
movement impulses
*Postcentral gyrus*
Reception area for pain,
temperature touch, and
pressure impulses

Posterior cerebral artery → *Occipital lobe*
Reception, interpretation,
and recall of visual
information

An occlusion of any one of the major arteries produces symptoms related to the part of the brain that is affected. As an example, if a person is suspected of hav-

**TABLE 8–2.   *The Aorta and Its Branches***

| Region of Aorta | Branches | Areas Supplied |
|---|---|---|
| *Ascending aorta* (near the heart and inside the pericardial sac) | → R. coronary artery — <br> → L. coronary artery — | → Heart tissue |
| *Aortic arch* (immediately beyond the ascending aorta) | → Brachiocephalic (innominate) | |
| | → R. subclavian ——— | → R. upper arm |
| | → R. common carotid | |
| | → R. internal carotid ——— | → Brain, eye, forehead, and nose |
| | → R. external carotid ——— | → Thyroid, tongue, tonsils, ear, etc. |
| | → L. common carotid | |
| | → L. internal carotid ——— | → (Same as R. internal carotid) |
| | → L. external carotid ——— | → (Same as R. external carotid) |
| | → L. subclavian ——— | → L. upper arm |
| *Descending thoracic aorta* (below the heart and gives off branches to structures in the thoracic cavity) | Visceral branches ——— | → Pericardium, bronchi, esophagus, and mediastinum |
| | → Parietal branches ——— | → Chest muscles, mammary glands, and diaphragm |
| *Abdominal aorta* (below the diaphragm in the abdominal cavity) | → Celiac (only ½ inch long but gives off three branches) | |
| | → L. gastric ——— | → Stomach |
| | → Splenic ——— | → Spleen |
| | → Hepatic ——— | → Liver |
| | → Superior mesenteric ——— | → Most of the small intestine and first half of large intestine |
| | → Inferior mesenteric ——— | → Last half of large intestine |
| | → R. and L. phrenic arteries ——— | → Diaphragm |
| | → R. and L. adrenal arteries ——— | → R. and L. adrenal glands |
| | → R. and L. renal arteries ——— | → R. and L. kidneys |
| | → R and L. ovarian or testicular ——— | → Ovaries in female, testicles in male |
| | → Four pairs of lumbar ——— | → Heavy musculature of abdominal wall |
| *Abdominal aorta* (at the lumbar region) | → R. common iliac artery (extends into the pelvis area) | |
| | → Internal iliac ——— | → Urinary bladder, rectum, and some reproductive organs |
| | → External iliac | |
| | → Femoral ——— | → R. and L. upper leg |
| | → L. common iliac artery ——— | → (Same as R. common iliac artery) |

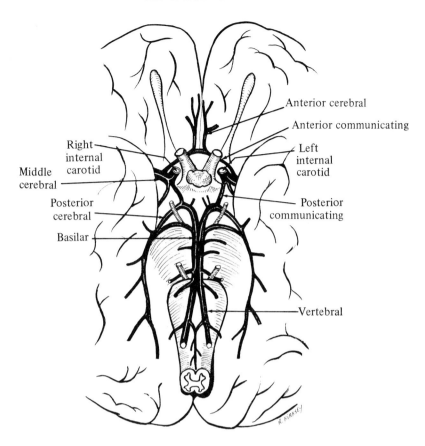

Right internal carotid

Middle cerebral

Posterior cerebral

Basilar

Anterior cerebral

Anterior communicating

Left internal carotid

Posterior communicating

Vertebral

**Figure 8-11.** A view of the brain from below shows the circle of Willis, which is essential for bringing blood to the brain cells.

ing a stroke and complains of visual disturbances, then possibly the posterior cerebral artery is occluded.

## Major Veins of Systemic Circulation

Veins (except for the pulmonary veins) return unoxygenated blood rich in $CO_2$ and other waste compounds from capillaries to the heart (Figure 8–12). The systemic veins drain blood from the tissues that were supplied by the systemic arteries. For the sake of study the systemic veins can be divided into three groups:

**SUPERFICIAL VEINS.** Most arteries tend to be found in deep areas of the body, whereas many veins are found near the surface. The two pairs of extremities are drained by some important superficial veins:

• *Cephalic.* Figure 8–12 shows that this vein originates in the hand on the thumb side and ascends along the lateral side of the forearm. Inferior to the elbow, the cephalic vein gives rise to a median cubital vein that connects to the basilic vein. The **median cubital** vein often is used for removing blood from a patient and for intravenous infusions.

• *Saphenous veins.* The great and small saphenous veins (Figure 8–12), and their many tributaries, help to drain blood from the lower legs. These two veins are important clinically because often they become varicose (unnaturally swollen). The **great saphenous** is the longest vein in the body. It begins in the medial anterior superficial tissues of the foot and continues up the medial side of the leg. It empties into the femoral vein near the groin. The **small saphenous** begins in the lateral superficial tissues of the foot and passes superiorly in the posterior region of the leg. It empties into the popliteal vein in the posterior region of the knee.

Varicose veins is a condition where superficial veins become dilated or swollen. People who are on their feet a lot or obese often experience this

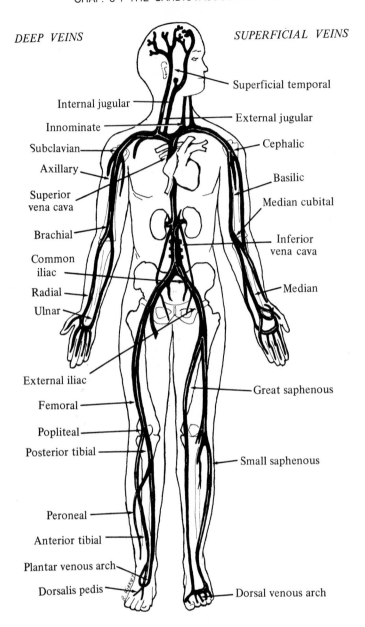

**Figure 8-12.**    Major veins of the body.

condition in veins in their lower legs. Varicose veins in the rectum are called hemorrhoids.

**DEEP VEINS.** These veins tend to be located parallel to arteries and usually have the same names as the artery next to them. They drain blood from deeper tissues and have many connections with superficial veins.

- *Upper extremities.* **Brachial** (upper arm), **axillary** (continuation of brachial into the axillary, armpit area), **subclavian** (continuation of axillary through shoulder region to superior vena cava).

- *Lower extremities.* **Anterior tibial, posterior tibial, popliteal, femoral, external iliac.**

**CRANIAL VENOUS SINUSES.** The word **sinus** means "a space" or "a hollow." In the skull there are several spaces that drain venous blood from the brain to the heart. These sinuses, located between the two layers of dura mater, drain blood from the orbital and cranial cavities. None of these cranial venous sinuses possesses valves like those found in the veins.

It was stated earlier that veins carry blood from capillaries to the heart. Not all the systemic veins discussed earlier open into the heart. Only two systemic veins, the **superior** and **inferior venae cavae,** open into the right atrium of the heart. The superior vena cava (Figure 8–12) receives blood from the head, neck, upper extremities, and chest and then enters the right atrium. The **inferior vena cava** is much longer than the superior vena cava, and it returns blood to the right atrium from parts of the body below the diaphragm. The inferior vena cava originates in the lower abdomen with the union of two **common iliac veins** and then moves superior along the dorsal (posterior) surface of the abdomen, through the liver, diaphragm, and lower thorax to finally enter the right atrium. The inferior vena cava receives the following veins:

- **Lumbar veins:** Four pairs of these drain the dorsal part of the trunk and spinal cord.
- Two **testicular (spermatic)** or **ovarian veins:** Testicular veins drain the testes of a male, and ovarian veins drain ovaries of a female.
- Two **renal veins:** Each kidney is drained by a renal vein.
- **Hepatic vein:** A hepatic vein drains blood from the liver into the inferior vena cava.

## HEPATIC PORTAL SYSTEM

The **hepatic portal system** involves veins only. The veins carry blood from the digestive organs to the liver, before the blood enters the inferior vena cava (Figure 8–13).

Veins from the spleen, stomach, intestines, pancreas, and gallbladder join to form the portal vein, which

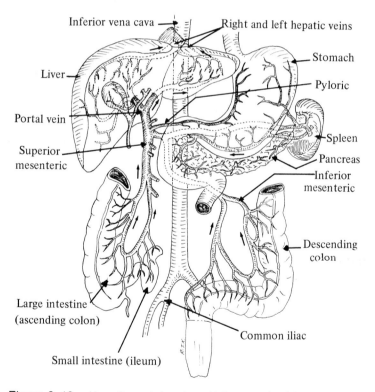

**Figure 8-13.** Hepatic portal system. Veins carrying blood from the stomach, intestines, spleen, and pancreas come together to form the portal vein. The portal vein enters the liver and gives off branches to sinusoids. Right and left hepatic veins drain blood from the liver into the inferior vena cava. Arrows indicate direction of flow.

enters the inferior surface of the liver. The portal vein gives off many branches that form spaces called sinusoids. The sinusoids are equivalent to capillaries. The portal artery brings oxygenated blood to the liver and gives off branches that ultimately join the sinusoids. Venous and arterial blood mix together in the sinusoids. Small veins drain the sinusoids and ultimately form hepatic veins that enter the inferior vena cava.

The main function of the hepatic portal unit is to inspect, cleanse, remove, and modify materials in the blood before it enters the general circulation. The blood coming to the liver from the digestive organs is rich in digestive products (proteins, fats, and carbohydrates) as well as bacteria. Phagocytic cells, called **Kupffer cells,** line the sinusoids and destroy the bacteria in the blood by phagocytosis. Normal liver cells in the sinusoids remove large amounts of proteins and glucose from the blood. As much as two-thirds of the glucose and one-half of the proteins are removed in the sinusoids. More detail concerning these functions will be presented in Chapter 19. This system is very important since it brings blood to the liver, which then removes bacteria, glucose, and proteins from blood before it enters the general circulation. It is important that the bacteria be removed from the blood to prevent their spread and

septicemia. It is important that most of the glucose be removed so that it will not upset the normal level of glucose already in the general circulation. The removal of proteins is important for the same reasons. The liver gradually releases glucose and proteins into the general circulation as they are needed.

## PULMONARY SYSTEM

The **pulmonary system** transports unoxygenated blood, rich in $CO_2$, from the heart to the lungs, exchanges $CO_2$ for $O_2$ and returns the oxygenated blood to the heart (Figure 8–14). The pulmonary unit originates in the right ventricle of the heart with the pulmonary trunk. The right ventricle pumps blood into the pulmonary trunk. The pulmonary trunk leaves the right ventricle and divides into right and left pulmonary arteries. The pulmonary arteries go to the right and left lung, finally forming pulmonary capillaries that surround alveoli (air sacs). The RBCs exchange $CO_2$ for $O_2$ through the alveoli of the lungs. The blood, now oxygenated, returns to the left atrium of the heart through pulmonary veins. Four pulmonary veins, two from each lung, carry

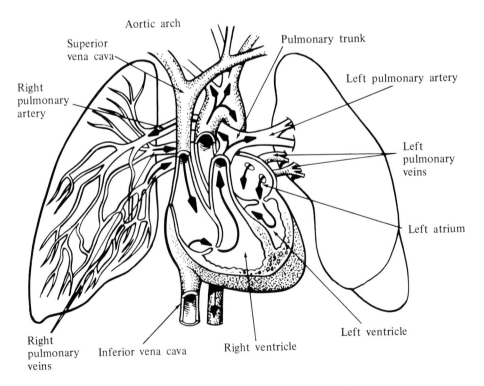

**Figure 8–14.** The pulmonary system consists of right and left pulmonary arteries, which carry deoxygenated blood to the lungs. Pulmonary veins carry oxygenated blood from the lungs to the left atrium.

oxygenated blood into the left atrium through the posterior wall.

### Important Point

Previously, we said that arteries carry blood away from the heart and, with one exception, carry oxygenated blood. The pulmonary trunk and arteries are the exception since they transport unoxygenated blood to the lungs. We also previously stated that veins carry deoxygenated blood to the right atrium, but the pulmonary veins carry oxygenated blood to the left atrium from the lungs. The pressure in the pulmonary system is only one-sixth that of the pressure in the aorta.

The pulmonary unit carries deoxygenated blood to the lungs where $CO_2$ is exchanged for $O_2$ and the blood is returned to the heart. The oxygenated blood is pumped to all the tissues by the left ventricle.

## 3  BLOOD PRESSURE

As blood is pumped through the heart and vessels, it is under pressure. This pressure is created because the diameters of the arteries into which the blood is pumped are small enough that blood encounters resistance. Pressure is created as the heart contracts and overcomes the resistance, thereby pushing blood into arteries. Blood pressure is present throughout the blood vessels, since their size creates resistance to the flow of blood.

Blood pumped under fairly high pressure (but not too high) is desirable so that it can reach all the tissues. Blood pressure at the heart is higher than in the tissues; therefore, blood flows from a high pressure area (heart) to a low pressure area (capillaries). Also, as blood reaches the capillaries, the movement of nutrients out of the arterial end of capillaries results from blood pressure. Blood pressure or hydrostatic pressure is high enough so that the nutrients are pushed out of the capillaries.

Since fluids flow from an area of high pressure to an area of low pressure, this explains why blood flows from arteries to capillaries. It also explains why blood flows from capillaries to veins, and from veins back to the heart. Blood pressure is high on the left side of the heart where the aorta leaves, but it is low on the right side where the veins bring blood back to the heart.

Blood pressure is measured and expressed in terms of millimeters of mercury (mm Hg) above the atmospheric pressure (760 mm Hg is the pressure of air surrounding our bodies). For example, if someone's blood pressure is 100 mm Hg, it is actually 100 mm Hg above normal atmospheric pressure, or 860 mm Hg. All parts of our body are subjected to atmospheric pressure (760 mm Hg). Normal blood pressure always is above 760 mm Hg. This is vital since blood flows from an area of high pressure to an area of low pressure. If blood pressure is equal to atmospheric pressure, little, if any, movement of blood will occur.

## ARTERIAL PRESSURE

Arterial pressure is created when blood is pumped against arterial walls. Arterial pressure is highest in the arch of the aorta immediately after it leaves a contracted left ventricle. This pressure, normally 115 to 120 mm Hg, is called **systolic pressure** (Figure 8-15) and it results from **ventricle systole.** After the blood leaves the heart the ventricles relax (**diastole).** The arteries stretch as they receive blood from the ventricles, and they recoil as they move the blood. The recoil of the arteries creates **diastolic pressure,** normally 75 to 80 mm Hg.

Arterial pressure drops as the arteries divide into smaller and smaller branches until they form **arterioles** (small arteries immediately prior to a capillary). In the arterioles the blood pressure (Figure 8-15) is about 30 mm Hg; but as the arterioles spread into the capillary (an even greater space), the pressure drops to about 20 mm Hg. This drop in pressure results from the blood now passing through a greater area than was present in the arterioles.

### Arterioles and Peripheral Resistance

**Arterioles** are the small arteries immediately prior to the capillaries. They branch diffusely (Figure 8-16) into a number of capillaries, finally creating a fantastic, spreading network that permeates every organ of the body. Where arterioles enter capillaries, tiny rings of smooth muscles, **precapillary sphincters,** open and close to regulate the amount of blood that flows into a capillary bed. Blood flow is not uniform for all tissues but depends on the tissue needs. This alternate opening and closing of the sphincters helps to control blood pressure by alternately increasing resistance to blood flow when closed, and decreasing resistance when open. It is fortunate that all the precapillary sphincters are not open at the same time since this would cause a drastic drop in blood pressure. The pressure could drop so low that it would be difficult to move blood out of the capillaries.

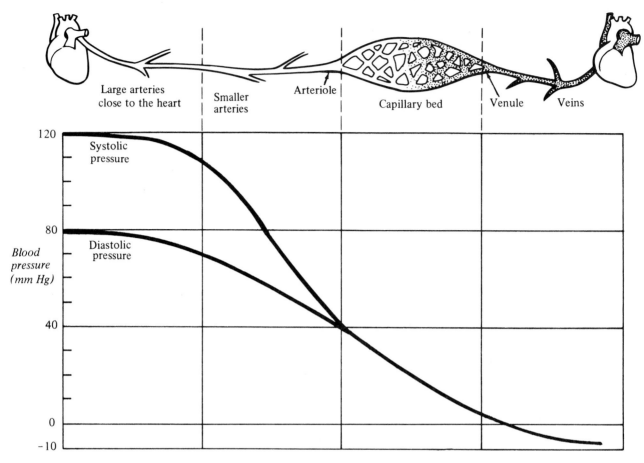

**Figure 8-15.** Blood pressure in arteries and veins. Blood pressure is quite high in vessels near the heart, and it decreases rapidly as blood moves into capillary beds. Blood pressure continues to drop as blood moves through veins into the right atrium of the heart. [Adapted from *Anatomy and Physiology,* Unit 6 Cardiovascular System Overhead Transparencies (Robert J. Brady Co., Bowie, Md.)]

## DETERMINATION OF BLOOD PRESSURE

This measurement is important in determining how the heart and circulatory system are functioning. Figure 8-17 shows the instrument, a **sphygmomanometer,** most commonly used for measuring blood pressure. The measurement consists of wrapping a cuff around the upper arm just superior to the elbow. The cuff then is inflated to a pressure that compresses the brachial artery while the radial pulse is being palpated. This pressure on the brachial artery will prevent any blood from being pumped through that part of the artery and no pulse can be heard through a stethoscope placed over the artery. By gradually releasing the pressure on the cuff and simultaneously watching the pressure gauge and listening for sounds, the systolic and diastolic pressures can be measured. When the first sounds are heard, the pressure should be noted. This is the **systolic pressure** (pressure created by the left ventricle pumping blood into the aorta). As the pressure on the cuff continues to be released, a second pressure is noted when the sounds cease. This is the **diastolic pressure** (pressure created by contraction and recoil of arteries). These two pressures are usually recorded as:

$$\frac{120 \text{ mm Hg}}{80 \text{ mm Hg}}$$
(systolic pressure) point at which sounds are first heard
(diastolic pressure) point at which sounds first cease

These values are considered to be an average reading for a person at rest, but it can vary from 90 to 140 for systolic pressure and 50 to 90 for diastolic pressure and still be considered normal.

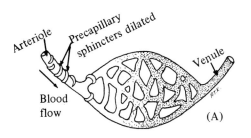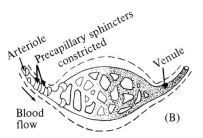

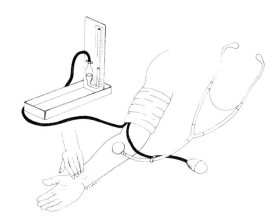

**Figure 8-16.** (A) Precapillary sphincters dilated, which allows blood to flow into capillary bed. (B) Precapillary sphincters constricted, which restricts flow of blood into capillary bed.

**Figure 8-17.** Sphygmomanometer used in measuring blood pressure.

Clinically, diastolic pressure often is considered more important than systolic pressure because it indicates the pressure or strain that the arteries are under. Also it is indicative of the amount of resistance in the peripheral vessels since diastolic pressure rises or falls with peripheral resistance. For example, if arteriosclerosis is developing, peripheral resistance increases, which causes an increase in diastolic pressure.

## FACTORS INVOLVED IN MAINTENANCE OF ARTERIAL BLOOD PRESSURE

To effectively keep blood moving through the tissues a high blood pressure must be maintained. Arterial blood pressure is directly affected by the ease with which blood flows through the arteries. The easier it is for the blood to flow, the lower the pressure will be. The harder it is for the blood to flow, the higher the pressure will be.

Several factors increase and decrease the flow of blood through arteries and thereby maintain arterial blood pressure.

### Rate of Cardiac Contractions

If the atria and ventricles are contracting rapidly, blood pressure increases, and vice versa. If the arterial blood pressure dropped to around 90 mm Hg, a reflex acceleration would occur in the rate of heart contractions to help restore normal pressure. Likewise, if the blood pressure of a resting person increased to 140 mm Hg, a reflex decrease would occur in the rate of heart contractions.

### Elasticity of Arteries

The tunica media layer of arteries, with its elastic tissue, allows arteries to dilate and constrict, which helps to move blood and maintain blood pressure. This property of arteries is responsible for diastolic pressure. If the arteries lose some of their elasticity, as occurs with arteriosclerosis, the diastolic pressure rises. The arteries then are like rigid tubes, and they are not able to help the heart maintain normal blood pressure.

### Peripheral Resistance

The resistance to blood flow in the arterioles is called **peripheral resistance.** Constriction of the precapillary sphincter muscles restricts the flow of blood into capillary beds. This acts to increase the pressure in the arterioles and arteries behind them. When the precapillary sphincter muscles dilate, they allow blood to easily pass into the low pressure region in the capillary beds and veins.

The peripheral resistance, maintained by constriction and dilation of precapillary sphincter muscles, is important in maintenance of blood pressure and blood flow. If all the precapillary sphincter muscles were to open at the same time, blood would flow into all the capillary beds, and blood pressure would drop tremendously. This also would cause blood to pool in the capillaries and reduce the flow of blood through vital organs, such as the brain, kidneys, liver, and lungs, resulting in a shock condition. To prevent this drop in pressure, not all the precapillary sphincters are open at one time. The only precapillary sphincters and capillary beds that are open at any one time are those where the blood is needed the most. The others are closed, which helps to maintain blood pressure at a high level and helps in the flow of blood.

### Blood Volume

The quantity of blood in the vessels directly affects blood pressure. The greater the quantity, the higher the pressure, and vice versa. If a person loses blood by hemorrhaging, blood pressure will drop. Likewise, if the amount of blood increases due to conditions such as **polycythemia** (large number of red blood cells) and **leukocytosis** (large number of white blood cells), blood pressure rises.

### Blood Viscosity ( Thickness)

The thicker that blood becomes, the more difficult it is for blood to flow. This causes an increase in blood pressure as the heart and arteries work harder to move the blood. The quantity of red blood cells and plasma pro-

teins determines the viscosity of blood. Polycythemia increases blood viscosity as well as blood volume. Anemia (decrease in red blood cells and hemoglobin) lowers blood viscosity and, thereby, blood pressure.

## FACTORS THAT CAN AFFECT ARTERIAL BLOOD PRESSURE

The previous factors are important in the maintenance of blood pressure. Other factors can affect blood pressure, but are not thought of as being involved in the normal maintenance of blood pressure. These factors are discussed next.

### Exercise

This factor, more than any other, greatly affects blood pressure. When someone increases physical exertion beyond the normal amount, all activities of the body are increased greatly; therefore, the rate of blood flow needs to be increased to the organs and tissues. This causes a reflex increase in the cardiac rate and blood pressure to as much as 150 to 180 contractions per minute and 180 to 200 mm Hg.

### Weight

People who are overweight have a greater amount of adipose tissue to circulate blood through than do people of normal weight. This requires the heart and arteries to work harder and often results in an increase in blood pressure. The increased adipose tissue often localizes in arteries, increasing atherosclerosis. This will narrow the lumen of arteries and increase blood pressure.

### Emotion

Distinct changes in a person's emotions from external stimuli that arouse fear, anger, and excitement can greatly increase blood pressure. Sympathetic nerves reflexly accelerate the rate of heart contractions and increase peripheral resistance.

### Age

The blood pressure of most adults remains about the same until a person is about 60 years of age. The arteries in a person gradually lose their elasticity over the years. At about 60 years of age, the loss of elasticity often is great enough to cause an increase in blood pressure. In some people hardening of the arteries occurs at a faster rate than in others; therefore, it is possible for a 40-year-old person to be 65 insofar as the condition of the arteries is concerned.

## ARTERIAL PULSE

The **arterial pulse** is defined as the alternate expansion and recoil of an artery. The arterial pulse is caused by the heart intermittently pumping blood into the arteries. The aorta bulges as it receives blood from the left ventricle during ventricular systole, and the aorta recoils as blood is pushed on through it. This alternate expansion and recoil of the aorta continues through the **brachial artery** in the upper arm and is finally measured in the **radial artery** in the lower arm.

The pulse is indicative of heart and arterial action; therefore, it is noted several times a day on hospitalized patients. The radial artery is the most common site for measuring pulse; since it crosses over the radius bone, it is possible to compress it against the bone and feel the pulsations.

### Effects of Gravity on Venous Flow

Gravity interferes with the flow of blood through veins from the lower parts of the body, especially when one is in the upright position. Several factors help move venous blood back to the heart:

**MUSCLE CONTRACTION.** Blood is helped along in veins that are located within and near skeletal muscles. When the muscles contract, they compress the veins and push the blood upward.

**VALVES.** Valves located along the length of veins (Figure 8–9) open to allow blood to flow upward, but close to prevent blood from flowing downward.

**DECREASING BLOOD PRESSURE IN VEINS TOWARD THE HEART.** The continuous decrease in venous pressure reaches its lowest point where veins enter the heart. The low pressure at the heart helps to pull blood upward from higher pressure areas, in the lower trunk and extremities.

**INSPIRATION MOVEMENTS.** During inspiration (breathing air in) a negative pressure is created in the thoracic cavity. This negative pressure acts to pull blood

upward from the higher pressure areas, located in the lower parts of the body.

## REGULATION OF BLOOD PRESSURE AND FLOW

The activities of the body's tissues will vary considerably during a day; therefore, adjustments of the blood pressure and blood distribution to the various body tissues must continually be made to meet these changing needs.

The nervous system is primarily responsible for these changes in that it transmits visceral efferent (motor) impulses to the heart and blood vessels to regulate their activities. There are two reflex centers in the brain, **cardiac** and **vasomotor,** that initiate these impulses. These two centers are stimulated by various afferent (sensory) nerve impulses and by chemical substances in the circulating bloodstream.

### Cardiac Reflex Center

The **cardiac reflex center,** located in the medulla of the brain (Figure 8–18), controls the rate and force of the heartbeat. This center contains both an area that speeds up the heart (cardio-accelerator) and an area that slows down the heart (cardio-inhibitory). The cardio-accelerator area receives sensory impulses that indicate the heart rate should be speeded up. The area responds by sending motor impulses along sympathetic fibers to the SA node in the heart, which increases the rate of heart contractions. The cardio-inhibitory area receives impulses that indicate the heart should be slowed down; it responds by sending impulses along parasympathetic fibers to the SA node, which slows the heart. Increasing the heart rate increases blood pressure and distribution of blood; decreasing the heart rate decreases blood pressure and distribution of blood.

### Vasomotor Reflex Center

The **vasomotor reflex center,** located in the medulla of the brain (Figure 8–18), regulates dilation (vasodilation) and constriction (vasoconstriction) of blood vessels. **Vasodilation** is an increase in the diameter of blood vessels, thereby increasing blood flow. **Vasoconstriction** is a decrease in the diameter of blood vessels, thereby decreasing blood flow. When the vasodilator center receives a sensory impulse indicating that dilation of

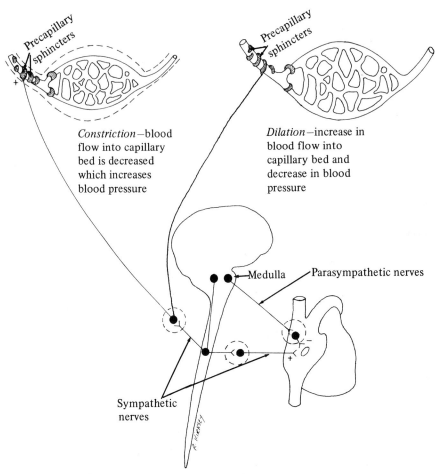

*Precapillary sphincters*

*Constriction*—blood flow into capillary bed is decreased which increases blood pressure

*Dilation*—increase in blood flow into capillary bed and decrease in blood pressure

Medulla

Parasympathetic nerves

Sympathetic nerves

**Figure 8-18.** Blood pressure is regulated by the cardiac and vasomotor reflex centers in the medulla of the brain.

blood vessels is necessary, it inhibits any further sympathetic nerve impulse transmission to the arterioles (precapillary sphincters). As a result, they dilate and allow more blood to flow through capillaries in that region. The vasoconstrictor area, when stimulated in the appropriate way, transmits sympathetic impulses to arterioles, which constrict and decrease the flow of blood through capillaries in that area.

A question arises: How do these cardiac and vasomotor centers receive sensory impulses that cause them to send out the appropriate motor impulses? Special receptor cells send sensory impulses to these centers, and they will be discussed shortly.

### Rate of Blood Flow

The rate of blood flow controls the amount of nutrients and wastes exchanged between the capillaries and tissues. If the rate of blood flow is seriously decreased, the affected tissues become **ischemic** (lack of blood flow to a part of the body) and malnourished. What factors affect the rate of blood flow? Does blood flow at different rates in the various vessels?

**FACTORS AFFECTING RATE OF BLOOD FLOW.** The rate of flow of any fluid, including blood, through vessels is determined by

$$\text{Flow} = \frac{\text{pressure}}{\text{resistance}}$$

FACTORS THAT DETERMINE RESISTANCE

- Viscosity of blood
- Length of vessels
- Cross-sectional area of vessels

This means that in blood vessels where the pressure is high and resistance is low the rate of flow will be faster.

Likewise, in vessels where pressure is low and resistance is high the rate of flow will be slower.

**RATE OF BLOOD FLOW THROUGH THE DIF-FERENT VESSELS.** Previously the question was asked whether blood flows at different rates in the various vessels. The answer is yes. Now we will study how the differences in pressure and resistance are responsible for the different rates of flow. Also, we will study the importance of the rate of blood flow in each of the different vessels.

Notice in Table 8–3 that the resistance in arteries is considerably less than that in veins and capillaries. As a result of this plus the high pressure, the rate of blood flow in arteries is very high. The importance of this is that oxygenated blood, rich in nutrients, is rapidly circulated to the tissues. When the blood reaches the capillaries, the resistance is quite high and the pressure is at a medium level. These two factors result in a very slow rate of flow through the tissues. This slow rate of flow is very important since it allows for an efficient exchange of nutrients and wastes between the capillaries and tissues. The reason the capillaries have such a high cross-sectional area can be seen in Figures 8–15, 8–16, and 8–17. The arterioles, which enter the capillary beds, branch extensively to form the capillary beds. This extensive branching increases the cross-sectional area and, therefore, tremendously increases the resistance of capillaries.

After the blood moves through the capillaries, it moves into the veins, where the resistance is greater than arteries but the pressure lower. The result is that the rate of flow is lower than that in arteries but higher than that in capillaries. The importance of this is that deoxygenated blood, rich in wastes, moves fairly rapidly from the tissues back to the heart. The heart will then pump this blood through the pulmonary system for exchange of $CO_2$ for $O_2$.

## PRESSORECEPTOR AND CHEMORECEPTOR CELLS

Special sensory receptor cells detect changes in the blood pressure and chemical composition of blood, which they transmit to the cardiac and vasomotor reflex center.

### Pressoreceptor Cells

**Pressoreceptor cells** are sensitive to changes in blood pressure and are located in the walls of the aortic arch, bifurcation of carotid arteries, and superior and inferior venae cavae (Figure 8–19).

### Chemoreceptor Cells

**Chemoreceptor cells** detect changes in the chemical composition of blood and are located in the aortic arch and the bifurcation of common carotid arteries (Figure

**TABLE 8–3.**  *Rate of Blood Flow in Blood Vessels, Pressure, Resistance, Etc.*

|  | Pressure | Resistance (Cross-Sectional Area) | Rate of Flow (cm/sec) | Importance |
|---|---|---|---|---|
| Arteries | High 32 to 120 mm Hg | Aorta, 2.5 cm² Arteries, 20 cm² Arterioles, 40 cm² | 40 10 to 40 0.1 to 10 | To rapidly carry oxygenated blood from heart to capillaries in tissues for exchange |
| Veins | Low 12 to –10 mm Hg | Vena cavae, 8 cm² Veins, 80 cm² Venules, 250 cm² | 5 to 20 0.3 to 5 0.3 | To carry deoxygenated blood rich in wastes fairly fast back to heart |
| Capillaries | Medium 12 to 32 mm Hg | 2500 cm² | Less than 0.1 | Slow rate allows for very efficient exchange of nutrients and wastes between capillaries and tissues |

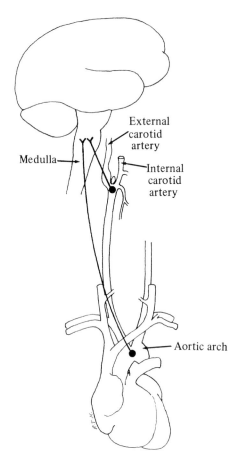

**Figure 8-19.** Pressoreceptor and chemoreceptor cells. These specialized cells, located in the aortic arch and bifurcation of the carotid arteries, are sensitive to chemical and pressure changes in the blood. Sensory impulses are sent to the cardiac and vasomotor reflex centers in the medulla.

8-19). The concentration of carbon dioxide, oxygen, lactic acid, and certain hormones is important in regulating the beat of the heart and action of blood vessels.

### Functions of Receptor Cells

Examples of how the receptor cells work in coordination with the cardiac and vasomotor reflex centers are as follows:

**CHANGE IN BLOOD PRESSURE.** If something happens to cause blood pressure to rise above normal levels, the pressoreceptor cells in the aortic arch and carotid arteries are stimulated and they send sensory impulses to the cardiac and vasomotor reflex centers. These centers, in the medulla, transmit parasympathetic impulses to the heart, slowing it down, and inhibit sympathetic impulses to the arterioles, resulting in vasodilation (Figure 8–18). Slowing the heart and dilating the blood vessels reduces the blood pressure back to its normal level. Dilating the blood vessels decreases the resistance to blood flow and lowers the blood pressure.

If something happens to cause a sudden drop in blood pressure, the pressoreceptors stimulate the cardio-acceleration and vasoconstriction centers in the medulla. The cardio-acceleration center transmits impulses along sympathetic nerves to the SA node, which increases the rate of heart contractions (Figure 8–18). The vasoconstriction center transmits sympathetic impulses to blood capillaries, causing them to constrict. These two actions help to return the blood pressure to its normal level.

**CHANGE IN CHEMICAL COMPOSITION.** If the concentration of oxygen or carbon dioxide changes significantly, chemoreceptor cells are stimulated and send impulses to the vasomotor and cardiac reflex centers. Chemoreceptor cells are located in the aorta and carotid arteries (Figure 8–19). These receptors are stimulated by changes in oxygen and carbon dioxide. For example, if the concentration of oxygen drops considerably, these receptors are stimulated, and they send impulses to the cardio-accelerator center in the medulla. This center transmits sympathetic impulses that accelerate the heartbeat. The vasoconstrictor center in the medulla receives the same impulses and transmits sympathetic impulses to arterioles, which constrict. These two reflex actions serve to increase the rate of heartbeat and blood pressure level. Increasing the rate of the heart pumps blood to the lungs more rapidly, and $CO_2$ is exchanged for $O_2$. Increasing blood pressure helps to push $O_2$ and nutrients out of capillaries into the cells faster and helps to increase the rate at which blood moves through the body.

# SUMMARY

### The Cardiovascular System
A. Composed of heart, arteries, capillaries, and veins; closed system that pumps blood throughout body.

B.  Anatomy of the heart
  1.  Wall of heart is composed of three layers: epicardium, protects heart against friction; myocardium, muscular layer that contracts and moves blood through heart; endocardium, inner lining of heart and protects myocardium.
  2.  Atria and ventricles: two upper chambers are atria; function, receive deoxygenated blood and pump it to the ventricles; ventricles, two lower chambers; function, pump oxygenated blood to tissues.
  3.  Heart valves: two types in heart, atrioventricular and semilunar; one-way valves in that they allow blood to flow through but close to prevent blood from flowing back through.
      a.  Atrioventricular: located between atria and ventricles; tricuspid, located between right atrium and ventricle; mitral, located between left atrium and ventricle.
      b.  Semilunar: located at entrance to aorta and pulmonary trunk.
C.  Blood supply to the heart
  1.  Coronary arteries branch off aorta and supply oxygenated blood to myocardium; coronary veins transport deoxygenated blood from myocardium into right atrium.
D.  Cardiac cycle and regulation of heart contractions
  1.  Cardiac cycle consists of diastole and systole; systole is contraction of chambers and diastole is relaxation of chambers; atria systole and ventricular diastole occur simultaneously; chambers fill with blood during diastole.
  2.  Heart sounds occur when valves open and close. Lub, first sound heard through stethoscope, results from atrioventricular valves closing; dup, second sound heard, results from closing of semilunar valves.
E.  Abnormalities of the heart that affect cardiac cycle
  1.  Rheumatic fever: streptococcal infection that spreads to valves from joints; toxins especially affect mitral valve, resulting in narrowing of valve or mitral stenosis.
F.  Regulation of rhythmic heart contractions
  Contractions of heart are regulated by autonomic nervous system. Transmission of impulses through heart involves two nodes and nerve bundles:
  1.  SA node: knot of cardiac tissue in right atrium; initiates heartbeat and sets rhythm; called pacemaker.
  2.  AV node: modified tissue at junction of right atrium and ventricle; receives impulses from atria and conducts them into atrioventricular bundle.
  3.  Atrioventricular bundle: nerve bundle that extends from AV node through ventricular system to Purkinje fibers.
  4.  Purkinje fibers: nerve fibers that extend from atrioventricular bundle into ventricles.
G.  Nervous control of heart
  1.  Electrocardiogram (ECG): measurement of heart activity; P wave, spread of nerve impulse from SA node through atria; Q, R, S wave, spread of nerve impulse through ventricles; T wave, repolarization or recovery phase of ventricles.
H.  Effect of ions on nervous control of heart
  1.  Effects of potassium ions ($K^+$): hyperkalemia or elevated level of potassium ions can result in cardiac arrest.
  2.  Effects of calcium ions ($Ca^{2+}$): blood calcium level above normal is called hypercalcemia; results in spastic contractions of myocardium.
I.  Volume of blood pumped through the heart
  1.  Stroke volume: amount of blood pumped out of a ventricle with each contraction; 70 ml is average.
  2.  Cardiac output: amount of blood pumped from a ventricle each minute; average is 5040 ml/min.
J.  Arteries
  1.  Transport oxygenated blood from heart to capillaries.
  2.  Arterial walls composed of three tissue layers:
      a.  Tunica externa: connective tissue layer; gives strength to artery.

      b. Tunica media: middle layer composed of smooth muscle and elastic tissue; allows dilation and constriction.

      c. Tunica interna: innermost layer composed of simple squamous tissue.

K. Veins

  1. Transport deoxygenated blood from capillaries to heart.

  2. Same three tissue layers as artery but thinner; less elastic and under lower pressure than arteries; valves present help to prevent backflow of blood.

L. Capillaries

Microscopic vessels; consist of single layer of simple squamous tissue; connect arteries to veins and allow exchange of nutrients and wastes.

  1. Size and distribution of capillaries: size is regulated by precapillary sphincter muscles; numbers of capillaries in tissues varies according to metabolic activity of the tissue (e.g., the more active the tissue, the greater the number of capillaries).

## The Circulatory System

Circulatory system is divided into three units: systemic, hepatic portal, and pulmonary.

A. Systemic: transports blood to and drains blood from all parts of body except air sacs (alveoli) of the lungs; Table 8–2 gives the major arteries of the systemic unit; Figure 8–11 presents the major veins of the systemic unit.

B. Hepatic portal system: consists of veins that drain digestive products from digestive organs into liver through hepatic portal veins; function of system is to inspect, cleanse, remove, and modify materials in blood before it enters general circulation.

C. Pulmonary system: transports unoxygenated blood from heart to lungs where it exchanges $CO_2$ for $O_2$ and returns oxygenated blood to heart.

## Blood Pressure

A. Arterial pressure: pressure of blood in arteries; systolic pressure results from contraction of ventricles; diastolic pressure results from recoil contraction of arteries.

  1. Arterioles and peripheral resistance: arterioles are small arteries; located at entrance into capillary bed; precapillary sphincters open and close entrance into capillaries and thereby regulate amount of blood entering capillary bed.

B. Determination of blood pressure: determined by the instrument sphygmomanometer; systolic pressure, pressure created by contraction of ventricles and can vary from 90 to 140 mm Hg; diastolic pressure, pressure created by contraction and recoil of arteries and varies from 50 to 90 mm Hg.

C. Factors involved in maintenance of arterial blood pressure

  1. Rate of cardiac contractions: increase in rate of contractions equals increase in blood pressure, and vice versa.

  2. Elasticity of arteries: decrease in elasticity equals an increase in blood pressure.

  3. Peripheral resistance: increase in resistance at precapillary sphincters increases pressure, and vice versa.

  4. Blood volume: increase in blood volume increases blood pressure, and vice versa.

  5. Blood viscosity (thickness): the thicker the blood, the higher the pressure, and vice versa.

D. Factors that can affect arterial blood pressure

  1. Exercise: increase in weight increases blood pressure due to extra adipose tissue and possible atherosclerosis.

  2. Weight: increase in weight increases blood pressure due to extra adipose tissue and possible atherosclerosis.

  3. Emotion: increase in emotion increases blood pressure.

  4. Age: increase in age decreases elasticity of arteries and thereby increases blood pressure.

E. Arterial pulse: pulse is the alternate expansion and recoil of an artery; indicates number of times heart contracts and strength indicates condition of the artery.

F. Effects of gravity on venous flow: flow of blood upward through veins is aided by several factors, muscle contractions, valves, decreasing blood pressure, and inspiration movements.

G. Regulation of blood pressure and flow
   1. Cardiac reflex center: located in medulla oblongata; contains cardio-accelerator and cardio-inhibitory areas that reflexly accelerate or inhibit heart rate and blood pressure.
   2. Vasomotor reflex center: located in medulla and includes vasoconstriction and vasodilation areas; control diameter of blood vessels at precapillary sphincters.

H. Rate of blood flow = pressure/resistance; rate of flow in arteries is fast, distributes blood rapidly to tissues; rate of flow in capillaries is slow, allows efficient exchange of nutrients.

I. Pressoreceptor and chemoreceptor cells are located in aortic arch, bifurcation of carotid arteries; detect changes in blood pressure and concentrations of oxygen and carbon dioxide, respectively, and transmit changes to medulla.

## The Cardiovascular System

True (A) or false (B). Questions 1 to 4.

1. The layers of the heart from the inside to the outside are endocardium, myocardium, and epicardium.

2. The right side of the heart pumps unoxygenated blood to the lungs.

3. The pathway that a nerve impulse travels as it passes through the heart is:
     SA node → bundle of His → AV node → Purkinje fibers

4. A cardiac cycle consists of a contraction (systole) and relaxation (diastole) period.

5. Which of the following is(are) correctly paired?
   1. P wave — measures atria contraction
   2. T wave — ventricles contracting
   3. Q, R, S wave — spread of impulse through ventricles
   4. ECG — electroencephalogram
   (a) 1, 2, 3     (b) 1, 3     (c) 2, 4     (d) 4     (e) All of these

6. Which of the following is(are) correctly paired?
   (a) Systemic unit — transports blood to all parts of body except air sacs
   (b) Hepatic portal — transports unoxygenated blood to lungs
   (c) Pulmonary system — cleanses, removes wastes, and modifies materials in blood
   (d) (a), (b)
   (e) (b), (c)

7. Which of these factors is(are) involved in maintenance of blood pressure?
   1. Rate of cardiac contractions     3. Blood viscosity
   2. Peripheral resistance     4. Exercise
   (a) 1, 2, 3     (b) 1, 3     (c) 2, 4     (d) 4     (e) All of these

Matching. Questions 8 to 12.

8. arterial pulse     **A.** sensitive to changes in blood pressure

9. cardiac reflex center     **B.** rate of blood flow is slow for exchange of wastes and nutrients

10. capillaries     **C.** indicative of number of times that heart contracts

11. vasomotor reflex center     **D.** controls diameter of blood vessels at precapillary sphincters

12. pressoreceptor cells     **E.** located in medulla and can increase or decrease heart rate

# Chapter 9

# SKIN

After reading and studying this chapter, a student should be able to:

1. Describe the structure of the epidermis.
2. Write a description of the location and types of tissues in the dermis.
3. Recognize a description of the structure and function of sweat and sebaceous glands, nails, and hair.
4. Discuss the protection, temperature regulation, sensory reception, and synthesis of vitamin D functions of the skin.
5. Describe the four changes involved in inflammation of tissues.
6. Differentiate among labile, stable, and permanent cells.

*The skin often is referred to as the integumentary system, since it is composed of a variety of organs such as nerves, blood vessels, sweat and oil glands. This system exhibits the structure-function concept quite well. The structure of the skin is what makes it the first line of defense against chemical and mechanical injuries.*

# 1  STRUCTURE OF THE SKIN

The skin is composed of two layers of tissues, **epidermis** and **dermis.**

## *EPIDERMIS*

The **epidermis** is the outer layer, and it is composed of strata or layers of epithelial tissue (Figure 9–1). The epithelial tissue actually is **keratinized stratified squamous** epithelial tissue. The thickness of the epidermis varies from area to area of the body. It is thickest in areas that are exposed to constant wear and tear, such as the palms of the hands and soles of the feet. The thicker and thinner areas of the skin are composed of four strata (Figure 9–1). The strata named in order from the outside to the inside are **stratum corneum, stratum lucidum, stratum granulosum,** and **stratum germinativum.**

Only one of the strata, **stratum germinativum,** is composed of living cells; the other strata are composed of dead keratinized cells. The outermost stratum, stratum corneum, constantly is being rubbed off. Stratum germinativum cells undergo mitosis quite rapidly to replace the lost stratum corneum cells. Each generation of cells is pushed upward as succeeding generations are produced. The cells gradually die as they move up through the strata, and the protoplasm undergoes changes called **keratinization.** There is no blood supply to the stratified epithelial tissue cells once they are pushed up from the stratum germinativum layer. This lack of blood is what causes the cells to gradually die and undergo keratinization. These changes are such that the protoplasm is changed into a protein called **keratin.** The process is complete when the cells reach the top stratum, stratum corneum. Keratin is water resistant; therefore, the stratum corneum, is a waterproof layer of cells that prevents large amounts of water from entering and leaving the body. These cornified, horny cells are constantly being shed or rubbed off. The rate at which cells are produced in the stratum germinativum is equal to the rate at which stratum corneum cells are lost.

**Melanin** or skin pigment is contained in stratum germinativum cells. The coloration of skin depends upon the amount of melanin present. Dark-skinned people have large amounts of melanin whereas light-skinned people have small amounts. Melanin is produced by cells called **melanocytes** and they are stimulated by sunlight. The ultraviolet rays of sunlight activate melanocytes so that they spread out. The spreading out of the melanocytes results in a browner color being produced, or a suntan. People who have freckles simply have areas that are composed of irregular clumps of melanin. Freckles are an inherited permanent trait and are present in the stratum germinativum. Creams and lotions are not effective in removing or covering up freckles because cosmetics cannot penetrate through the strata to the stratum germinativum.

## *DERMIS*

The **dermis** (Figure 9–1) is the layer under the epidermis. It is considered the true skin, and it is firmly attached to the epidermis. The ridges and valleys of the epidermis are what produce each person's characteristic fingerprints; these ridges actually originate in the

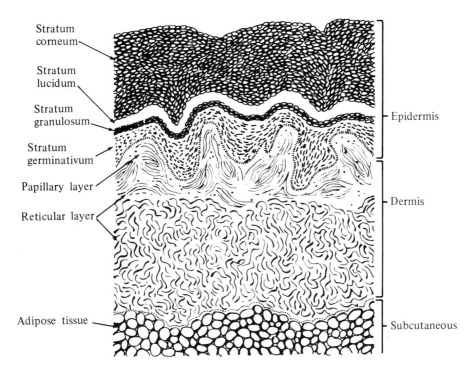

Stratum corneum

Stratum lucidum

Stratum granulosum

Stratum germinativum

Papillary layer

Reticular layer

Adipose tissue

Epidermis

Dermis

Subcutaneous

**Figure 9-1.** Layers of the skin. The epidermis and the strata making it up are shown, along with the dermis and the subcutaneous layer of tissue under the skin.

dermis. These structures firmly attach the dermis to the epidermis. The area of the dermis in which the ridges and valleys are located is called the **papillary layer.** The area below the papillary layer is called the **reticular layer.** Dense connective tissue and elastic connective tissue make up the reticular layer. In addition the dermis is well supplied with blood vessels, nerves, sweat glands, oil glands, and hairs (Figure 9-2). The dense connective tissue gives the skin strength and the elastic connective tissue gives the skin extensibility and elasticity. These two properties are vividly exhibited in pregnant women and obese people. In both cases the skin is stretched, but it will contract back to its normal shape and size when the baby is born and/or the weight is lost. As one grows older the amount of elastic tissue diminishes, and fat is lost from the subcutaneous tissue. These losses ultimately result in wrinkles.

Immediately below the dermis is the **subcutaneous tissue** or **superficial fascial membrane.** This tissue is composed primarily of adipose cells and is not part of the skin. Blood vessels, lymph vessels, nerves, hair follicles, and sweat glands either are located here or pass through this tissue.

# 2  DERIVATIVES OF THE SKIN

The sweat glands, sebaceous glands (oil glands), nails, ceruminous glands, hair, and arrector pili muscles all result from specialization of cells in the skin.

## SWEAT GLANDS (SUDORIFEROUS GLANDS)

**Sweat glands (sudoriferous glands)** are distributed extensively over the body but are more numerous in the axillae, forehead, soles of the feet, and palms of the hands. Sweat glands are composed of epithelial tissue that has grown downward into the dermis and subcutaneous tissue. The epithelial tissue specializes into glandular tissue, which forms sweat. Each gland is composed of a tube that is extremely coiled at the bottom. The portion of the gland that connects the coiled tube to the surface of the skin is the excretory duct. The excretory duct opens onto the skin surface by a pore opening. The coiled end (Figure 9–2) can be located both in the dermis and subcutaneous tissues. Capillaries surround the coiled end, and sympathetic nerves from the autonomic nervous system innervate the capillaries.

As the internal body temperature rises above a certain level, the heat receptor cells in the skin are stimulated. They send sensory impulses to the hypothalamus in the brain, which integrates the sensory impulses and sends motor impulses to the sweat glands. This results in water and salts being produced by the glands in increased quantities. The water and salts move up the excretory ducts of the sweat glands to the surface of the skin, where the water evaporates. The evaporation of water is a process of converting water from a liquid state to a gaseous state and requires heat. Since heat is used up in this conversion process it functions to lower the body temperature.

## SEBACEOUS GLANDS

**Sebaceous glands (oil glands)** are composed of epithelial tissue and open into the hair follicles (Figure 9–2). They are distributed everywhere on the body except the palms of the hands and soles of the feet. Sebaceous glands secrete an oily substance called **sebum**

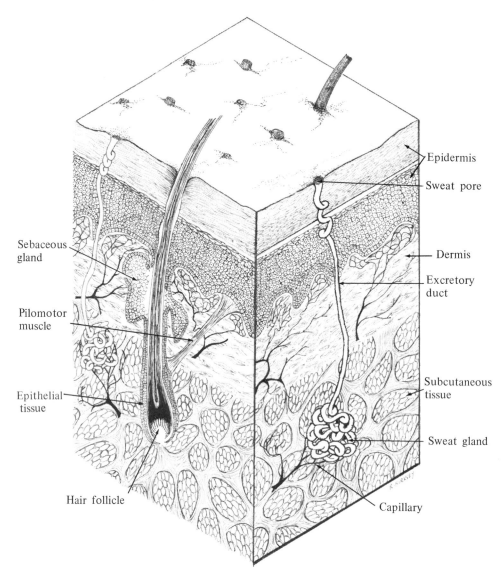

**Figure 9-2.**  The structure and location of skin derivatives.

(oil). Unlike sweat glands, sebaceous glands do not have their own ducts. Sebum passes through hair follicles up to the skin surface, where it helps to both waterproof and prevent drying of the skin. If dirt particles block the openings of the sebaceous glands, sebum accumulates and is oxidized, resulting in blackheads. The sebaceous glands are usually quite active during the teen years, and as a result blackheads also are quite prevalent. Sebaceous glands can become infected by pus-producing microorganisms, resulting in acne.

## NAILS

**Nails** (fingernails and toenails) are composed of modified, keratinized epithelial tissue. The new cells are produced by the stratum germinativum, which is located in the nail root. The body of the nails extends out and covers the nail bed, which is really dermis. The nail bed is well supplied with blood vessels, which give it its typical pink appearance. The white crescent-shaped structure is the **lunula,** below which is the nail root.

## HAIR

**Hair** (Figure 9–2) and hair follicles result from epithelial tissue that has grown downward into the dermis and subcutaneous layers. The epithelial tissue develops into specialized tissue that can produce hair cells. The deepest region of a hair follicle is the root. The production of new hair cells takes place in the root by means of mitosis. The upward movement of new hair cells occurs through the hair shaft as new generations of cells are produced.

Two sebaceous glands are attached to each hair shaft along with a small bundle of smooth muscle tissue, **arrector pili** muscle or **pilomotor muscle.** The other end of each pilomotor muscle (Figure 9–2) attaches to the papillary layer of the dermis. The muscle contracts from the shaft toward the papillary layer attachment, and contraction pulls the hair into an upright position. This ultimately results in hair standing on end and "goose bumps." This process serves a purpose we will discuss shortly.

## CERUMINOUS GLANDS

**Ceruminous glands** are located in the dermis along the length of the canal (external auditory means) leading into the middle ear. The glands secrete a waxy substance that commonly is called ear wax. The wax helps to prevent the tympanic membrane (eardrum) from drying out.

# 3 FUNCTIONS OF THE SKIN AND DERIVATIVES

The skin has several functions, three of which are quite important: protection, temperature regulation, and sensory reception. Another function is the production of vitamin D.

## PROTECTION

The keratinized stratum corneum layer helps prevent microbes from penetrating to the deeper strata and tissues. Sweat and sebum both have antibacterial properties that normally prevent bacteria from penetrating the epidermis. In Chapter 3 you learned that microorganisms normally are found on the skin and are called **normal flora.** The anatomic barrier, sweat and sebum of the skin, prevents these microorganisms from penetrating the skin and becoming pathogenic. The normal flora decompose the sweat and sebum secretions, which results in body odor.

The keratin protein compound (fibrous protein) in the stratum corneum waterproofs the skin and prevents excessive entrance and loss of fluids through the skin. This waterproofing is very important in maintaining homeostasis of the body. Without this waterproof barrier, fluids could both evaporate and enter the body in excessive quantities. This waterproof covering is what allows you to enjoy swimming in fresh water and in salt water and still maintain a normal level of body fluids. When you are swimming in fresh water, the concentration of solutes and of osmotic pressure inside the body is greater than that in the fresh water. Therefore, the higher osmotic pressure tries to pull water into the body. The waterproof skin prevents the internal osmotic pressure from pulling water inside. When you are swimming in salt water, the osmotic pressure is greater in the salt water than in the body; therefore, the salt water attempts to pull water out of the body. The waterproof epidermis prevents water from osmosing out of the body and causing dehydration of tissues.

## TEMPERATURE REGULATION

It is important that body temperature be maintained fairly close to 37°C. The skin and its derivatives act as excellent temperature-regulating devices. The sweat glands increase their secretion of sweat when the internal temperature rises. The sweat evaporates from the surface of the skin and this acts to cool the body temperature.

The blood capillaries under the epidermis also help to regulate body temperature. Excess heat produced by chemical reactions is carried throughout the body by the blood. The heat radiates from the epidermal capillaries through the skin and out of the body. If the body temperature rises, the vessels dilate (vasodilation), and more heat is lost; but if the body temperature drops, the vessels constrict in diameter (vasoconstriction), and less heat is lost.

## SENSORY RECEPTION

The skin contains many specialized sensory receptor cells. These cells are specialized for certain stimuli— heat, cold, pain, touch, and pressure. These sensory receptors carry information about the external and internal environment of the body to the sensory integrating areas of the brain.

The motor areas of the brain send out motor impulses to the various parts of the body, which respond in a way that results in the body adjusting itself to environmental conditions. An example of this sequence of events is an increase in body temperature. Heat receptor cells are stimulated as the temperature rises, and they send afferent (sensory) impulses to the heat control center in the hypothalamus.

The sensory receptor cells are very important since they have to detect changes in the environment and notify the proper areas of the brain so that the appropriate corrective responses can be made. If the skin did not contain many receptor cells, it would be quite difficult for the body to maintain homeostasis.

## SYNTHESIS OF VITAMIN D

The ultraviolet rays of the sun interact with **cholesterol** (steroid compound, Chapter 2) to form vitamin D, which is important for proper bone development.

## 4  INFLAMMATION

The next great defense the body has against infection, after the skin, is the process called **inflammation.** Many irritants, in addition to bacteria, can cause inflammation. For example, cuts, blows, chemicals, fire, and friction all can result in inflammation. The symptoms of inflammation are redness, heat, swelling, and pain. The microscopic changes that cause these symptoms and their importance are as follows:

### REDNESS

**Redness** is caused by dilation of arterioles, venules, and capillaries (Figure 9–3). The dilation of these vessels results from the release of various chemicals in the damaged area, one of which is **histamine.** Histamine stimulates arteriolar dilation. The importance of this event is that dilation of the blood vessels brings a large volume of blood (rich in nutrients for phagocytosis and wound healing) to the damaged area.

### HEAT

The **heat** symptom results from an increased flow of blood to the damaged area; thus, an increased amount of heat radiates from the region.

### SWELLING

The **swelling** results from histamine and other chemicals increasing the permeability of blood capillaries. This permeability change allows large amounts of fluids and WBCs to move out of the capillaries (Figure 9–3). The increase in fluids results in localized edema or swelling.

Certain chemicals cause localized clotting of the fluids in the injured area. Clotting acts to wall off the injured area, and this is important to prevent the spread of bacteria and fluids to surrounding tissues.

A large number of WBCs (neutrophils and monocytes) move by **diapedesis** out of the capillaries to the region of injury. They act to phagocytize any bacteria that might be present. Some WBCs will be de-

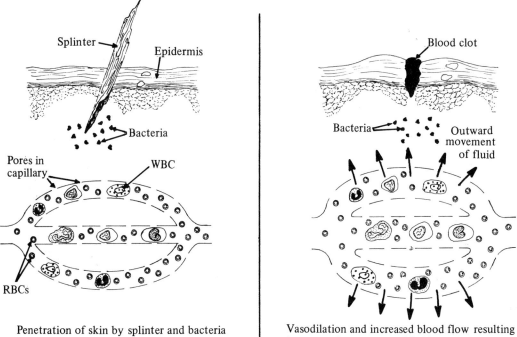

Penetration of skin by splinter and bacteria

Vasodilation and increased blood flow resulting in outward movement of fluids and edema

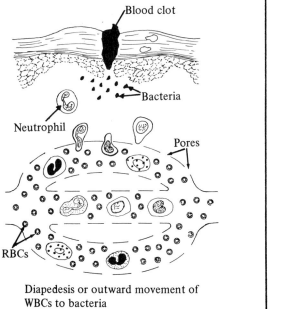

Diapedesis or outward movement of WBCs to bacteria

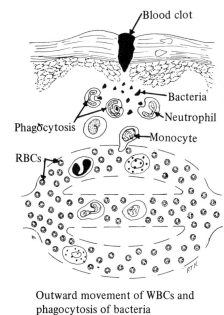

Outward movement of WBCs and phagocytosis of bacteria

**Figure 9–3.** Stages of inflammation.

stroyed along with bacteria. Their remains form what is called pus.

## PAIN

The **pain** symptom cannot be explained exactly, but it is thought that the increased amount of fluid and blood in the injured area acts on nerve endings to produce pain.

If bacteria move into lymph capillaries and are carried away from the inflamed area by lymph vessels, they will be destroyed by phagocytes in lymph nodes.

Inflammation is a temporary means of protecting the body. Following inflammation wound healing occurs,

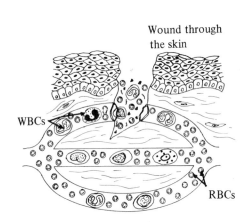

A wound through the skin results in bleeding

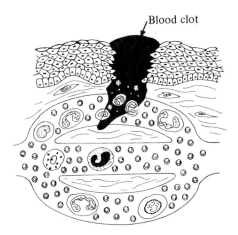

Inflammation of the capillary; formation of blood clot and growth of epithelial tissue

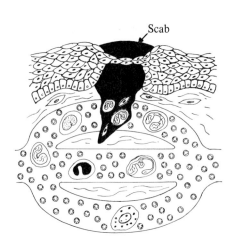

Production of new epithelial tissue and repair of capillary beneath scab

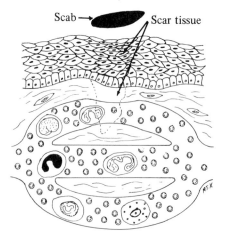

Sloughing off of scab; connection of blood capillaries; and formation of scar tissue

Figure 9-4.    Stages in the process of wound healing.

which is necessary to permanently repair damaged tissue and thereby restore permanent protection.

# 5 WOUND HEALING

## CELL REPLACEMENT

Wound healing occurs in some tissues and not in others. The replacement of destroyed cells, or wound healing, can only occur in tissues that have the capacity to divide by mitosis. Cells of the body can be placed into three groups, depending upon their ability to replace damaged cells: labile, stable, and permanent.

**Labile** (not fixed) cells retain the ability to divide by mitosis throughout life. Examples of where these cells are found are as follows:

1. Epithelial tissue:  Epidermis
Lining of oral cavity
Lining of respiratory tract
Lining of male and female genital tracts
Lining of ducts
Bone marrow

2. Lymphoid tissues:  Lymph nodes
Spleen
Tonsils

The epithelial tissues are exposed to a great deal of friction; therefore, the cells constantly slough off and are replaced. The epithelial lining of the small intestine is exposed to friction and chemical reactions. As a result the entire lining is replaced every few days.

**Stable cells** have the ability to reproduce, but do not under normal conditions. These cells are not continuously being lost and replaced. If these cells are damaged, they will replace themselves. An example is liver tissue.

**Permanent** cells that cannot reproduce include smooth, skeletal, and cardiac muscles. Some evidence indicates that muscle tissue may be able to reproduce. Also nerve tissue in the central nervous system cannot reproduce. Repair to muscle tissue does not involve regeneration of muscle cells but rather replacement with scar tissue. The scar tissue fills in the damaged areas, thereby protecting the deeper tissues from infection. However, the scar tissue lacks contractile ability and will slightly hinder contraction of the muscles.

### Steps Involved in Wound Healing

Figure 9–4 shows a wound through the epidermis into the dermis of the skin. The steps involved in healing this wound are as follows:

1. Inflammation and all activities associated with inflammation occur.
2. The blood clot that is formed during inflammation will fill the gap between the cut edges of the epidermis. This stops the bleeding from the wound and brings in the WBCs that phagocytize bacteria.
3. After clotting has occurred, the epithelial cells and fibroblasts (connective tissue cells that form collagenic fibers and matrix) begin to grow and reproduce rapidly (Figure 9–4). The production of new cells results in a bridge being formed across the injured area. This helps to give strength to the injured area.
4. Continuous production of epithelial and connective tissue continues under the scab. The damaged capillaries begin to form branches (Figure 9–4).
5. The scab sloughs off and the repair of the wond is complete. Scar tissue is all that is left at the site of the injury.

# SUMMARY

### Structure of the Skin
A. Epidermis
1. Outer layer composed of strata of dead keratinized squamous epithelial tissue; no blood supply; stratum germinativum only living layer and contains melanocytes that produce the pigment called melanin.

B. Dermis
    *1.* Composed of reticular and papillary layers; dense and elastic connective tissue gives dermis strength and elasticity.

## Derivatives of the Skin

A. Sweat glands (sudoriferous glands)
    *1.* Composed of modified epithelial tissue; glands located in dermis or subcutaneous tissue; ducts connect glands to skin surface; sweat produced by glands moves to skin surface where it evaporates; conversion of water from liquid to gaseous state uses up heat and lowers body temperature.

B. Sebaceous glands
    *1.* Attached to sides of hair follicles; secrete sebum, which moves up hair follicles; sebum waterproofs skin and prevents drying of skin and hair.

C. Nails
    *1.* Fingernails and toenails grow from stratum germinativum; protect tips of fingers and toes.

D. Hair
    *1.* Composed of specialized epithelial tissue; deepest region is the root where new hair cells are formed; arrector pili muscles are attached to hair shafts and, when contracted, pull hairs upright.

E. Ceruminous glands
    *1.* Located along external auditory meatus; secrete ear wax, which helps to prevent the tympanic membrane (eardrum) from drying out.

## Functions of the Skin and Derivatives

A. Protection
    *1.* Keratin in stratum corneum helps to protect body against invasion of bacteria and loss or gain of liquid.

B. Temperature regulation
    *1.* Evaporation of sweat uses up heat and therefore lowers body temperature.
    *2.* Blood vessels in the dermis regulate temperature by dilating or constricting blood vessels, thereby increasing or decreasing heat loss.

C. Sensory reception
    *1.* The dermis is the site of many receptor cells, sensitive to certain stimuli—heat, cold, pain, touch, and pressure; these cells make it possible for the brain to be aware of changes in the internal and external environment, thereby maintaining homeostasis.

D. Synthesis of Vitamin D
    *1.* Synthesis of vitamin D results from ultraviolet rays of sun converting cholesterol to vitamin D.

## Inflammation

A defense against invasion of bacteria; involves several changes:

A. Redness: vasodilation of blood vessels in dermis; importance is increased blood flow to injured area, which promotes healing.

B. Heat: results from vasodilation.

C. Swelling: results from histamine increasing permeability of blood vessels; important because large number of white blood cells (WBCs) move out of blood vessels and phagocytize bacteria.

D. Pain: thought to result from increased fluid stimulating pain receptor cells.

**Wound Healing**

A. Cell replacement

Three groups of cells based on ability to replace themselves if injured:

1. Labile: retain ability to divide throughout life; examples, epithelial and lymphoid.
2. Stable: ability to reproduce but do not under normal conditions; if tissue is injured, then cells can replace damaged ones; example, liver.
3. Permanent: cells cannot reproduce or replace themselves if injured; examples, smooth, skeletal, and cardiac muscles, and nerve tissue.

B. Steps Involved in Wound Healing

Five steps involved in wound healing are illustrated in Figure 9-4.

## The Skin

Matching. Questions 1–5.

1. stratified epithelial tissue    A. functions of dermis
2. stratum germinativum    B. produce pigment
3. dense connective tissue    C. epidermis
4. melanocytes    D. located in dermis
5. extensibility and elasticity    E. produces new cells

True (A) or false (B). Questions 6 to 9.

6. Sweat glands are modified dermis tissue.
7. Sweating lowers body temperature by dilation of blood vessels in dermis.
8. Sebaceous glands secrete sebum, which travels up to the skin surface and helps waterproof skin.
9. Hair is modified epidermal tissue, and arrector pili muscles pull them up when it is cold.
10. Which of the following are functions of the skin?

    1. Protection    3. Temperature regulation
    2. Elasticity    4. Inflammation

    (a) 1, 2, 3    (b) 1, 3    (c) 2, 4    (d) 4    (e) All of these

11. Which of the following is (are) *not correctly* paired?

    (a) Increase in body temperature — vasodilation of blood vessels in dermis
    (b) Sensory reception — sensory receptor cells in dermis
    (c) Labile cells — reproduce only when damaged
    (d) Inflammation — redness, heat, swelling, and pain
    (e) None of these

# Chapter 10

# LYMPHATIC SYSTEM

After reading and studying this chapter, a student should be able to:

1. Give the location and function of lymph capillaries.
2. Describe the anatomy and functions of lymph nodes.
3. Write a description of the location, anatomy, and functions of the spleen.
4. Name the three tonsils and give their functions.
5. Recognize a description of the location and functions of the thymus gland.
6. Give the location and function of Peyer's patches.

*The lymphatic system is composed of lymph organs such as the lymph nodes, tonsils, and spleen. The lymphatic system is closely associated with the cardiovascular system, since it is made up of vessels that collect and circulate fluid (lymph).*

# 1  LYMPH CAPILLARIES

**Lymph capillaries** originate as open-ended vessels in close association with blood capillaries. They drain water, proteins, microbes and other foreign materials from interstitial spaces into lymph vessels. Lymph vessels ultimately drain fluid into the blood stream, thereby returning to the blood important proteins that leaked out of blood capillaries.

# 2  LYMPH NODES

**Lymph nodes** are oval-shaped bodies (Figure 10–1) composed of lymph tissue surrounded by a fibrous capsule. They are located along the lymph vessels; however, they tend to be found in large masses in certain areas of the body, such as the cervical, axillary, and inguinal areas.

Each node is composed of numerous compartments (Figure 10–2) filled with white blood cells called **lymphocytes.** Each node receives lymph from several vessels called *afferent* vessels. The lymph drains through the compartments where the phagocytic cells phagocytize microbes and other foreign materials. The lymph that drains from the nodes, in one or two *efferent* vessels, has been filtered or purified of microbes. Lymph nodes have some other protective functions, which are discussed next.

## FILTRATION

**Filtration** of microbes, carbon particles, pathogenic organisms, and dead blood cells occurs in the compartments of lymph nodes. The phagocytic cells that carry

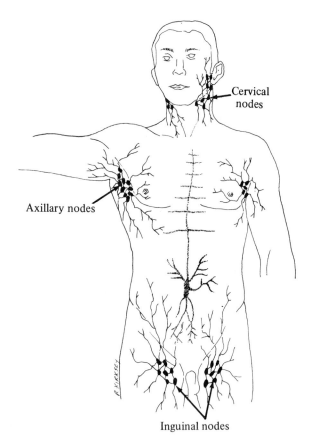

**Figure 10–1.**  Location of lymph nodes. The inguinal, axillary, and cervical regions are where most of the lymph nodes are concentrated.

out phagocytosis are part of the **reticuloendothelial system (RES).** This is an important protective function, because if microbes and pathogenic organisms are not filtered out, they will be carried into the bloodstream by the lymph. Once in the bloodstream they will be circulated throughout the body, thereby causing septicemia.

Notice in Figure 10–1 that there are masses of lymph nodes located in regions where normally there are large

226

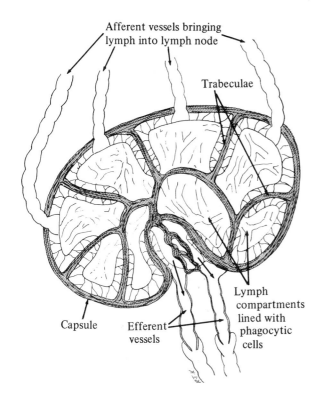

Figure 10-2. Internal structure of lymph node, showing the drainage of lymph through afferent vessels into compartments (lined with phagocytic cells) and into efferent vessels.

numbers of microbes found on the surface of the skin. For example, the axillary, cervical, and inguinal areas are where large populations of bacteria normally are found. The large masses of lymph nodes in these areas filter out bacteria that may gain entrance to the body.

## MANUFACTURE OF LYMPHOCYTES

Manufacture of lymphocytes by lymph nodes occurs within the many compartments. Lymphocytes are white blood cells that play an active role in manufacturing antibodies. The lymphocytes are carried by lymph vessels into the bloodstream.

## MANUFACTURE OF ANTIBODIES

Manufacture of antibodies in the lymph nodes occurs by T-cells (Chapter 3). The production of antibodies by T-cells occurs when antigens (foreign proteins such as bacteria) are carried into the lymph nodes. When antigens enter the lymph nodes, they stimulate the T-cells

to produce antibodies (immunoglobulins, Igs). The antibodies immediately attack the antigens in the lymph nodes, thereby inactivating them. The antibodies are carried by the lymph into the bloodstream where they circulate and inactivate specific antigens in the bloodstream.

The immunity that the T-cells produce is called **cellular immunity** as opposed to the **humoral immunity** that the B-cells produce (Chapter 3). The cellular immunity that the T-cells give the body is responsible for the rejection of transplants. T-cells remain in lymphoid tissue and continue to form new T-cells for months or years.

## 3  SPLEEN

The spleen is slightly inferior to the diaphragm in the left hypochondriac region of the abdomen (Figure 10-3). The spleen is approximately 7.6 cm wide and 14.0 cm long. The outside is covered by a fibrous capsule, and the interior is well endowed with hollow spaces called **sinusoids.** Inside the capsule also is found **splenic pulp,** red and white. The white pulp is composed of normal lymphocyte tissue. It contains plasma cells that produce antibodies when antigens invade this area. White pulp also produces lymphocytes. The red pulp is composed of reticular fibers, and it contains large numbers of red blood cells and reticuloendothelial cells that act as phagocytes.

The splenic artery enters the hilum of the spleen and divides into many, many branches. The branches carry blood to capillaries, which connect to venous sinuses. Some blood passes into red pulp and then into the venous sinuses. The venous sinuses carry blood into small veins, which ultimately carry blood into the splenic vein, which drains blood from the spleen into the inferior vena cava. The filtration of the blood through the venous sinuses and red pulp acts to remove bacteria since both the venous sinuses and red pulp contain large amounts of phagocytic cells.

The protective functions of the spleen include the following:

**Production of lymphocytes and T-cells** is an important protective function. Lymphocytes move into the blood and circulate throughout the body. They act as precursors for the production of various cells, especially T-cells. T-cells function to produce immunoglobulins in the spleen as well as in the lymph nodes.

**Removal of old worn-out red blood cells** takes place in the spleen. RBCs last approximately 90 to 120 days,

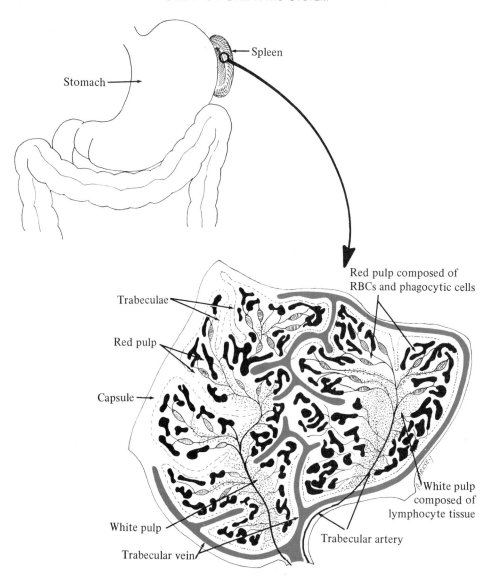

**Figure 10-3.** The position of the spleen is shown above. The inner contents of the spleen are shown below.

at which time they are broken down. The iron is removed from the RBCs and released into the bloodstream. Worn-out hemoglobin molecules are converted to a pigment, **bilirubin,** which is circulated through the blood to the liver.

**Filtration of bacteria** occurs as a result of the interaction of phagocytic cells that line the venous sinuses and red pulp.

**Storage and release of blood** into the general circulation is another function. For example, if you have ever run for a period of time and noticed a pain on your left side, this probably was the spleen contracting and releasing blood into the general circulation. The extra

blood is needed to maintain the increased physiologic activities of the body brought on by running.

## 4   TONSILS

The tonsils are three patches of lymphoid tissue located in the pharynx. They are located in the moist mucous membrane where they filter out microorganisms that enter the respiratory tract.

The **pharyngeal tonsil** is located on the posterior wall of the nasopharynx (Figure 10–4). Inflammation or

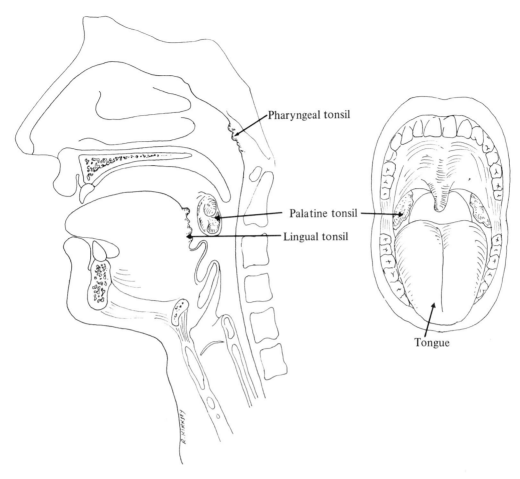

**Figure 10–4.** The three patches of lymphoid tissue called tonsils.

enlargement of this tonsil often occurs during childhood, at which time it might be removed. This tonsil also is referred to as **adenoids** when it is inflamed.

The **palatine tonsils** are two round masses of lymphoid tissue located on each side of the oropharynx (Figure 10–4). **Tonsilitis** generally refers to inflammation of the palatine tonsils. This generally occurs when they are filtering out bacteria.

The **lingual tonsils** are located inferior to the tongue (Figure 10–4). The three groups of tonsils function to filter bacteria and produce lymphocytes.

## 5 THYMUS GLAND

The **thymus gland** is located in the mediastinum (Figure 10–5) slightly superior to the aortic arch. The shape is similar to that of the thyroid since it is composed of two lobes. It is grayish-pink in color. Immediately after birth until about age 12, the thymus is large and active. After this time it gradually degenerates.

Until recently the functions of the thymus were a mystery. Researchers still do not agree as to the exact functions of the thymus. One theory is that the thymus is large and active during the final stages of fetal development in the mother's uterus. During this time it produces cells (T-cells) that are precursors to plasma cells. These precursors are emptied into the bloodstream and carried to the lymph nodes where they are stored in the various compartments. These precursors develop into plasma cells when they are stimulated by antigens.

Another theory is that the thymus acts as an endocrine gland to secrete a hormone, **thymosin.** The target organs of this hormone are the lymph nodes and spleen (Figure 10–5). Thymosin acts to stimulate the development of T-cells in these organs into plasma cells that can produce **Igs (immunoglobulins).**

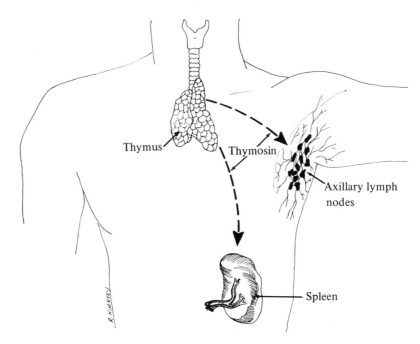

**Figure 10-5.** The anatomy and location of the thymus. The secretion of the hormone thymosin and its target organs also are shown.

This is the first lymphatic organ to develop. The thymus can be thought of as the master lymphatic organ since it does seem to control the development of lymphocytes and plasma cells in the lymph nodes and spleen. It plays a major role in the development of immunity in a newborn child until about 12 years of age, when it begins to degenerate.

## 6  PEYER'S PATCHES

**Peyer's patches** are clumps of lymphatic tissue located within the walls of the terminal portion of the small intestine (ileum). They filter out bacteria and foreign particles that reach this point in the small intestine.

## SUMMARY

**Lymph Capillaries**
A. Originate as open-ended vessels in close association with blood vessels.
B. Drain water, proteins, microbes, and other foreign materials from interstitial spaces into blood.

**Lymph Nodes**
A. Oval-shaped bodies composed of lymph tissue; located along lymph vessels; composed of compartments filled with lymphocytes; lymph drains into nodes through afferent lymph vessels; drains out through efferent vessels.
B. Functions
   1. Filtration: microbes, pathogenic organisms, and dead blood cells are filtered out from lymph.
   2. Manufacture of lymphocytes: each compartment makes lymphocytes that are released into lymph.

3. Manufacture antibodies: antibodies are made by T-cells in nodes when antigens are present in lymph.

### Spleen

A. Inferior to diaphragm in left hypochondriac region; interior composed of sinusoids that contain phagocytic cells and lymphocyte-producing tissue; lymph does not drain through spleen.
B. Functions
   1. Production of lymphocytes.
   2. Removal and destruction of old worn-out RBCs.
   3. Filtration of bacteria.
   4. Storage and release of blood.

### Tonsils

A. Three patches of lymphatic tissue in the pharynx: pharyngeal, palatine, and lingual.
B. Functions: filter bacteria that enters mouth; produce lymphocytes.

### Thymus Gland

A. Located in mediastinum superior to aortic arch; composed of two lobes.
B. Functions
   1. Produces T-cells that are carried to lymph nodes and develop into plasma cells.
   2. Secretes thymosin hormone. Travels to lymph nodes and stimulates development of T-cells into plasma cells.

### Peyer's Patches

A. Clumps of lymphatic tissue; located within walls of ileum region of small intestine.
B. Function: filter bacteria and foreign particles.

## Lymphatic System

1.  Lymph capillaries are located _____ and function to _____.
    (a) as connections between arteries—allow exchange of lymph and veins
    (b) as connections between lymph vessels—pick up waste material
    (c) as open ended vessels near blood capillary vessels—drain various materials from tissues
    (d) None of these

2.  Lymph nodes function to:
    1. Filter material from lymph  3. Make antibodies
    2. Make lymphocytes           4. Store and release blood
    (a) 1,2,3,  (b) 1,3,  (c) 2,4  (d) 4  (e) All of these

3.  The spleen is located _____ and functions to _____.
    (a) superior to diaphragm—produce lymphocytes, destroy RBCs
    (b) superior to stomach—remove and destroy RBCs
    (c) inferior to diaphragm—produce lymphocytes, destroy RBCs, and filter bacteria
    (d) None of these

4.  The tonsils consist of a paired mass of tissue in the pharynx that filters bacteria.
    True (A) or false (B).

5.  The thymus gland is located _____ and functions to _____.
    (a) superior to aortic arch—filter lymph
    (b) inferior to aortic arch—produce T-cells
    (c) inferior to aortic arch—secrete thymosin
    (d) superior to aortic arch—secrete thymosin

6.  Peyer's patches are located in the ileum region of the small intestine where they filter bacteria.    True (A) or false (B).

# Chapter 11

# SENSORY RECEPTORS AND SENSE ORGANS

After reading and studying this chapter, a student should be able to:

1. Name the four characteristics of stimuli (sensations).
2. Distinguish among somatic, visceral, and referred pain.
3. Name and give the function of the three layers of tissue that compose the eye.
4. Distinguish between rods and cones as to locations and functions.
5. Describe the rhodopsin cycle that occurs in rods.
6. Name the refractive media (in sequence) from the front to the back of the eye.
7. Describe the accommodation changes to the lens and iris for near and for distant vision.
8. Recognize a written description of hyperopia and myopia.
9. Write a description of the anatomy and functions of the middle ear.
10. Discuss the structure and function of the organ of Corti.
11. Trace the path that sound waves follow from the external ear until they are converted to nerve impulses in the organ of Corti.
12. Distinguish between static and dynamic equilibrium as to organs involved and changes within them.
13. Describe taste buds and the four primary tastes.
14. Describe how smell impulses are initiated.

*In Chapter 5 we discussed the fact that nerve impulses originate at receptor cells and are carried to specific areas of the brain. The brain is important here since this is where the impulses are interpreted as being pleasant or unpleasant; however, the sensory endings and sense organs are important also. They are specialized to receive internal and external stimuli (senses). These stimuli (senses) allow one to experience and appreciate beautiful things as well as to avoid danger. Humans would not be able to maintain homeostasis and to survive very long without all their sensory receptor endings and sense organs.*

# 1  LOCATION AND CLASSIFICATION OF SENSORY RECEPTOR CELLS

These endings and organs are located at the peripheral ends of sensory dendrites (Figure 11–1). The receptors and stimuli are classified as **cutaneous** (skin), **visceral** (internal organs), **olfactory** (smell), **gustatory** (taste), and **visual, auditory,** and **position.** The receptor cells receive various forms of stimuli and convert them to nerve impulses that are transmitted to the brain. The receptor cells transform energy from the form in which they receive it into electrical energy. This transformation is critical because electrical energy is needed to transmit nerve impulses in the body. Each receptor is specialized to transmit a specific stimulus. For example, gustatory (taste) receptors transmit taste stimuli, and visual receptors transmit visual stimuli. Each receptor

continues to transmit these impulses despite the type of stimulus applied. This is the reason you see stars or hear ringing noises when you sustain a hard blow to the eyes or ears.

# 2  CHARACTERISTICS OF STIMULI (SENSATIONS)

## INTENSITY

Some stimuli of the same class are more intense than others. Two criteria determine intensity of stimuli: the number of receptor cells stimulated, and the frequency (rate) at which the sensory nerves transmit impulses. For example, if someone hits you hard on the arm, many touch receptor cells are stimulated, and the fre-

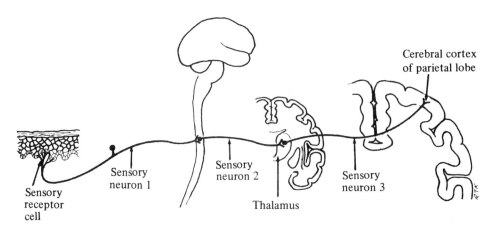

Figure 11–1.   Neurons and pathway of sensory impulses. All general sensory impulses (pain, temperature, touch, and pressure) originate at specialized receptor cells. The impulses then are relayed by three neurons to the cerebral cortex of the parietal lobe.

quency of the impulses being carried to the brain is greater than if someone touches you lightly on the arm.

## AFTERIMAGES

Often we seem to be conscious of sensations after the stimuli have stopped. These persistent sensations are called afterimages. For example, if you look at a bright light and then close your eyes, you probably will still see a bright spot, the afterimage of the light bulb.

## PROJECTION

Stimuli are registered and interpreted in the brain only as to the type, intensity, and origin; however, we always project the stimuli back to their source. For example, if someone touches a hot stove with his hand, he withdraws his hand and looks at it to see if it's burned. The sensation of his hand being hot was registered in the individual's brain and not in his hand, but the hot sensation was projected back to his hand. This characteristic allows the person to locate the stimulus and remove his hand. Projection is considered an important protective characteristic, since it allows a person to locate a stimulus and take appropriate actions to protect himself.

## ADAPTATION

Adaptation refers to a person being unaware of stimuli being received and transmitted by sensory receptor cells. Adaptation typically occurs when stimuli are of constant intensity over a prolonged period of time. For example, when a person first applies perfume or cologne to the body, he or she is quite aware of the aroma. After a few minutes the person probably cannot detect the aroma since the olfactory receptor cells have adapted to it. The wearing of clothes and contact lenses are examples of touch receptor cells adapting to touch stimuli of constant intensity over a prolonged period of time.

Not all receptor cells adapt as quickly as others. The receptors that detect potentially harmful stimuli adapt slowly. Pain and proprioceptor cells (detect sense of body position and movement) adapt quite slowly; touch, smell, and temperature cells adapt rapidly.

# 3 CUTANEOUS (SKIN) RECEPTORS AND SENSES

The skin is sensitive to many different stimuli (senses), such as touch, pressure, heat, cold, and pain. The numbers of receptors for these senses and their distribution in the skin varies. Pain receptors are found in large quantities, widely distributed over the body, compared to temperature receptors. As a result of the quantity and distribution of these receptors, some areas of the skin are more sensitive to certain stimuli than others.

## TOUCH AND PRESSURE

The receptors for touch can be found around hair follicles and in the papillary layer of the skin (Figure 11-2). The receptors for pressure are located below the skin and membranes and close to tendons and joints. Touch and pressure sensations are similar yet different. Pressure sensations are spread more widely and are of stronger intensity than are those of touch.

## TEMPERATURE (HEAT AND COLD) RECEPTORS

Changes in internal and external temperature are detected by temperature receptors (Figure 11-3). The sensory impulses are carried to the general sensory area of the parietal lobe. Motor impulses from the frontal lobe are sent to effectors to maintain or restore normal body temperature (37°C).

The mucous membranes lack temperature receptor cells, except in the rectum and mouth. This is the reason that a person who eats or drinks hot foods does not feel heat in the stomach and intestines; temperature receptor cells are absent from the mucous membranes in these regions.

## PAIN RECEPTORS AND TYPES OF PAIN

Pain receptors are distributed widely throughout the skin, mucous membranes, skeletal muscles, and internal organs (Figure 11-4). Pain receptors differ from others in two important ways. First, they can be stimulated by any stimulus that is very intense; the others respond only to specific stimuli. This nonspecific characteristic

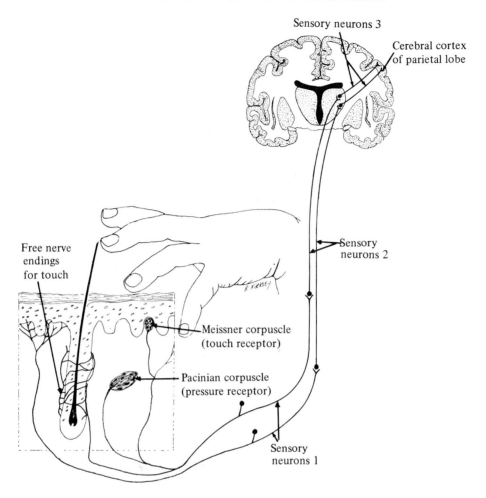

**Figure 11-2.** Receptors for touch and pressure. Touch stimuli can be detected by free nerve endings around hairs as well as by Meissner corpuscles. Pressure stimuli are detected by Pacinian corpuscles.

is important since all stimuli, if they were intense, could damage body tissues. Second, there is little adaptation of pain receptors to continuous stimulation. This is a protective characteristic in that the brain is constantly aware of the pain until whatever is causing the problem has been remedied.

Three types of pain commonly occur in the body: **somatic, visceral,** and **referred.** Somatic pain originates in the skin, skeletal muscles, and joints. Visceral pain originates in the smooth muscles of all visceral organs. Referred pain originates in the visceral organs, but the brain interprets the pain and projects the stimuli back to areas of the skin. Visceral pain nerves carry pain impulses from the visceral organs into the spinal cord. Here pain nerves from the visceral organs and the skin synapse with association (central) neurons. Some visceral impulses have their own private pathway to the

brain, but others share pathways to the brain with skin neurons. The visceral pain impulses that are carried on the common pathway with skin impulses are interpreted as coming from the skin. The brain projects the stimuli back to certain areas of the skin rather than to the proper visceral organs. The pain associated with **angina pectoris** is an example of referred pain. Angina pectoris is actually pain in the heart resulting from a lack of oxygen to the cardiac muscles. The brain interprets and projects the source of pain to the left shoulder and arm. The explanation for this is simply that the pain nerves from the heart and left shoulder–arm are carried on a common pathway to the brain. Some examples of referred pain are pneumonia, which is projected as abdominal pain, and kidney pain, which is projected to the lower lateral portion of the buttocks or to the entire lumbar area of the back.

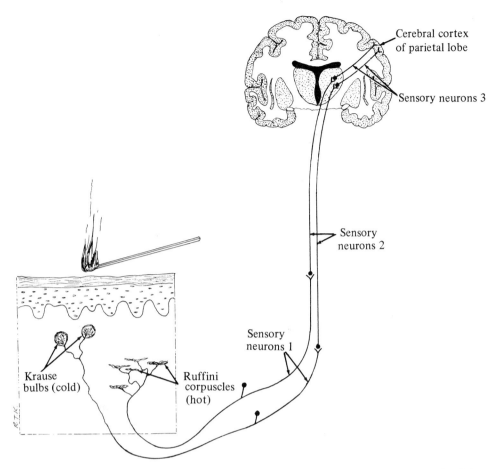

**Figure 11-3.** Temperature receptor cells. Cold temperature stimuli are received by Krause bulbs. Hot temperature stimuli are received by Ruffini corpuscles.

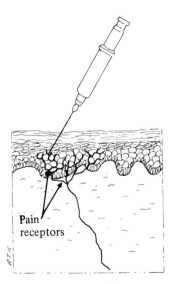

**Figure 11-4.** Pain receptors are free nerve endings. They can be stimulated by any intense stimulus. If an injection hurts, it indicates stimulus of pain receptor cells, whereas if it does not hurt, it indicates they were not stimulated.

## *PROPRIOCEPTORS*

Proprioceptors are located in muscles, tendons, and joints; they are stimulated by movement of these structures (Figure 11–5). They signal the brain as to the position and degree of contraction of the limbs and the body as a whole. These proprioceptors play an important role in reflexes.

## 4  SPECIALIZED SENSE ORGANS

The special senses of vision, smell, hearing, and taste are detected by receptor cells in sense organs. These senses are stimulated at specific points on the body, in contrast to the other senses, which have many stimulation points.

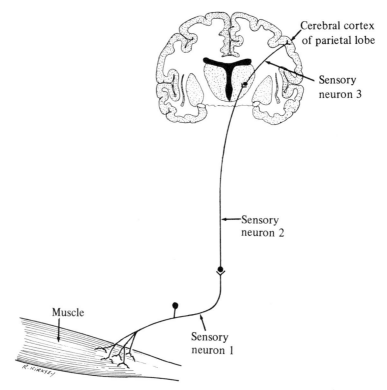

**Figure 11-5.** Proprioceptors are in muscles, tendons, and joints. They are stimulated by movement of these parts of the body.

## VISUAL SENSE ORGAN: EYE

The eye contains visual receptor cells that receive and convert **radiant energy** into nerve impulses (**electrical energy**). The visual impulses are carried to the occipital lobe and interpreted as a visual image. Associated structures that enable the eye to function as a visual sense organ will be discussed first.

### Protective Structures

**EYE SOCKET.** The eyeball is protected by a bony socket (the orbit), formed by cranial and facial bones. The socket also contains a large amount of adipose tissue, muscles, nerves, and blood vessels. The adipose tissue cushions the eye against blows.

**EYELIDS (PALPEBRAE).** Eyelids are movable curtains anterior to the eyeball (Figure 11-6). They protect the eye from dust, foreign objects, blows, and light. Eyelashes project outward from the eyelids and help prevent the entrance of foreign objects. Sebaceous glands are attached to the bases of the eyelashes and secrete sebum, which helps to waterproof and prevent entrance of microbes. A sty results from inflammation of these glands.

The **conjunctiva,** a mucous membrane, lines the eyelids and covers the exposed surface of the sclera and cornea. In a newborn child this membrane is protected from entrance of gonococci organisms by the addition of a few drops of silver nitrate ($AgNO_3$). The gonococci organisms can enter the conjunctiva as the infant passes through the mother's vagina during birth. If the eyes are infected, blindness (**ophthalmia neonatorum**) can result. **Conjunctivitis** (pink-eye) is inflammation of the conjunctiva.

**LACRIMAL APPARATUS.** The eyes must be kept moist at all times to keep the tissues from drying out and to remain clean. The lacrimal apparatus consists of structures that secrete and drain tears from the eyes.

The lacrimal gland (Figure 11-6) is almond shaped and is located under the eyelids at the superior lateral edge of the eye. The gland secretes tears that contain a bacteria-killing enzyme, **lysozyme.** The tears flow medially across the eye and drain into lacrimal canals that carry the tears into the lacrimal sac. The nasolac-

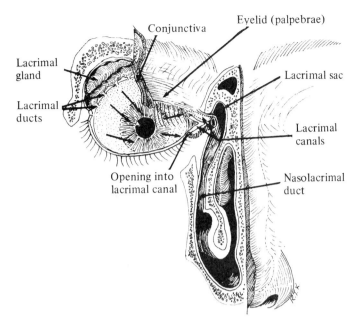

**Figure 11-6.** The eyelids and underlying conjunctiva are shown. The lacrimal gland secretes tears that flow down and across the eye. The tears enter lacrimal canals that carry them to the nasolacrimal duct and ultimately into the nasal cavity.

rimal duct carries tears from the sac into the nasal cavity.

The tears prevent the outer surface of the eye (cornea) from drying out. If it did dry out, the tissue would become cornified like epidermis. This would hinder the formation of visual impulses.

In addition, the tears remove dirt, organisms, and any other foreign material from the eye.

### Movement of Eye

The eye has to be moved in various directions to receive various light rays. The muscles that move the eye are **extrinsic muscles** (attached to outer surface of eye), and there are six pairs of these skeletal muscles (Figure 11-7). The superior, inferior, medial, and lateral rectus muscles, plus the superior and inferior oblique muscles, all rotate the eye in every possible direction. Cranial nerves III (oculomotor), IV (trochlear), and VI (abducens) transmit somatic, efferent impulses to these muscles, which result in eye movements.

### Layers (Coats) of Tissue

Three layers (coats) of tissue compose the eye: **sclera**, **vascular**, and **retina**.

**SCLERA.** The **sclera** (Figure 11-8) is the outer layer (white of the eye). This coat is composed of tough, fibrous tissue. The cornea is a clear transparent region of the sclera, located anteriorly. It has no blood supply.

The sclera protects and supports the deeper tissues. The exposed area of the sclera is covered by a continuation of the conjunctiva from under the eyelids. The transparent cornea is the area through which light rays enter the eye. An interesting point about the cornea is that it can be transplanted quite well since it lacks a blood supply. This means that it initiates little, if any, antigen–antibody reaction and, therefore, little tissue rejection. Tissue rejection essentially involves incompatible antigen–antibody reactions. The cornea not only allows light rays to enter but also refracts them.

**VASCULAR LAYER.** The **vascular layer** is the middle layer of the eye. It is quite vascular (many blood vessels) and strongly pigmented. The vascular layer is complex because it is divided into three important regions: ciliary body, choroid, and iris.

The **ciliary body** (Figure 11-9), in the vascular layer, is composed of the ciliary muscle and ciliary processes. The ciliary muscle is like a circular curtain with a hole in the center and is composed of circular and radial smooth muscle fibers. The **suspensory ligament** (Figure 11-9) connects the ciliary muscle fibers to the

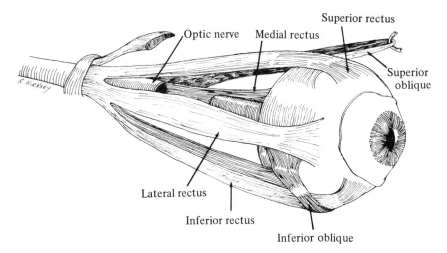

**Figure 11-7.** Extrinsic muscles and movement of the eye. There are six pairs of muscles that attach to the eye and move it in various directions. [Adapted from *Dorland' Illustrated Medical Dictionary*, 25th edition (Philadelphia: W. B. Saunders Co., 1974)]

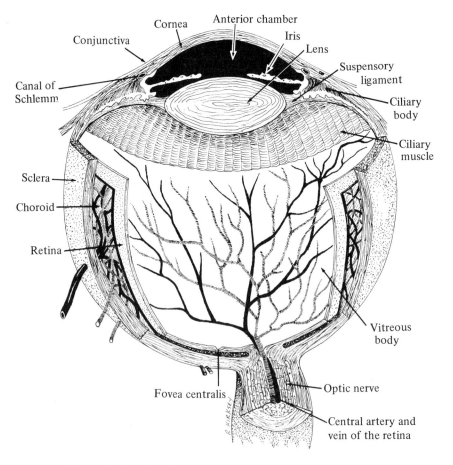

**Figure 11-8.** The three layers and various parts of the eye.

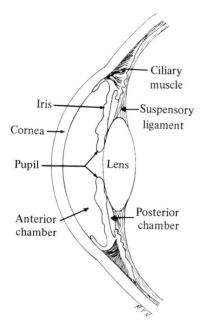

**Figure 11-9.** Sagittal view of eye. The attachment of the suspensory ligaments to the lens is shown.

lens. The ciliary muscle and ligament hold the lens in place and change its shape when focusing on near or distant objects. This process will be described in more detail.

The **iris,** anterior to the ciliary body, is the colored part of the eye. Two groups of smooth muscles make up the iris, circular (sphincter) and radial (dilator) (Figure 11-10). In the center of the iris is a hole called the **pupil.** The iris regulates the amount of light that enters the pupil. The **circular (sphincter)** muscles contract and decrease the diameter of the pupil, thereby decreasing the

amount of light entering the pupil. The **radial (dilator)** muscles contract and increase the diameter of the pupil, thereby increasing the amount of light entering the eye.

The **choroid** region furnishes blood to the other layers of the eye. Not only is the iris pigmented, but the posterior region of the choroid is dark brown in color. This pigmented area prevents reflection by absorbing light that has hit and passed through the retina.

**RETINA.** The retina (Figure 11-11) is the innermost layer of the eye and contains the receptor cells for vision, **rods** and **cones.** These cells are named for their appearance (Figure 11-12) and are located near the choroid region. Light rays pass through the eye, hit the retina, and pass through two layers of neurons before being absorbed by the rods and cones.

Approximately 7 million cones and 100 million rods are distributed throughout the retina. The cones are found primarily in the **fovea centralis,** which is in the center of the **macula lutea** (Figure 11-11). The macula lutea is a yellowish area in the center of the retina, and a small depression in the center is the fovea centralis.

Since there is such a large concentration of cones in the fovea centralis, it is the point of most acute vision. There are no rods at this point. Rod distribution increases from the macula lutea out to the periphery of the retina.

The rods and cones transform radiant light energy into visual nerve impulses, which are carried to the occipital lobe. The transformation process is an example of the first law of thermodynamics and occurs when pigments are chemically changed as they absorb light rays.

The **rhodopsin cycle** that occurs in rods is shown in Figure 11-13. **Rhodopsin** is a visual purple pigment

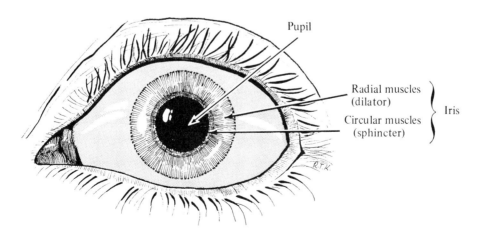

**Figure 11-10.** Pupil and iris of the eye. The circular (sphincter) and radial (dilator) muscles are shown in the iris.

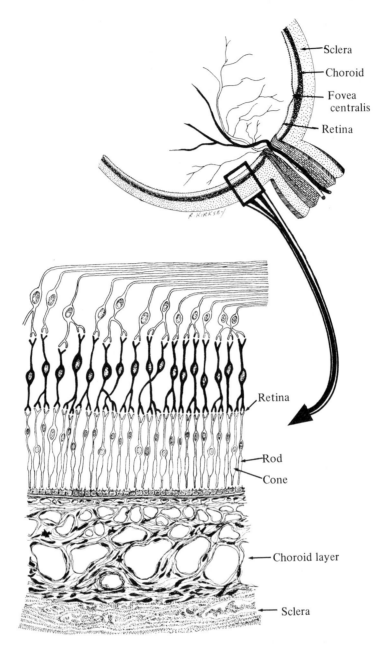

Sclera

Choroid

Fovea
centralis

Retina

Retina

Rod

Cone

Choroid layer

Sclera

**Figure 11-11.** An enlarged view of the retina, rods, and cones is shown. The fovea centralis also is shown.

that is very sensitive to light. As light strikes the rhodopsin molecules, they are broken down into (decomposition reaction) **retinene** and **scotopsin**. This chemical decomposition somehow initiates a nerve impulse in the rod. The vital resynthesis of rhodopsin can occur in the dark only and requires vitamin A. Retinene and scotopsin combine slowly to reform rhodopsin in the dark if an adequate amount of vitamin A is present. Retinene and vitamin A are related, and if vitamin A is not present in large enough quantities, rhodopsin can-

not be resynthesized. A lack of vitamin A may result in poor vision in dim light or **night blindness.** Rods function in dim light, or they are used for night vision. They can detect movement of objects, but not color or detail. The detection of color and detail is made possible by the cones.

When one walks from bright light into a darkened room, one can see very little at first. Usually within a few minutes, however, one can see quite well. The time lapse for adaptation to night vision results from the

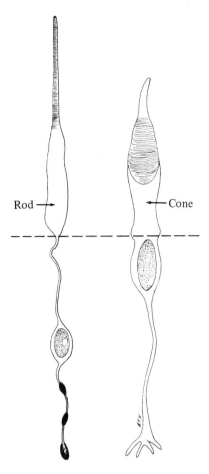

Figure 11-12. An enlarged view of a rod and a cone.

combination of cones that are stimulated. For example, you perceive white when an equal number of the three types of cones are stimulated. The color black is perceived when no cones are stimulated. Other colors realized result from the percentage of the three types of cones that are stimulated.

There are various types of color blindness, such as red–green color blindness, all of which are caused by the absence or malfunction of certain cones. Color blindness is a sex-linked inherited trait.

## PHYSIOLOGY OF VISION

The fovea centralis is the point of most acute vision due to the large concentration of cones. This means that when light rays enter the eye they are refracted (bent) so that they will hit the fovea centralis (Figure 11-14). Three processes are involved in focusing the light rays on the fovea centralis:

1. **Refraction (bending) of light rays:** various internal structures refract light rays so that they will hit the fovea centralis.
2. **Accommodation of lens and iris:** the lens and iris change shape and size as the eyes focus on near and distant objects (Figure 11-14).
3. **Convergence and divergence of the eyes:** movement of the two eyeballs inward and outward as they focus on near and distant objects.

time it takes for the resynthesis of rhodopsin. Similarly, when one walks into bright light from a darkened room, one can see little at first. This adaptation to daylight vision involves a change from rods to cones initiating nerve impulses.

Cones also contain photosensitive pigments that are changed (decomposition reaction) when they absorb light. Brighter light is needed to change pigments in the cones; therefore, they are responsible for daylight and color vision.

### Young–Helmholtz Theory of Color Vision

The most widely accepted theory for color vision is the Young–Helmholtz theory. According to this theory there are three different types of cones: red cones containing pigment that absorbs red rays; green cones containing pigment that absorbs green rays; and blue cones containing pigment that absorbs blue rays.

The color you perceive depends on the number and

### Refraction of Light Rays

Many light rays enter the eye at such an angle that they would never hit the fovea centralis unless they were refracted (Figure 11-14). Several structures are involved in the refraction process, and they are discussed in order from outside the eye toward the retina.

The **cornea** (Figure 11-15) is the anterior transparent region of the sclera. Initially, light rays are refracted as they pass through the cornea.

The **aqueous humor** (Figure 11-15) is a fluid that is secreted from arterial capillaries, in the ciliary body, into the posterior chamber. It moves through the pupil into the anterior chamber. Aqueous humor is absorbed through the **canal of Schlemm** into the venous capillaries of the ciliary body. The rate of aqueous humor production is equal to the rate of its absorption. The aqueous humor refracts light rays after they pass through the cornea. It also furnishes nutrients to the cornea, which lacks a blood supply, and removes wastes.

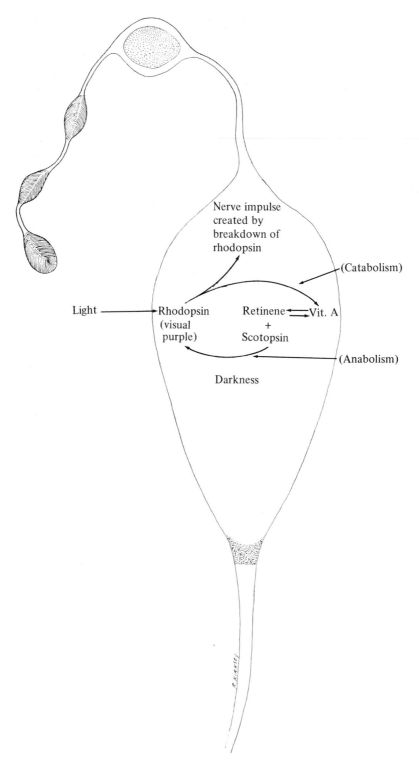

**Figure 11-13.** Rhodopsin cycle in a rod. When light strikes the rods, it causes rhodopsin to be broken down to retinene and scotopsin, which initiates a nerve impulse. Rhodopsin is resynthesized in the darkness when retinene, scotopsin, and vitamin A combine.

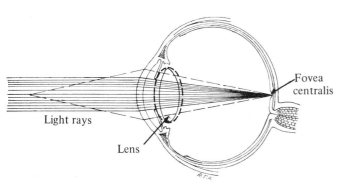

Figure 11-14. Refraction of light rays. Light rays entering the eye must be refracted so that they hit the fovea centralis (the point of most acute vision).

Glaucoma is an abnormal condition where intraocular pressure increases due to the amount of aqueous humor produced being greater than that being absorbed. The increase in aqueous humor pushes the vitreous humor backward into the retina, possibly decreasing blood flow and causing death of the retina. If this condition is not corrected, it results in blindness.

The **lens** is a very tough elastic structure that is held in position by suspensory ligaments from the ciliary body (Figure 11-15). The lens changes shape by the contraction and relaxation of the **ciliary muscles.** The change in shape affects the amount of light refraction that the lens is able to produce.

A cataract is a condition characterized by opaqueness of the lens. The faulty lens can be surgically removed and corrective lens are then worn.

Presbyopia or old age vision is a condition that occurs as one grows older. As one ages, the lens loses fluid, resulting in decreased elasticity; this results in decreased ability to focus on near objects, (farsightedness).

**Vitreous humor (body)** is a thick fluid that has the consistency of gelatin. It is located in the posterior compartment of the eyeball and behind the lens. The vitreous humor refracts light rays slightly before they hit the fovea centralis, helps to maintain the shape of the eyeball, and helps to maintain the retina in the proper posi-

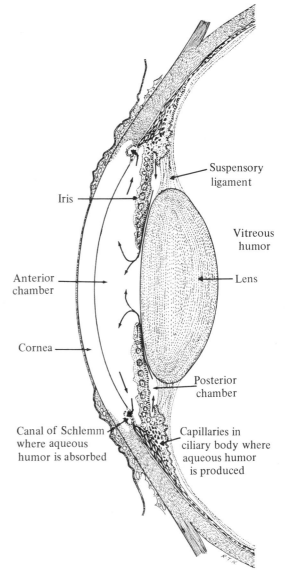

Figure 11-15. Production, flow, and absorption of aqueous humor. Capillaries in the ciliary body produce aqueous humor, which flows from the posterior chamber into the anterior chamber and into the canal of Schlemm.

tion. Vitreous humor is not constantly being produced and absorbed; therefore, any loss normally cannot be replaced by the eye.

### Accommodation of Lens and Iris

Accommodation is the second process that is vital for focusing light rays on the fovea centralis. This process involves changing the size of the pupil and the shape of the lens. The degree to which light rays need to be refracted depends on whether the object is close or far away. The amount of light needed to form an image also varies with the distance the object is from the eyes.

**ACCOMMODATION FOR NEAR VISION.** If an object is within 20 feet of the eyes, the pupil and lens undergo the following accommodation changes.

1. **Pupil constricts:** a reduced amount of light is needed for near vision; therefore, the sphincter (circular) muscles of the iris contract due to parasympathetic nerve impulses and reduce the size of the pupil (Figure 11–16).
2. **Lens bulges:** the lens has to bulge to become more convex for near vision. This bulging gives the lens

more refractive power. The bulging of the lens occurs when the ciliary muscle contracts and relaxes tension of the suspensory ligaments attached to the lens (Figure 11–16). The lens is elastic, and it bulges as the tension is released.

The accommodation changes for near vision are

Contraction of sphincter (circular muscle) → Decreased size of pupil → Reduced amount of light entering eye

Contraction of ciliary muscle → Decreased tension on suspensory ligaments attached to the lens → Bulging of lens makes it more convex and gives it more refractive power

**ACCOMMODATION FOR DISTANT VISION.** If an object is farther than 20 feet from the eyes, two accommodation changes to the pupil and lens occur:

1. **Pupil dilates:** an increased amount of light is needed for distant vision; therefore, the dilator (radial) muscles of the iris contract due to sympathetic nerve impulses and increase the size of the pupil (Figure 11–17).
2. **Lens flattens out:** for distant vision the refractive power of the lens has to decrease; therefore, it has to flatten out. The flattening of the lens occurs when the ciliary muscle relaxes and increases tension on the suspensory ligaments, which are attached to the lens (Figure 11–17).

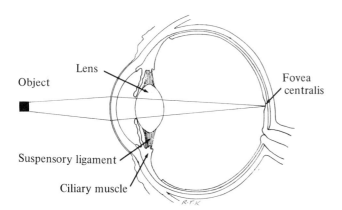

**Figure 11–16.** Accommodation for near vision. To see objects close to the eyes, the lens must bulge. This occurs when the ciliary muscle contracts and relaxes tension on the suspensory ligaments, allowing the lens to bulge.

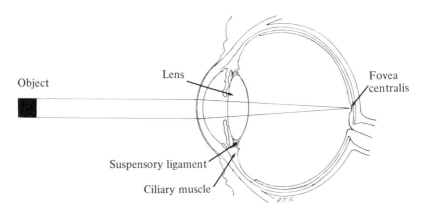

**Figure 11–17.** Accommodation for distant vision. To see objects far away from the eyes, the lens must flatten out. This occurs when the ciliary muscle relaxes and increses tension on the suspensory ligaments, causing the lens to flatten.

The accommodation changes for distant vision are

| Contraction of | → | Increased size of | → | Increased |
|---|---|---|---|---|
| radial (dilator) | | pupil | | amount of light |
| muscles | | entering the eye | | |

| Relaxation of | → | Increased tension | → | The lens flattens |
|---|---|---|---|---|
| ciliary muscles | | on suspensory | | out which re- |
| | | ligaments at- | | duces its refrac- |
| | | tached to the lens | | tive power |

## Convergence and Divergence of the Eyeballs

Convergence (medial movement) and divergence (lateral movement) of the eyeballs is the third process that is involved in light rays being focused on the fovea centralis. When one is focusing on a near object, the eyes must converge, whereas they diverge when focusing on distant objects.

## NORMAL VISION AND ABNORMAL CONDITIONS

**Normal vision** is termed **emmetropic vision** and is often referred to as 20/20 vision. Normal and abnormal sight is determined by looking at the **Snellen chart** (Figure 11–18). A person normally is 20 ft from the chart, and if he or she has normal vision, can identify a line of letters labeled 20. The designation 20/20 means:

$$\frac{20 \text{ (feet from the chart)}}{20 \text{ (labeled line of letters)}}$$

Notice that 20/20 = 1; therefore, a person with normal eyesight could stand 100 ft from the chart and read line 2, which also is labeled 100 or 100/100 = 1. If the person stood 15 ft from the chart and could read line 9, which also is labeled 15 or 15/15 = 1, that person would have normal vision.

## Farsightedness

**Farsightedness (hyperopia)** is a condition in which a person can clearly see objects far away, but objects close to the eyes appear blurry. Objects close to the eyes cannot be seen clearly because the image is focused behind the retina. The cause is either that the eyeball is too short or the refractive power of the lens is too weak (Figure 11–19). If the eyeball has shortened, the image is focused behind the retina. This occurs because the refracting structures still focus the image at the original position of the retina. A weakened refractive power of

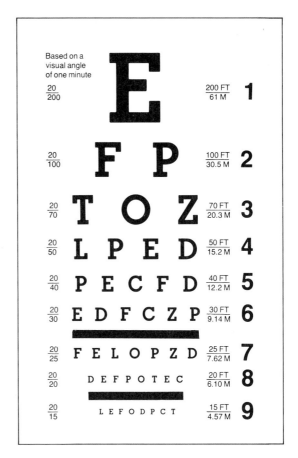

**Figure 11–18.** Snellen chart. This chart is used to determine if a person has normal 20/20 vision. Normally, a person stands 20 ft from the chart and should be able to read line 8, marked 20/20.

the lens results from an inability of the lens to accommodate or bulge for near vision. Lenses gradually lose their ability to accommodate for near vision as they lose elasticity with age (**presbyopia**). Hyperopia can be corrected by the use of biconvex lens (Figure 11–19).

## Nearsightedness

**Nearsightedness (myopia)** is a condition in which a person can clearly see objects close to the eyes, but objects far away appear blurry. Objects far from the eyes cannot be seen clearly because the image is focused in front of the retina (Figure 11–19). The cause is that the eyeball is too long, or the refractive power of the lens is too strong. If the eyeball has lengthened, the image is focused in front of the retina. This occurs because the refracting structures still focus the image at the original position of the retina. If the refractive power of the lens is too strong, the image is focused in front of the retina.

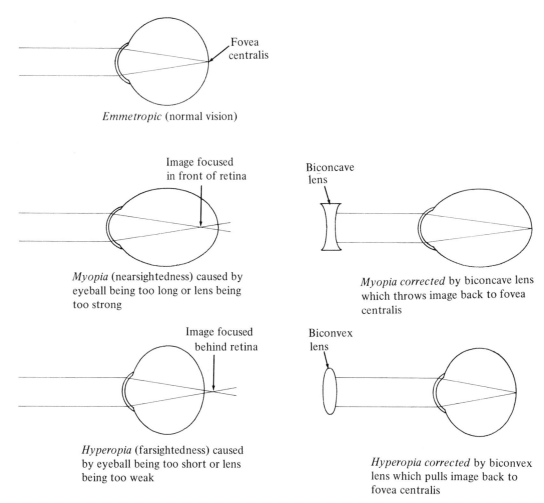

**Figure 11-19.** Emmetropia (normal vision), myopia (nearsightedness), and hyperopia (farsightedness). The three types of vision and the types of lens to correct abnormal vision are shown.

Nearsightedness is corrected by the use of biconcave lens (Figure 11–19).

### Astigmatism

**Astigmatism** (Figure 11–20) is a condition in which there is unequal curvature of the cornea, causing an image to be focused unequally on the retina. Astigmatism often accompanies myopia and hyperopia.

## RETINAL EXAMINATION

A doctor uses an instrument called an ophthalmoscope to look into a patient's eye when performing an examination. The doctor looks through the eye into the retina and studies the **macula lutea, fovea centralis, optic disk,** and the **blood vessels** that radiate out from the optic disk (Figure 11–21). The optic disk is a pale pinkish disklike structure on the nasal side of the fovea centralis. This is an important point to study since the blood supply to the retina enters through the optic nerve and radiates out from the optic disk. The appearance of the retinal vessels is valuable in diagnosing problems. For example, if a person has high blood pressure, diabetes mellitus, or glomerulonephritis (inflammation of glomerulii in the kidneys), the appearance of the retinal blood vessels changes considerably. If a person has glaucoma, the high intracranial pressure can obstruct the drainage of blood from the retina, which drains through the optic disk. The high pressure and obstruction of blood flow cause the optic disk to redden and swell. This condition is called **choked disk** or

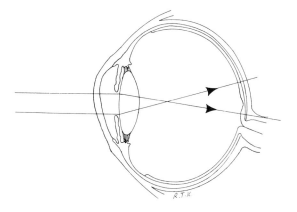

**Figure 11-20.** Astigmatism. If the lens or cornea has an unequal curvature, the image will not be focused properly on the fovea centralis.

**papilledema** and is quite visible to an examiner using an ophthalmoscope.

## HEARING AND EQUILIBRIUM SENSE ORGAN: THE EAR

The ear is concerned with two senses, hearing and equilibrium. It contains specialized receptors for both hearing and equilibrium. The ear is divided into three parts: external, middle, and inner. The external and middle parts of the ear transform sound waves to vibrations and conduct them to the receptors in the inner ear. We will first discuss hearing and then equilibrium.

### The External Ear

The **external ear** (Figure 11-22) is the only visible part of the ear. It is composed of elastic cartilage covered with skin that is called the **auricle** or **pinna.** Extending inward from the auricle to the **tympanic membrane** is a canal, the **external acoustic meatus.** The canal is approximately 1 inch long and is lined with ceruminous glands, which secrete cerumen (earwax). The auricle and external acoustic meatus act to collect and direct sound waves to the tympanic membrane (eardrum).

### The Middle Ear

The **middle ear** (Figure 11-22) is a small air cavity that contains three small bones (ossicles). The lateral wall is the tympanic membrane and the medial wall separates the middle ear from the inner ear. The medial wall consists of two openings, the **round** and the **oval windows,** each of which is covered with a membrane. The air cavity is lined with a mucous membrane, which extends from the middle ear to the upper part of the throat (nasopharynx) by way of the auditory or eustachian tube (Figure 11-22).

The air cavity from the nasopharynx to the middle ear is beneficial since it allows one to equalize the air pressure outside the body with that inside the middle ear. When you change altitudes, the air pressure outside the body changes, but the middle ear pressure does not. These two pressures have to be equalized to prevent rupturing of the tympanic membrane. Equalization is

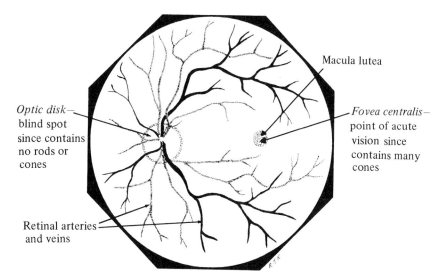

Macula lutea

Optic disk—
blind spot
since contains
no rods or
cones

Fovea centralis—
point of acute
vision since
contains many
cones

Retinal arteries
and veins

**Figure 11-21.** Internal parts of the eye as seen with an ophthalmoscope. The appearance of the retinal vessels and optic disk is important in diagnosing glaucoma, glomerulonephritis, and diabetes mellitus.

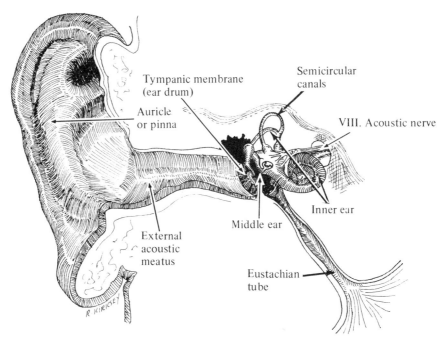

**Figure 11-22.**   The external, middle, and inner ears compose the sensory organ called the ear.

accomplished by yawning or swallowing, which allows air to enter through the eustachian tube. The eustachian tube can be detrimental since it serves as a passageway for microorganisms to the middle ear. When a person has an infection, it is not uncommon for microorganisms to move from the nose and throat into the middle ear, resulting in a middle ear infection.

Three small bones called **ossicles** extend from the tympanic membrane across the middle ear to the oval window (Figure 11–23). These bones are named according to their shape: **malleus** (hammer), **incus** (anvil), and **stapes** (stirrups). The malleus is attached to both the tympanic membrane and the incus; the incus is attached to the stapes. The stapes also is attached to the oval window. The ossicles articulate with each other in such a way that they can move freely.

**FUNCTIONS OF TYMPANIC MEMBRANE AND OSSICLES.**   Sound waves hit the tympanic membrane and cause it to start vibrating (Figure 11–23). The tympanic membrane then changes sound waves into mechanical vibrations. The malleus, incus, and stapes now begin to vibrate at the same rate as the tympanic membrane. The stapes finally transfers the vibrations to the oval window by a rocking motion. The oval window is an entrance into the inner ear.

The ossicles can amplify (increase) and decrease the amplitude of a sound wave. Normal sound waves hitting the tympanic membrane must be amplified by the ossicles. This is necessary because the sound waves are transmitted from a large surface area (tympanic membrane) to a small surface area (oval window). To stimulate movement of the oval window and fluid in the inner ear, normal sound waves have to be amplified about 20 times. However, if high-amplitude sounds enter the middle ear, they can be decreased to prevent damaging the inner ear. The reduction in amplitude is accomplished by two small muscles attached to the ossicles. High-amplitude sound waves stimulate contraction of these muscles. Their contractions reduce the vibrations of the ossicles and thereby reduce the amplitude of the sound waves before they enter the inner ear.

**FUNCTIONS OF THE MIDDLE EAR.**   The middle ear changes sound waves to mechanical vibrations and transfers them to the oval window, which is an entrance into the inner ear. It also equalizes the internal air pressure on the tympanic membrane with that of the outside air pressure (by the eustachian tube) to prevent rupturing of the membrane. The middle ear has the capability to reduce the intensity of loud noises to protect the inner ear.

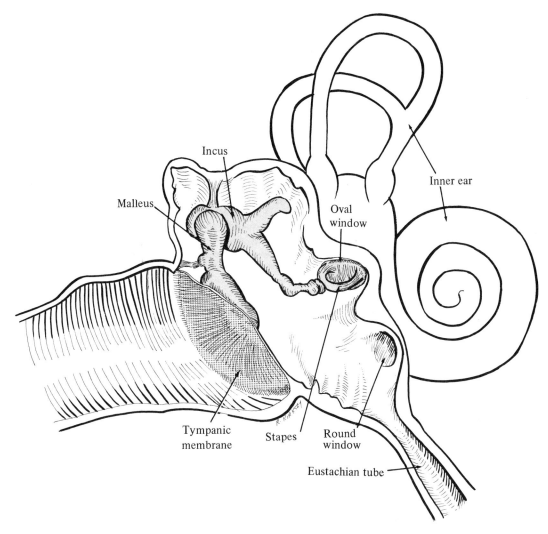

**Figure 11-23.**  The malleus, incus, and stapes of the middle ear.

Otitis media is a common infection of the middle ear. It results from microorganisms spreading from the pharynx into the middle ear through the eustachian tube. The infection results in inflammation of the mucous membrane and a buildup of pus. Transmission of impulses through the ossicles can be affected.

### The Inner Ear

The **inner ear** (Figure 11-24) is very important since this is the area in which the receptors for hearing and equilibrium are located. This area has a very compli-

cated shape; therefore, it is called a **labyrinth.** The inner ear is composed of the bony and membranous labyrinths (Figure 11-24). The bony labyrinth is a series of hollow bony canals that contain a fluid called **perilymph.** The bony labyrinth is divided into three structures: **cochlea, vestibule,** and **semicircular canals.** The membranous labyrinth has four divisions: **cochlear duct** (within the cochlea), **utricle** and **saccule** (within the vestibule), and **semicircular ducts** (within the semicircular canals). The membranous labyrinth contains endolymph fluid. We will discuss the cochlea and cochlear duct first since this is where the receptors for hearing are located.

**COCHLEA AND COCHLEAR DUCT.** The word **cochlea** means snail, and this is what the bony cochlea

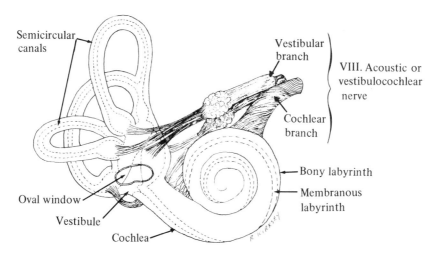

**Figure 11-24.**   The cochlea, vestibule, and semicircular canals make up the inner ear.

looks like (Figure 11–24). It is shaped like a spiral that is wound $2\frac{1}{2}$ times around a central core.

Inside the cochlea is the membranous cochlear duct, which is somewhat triangular shaped (Figure 11–25). It is similar to a shelf in that it divides the bony cochlea into an upper compartment (**scala vestibuli**) and a lower compartment (**scala tympani**). The scala vestibuli and scala tympani contain perilymph, and the hollow cochlear duct between them contains endolymph.

The roof of the cochlear duct is the **vestibular membrane (Reissner's membrane),** and the floor is the **basilar membrane.** Attached to the basilar membrane is the spiraling **organ of Corti** (Figure 11–26), which contains the receptor cells for hearing. The organ of Corti is composed of supporting cells and hair cells. The **tectorial membrane,** which sits atop the cilia, is attached at one end and free at the other. Each hair cell contains a sensory dendrite from the cochlear branch of the **vesti-**

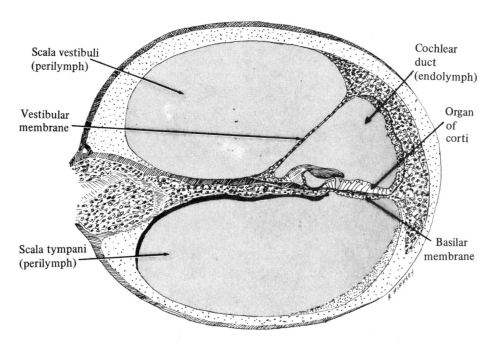

**Figure 11-25.**   Section through the cochlea, showing the three compartments of the cochlea and the fluid they contain. The organ of Corti in the cochlear duct also is shown.

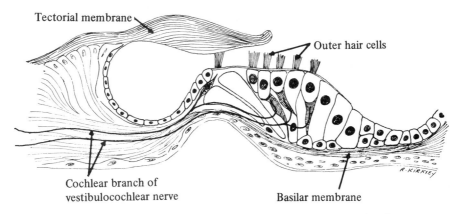

Figure 11-26.    Organ of Corti. Receptor cells for hearing are contained in the organ of Corti. The bending of hair cells against the tectorial membrane initiates nerve impulses, which are carried by the cochlear branch of the vestibulocochlear nerve to the temporal lobe.

bulocochlear cranial nerve (acoustic, VIII). These dendrites converge and give rise to axons that continue to the temporal lobe of the cerebral cortex. Nerve impulses are initiated when the hair cells are bent against the tectorial membrane. The process by which these hair cells are bent will be discussed next.

To better understand the transmission of sound vibrations through the inner ear, refer to Figures 11-26 & 11-27 as you read this material. The vibrations of the stapes, which is attached to the oval window, cause wave movements of perilymph in the scala vestibuli (Figure 11-27). The wave movements of the perilymph

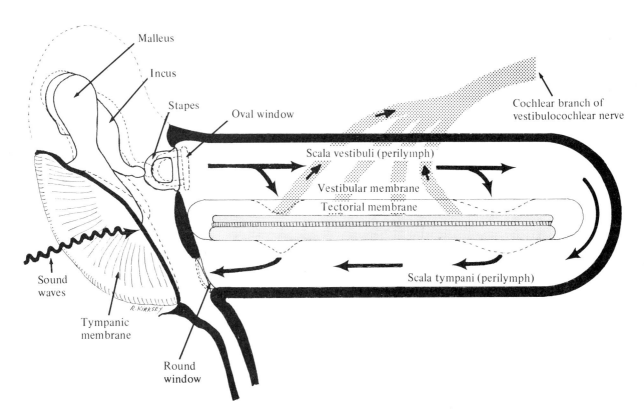

Figure 11-27.    Summary of sound wave transmission and initiation of nerve impulses. The pathway of sound waves is shown, as well as initiation and transmission of sound impulses.

travel through the scala vestibuli compartment and then through the **helicotrema** (a small opening) into the scala tympani compartment. The perilymph in the scala tympani now begins to move and causes the basilar membrane (Figure 11-26) to move at the same rate. The movement of the basilar membrane causes the attached hair cells (Figure 11-26) to be bent against the tectorial membrane. The bending of the hair cells against the tectorial membrane initiates nerve impulses. The perilymph movement in the scala vestibuli also can set the vestibular membrane into motion, causing movement of the **endolymph** in the cochlear duct (Figure 11-25). The endolymph ultimately causes the basilar membrane to move and the hair cells to be bent against the tectorial membrane.

The movement of the perilymph in the scala tympani finally ceases when it expends itself against the round window. The round window is located at the beginning of the scala tympani, and it absorbs the movement of the perilymph; therefore, the stimuli that initiate sound impulses die at the round window.

**VESTIBULE, SEMICIRCULAR CANALS, AND EQUILIBRIUM.** Two divisions of the bony and membranous labyrinth are involved with equilibrium. The sense of equilibrium actually involves two senses, a sense of **static equilibrium** and a sense of **dynamic equilibrium.** Each results from activities in different regions of the inner ear. **Static equilibrium** refers to the position of the body (mainly the head) in relation to the ground. **Dynamic equilibrium** refers to the maintenance of body position (mainly the head) in response to sudden movements.

**STATIC EQUILIBRIUM.** Static equilibrium is maintained by the vestibule. The vestibule lies between the cochlea and the semicircular canals (Figure 11-28). It contains two membranous sacs, **utricle** and **saccule,** which contain the fluid endolymph. Both ends of each semicircular canal open into the utricle. The floor of the utricle contains many hair cells, which are dendrites from the vestibular branch of the vestibulocochlear nerves (acoustic, VIII).

Particles of calcium carbonate ($CaCO_3$), called **otoliths,** are entangled in the hair cells. The otoliths are influenced by gravity. When the head and body change position, the otoliths move and bend hair cells in the direction of the pull of gravity. The bending of the hair cells initiates nerve impulses that are initially carried to the cerebellum and to the cerebral cortex. They cause the individual to recognize a change in the position of the head and body. These nerve impulses are important in maintaining and restoring posture.

**DYNAMIC EQUILIBRIUM.** The three canals of the inner ear that play a major role in helping to maintain the position of the body in response to sudden movements are the **semicircular canals.**

There are three semicircular canals and all contain a membranous semicircular duct (Figure 11-28). They are arranged at right angles to each other. Another way to describe their arrangement is that of a chair with side

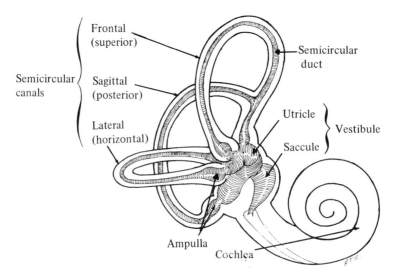

**Figure 11-28.** Vestibule and semicircular canals. The membranous labyrinth is the shaded area. The bony labyrinth is the white area outside the membranous labyrinth.

arms, with the back, seat, and arms of the chair at right angles to one other. Each canal is in a different plane: lateral (horizontal), frontal (superior), and sagittal (posterior). Each semicircular duct begins and ends at the utricle, and one end has an enlarged area called the **ampulla.** Hair receptor cells line the ampulla, and their

tips are covered by a gelatinous material containing otoliths. The hair cells contain dendrites from the vestibular branch of the vestibulocochlear nerve (acoustic, VIII). The hair cells are bent by movement of the endolymph, and nerve impulses are initiated. Only sudden changes in movement, such as rapid accelera-

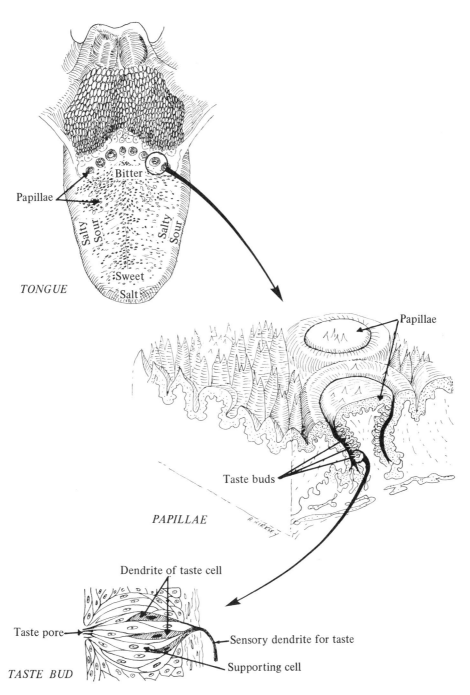

Figure 11-29.  Tongue, papillae, and taste bud. The four types of papillae are shown distributed around the tongue. An enlarged view of a papilla along with a taste bud is shown.

tion or deceleration, can initiate nerve impulses. Since the semicircular canals lie in different planes, no matter what plane the body is in, at least one semicircular duct will initiate nerve impulses if the body undergoes sudden movements. The sensory impulses are carried initially to the cerebellum and then to the cerebral cortex, which sends out motor impulses to muscles to correct for these sudden movements.

## TASTE SENSE ORGAN: TONGUE

Taste is classified as a chemical sense because of the fact that receptor cells are stimulated by chemical solutions. A substance has to be dissolved or be in solution before it can arouse a sensation of taste.

**Taste buds** (Figure 11-29) are the receptors for taste and are located primarily in the **papillae** of the tongue. Each taste bud is somewhat oval in shape and has a pore opening onto the tongue surface. Dissolved solutions enter the pore and stimulate dendrites in the taste buds. The dendrites converge and give rise to axons that course through the glossopharyngeal (IX) and a branch of the facial (VII) cranial nerves to the temporal lobe of the cerebral cortex.

There are four types of taste buds and four primary tastes: sweet, sour, salt, and bitter. These different taste buds are not distributed equally in all areas of the tongue. For example, Figure 11-29 shows that the back of the tongue is sensitive to bitter taste; the lateral surface of the tongue is sensitive to salty and sour tastes; the tip of the tongue is sensitive to sweet tastes. Humans are able to experience many tastes other than the four primary tastes. Other tastes probably result from blending of the primary four and the sense of smell. The sense of smell is quite important in experiencing taste. The importance is demonstrated when one has a cold, and the food tastes abnormal since it cannot be smelled properly.

## SMELL SENSE ORGAN: NOSE

The sense of smell is a chemical sense and gaseous substances must dissolve in mucus to stimulate olfac-

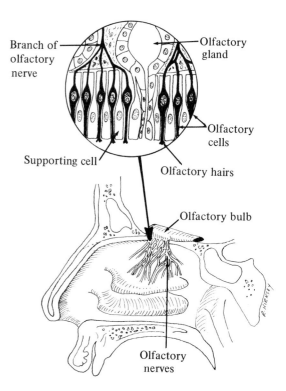

**Figure 11-30.** Olfactory cells have cilia that protrude into the olfactory cavity. Substances that dissolve in mucus stimulate the hair cells and initiate nerve impulses for smell.

tory receptor cells. Olfactory cells (Figure 11-30) are the receptors for the sense of smell and are located in the upper part of the nasal cavity. They are elongated cells with cilia protruding into the olfactory cavity. Nerve fibers leave the olfactory cells and pass upward to form the olfactory cranial nerve (I).

### Adaptation and Fatigue of the Sense of Smell

The olfactory receptor cells adapt and fatigue rapidly to persistent odors. This means that the receptors lose their ability to detect a specific odor that persists for several minutes; however, a new odor can be detected at once. For example, when perfume is applied the smell is quite evident. After a few minutes, the wearer cannot detect the smell; however, the smell probably can be detected by others.

# SUMMARY

### Location and Classification of Sensory Receptor Cells
A. Sensory receptors are classified as cutaneous, visceral, olfactory, gustatory, visual, auditory, and by position.

## Characteristics of Stimuli (Sensations)

A. Intensity: number of receptor cells stimulated and frequency of impulses determine intensity.
B. Afterimages: conscious of sensations after stimuli stops.
C. Projection: brain projects stimuli back to source.
D. Adaptation: person becomes unaware of constant stimuli.

## Cutaneous (Skin) Receptors and Senses

A. Touch and pressure: located around hair follicles and below skin for touch and pressure, respectively.
B. Temperature (heat and cold) receptors: detect changes in body temperature and transmit impulses to brain.
C. Pain receptors and types of pain: pain receptors distributed widely; can be stimulated by any stimulus that is intense; three types of pain: somatic, visceral, and referred.
D. Proprioreceptors: located in muscles, tendons, and joints; stimulated by movement of these structures and signal brain as to position and degree of contraction of limbs.

## Specialized Sense Organs

A. Visual sense organ: eye
  1. Protective structures: eye socket, eyelids, and lacrimal apparatus all function to protect the eyeball.
  2. Movement of eye: six pairs of extrinsic skeletal muscles are attached to external surface of eye; function to move eyes in various directions.
  3. Layers (coats) of tissue
     a. Sclera: outer coat; composed of fibrous tissue that protects eye; cornea is transparent region and functions to refract light rays.
     b. Vascular: (1) Ciliary body, composed of ciliary muscles and ligaments attached to lens; function, changes shape of lens for focusing light rays. (2) Iris, composed of circular and radial smooth muscles; function, dilates and constricts size of pupil and thereby regulates amount of light entering eye. (3) Choroid, brown pigmented region that absorbs light.
     c. Retina: contains receptor cells, rods and cones, for vision; fovea centralis, point of acute vision and where cones are located; rods contain rhodopsin that is broken down by light and initiates nerve impulse; rods initiate nerve impulses in dim light; cones contain pigments that function in bright light and color vision.
B. Physiology of vision
  1. Refraction of light rays: Cornea, aqueous humor, lens, and vitreous humor refract light rays (in this sequence) so that they hit the fovea centralis.
  2. Accommodation of lens and iris. Accommodation for objects within 20 ft of the eyes are constriction of pupil and bulging of lens; accommodation for objects farther than 20 ft from the eyes are dilation of pupils and flattening of lens.
C. Normal vision and abnormal conditions
  1. Normal vision (emmetropic): designated as 20/20.
  2. Farsightedness (hyperopia): person can see objects clearly far away only; results from eyeball being too short for refractive media; corrective lenses refract light rays to hit retina.
  3. Nearsightedness (myopia): person can see objects clearly close to eyes only; results from eyeball being too long for refractive media.
  4. Astigmatism: cornea has an unequal curvature, thereby not refracting light rays properly onto retina.
D. Retinal examination: eye examination with an ophthalmoscope shows the macula lutea, fovea centralis, optic disk, and blood vessels radiating from optic disk.

    E. Hearing and equilibrium sense organ: the ear
        *1.* External ear: composed of auricle and external acoustic meatus; function, collects and directs sound waves to tympanic membrane.
        *2.* Middle ear: composed of three bones (ossicles): malleus, incus, and stapes; lateral wall consists of tympanic membrane and medial wall separates middle from inner ear; nasopharynx connects pharynx to middle ear. Functions: (1) changes sound waves to mechanical vibrations and transmits them to inner ear; (2) equalizes internal air pressure on tympanic membrane with that of the outside air pressure to prevent its rupture.
        *3.* Inner ear: composed of (a) cochlea, contains organ of Corti, which initiates sound impulses; (b) vestibule, saccule, and utricle regions contain hair cells and otoliths, which initiate static equilibrium impulses when position of head is changed; (c) semicircular canals, three canals contain fluid that stimulates hair cells in ampulla when sudden changes in movement occur.
    F. Taste sense organ: tongue
        *1.* Taste buds, receptors for taste; four types sensitive to primary tastes: sweet, sour, salt, and bitter; taste impulses conducted over glossopharyngeal (IX) and facial (VII) nerves to temporal lobe.
    G. Smell sense organ: nose
        *1.* Olfactory receptor cells are stimulated by gaseous particles; smell impulses conducted over cranial nerve (I) to the smell association area in the cerebral cortex.

### Sensory Receptors and Sense Organs

1. The characteristics of stimuli (sensations) are:

   1. Intensity     3. Projection
   2. Afterimages   4. Adaptation

   (a) 1, 2, 3     (b) 1, 3     (c) 2, 4     (d) 4     (e) All of these

2. Which of the following is (are) incorrectly paired?

   (a) Sclera — protection
   (b) Ciliary body — changes shape of lens
   (c) Iris — initiates visual nerve impulses
   (d) Retina — contains rods and cones
   (e) None of these

3. Accommodation for near vision involves:

   (a) Constriction of pupil and flattening of lens
   (b) Dilation of pupil and bulging of lens
   (c) Constriction of pupil and bulging of lens
   (d) None of these

Questions 4 to 10 are (A) true or (B) false.

4. Myopia is nearsightedness and results from eyeball being too long.

5. Hyperopia results from the cornea having an unequal curvature.

6. Middle ear transmits mechanical vibrations to tympanic membrane.

7. Organ of Corti is located in scala vestibuli and initiates sound impulses when oval window contacts hair cells.

8. Dynamic equilibrium impulses result from movement of fluid within ampulla of semicircular canals.

9. The tongue contains taste buds that are sensitive to four primary tastes.

10. Olfactory receptor cells are stimulated by gaseous particles that dissolve in mucus.

# Chapter 12

# BONES AND THE SKELETAL SYSTEM

After reading and studying this chapter, a student should be able to:

1. Describe the regions of a long bone and give the location and function of spongy and compact bone.
2. Describe the functions of periosteum, endosteum, articular, and epiphyseal cartilages.
3. Distinguish among first-, second-, and third-class levers.
4. Write a description of endochondral and intramembranous ossification.
5. Recognize a description of the steps involved in growth of length and circumference of bones.
6. Give the functions of collagen and calcium salts.
7. Describe the location and function of haversian system components.
8. Give the location and function of yellow and red marrow.
9. Describe the four stages of bone repair.

# 1 CLASSIFICATION AND STRUCTURE OF BONES

The bones that make up the axial and appendicular skeletons are classified according to their shape into long, short, flat, and irregular bones.

## LONG BONES

Long bones are longer than they are wide. Figure 12-1 shows a long bone consisting of two different regions. The **diaphysis** (shaft), composed of compact bone, has a round hollow cavity lengthwise through its center. The hollow space is called the **medullary cavity,** and it contains yellow bone marrow (fatty tissue) plus arteries, veins, and nerves.

Each end of the bone is called an **epiphysis.** The outer region is compact bone, and the inner region is spongy bone. The spongy bone in the proximal epiphyses of certain adult long bones contains red bone marrow. Notice that the epiphyses are broader than the shaft. This extra width enables them to articulate with other bones better and to furnish a greater surface area for muscle attachment.

The entire shaft has a slight curvature, which gives it added strength to support weight and absorb jolts. The compact bone is very strong bony tissue; the strength of a long bone is in the shaft and is derived from the compact bone and the slight curvature. The spongy bone in the epiphyses, plus the hollow shaft, gives lightness to a bone. If long bones were solid, your weight would be considerably heavier, and your skeletal muscles would have to be larger to move the heavy bones.

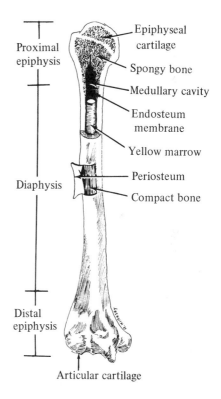

**Figure 12-1.** The regions and parts of a long bone are shown with a sagittal section of the proximal epiphysis.

## SHORT BONES

Short bones are somewhat cubical in shape. They have a thin outer layer of compact bone and an inner region of spongy bone. The wrist and ankle bones are examples.

## FLAT BONES

Flat bones are thin with spongy bone sandwiched between compact bone. Examples are ribs and sternum (breast bone).

## IRREGULAR BONES

Irregular bones have no definite shape. Spongy bone composes the inner region and is surrounded by a thin layer of compact bone. Ossicles (malleus, incus, stapes), vertebrae, and the lower jaw are examples.

## 2   BONE MEMBRANES AND CARTILAGES

Membranes and cartilages play important roles in the structure and function of bones.

## PERIOSTEUM MEMBRANE

The **periosteum membrane** covers the surface of bones except at joints. It is very tough and is composed of fibrous connective tissue. The periosteum membrane (Figure 12–1) has several important functions.

Bone formation occurs inward from the inner layer of the periosteum. New bone cells are produced in such a way as to increase the circumference (distance around the outer surface) of bones. If a bone is fractured, the periosteum plays an important role in the healing process.

The periosteum membrane serves as a point of attachment for muscle tendons and bone ligaments. The movement of bones is enhanced by the firm attachment of muscle tendons to the periosteum. Bones are connected to each other by ligaments that attach to the periosteum.

The periosteum membrane is the entrance point for blood vessels. Nutrient arteries, which carry nutrients into the bone tissue, enter through the periosteum.

## ENDOSTEUM MEMBRANE

The **endosteum membrane** (Figure 12–1) lines the **medullary cavity.** Osteoclasts (bone-destroying cells) are contained in this membrane. These cells destroy

bone tissue making up the inner surface of the shaft. The thickness of the shaft really does not change, since the rate of bone destruction equals the rate of bone formation by the osteoblast cells in the periosteum.

## ARTICULAR CARTILAGE

The **articular cartilage** (hyaline cartilage) covers the articular surface (Figure 12–1) of the epiphyses. The articular surface is where two bones articulate or rub against each other. The articular cartilage reduces friction and prevents the wearing away of bone tissue.

## EPIPHYSEAL CARTILAGE

The **epiphyseal cartilage** (Figure 12–1) is located in the epiphyses of long bones. It produces cartilage cells that ossify into bone tissue; therefore, it increases the length of long bones.

## 3   BONE MARKINGS

Bones have many projections, openings, and depressions that are important. They can be used as reference points to locate muscles and nerves. Many of the projections increase bone surface area for attachment of muscle tendons, which facilitate muscles moving bones. Examples and descriptions of some of these markings are as follows:

1. **Trochanter:** a large prominence (process) to which muscle tendons attach. The greater and lesser trochanters of the femur are examples.
2. **Condyle:** a rounded projection that articulates with another bone. The occipital condyles on the inferior surface of the skull articulate with the atlas vertebra. They enable a person to move the head.
3. **Crest:** a narrow ridge of bone to which muscles attach. The iliac crest is the superior border of the hipbone. It can be used as a reference point in X-rays and in locating an injection site in the buttocks.
4. **Head:** a rounded projection that extends from a neck region of a bone and articulates with another bone. The head of the humerus articulates with a cavity in the scapula.
5. **Tubercle:** a small rounded process that increases sur-

face area for muscle attachment. The greater tubercle is located at the proximal end of the humerus.

6. **Process:** a sharp bony projection to which muscles can attach. The vertebrae in the neck (cervical vertebrae) have long spinous processes.

7. **Foramen:** an opening in a bone through which structures pass. Blood vessels, nerves, and the spinal cord are examples of structures that pass through foramina. The **foramen magnum** is an opening in the base of the skull. The spinal cord passes through the foramen magnum and joins the brain.

8. **Fossa:** a shallow concave depression that can articulate with a head or condyle of another bone. The **acetabular fossa** in the pelvic bone articulates with the head of the femur.

9. **Sinus:** a cavity located within a bone that serves to decrease the weight of a bone. A sinus cavity is lined with a mucous membrane; sinusitis involves inflammation of the mucous membranes lining the sinuses.

# 4  BONES ACTING AS LEVERS

A lever is a rigid bar that is used to help move something, or we use it to help us perform work. We use levers many times a day. Some examples are a bottle opener removing a bottlecap; the claw end of a hammer pulling out a nail; a wheelbarrow transporting a load of dirt; and scissors cutting out a dress pattern. The lever in each of these examples reduces the amount of work required to perform the indicated action. The human body contains many levers (bones) that enable it to accomplish various work activities—running, walking, lifting, grasping, climbing, breathing, and throwing.

## COMPONENTS OF A LEVER

The movement of each lever involves three components:

1. **Fulcrum:** the joint at which the movement takes place. For example, the elbow joint is the point where movement between the upper and lower arm occurs.

2. **Resistance:** the weight of the body part that is moved, plus any weight that the part may be supporting. For example, if the lower arm was moved, the resistance would be the weight of the lower arm.

3. **Force or power:** the muscles that contract and move the lever. For example, the biceps brachii muscle flexes the lower arm (forearm).

## CLASSES OF LEVERS

Levers are grouped into three classes depending on the locations of the fulcrum, resistance, and force or power.

### First-Class Lever

The fulcrum (joint) is located between the power source and the resistance in a first-class lever (Figure 12–2A). An example is a **hemostat** (a surgical instrument used to arrest flow of blood) (Figure 12–2B). The material is the resistance, and the fingers serve as the power. In the body the lower arm (forearm), when extended by the **triceps brachii** muscle, is also an example of a first-class lever. The elbow joint is the fulcrum, the lower arm is the resistance, and the triceps brachii is the power source.

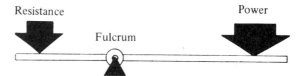

**(A)**  First class lever is characterized by the fulcrum being located between the resistance and the power.

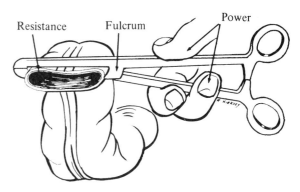

**(B)**  A hemostat is a first class lever with the fulcrum being located between the power and the resistance.

Figure 12–2.  First-class lever.

## Second-Class Lever

The resistance is between the power and the fulcrum in a second-class lever (Figure 12–3A). The wheelbarrow (Figure 12–3B) is an example with load (resistance) located between the handle (power) and the wheel (fulcrum). There is disagreement among experts as to whether there are any second-class levers in the body. One example that is given is the use of the feet and the lower leg muscle (gastrocnemius) to rise and stand on tiptoes. The resistance is the body weight; power is the gastrocnemius muscle of each lower leg; and the fulcrum is the ball of each foot.

## Third-Class Lever

The power is between the resistance and the fulcrum in a third-class lever (Figure 12–4A). A pair of **forceps** (Figure 12–4B) is an example with the fingers acting as the power and the joined ends acting as the fulcrum. An

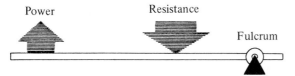

**(A)** A second class lever is characterized by the resistance being located between the power and the fulcrum.

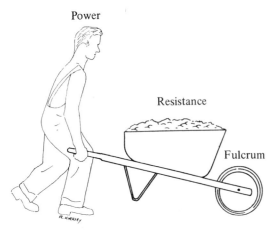

**(B)** A wheelbarrow is an example of a second class lever with the resistance located between the fulcrum and power.

**Figure 12–3.**   Second-class lever.

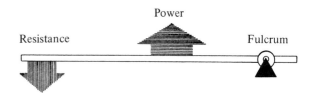

**(A)** A third class lever is characterized by the power being located between the fulcrum and the resistance.

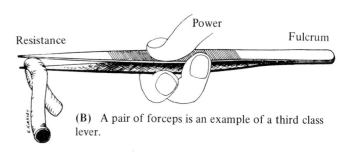

**(B)** A pair of forceps is an example of a third class lever.

**Figure 12–4.**   Third-class lever.

example of a third-class lever in the body is the flexion of the lower arm by the **biceps brachii** muscle. The power is the point where the biceps brachii muscle attaches to the radius bone; resistance is the lower arm and any weight it might be supporting; the elbow joint acts as the fulcrum.

A lever can be grouped into more than one of these classes, depending on how it is moved. The forearm, for example, can be a first- or third-class lever depending on the movement (flexion or extension).

First-class levers, in the body, primarily help to maintain or restore equilibrium; extension of the lower arm to brace yourself when falling is an example. Second-class levers basically help to reduce power; rising on the toes acts to reduce the power required to move some loads. Third-class levers are basically used for speed and range of movement; a pitcher throwing an overhand fastball is an example.

The movement of body parts rarely involves a single lever. Generally, movement involves several levers or a system of levers functioning together. There are many kinds of movements that levers can undergo. The fulcrum (joint) is the point at which levers move, and the structure of each joint determines what kind of movements are possible. The structure and classification of joints will be covered later in this chapter.

# 5  FORMATION OF BONE TISSUE

The formation of hard bone tissue begins in a fetus, which is developing within the mother's uterus, at the end of about the eighth week. At this point the skeleton is composed of pliable cartilaginous bones. These cartilaginous bones act as patterns for the ossification and calcification of the hyaline cartilage to hard bone tissue. **Ossification** (bone formation) essentially is synthesis of organic bone matrix by bone-forming cells (osteoblasts). There are two ways in which ossification, or bone formation, occurs: **intramembranous** and **endochondral** ossification.

## *ENDOCHONDRAL OSSIFICATION*

Most of the 206 bones in the skeleton undergo this process except the bones of the face, flat bones of the skull, hyoid, and clavicle. Endochrondral ossification involves the formation of ossification regions in the center of the diaphysis and epiphyses (Figure 12–5). In these ossification regions the hyaline cartilage cells enlarge and then die, leaving a hollow cavity. Blood vessels remove the hyaline cartilage debris and at the same time bring in **osteoblasts** or bone-forming cells. The osteoblasts begin to secrete collagenic fibers (protein material) into the intercellular space matrix. Following the secretion of collagen, inorganic calcium salts are brought by the blood to the matrix. These calcium salts primarily in-

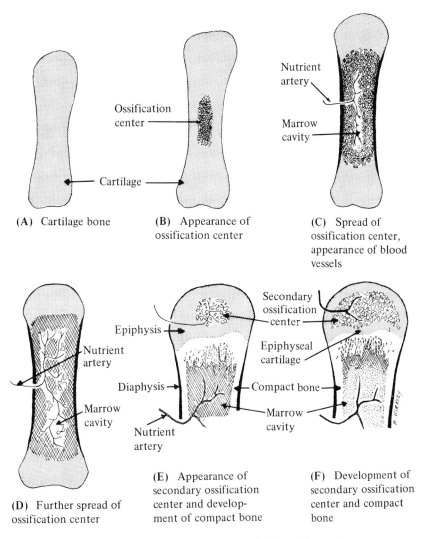

(A) Cartilage bone

(B) Appearance of ossification center

(C) Spread of ossification center, appearance of blood vessels

(D) Further spread of ossification center

(E) Appearance of secondary ossification center and development of compact bone

(F) Development of secondary ossification center and compact bone

**Figure 12-5.**   Stages in endochondral bone formation.

clude calcium phosphate, $Ca_3(PO_4)_2$; calcium carbonate, $CaCO_3$; and calcium fluoride, $CaF_2$. The deposition of the calcium salts in the matrix is called **calcification.** It is this process that actually makes the matrix and the entire bone "hard." These processes continue until all the hyaline cartilage has been replaced with hard bone, except for a thin strip of cartilage at each end between the **diaphysis** and **epiphysis.** This thin strip is called the **epiphyseal cartilage,** and it is essential for further increase in the length of bones.

## INTRAMEMBRANOUS OSSIFICATION

The bones of the face, flat bones of the skull, hyoid, and clavicle are formed by **intramembranous ossification.** As the name indicates, this process occurs within membranes. It begins at the end of approximately the eighth week of development, or during the fetal stage of development of a child. The process is initiated when osteoblasts move into the center of fibrous connective tissue membranes. The osteoblasts secrete collagenic fibers into the matrix, which is followed by calcification.

Calcification differs from ossification. Ossification involves the laying down of collagenic fibers, which could be compared to iron reinforcing rods that are laid down prior to pouring concrete in a mold. Calcification could be compared to the pouring of concrete over reinforcing rods (collagenic fibers) in a mold. The concrete is actually what gives a structure its "hardness" and that is what calcification does for a bone. Iron reinforcing rods (collagenic fibers) help reinforce a structure and prevent it from being brittle. This is what collagenic fibers do to bones.

Intramembranous ossification radiates from the center toward the edges of a membrane. The bone formation or ossification does not reach the far edges of the membranes that join each other because the membranes continue to grow. At birth, **fontanels** or membranous soft spots are present where the far edges of skull bones join each other.

---

## 6  GROWTH IN LENGTH AND CIRCUMFERENCE OF BONES

---

After a child is born the bones continue to grow in length and circumference for several years. These growth processes take place in two different regions of a bone.

## GROWTH IN LENGTH

A bone grows in length as a result of the epiphyseal cartilage (Figure 12-6). The epiphyseal cartilage produces new layers of cartilage cells that die and are invaded by **osteoblasts.** The osteoblasts produce organic collagen, and calcification follows. The layers of calcified bone tissue increase the length of the bone. The epiphyseal cartilage is stimulated to produce new cartilage cells by the **somatotrophic hormone** (growth hormone). If a lower than normal amount of somatotrophic hormone is secreted (hyposecretion) by the anterior pituitary, bones do not grow at their normal rate and **dwarfism** can result. If a greater than normal amount of somatotrophic hormone is secreted (hypersecretion) during the growing years, **gigantism** can result. Both of these conditions are characterized by a proportionate increase or decrease in bone growth. Bones continue to grow in length until a person reaches about 18–20 years of age, at which time the level of the somatotrophic hormone decreases, and the epiphyseal cartilage ossifies.

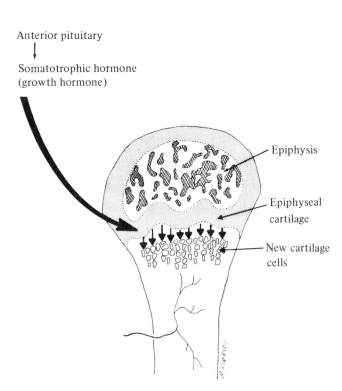

Anterior pituitary

Somatotrophic hormone
(growth hormone)

Epiphysis

Epiphyseal
cartilage

New cartilage
cells

**Figure 12-6.**  Growth in the length of a bone results from somatotrophic hormone stimulating the epiphyseal cartilage to produce new cartilage cells, which die and are invaded by osteoblasts.

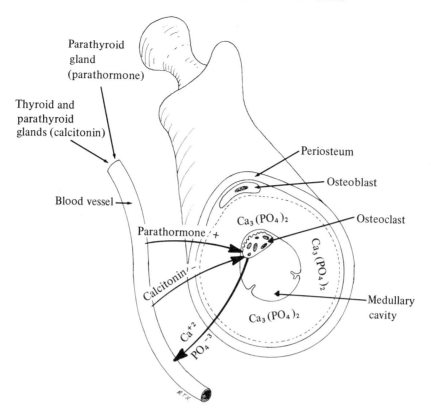

**Figure 12–7.** Growth in circumference of a bone results from activities of osteoblasts and osteoclasts. The influence of parathormone and calcitonin hormones on osteoclasts is shown.

## GROWTH IN CIRCUMFERENCE

A bone grows in circumference as a result of the actions of **osteoblast** and **osteoclast** cells. Osteoblasts in the inner layer of the periosteum (Figure 12–7) lay down new bone tissue on the external surface of bone. Inside the medullary cavity, osteoclasts (bone-eating cells) break down bone tissue at approximately the same rate as osteoblasts produce new bone tissue. This means that the inner circumference of the medullary cavity is increased as well as the outer circumference of the bone; however, the thickness of the bone does not change appreciably.

The exact manner in which the osteoclasts break down bone tissue is not known. One theory is that **parathormone** (a hormone released by the parathyroid gland) stimulates osteoclasts to release an enzyme that breaks down the bone matrix. As the matrix is broken down, calcium ($Ca^{2+}$) ions and phosphate ($PO_4^-$) ions are released into the blood (Figure 12–7). If too much parathormone is released, an excessive amount of $Ca^{2+}$ is released into the blood, resulting in **hypercalcemia.**

Since the strength of a bone is dependent upon calcium salts, the bone becomes very weak and fractures easily as it loses excessive amounts of calcium. The hormone, **calcitonin** (also released by the parathyroid plus the thyroid gland), works with parathormone to regulate the level of blood calcium. Calcitonin inhibits the activities of osteoclasts, thereby keeping the bone matrix intact and lowering the level of $Ca^{2+}$ in the blood. These hormones, parathormone and calcitonin, are antagonistic and, if functioning normally, they maintain a normal level of calcium in the blood.

## 7 IMPORTANCE OF COLLAGEN AND CALCIUM SALTS

The matrix of bone tissue is just like the other types of connective tissue in that it is composed of amorphous and fibrous material. However, bone matrix is different from the matrix of other types of connective tissue in that it is very hard. The inorganic calcium salts that are deposited during calcification give bone its strength. The organic collagen protein material secreted by osteoblasts prevents bones from being brittle. Two-thirds of the matrix (in adults) is composed of inorganic calcium salts; however, the organic collagen is important also. The relative importance of collagen and calcium salts can be seen by comparing the bones of young and elderly people. The bones of young children primarily contain collagen, making them flexible but not brittle. This is the reason young children seem to be able to endure numerous falls to the floor and ground without breaking any bones. As people get older more bone strength is required; therefore, inorganic materials increase as organic materials decrease. The bones of elderly people are quite brittle and break easily because of a lack of organic collagen.

The matrix of bone tissue is maintained by **osteocytes,** which are mature osteoblasts. In other words, os-teoblasts are young bone cells that lay down bone tissue, and then they mature into osteocytes. The manner in which blood brings nutrients to bone cells and carries waste away will be discussed next.

# 8   THE HAVERSIAN SYSTEM

Bone tissue is no different from other tissues in that the cells must receive nutrients and give off wastes. Blood delivers nutrients to and carries wastes away from all body cells, including bone cells. Blood is carried throughout compact bone tissue by **haversian systems.** Each haversian system is composed of the following components: lacunae (contain osteocytes), haversian canal, canaliculi, and lamellae.

**Lacunae** are minute, fluid-filled cavities within compact bone (Figure 12–8). Osteocytes are found in the

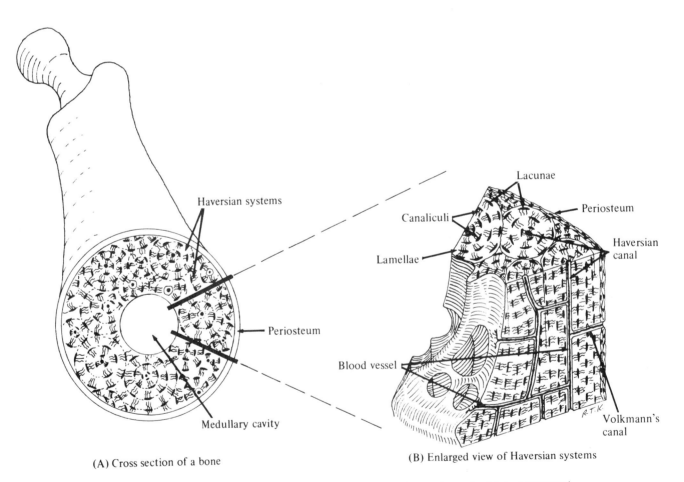

(A) Cross section of a bone

(B) Enlarged view of Haversian systems

**Figure 12-8.**   Haversian system. (A) Cross section of a bone shows that it is composed of many haversian systems. (B) The component parts of haversian systems are shown.

lacunae. The other haversian system components function to carry blood (with nutrients) to and wastes away from the lacunae and osteocytes.

The **haversian canal** is the central canal of a haversian system, and it runs lengthwise (Figure 12–8) through compact bone. Arteries and veins course lengthwise through compact bone in haversian canals.

**Canaliculi** are small canals that radiate from the haversian canals and connect to the lacunae (Figure 12–8). The canaliculi also connect lacunae to lacunae. These small canals carry nutrients and wastes both from the haversian canal to the osteocytes (contained in lacunae) and back to the haversian canal. Canaliculi also carry nutrients and wastes from lacunae to lacunae.

The **lamella** (Figure 12–7) is a concentric layer of bone tissue. Each haversian system is composed of several lamellae, usually five or fewer.

Blood vessels penetrate the periosteum membrane through Volkmann's canals, which then join haversian canals at a perpendicular angle. Many small blood vessels called periosteal vessels enter and leave bones through Volkmann's canals. Larger blood vessels called **nutrient** or **medullary** vessels enter bones and join the medullary cavities of bones. They ultimately interconnect with the haversian canals.

## 9  BONE MARROW

Bones contain a tissue called **bone marrow.** Adult bones contain two types of marrow: yellow and red.

### YELLOW MARROW

**Yellow marrow** is found in the medullary cavity of long bones. It is composed of adipose tissue, which serves as a reserve source of energy for the osteocytes.

### RED MARROW

**Red marrow** is found in many fetal and young bones, but in the adult it is restricted to the proximal epiphyses of the femur and humerus, as well as the vertebrae, sternum, ribs, and cranial bones. Red marrow is composed of connective tissue and cells that carry out the following functions:

- Red blood corpuscle (RBC) production.
- Red blood corpuscle destruction by phagocytes.
- Formation of granular white blood cells (WBCs).
- Formation of platelets.

## 10  BONE FRACTURES AND REPAIR

A break in the continuity of a bone is termed a bone fracture. The fracture can be either a partial or a complete break through the bone. A partial fracture often is only a fracture line on a bone and frequently occurs in skull bones. Some of the common types of fractures are listed next.

A **simple (closed) fracture** is one in which the broken bones do not penetrate through the skin. Since the skin is not broken there is no possibility of bacteria entering the tissues and setting up an infection.

In **compound (open) fractures** the broken bones penetrate through the skin. This presents more problems than the simple fracture because bacteria can enter through the skin and possibly create an infection. This requires treatment of the fracture and infection.

A **comminuted fracture** is one in which the bone is broken into more than two fragments.

A **greenstick fracture** is one in which some of the fibers break but others only bend. This fracture is similar to the splinter appearance of a green tree limb when it is broken. This fracture is common in young children because of the large amount of organic collagen in their bones. Older people have less organic collagen and more inorganic calcium in their bones. As a result their bones tend to be more brittle and break more easily.

The repair of a bone fracture involves all the processes of inflammation and wound healing. The stages involved in bone repair are shown in Figure 12–9 and discussed next.

Stage 1 is the same as the first stage involved in the repair of any tissue—formation of a blood clot. A blood clot forms between the broken ends of the bones and tissues approximately 6 to 8 hours after a fracture. The torn ends of the periosteum and endosteum supply osteoblasts to the area. Many cartilage-forming cells (chondroblasts) begin to appear in the fracture area. The clot along with all the osteoblasts and chondroblasts forms a **procallus.**

Stage 2 is characterized by gradual formation of

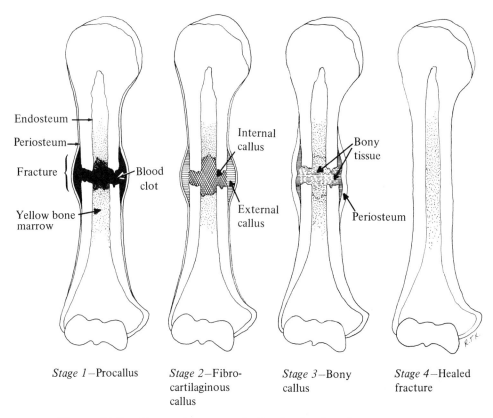

Figure 12-9. Stages of bone repair. For details of each stage see text.

young fibrous connective tissue, which then hardens to form the **fibrocartilaginous callus.** The callus forms a sleevelike structure around the fracture site and acts as a model for ossification and calcification.

Stage 3 is characterized by gradual replacement of the fibrocartilaginous tissue with a bony callus. The deep layers of the periosteum supply large numbers of osteoblasts that begin to secrete new bone tissue (ossification) from the outside of the callus inward. Calcifica-

tion follows ossification, as in bone growth, and finally a hard bony callus is formed that rigidly connects the ends of the fractured bone. As a protective measure, excess bony tissue is formed at the site of the fracture.

Stage 4 is characterized by gradual resorption of the excess bony tissue at the fracture site by osteoclasts. The resorption often is so thorough that it may be impossible to determine exactly where the fracture occurred.

## SUMMARY

**Classification and Structure of Bones**
A. Long bones: longer than they are wide; composed of diaphysis, epiphysis, and medullary cavity regions.
B. Short bones: somewhat cubical in shape; composed of outer compact and inner spongy bone; *Ex.*—wrist and ankle bones.
C. Flat bones: outer compact and inner spongy bone; *Ex.*—ribs and sternum.
D. Irregular bones: have no definite shape; composed of outer compact and inner spongy bone; *Ex.*—vertebrae.

## Bone Membranes and Cartilages

A. Periosteum: covers bone surfaces except at joints; composed of fibrous connective tissue. Functions: (1) new bone cells produced by inner layer, (2) point of attachment for tendons and ligaments.
B. Endosteum: lines medullary cavity; contains osteoclasts.
C. Articular: covers articular surface of epiphyses; reduces friction when bones articulate.
D. Epiphyseal: located in epiphyses of long bones; increases length of bones.

## Bone Markings

Many projections, openings, and depressions present in bones are important for attachment of muscles or to allow passage of nerves and blood vessels.

## Bones Acting as Levers

A lever is a rigid bar that is used to reduce the amount of work required to perform a job.
A. Components of a lever: (1) fulcrum, joint where movement of lever occurs; (2) resistance, weight of body part moved; (3) force or power, muscles that move levers.
B. Classes of levers: (1) first class, fulcrum in center between resistance and power, or RFP; *Ex.*—extension of forearm. (2) Second-class, fulcrum is at one end, power at the other end, and resistance is in the center, or PRF; (3) third-class, power is between resistance and fulcrum, or RPF.

## Formation of Bone Tissue

A. Endochondral ossification: involves ossification centers in diaphysis and epiphyses; cartilage cells die and are invaded by osteoblasts, which secrete matrix material; deposition of calcium salts or calcification follows; most bones formed by this process.
B. Intramembranous ossification: involves osteoblasts moving into center of fibrous connective tissue membranes, which secrete matrix material; deposition of calcium salts or calcification follows; process radiates from center of bones toward edges, but skull bones remain membranous or have fontanels.

## Growth in Length and Circumference of Bones

A. Growth in length: epiphyseal cartilage produces new cartilage cells in epiphyses due to stimulation by somatotrophic hormone; cells die and are invaded by osteoblasts, which produce matrix material; calcification or hardening of bone tissue follows; process continues until level of somatotrophic hormone decreases.
B. Growth in circumference: results from osteoclasts breaking down tissue inside medullary cavity; osteoblasts lay down new tissue under periosteum; osteoclasts stimulated by parathormone and inhibited by calcitonin; ultimate result is increase in circumference of bone.

## Importance of Collagen and Calcium Salts

A. Collagen: organic material secreted by osteoblast that reduces brittleness; decreases with age and main reason why bones of elderly are brittle.
B. Calcium salts: inorganic material deposited into matrix by blood; hardens matrix; amount increases as bone size increases.

## The Haversian System

Bone tissue interacts with haversian systems to receive and give off wastes; components and functions of haversian systems are:
A. Lacunae: cavities that contain osteocytes.
B. Haversian canal: central canal through which blood is transported the length of the bone.

C. Canaliculi: small canals carrying nutrient-rich blood from haversian canals to lacunae and blood with wastes to canals.

D. Lamella: concentric layer of bone tissue.

**Bone Marrow**

A. Yellow: located in medullary cavity of bones; composed of adipose tissue; reserve source of energy.

B. Red: extensively located in bones in young children; in adult is limited to proximal epiphyses of a few bones as well as vertebrae, sternum, ribs, and cranial bones. Functions: (1) RBC production, (2) RBC destruction, (3) granular WBC formation, (4) formation of platelets.

**Bone Fractures and Repair**

A. Fractures
   1. Simple: broken bones do not penetrate skin.
   2. Compound: broken bones penetrate skin.
   3. Comminuted: bone is broken into more than two fragments.
   4. Greenstick: some bone fibers break but others bend.

B. Bone repair involves four stages:
   1. Stage 1: formation of a blood clot.
   2. Stage 2: formation of a fibrocartilaginous callus.
   3. Stage 3: formation of bony callus.
   4. Stage 4: resorption of excess bony tissue at fracture site by osteoclasts.

## Bones and the Skeletal System

Matching. Questions 1–5.

1. epiphysis          A.   located in epiphysis and lightens bone
2. diaphysis          B.   shaft
3. medullary cavity   C.   gives strength to bones
4. compact bone       D.   flared region that articulates with another bone
5. spongy bone        E.   hollow cavity in diaphysis of bone

True (A) or false (B). Questions 6 to 9.

6. Periosteum covers outer surface of a bone and functions as a point of attachment for tendons and ligaments.

7. Epiphyseal cartilage is important for reducing friction between articulating bones.

8. Levers are important for jobs around the home but do not exist in the body.

9. The components of a lever include resistance, fulcrum, and power.

10. Which of the following is (are) correct for endochondral ossification?
    1. Primary ossification center in diaphysis
    2. Osteoblasts invade dead cartilage cells and secrete matrix
    3. Calcification involves deposition of calcium salts
    4. Occurs only in a few bones
    (a)   1, 2, 3       (b)   1, 3       (c)   2, 4       (d)   4       (e)   All of these

11. Growth in circumference of bone tissue involves:
    1. Osteoclasts laying down new tissue
    2. Osteoblasts breaking down tissue
    3. Parathormone inhibiting osteoblasts
    4. Calcitonin inhibiting osteoclasts
    (a)   1, 2, 3       (b)   1, 2       (c)   2, 4       (d)   4       (e)   All of these

12. A haversian system includes:
    1. Lacunae, contains osteocytes
    2. Haversian canal, connects to lacunae
    3. Lamella, concentric layer of bone tissue
    4. Canaliculi, canals that transport blood the length of bones
    (a)   1, 2, 3       (b)   1, 3       (c)   2, 4       (d)   4       (e)   All of these

13. Which of the following is(are) correct in reference to bone marrow?
    (a) Yellow, located in medullary cavity of long bones
    (b) Red, produces RBCs, WBCs, and platelets
    (c) Red, located in almost all bones of an adult
    (d) a, b, c
    (e) a, b

# Chapter 13

# MUSCLES AND MUSCULAR SYSTEM

After reading and studying this chapter, a student should be able to:

1. Describe the location and function of sarcolemma, sarcoplasm, sarcoplasmic reticulum, myofibrils, and sarcomere.
2. Describe the steps involved in contraction of a sarcomere.
3. Write the three chemical cycles of muscle contraction.
4. Differentiate among isotonic, isometric, tetanic, and summation contractions.
5. Discuss the location and function of origin, insertion, and body parts of a skeletal muscle.
6. Recognize a description of prime mover and antagonist muscles.
7. Define flexion, extension, abduction, adduction, supination, and pronation body movements.

# 1 MICROSCOPIC STRUCTURE OF SKELETAL MUSCLE TISSUE

A typical skeletal muscle, such as the biceps brachii, is composed of many elongated cells. These cells are multinucleated (many nuclei). Because of the length of each individual muscle cell, they are referred to as **muscle fibers** (Figure 13-1). Each muscle fiber is composed of cellular structures similar to those found in other cells, as well as structures found exclusively in muscle fibers. These structures are as follows.

**Cell membrane** or **sarcolemma** is the covering surrounding each muscle fiber (Figure 13-1).

**Cytoplasm** or **sarcoplasm** is surrounded by the sarcolemma. The chemical composition of sarcoplasm plays an important role in the contraction of muscles. The sarcoplasm contains about 75 percent water, 20 percent proteins, and 5 percent other chemical compounds. The proteins are primarily **actin** and **myosin,** which interact to form actomyosin during muscle contraction. Examples of compounds included in the 5 percent are carbohydrates (glucose and glycogen), lipids, inorganic salts, ATP (adenosine triphosphate), and phosphocreatine. These compounds, along with actin and myosin, will be considered in detail during discussion of the physiology of muscle contraction.

The **sarcoplasmic reticulum** (Figure 13-2) is a system of membranes that is similar to but not exactly the same as the endoplasmic reticulum (ER). A large number of calcium ions ($Ca^{2+}$) are stored in and released by the sarcoplasmic reticulum.

**Myofibrils** (Figure 13-1) are fine fibers, running lengthwise through muscle fibers. Figure 13-2 shows an end view of myofibrils. Notice how the actin molecules are arranged in a hexagonal manner around each myosin molecule. Actually, each actin molecule is chemically bonded to the myosin molecules as shown in Figure 13-3. The striated appearance that characterizes skeletal muscle tissue is the result of the arrangement of the actin and myosin proteins in the myofibrils. The dark regions are called A bands (Figure 13-3) and are composed of thick myosin protein filaments, overlapping and interconnected with actin protein filaments. The Z line is actually a membrane. Since these myofibrils are stacked on top of each other, the bands in each myofibril are continuous with those in the myofibrils above and below. This arrangement is responsible for the characteristic striated appearance of skeletal muscles.

A **sarcomere** is the region between two Z membranes in a myofibril (Figures 13-1 and 13-3). A sarcomere is called the **structural unit** of a skeletal muscle because it is composed of actin and myosin proteins. Also, it is the **functional unit** of a skeletal muscle because contraction results from activities that occur within each sarcomere. In other words, each sarcomere within a muscle contracts or shortens in length; therefore, all the sarcomeres acting together contract an entire skeletal muscle. The mechanism of how each sarcomere contracts will be discussed next.

# 2 PHYSIOLOGY OF MUSCLE CONTRACTION: SLIDING FILAMENT THEORY

For a sarcomere to contract or shorten, the two Z membranes must be moved closer to each other. The theory that explains how this occurs is called the **sliding filament theory.** Nerve impulses cross the neuromuscular junction by neuromuscular transmitters into the sarcolemma membrane, where they continue until they reach a Z membrane or T tubule.

The T tubule (Figure 13-1) carries impulses into the myofibrils. The nerve impulse stimulates the sarcoplasmic reticulum to release calcium ions ($Ca^{2+}$), which travel to bridge connections between myosin and actin

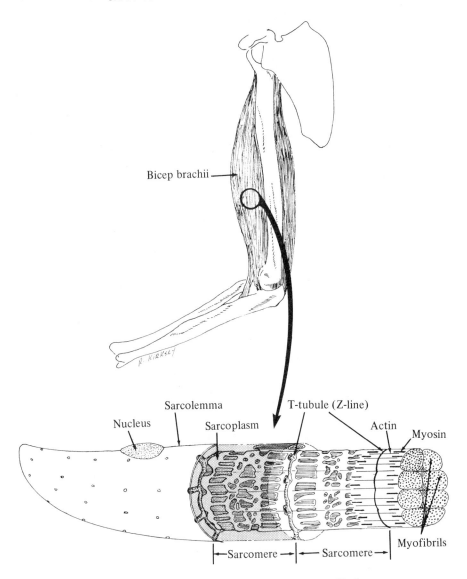

Bicep brachii

Nucleus
Sarcolemma
Sarcoplasm
T-tubule (Z-line)
Actin
Myosin
Myofibrils
Sarcomere
Sarcomere

*Enlarged view of a muscle fiber with myofibrils*

**Figure 13-1.** Microscopic structure of skeletal muscle. The biceps brachii muscle is shown above, and an enlarged view of the microscopic parts of a skeletal muscle is shown below.

protein filaments. The calcium ions stimulate ATP molecules to release energy, which causes the bridge attachments between myosin and actin to break and re-form and break and re-form. This alternate breaking and re-forming of the bridges slides the actin filaments toward the center of a sarcomere. Since actin filaments are attached to Z membranes, they are pulled closer together. This acts to shorten the length of a sarcomere. Once the nerve impulse ceases, the calcium ions move back into the sarcoplasmic reticulum and the cross-bridges break. This causes the actin filaments and Z membranes to go back to their original position, or the muscle relaxes.

# 3 CHEMISTRY OF MUSCLE CONTRACTION

## CHEMICAL CYCLES

The immediate source of energy required for muscle contraction is ATP (adenosine triphosphate). Each time one of the high-energy bonds in ATP is broken, energy is released, and this release of energy causes the myosin and actin protein bridges to break. The ATP molecules are broken down rapidly and have to be replenished to

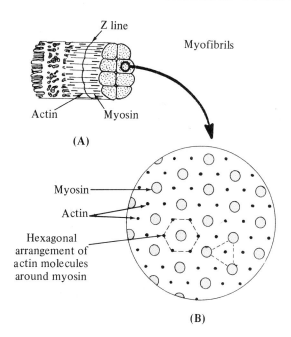

**Figure 13-2.** (A) End view of myofibrils; (B) arrangement of six actin molecules around each myosin molecule.

keep the muscles contracting. The resynthesis of ATP and other chemical reactions actually involve three chemical cycles. The three cycles are shown in Figure 13-4. The arrows in Figure 13-4 illustrate which compounds combine together with certain sources of energy to resynthesize ATP, phosphocreatine, and glycogen.

1. Cycle 1: This cycle involves the breakdown and resynthesis of ATP. The breakdown of ATP → ADP results when a high-energy bond is broken and energy is released. The energy is utilized to contract the sarcomeres of the muscle. The reformation of ATP is a synthesis (combination) reaction. Synthesis reactions require energy to combine two or more compounds into a more complex one. The energy necessary to combine ADP + PO → ATP comes from the breakdown of creatine phosphate in cycle 2 (Figure 13-4). ATP is in limited quantities in a muscle cell; therefore, it must be re-formed. Not all energy released by ATP is used for muscle contraction. Only about 25 percent of the energy released is used for muscle contraction. The other 75 percent is released as heat.

2. Cycle 2: The breakdown and resynthesis of creatine phosphate is involved in cycle 2 (Figure 13-4). Creatine phosphate is important for the re-formation of ATP. The breakdown of creatine phosphate releases energy necessary for the resynthesis of ATP. Much of the energy released radiates into the blood

and is used to help maintain body temperature. Creatine phosphate is vital, and the energy necessary to resynthesize it comes from cycle 3.

3. Cycle 3: Glycogen (polysaccharide) is broken down and resynthesized in cycle 3 (Figure 13-4). Glycogen is the ultimate source of energy for muscle contractions. It furnishes the energy necessary to resynthesize creatine phosphate (cycle 2); creatine phosphate furnishes energy to resynthesize ATP (cycle 1). Glycogen is resynthesized by combining 80 percent of the pyruvic acid molecules (Figure 13-4). The energy comes from the oxidation of 20 percent of the pyruvic acid molecules.

The resynthesis of glycogen occurs during normal, moderate activity when one is able to breathe in enough oxygen to oxidize 20 percent of the pyruvic acid. If a person greatly increases muscular activity, the production of lactic acid is also increased. At the same time, one cannot breathe in enough $O_2$ to break down the lactic acid; this creates an **oxygen debt.** The oxygen debt results in an accumulation of lactic acid. The oxygen debt is repaid by deep and rapid breathing, and in the presence of a large amount of $O_2$, lactic acid is converted back to glycogen. A large accumulation of lactic acid results in "muscle soreness and fatigue."

## PRODUCTION OF BODY HEAT

One of the functions of the skeletal muscular system is the production of heat. The energy liberated in each cycle of Figure 13-4 primarily is in the form of radiant heat energy. Only 20 to 30 percent of this radiant heat energy can be converted to mechanical energy, which is the form required to contract muscles and produce movement. The other 70 to 80 percent of the radiant heat energy is carried by the blood throughout the body. This heat is important since it maintains body temperature and speeds up chemical reactions that occur throughout the body.

# 4 PHYSIOLOGIC CHARACTERISTICS OF SKELETAL MUSCLES

Skeletal, smooth, and cardiac muscles all exhibit certain physiologic characteristics. However, only skeletal muscles will be discussed at this time. The physiologic characteristics exhibited by skeletal muscles are as follows.

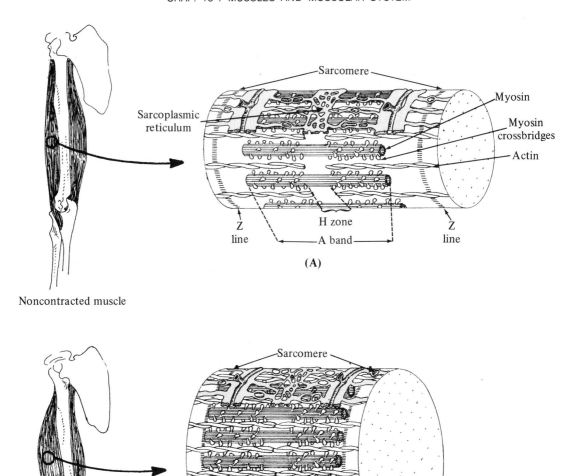

Noncontracted muscle

Contracted muscle

**Figure 13-3.** (A) Noncontracted muscle and relaxed sarcomere, (B) contracted muscle and shortened sarcomere.

## IRRITABILITY

Skeletal muscles are able to receive and respond to nerve impulses. In fact, nerve impulses are essential for muscle contractions. The sarcolemma transmits nerve impulses in the same manner as nerve membranes.

## CONTRACTILITY

Contractility is a unique physiologic characteristic of muscle tissue. Skeletal, smooth, and cardiac muscles all have the ability to contract or shorten. Skeletal muscles can undergo several types of contractions: tonic, isotonic, isometric, twitch, summation, tetanic, fibrillation, convulsions, and spasm.

### Tonic Contraction (Muscle Tone)

**Tonic contraction** occurs when only a few muscle fibers contract, rather than all the fibers within a muscle contracting. Since only portions of a muscle contract, no movement occurs, but the muscle is firm. During a normal day a person's skeletal muscles exhibit muscle

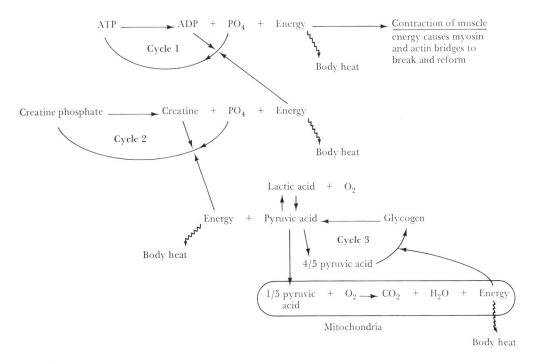

Figure 13-4. Three chemical cycles involved in the chemistry of muscle contraction.

tone. For example, to maintain posture the anterior and the posterior muscles have to exhibit muscle tone.

Muscles lose muscle tone as they are inactivated; this occurs quite often as people get older and use their muscles less. People who are incapacitated for long periods of time because of illness or injury also exhibit a loss of muscle tone.

## Isotonic Contraction

**Isotonic contractions** are those in which the tension in a muscle remains the same, but the muscle shortens and produces movement. All our normal body movements are isotonic contractions.

## Isometric Contraction

With **isometric contractions** the muscle length remains the same, but the muscle tension increases. This type of muscular contraction actually does not result in shortening of muscle fibers. For example, if one pushes against a rigid fixed bar, it will not move; however, a tremendous amount of heat energy is given off since none is converted to mechanical energy to move the rigid bar. Isometric contractions occur in the muscles that maintain posture. This type of contraction also occurs when

the arm and forearm are converted into a rigid rod to push something.

## Twitch Contraction

A **twitch contraction** is a response to a single stimulus. Figure 13-5 shows the three phases of a simple twitch contraction. The **latent period** is the time between the reception of a stimulus and the beginning of a muscle contraction. The latent period is thought to be the time it takes for an impulse to travel along a sarcolemma into a sarcomere to the myosin–actin crossbridges. The **contraction period** is the time required for a muscle to contract. This is the amount of time it takes for the actin protein filaments and Z membranes to be moved toward the center of the sarcomeres. The **relaxation period** is the time it takes a muscle to relax. In other words, this is the time required for the Z membranes and actin filaments to return to their normal position. There are no examples of simple twitch contractions in our normal body movements.

## Summation Contraction

If a muscle receives stimuli during the relaxation period, the strength of the second stimulus is added to the first, resulting in a stronger contraction. Figure 13-6

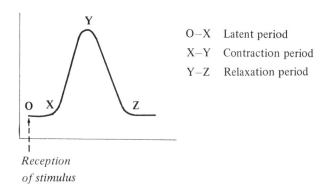

O–X    Latent period

X–Y    Contraction period

Y–Z    Relaxation period

**Figure 13-5.** The three phases of simple twitch contraction. See text for a discussion of each phase.

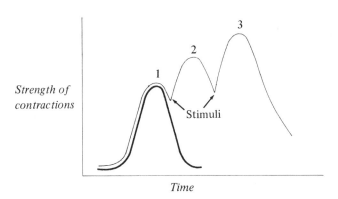

**Figure 13-6.** Two summation contractions are compared to a simple twitch.

shows a simple twitch contraction receiving a stimulus during the relaxation period. The next contraction is stronger than the first, and the third contraction is stronger than the second. This phenomenon of increasing strength of contractions is called **summation**. The stronger contractions result from stimulation of more motor units.

### Tetanic Contraction or Tetanus

**Tetanic contraction** or **tetanus** occurs when a muscle receives a series of stimuli in rapid succession (Figure 13-7). A muscle will undergo tetanic contractions only when the stimuli are received so rapidly that the muscle cannot start the period of relaxation. In other words, the stimuli are received so rapidly that a muscle remains in the period of contraction until the stimuli stop or until the muscle fatigues. Tetanus contractions produce smooth, sustained movement. Normal body movements result from tetanic contractions. If simple

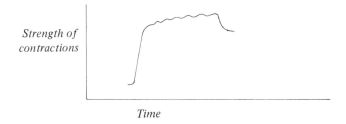

**Figure 13-7.** Tetanic contractions are shown with the muscle remaining in a state of contraction and not relaxing.

twitches were responsible for body movement, we would exhibit jerky, unsustained contractions.

### Fibrillation

**Fibrillation** is abnormal contraction of a muscle where individual muscle fibers contract in an uncoordinated manner. The muscle seems to quiver and no effective movement results. If fibrillation occurs in the ventricles of the heart, the condition is called **ventricular fibrillation**. The ventricles normally pump blood to the lungs and body as a whole; therefore, ventricular fibrillation prevents blood from being pumped to these areas, and death often follows quickly.

### Convulsions

**Convulsions** are abnormal contractions of groups of muscles. This is similar to fibrillation but involves groups of muscles rather than a single muscle.

### Spasm

A **muscle spasm** is a sudden involuntary contraction. It can occur in skeletal and smooth muscles. If the spasms are prolonged, the condition is called a **cramp**.

## 5   FUNCTIONAL PARTS OF A SKELETAL MUSCLE

Skeletal muscles are the source of power necessary to move bones. Each skeletal muscle is composed of three functional parts: origin, insertion, and action. The **origin** is the less movable end of the muscle and often is attached to a bone (Figure 13–8). Generally, the origin end remains motionless while the other end of the mus-

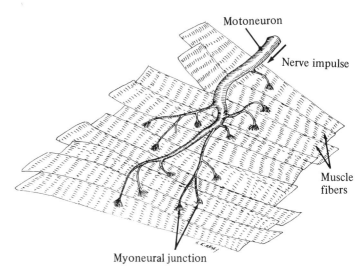

Figure 13-9.   A motor unit, which is composed of a moto-neuron and branches that innervate muscle fibers.

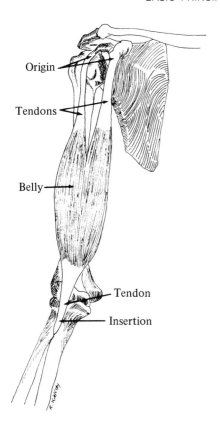

**Figure 13-8.**   Parts of a skeletal muscle showing the origin, insertion, and belly of a muscle. Tendons attach the origin and insertion to other structures.

cle (insertion) moves a bone. The **insertion** is the most movable end of the muscle and also is attached to a bone. The **body** is the thickest part of a muscle. It contains the functional units of the muscle, which work as a group to move the insertion end. When the belly contracts, the insertion end of the muscle is moved toward the origin. The origin and insertion ends of a muscle attach not only to bones but also to cartilage, skin, fasciae, and other muscles. The ends are connected to these structures by tendons, which are composed of fibrous connective tissue. Some tendons are white and shaped like cord; others resemble a flat broad sheet called **aponeurosis.**

# 6   MOTOR UNITS AND MYONEURAL JUNCTIONS

Each skeletal muscle is stimulated to contract by nerve impulses. Neurons that carry nerve impulses to skeletal muscles are called **somatic motoneurons.** The axon end

of a motoneuron enters a skeletal muscle and divides into many branches, which terminate on muscle fibers. The junction point between the nerve and the muscle fiber is called a **myoneural junction** (Figure 13-9). The nerve impulse is carried from the axon to the muscle fiber by **acetylcholine. A motor unit** is composed of one motoneuron and all the muscle fibers supplied by its branches (Figure 13-9). A skeletal muscle is composed of a tremendous number of muscle fibers; therefore, many motor units innervate a skeletal muscle.

# 7   BASIC PRINCIPLES OF SKELETAL MUSCLE ACTIONS

The basic principles of muscle actions are important to fully understand how levers are moved. These principles will be emphasized in the discussion of levers and the muscles that move them.

Muscles usually are not located over the bone or bones that they move. Generally, muscles are located superior or inferior to the bones that are moved.

Skeletal muscles tend to work in pairs. One member of the pair is the **prime mover (agonist),** and the other is the **antagonist.** The prime mover is the muscle that is responsible for the particular movement that a lever undergoes. For example, the biceps brachii is the prime mover for the flexion movement of the radius and ulna bones (forearm).

The antagonist is the muscle that produces the exact opposite movement of the prime mover. For example, an extensor muscle is the antagonist of a flexor muscle. The extension and flexion movements are antagonistic or exactly opposite movements. Coordinated movements cannot occur if the prime mover and antagonist contract simultaneously; therefore, the antagonist relaxes as the prime mover contracts. When the opposite movement is performed, the antagonist becomes the prime mover and the prime mover becomes the antagonist. For example, when flexing the forearm, the bi-

ceps brachii is the prime mover, and the triceps brachii is the antagonist (Figure 13–10); but when extending the forearm, the triceps brachii is the prime mover, and the biceps brachii is the antagonist.

The only time that prime movers and antagonists contract simultaneously is when a part of the body is held rigid, for example, when one uses the arms to push on some object.

Skeletal muscles produce movement by pulling rather than pushing. The insertion end of a muscle is pulled toward the origin. Usually the belly and origin of

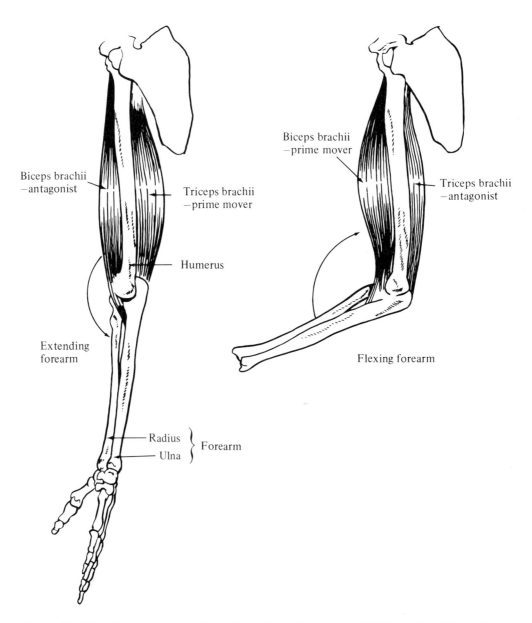

**Figure 13–10.** The prime mover (biceps brachii) and the antagonist (triceps brachii) are shown flexing the forearm. The triceps brachii and biceps brachii interact to extend the forearm.

a skeletal muscle are on one side of a fulcrum, and the insertion is on the other side.

Nervous stimuli are needed to contract skeletal muscles. The visceral (smooth) and cardiac muscles can contract without nervous stimuli, but the skeletal muscles cannot. Normally, inside the body, nerve impulses stimulate skeletal muscle contractions.

# 8 BODY MOVEMENTS

There are four types of movements that body parts undergo at joints: angular, circumduction, rotation, and special movements.

## ANGULAR

**Angular** movement changes the angle between bones by decreasing or increasing the angle between bones. There are four kinds of angular movement.

### Flexion

**Flexion** decreases the angle between two body parts by moving them closer together. Often this movement is used to withdraw the extremities from some unpleasant stimulus. The withdrawal of the hand from a hot plate (Figure 13–11) is an example of flexion.

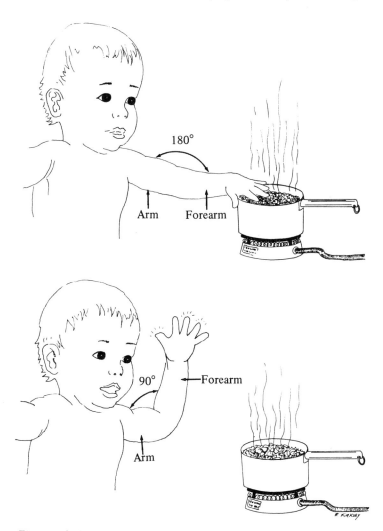

**Figure 13–11.** Flexion movement. When a child touches a hot object, the angle between the arm and forearm is 180°. The heat causes the child to flex the arm away, decreasing the angle between the arm and forearm to 90°.

## Extension

**Extension** increases the angle between two body parts by moving them farther apart. This movement returns a body part to its normal anatomic position after it has been flexed. The extension of the hand and lower arm to their normal position after withdrawing from the hot plate is an example. Extension of a part beyond the normal anatomic position is hyperextension.

## Abduction

**Abduction** is movement of a body part away from the midsagittal plane of the body. The sidestraddle hop ex-

ercise (Figure 13–12) is an example of the arms and legs simultaneously being abducted.

## Adduction

**Adduction** is a movement toward the midsagittal plane of the body or a body part. The sidestraddle hop exercise also involves moving the arms and legs back to the midsagittal plane of the body (Figure 13–12).

## CIRCUMDUCTION

**Circumduction** is movement of a body part through each angular movement in succession so that the part completes a circle.

## ROTATION

**Rotation** is the movement of a body part around a longitudinal axis without a change in position of the part. For example, when one shakes the head "no" (Figure 13–13), the head is being rotated around a part of the second cervical vertebra.

## SPECIAL MOVEMENTS

Special movements are movements that do not fit into any of the other types. **Supination** is movement of the forearm so that the palm is facing anteriorly and the radius and ulna bones of the forearm are parallel (Figure

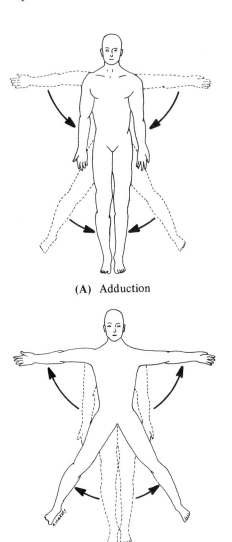

**(A)** Adduction

**(B)** Abduction

**Figure 13–12.** (A) Movement of the arms and legs to the midline is an adduction movement. (B) Movement of the arms and legs away from the midline is an abduction movement.

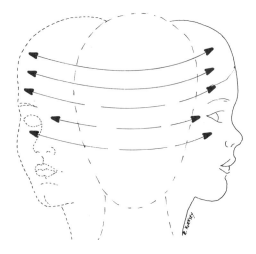

**Figure 13–13.** Rotation movement. When a person shakes the head no, the head is rotated.

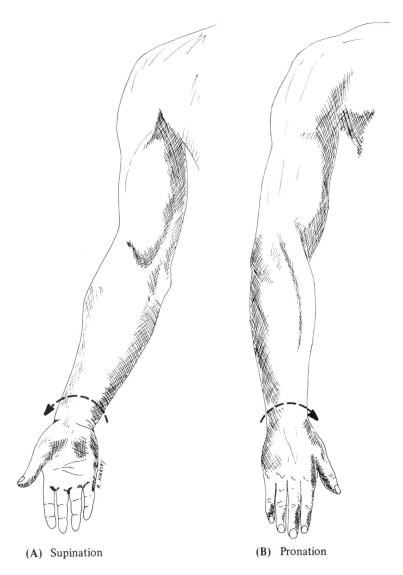

**(A)** Supination                    **(B)** Pronation

Figure 13-14.   Supination and pronation.

13-14A). Every time one turns the key in a car ignition to start the motor, a supination movement is performed.

**Pronation** is movement of the forearm so that the palm is facing downward with the radius crossed over the ulna bone (Figure 13-14B). When one turns the key in a car ignition to stop the motor, one performs a pronation movement.

---

# SUMMARY

---

### Microscopic Structure of Skeletal Muscle Tissue

A muscle fiber is composed of many cellular structures: (a) sarcolemma, cell membrane covering a muscle fiber; (b) sarcoplasm, cytoplasm within sarcolemma, composed of actin and myosin proteins; (c) sarcoplasmic reticulum, system of membranes that is identical to endoplasmic reticulum; (d) myofibrils, fine protein fibers composed of actin and myosin protein filaments; (e) sarcomere, a structural and functional unit of a skeletal muscle; located between two Z lines and composed of actin and myosin proteins; function, site where contraction or shortening of muscle fiber occurs.

### Physiology of Muscle Contraction: Sliding Filament Theory

A. Nerve impulse stimulates release of calcium ions ($Ca^{2+}$) from sarcoplasmic reticula.
B. $Ca^{2+}$ stimulates ATP to release energy at myosin–actin bridge connections.
C. Bridge attachments break and re-form.
D. Actin filaments slide toward center of sarcomere.
E. Z lines pulled closer together.
F. Sarcomere shortens.
G. Nerve impulse ceases.
H. $Ca^{2+}$ moves back into sarcoplasmic reticula.
 I. Actin filaments and Z lines slide back to their original position or sarcomeres lengthen.

### Chemistry of Muscle Contraction

A. Chemical cycles
  1. Cycle 1: involves decomposition of ATP with release of energy, followed by resynthesis of ATP; energy released is used to contract sarcomeres.
  2. Cycle 2: involves breakdown of creatine phosphate with release of energy, followed by its resynthesis; the energy released is utilized in synthesis of ATP.
  3. Cycle 3: involves breakdown and resynthesis of glycogen; breakdown releases energy that is used for resynthesis of creatine phosphate.

### Physiologic Characteristics of Skeletal Muscles

A. Irritability: ability to receive and respond to nerve stimuli.
B. Contractility: ability of muscles to contract or shorten; types of contractions are:
  1. Tonic contraction (muscle tone): some muscle fibers contract but others do not; helps maintain posture; tone decreases as muscles are inactivated.
  2. Isotonic contractions: tension in muscle remains same, but muscle produces movement; *Ex.* normal body movements.
  3. Isometric contractions: muscle length remains same but tension increases; *Ex.*—maintain posture.
  4. Twitch contraction: response to a single stimulus; involves latent, contraction, and relaxation periods.
  5. Summation contractions: phenomenon of increasing strength of contractions.
  6. Tetanic contractions: responses of a muscle when it receives a series of stimuli in rapid succession; muscle remains contracted and does not relax; produce smooth sustained movement.
  7. Fibrillation: abnormal, uncoordinated cardiac muscle contractions; ventricular fibrillation can be fatal.
  8. Convulsions: abnormal, uncoordinated contractions of groups of muscles.
  9. Spasm: sudden, involuntary contraction; if prolonged it is called a cramp.

### Functional Parts of a Skeletal Muscle

A. Origin: less movable end of muscle; often attached to bones by means of tendons.
B. Insertion: movable end of muscle that is attached to bones; insertion end moves toward origin.
C. Belly or body: contains functional units of muscle; responsible for contraction of muscle.

### Motor Units and Myoneural Junctions

A. Motor unit: composed of one motoneuron and all the muscle fibers supplied by its branches.
B. Myoneural junction: Junction between nerve and muscle fiber.

**Basic Principles of Skeletal Muscle Actions**

A.  Prime mover (agonist): muscle that moves a bone (lever).
B.  Antagonist: muscle that produces exact opposite movement of the prime mover; becomes prime mover when it contracts and produces opposite movement of original prime mover.

**Body Movements**

A.  Angular: movements that decrease or increase the angle between bones.
    *1.* Flexion: decreases angle between two body parts.
    *2.* Extension: increases angle between two body parts.
    *3.* Abduction: movement of body part away from middle of body.
    *4.* Adduction: movement of body part toward midline.
B.  Circumduction: movement of body part so that it completes a circle.
C.  Rotation: movement of a part around a longitudinal axis without a change in position.
D.  Special movements
    *1.* Supination: movement of palm so that it is facing anteriorly; turning a key to start a car motor is an example.
    *2.* Pronation: movement of palm so that it is facing downward; turning a key to stop car motor is an example.

## Muscles and Muscular System

Matching. Questions 1 to 5.

| | | | |
|---|---|---|---|
| **1.** | sarcolemma | A. | fine protein fibers |
| **2.** | sarcoplasm | B. | cell membrane covering a muscle fiber |
| **3.** | sarcoplasmic reticulum | C. | Cytoplasm within sarcolemma |
| **4.** | myofibrils | D. | structural and functional unit of a muscle |
| **5.** | sarcomere | E. | system of membranes in a muscle |

The following statements will be used to answer question 6.
1. $Ca^{2+}$ stimulates ATP to release energy at myosin–actin bridge connections.
2. $Ca^{2+}$ moves back into sarcoplasmic reticulum.
3. Nerve impulse stimulates release of $Ca^{2+}$ from sarcoplasmic reticula.
4. Sarcomere shortens.
5. Z lines pulled closer together.
6. Bridge attachments break and re-form.
7. Active filaments slide toward center.

**6.** Which choice below presents the steps involved in contraction of a sarcomere in the correct sequence?
(a)   3, 1, 6, 7, 5, 4, 2
(b)   3, 4, 1, 6, 7, 5, 2

**7.** Chemistry of muscle contractions involves:
1. Cycle 1: decomposition of ATP and release of energy.
2. Cycle 2: breakdown and resynthesis of glycogen.
3. Cycle 3: breakdown of glycogen releases energy that is used for resynthesis of creatine phosphate.
4. Decomposition reactions do not release energy.
(a)   1, 2, 3      (b)   1, 3      (c)   2, 4      (d)   4      (e)   All of these

True (A) or false (B). Questions 8 to 14.

**8.** Muscle tone contractions help maintain posture.

**9.** Isometric contractions help move the body.

**10.** Smooth, sustained movements result from isotonic contractions.

**11.** A motor unit consists of one motoneuron and all the muscle fibers supplied by its branches.

**12.** Flexion movements increase the angle between body parts.

**13.** Extension decreases the angle between body parts.

**14.** A prime mover muscle has actions opposite to an antagonist.

# Chapter 14

# LEVERS (BONES), MUSCLES, AND MOVEMENTS OF THE AXIAL SKELETAL SYSTEM

After reading and studying this chapter, a student should be able to:

1. Recognize the bones of the skull in a drawing.
2. Describe the locations and functions of fetal fontanels.
3. Give the function of sternocleidomastoid and semispinalis capitis muscles.
4. Write the names and number of vertebrae in each region of a vertebral column.
5. Name the four curves of the vertebral column.
6. Describe scoliosis, kyphosis, and lordosis.
7. Distinguish between true and false ribs.
8. Give the function of external and internal intercostals and the diaphragm.

*We will discuss the bones and movement of the axial skeleton in this chapter and then the appendicular skeleton in the next chapter. All the muscles of the body are illustrated in the anterior and posterior views in Figures 14–1 and 14–2. The **axial skeleton** derives its name from the fact that the 80 bones composing it are found in the midline of the body or close to it (Figure 14–3). These bones form the axis (a straight line) of the body, to which the appendicular skeleton attaches. The axial skeleton is rigid and moves little compared to the appendicular skeleton. It serves as a rigid structure to which the freely movable appendicular skeleton attaches. The parts of the axial skeleton will be discussed now.*

# 1  SKULL AND MUSCLES THAT MOVE IT

The skull is made up of 29 bones:

| | | |
|---|---|---|
| 1 frontal | 1 sphenoid | 2 maxillae |
| 2 parietal | 1 ethmoid | 1 mandible |
| 2 temporal | 2 nasal | 2 lacrimal |
| 1 occipital | 2 zygomatic | 1 vomer |
| 2 pataline | | 6 ossicle bones of the two middle ears (2 malleus, 2 incus, 2 stapes) |
| 2 inferior conchae | | |
| 1 hyoid | | |
| | | 29 total |

## GENERAL FEATURES OF THE SKULL

With the exception of the mandible (lower jaw) and the ossicles, the bones of the skull are immovable and thus provide excellent protection for the brain, eye, and ear. The immovable bones are united by jagged joints called sutures (Figure 14–4A). By drawing an imaginary line through the coronal or frontal suture, we obtain the **coronal plane**. The **sagittal suture** is the source of the **sagittal plane**.

The **frontal bone** (Figure 14–4) forms the anterior forehead region of the skull and the roof of the eye sockets. Within the frontal bone are the frontal sinus cavities, which are lined with mucous membranes. The sinuses communicate with the nasal cavity.

The two **parietal bones** (Figure 14–4) form the superior and lateral surfaces of the skull. They join medially at the sagittal suture. Each parietal bone lies over one of the two parietal lobes of the brain.

The two **temporal bones** form the lower lateral side of the skull. They house the middle and inner ear regions. A large opening in each temporal bone is the external auditory meatus. Each temporal bone lies over the corresponding temporal lobe of the cerebral cortex.

The **occipital bone** (Figure 14–4) forms the posterior surface and a portion of the base of the skull. The large **foramen magnum** is an opening in the occipital bone (Figure 14–4) through which the spinal cord attaches to the **medulla oblongata** of the brain. The occipital bone lies over the occipital lobe of the cerebral cortex. The occipital condyles are lateral to the foramen magnum, and articulate with the first cervical vertebra (atlas).

The **sphenoid bone** resembles a bat with its wings outstretched. It forms a portion of the floor of the skull and extends from one temporal bone to the other. It contains a depression, the sella turcica, which houses and protects the pituitary gland (master gland).

The **ethmoid bone** (Figure 14–5) forms most of the bony structure of the nasal cavity. The perforated cribiform plate is part of the ethmoid bone. Nerve branches from the olfactory receptor cells pass through the cribiform plate. The branches merge to form the olfactory nerve, which continues on to the temporal lobe of the cerebral cortex.

The two **nasal bones** (Figures 14–4 and 14–5) are oblong and thin and form the upper bridge of the nose. The lower portion of the nose is composed of cartilage.

The cheekbones are formed by the two **zygomatic bones**. Each bone also forms a portion of the orbital cavity. The zygomatic arch (Figure 14–4) is formed by the union of the zygomatic bone and the zygomatic process of the temporal bone.

The **maxilla**, the upper jaw bone (Figures 14–4 and 14–5), is formed from two bones (maxillae) that have fused together. It forms a portion of the eye sockets, hard palate, and lateral walls of the nasal cavities and

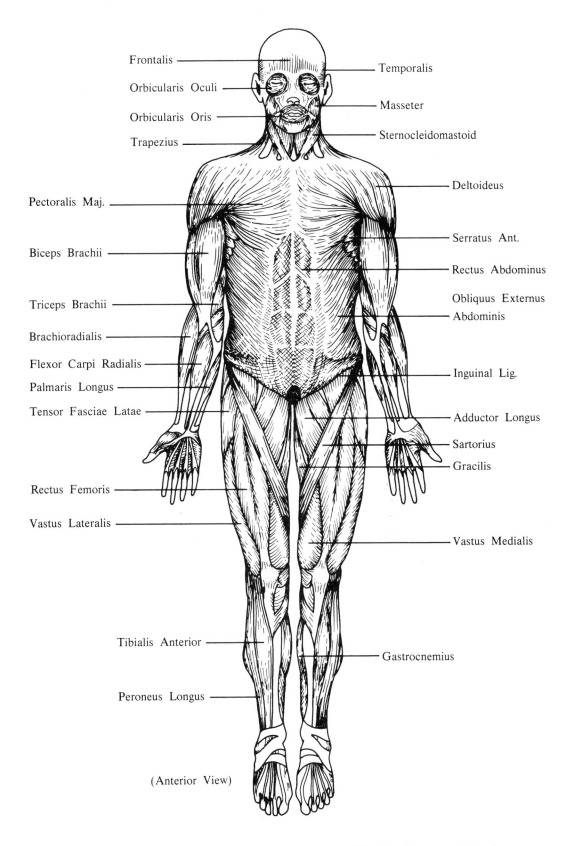

Frontalis

Orbicularis Oculi

Orbicularis Oris

Trapezius

Pectoralis Maj.

Biceps Brachii

Triceps Brachii

Brachioradialis

Flexor Carpi Radialis

Palmaris Longus

Tensor Fasciae Latae

Rectus Femoris

Vastus Lateralis

Tibialis Anterior

Peroneus Longus

(Anterior View)

Temporalis

Masseter

Sternocleidomastoid

Deltoideus

Serratus Ant.

Rectus Abdominus

Obliquus Externus
Abdominis

Inguinal Lig.

Adductor Longus

Sartorius

Gracilis

Vastus Medialis

Gastrocnemius

**Figure 14-1.** Anterior view of muscles of the body. (Reprinted by permission from *Anatomy and Physiology,* Unit 4, "The Muscular System." Bowie, Md.: Robert J. Brady Company)

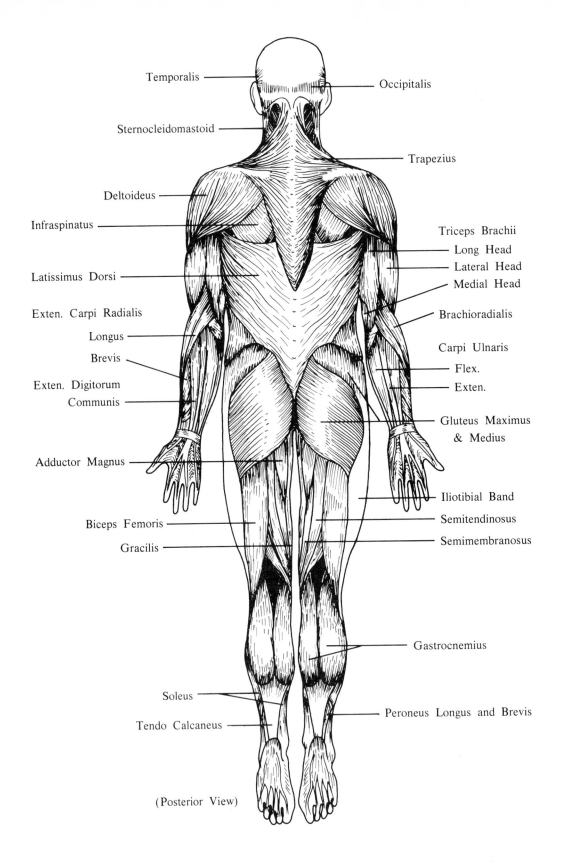

Temporalis

Occipitalis

Sternocleidomastoid

Trapezius

Deltoideus

Infraspinatus

Triceps Brachii
Long Head
Lateral Head
Medial Head

Latissimus Dorsi

Brachioradialis

Exten. Carpi Radialis

Carpi Ulnaris

Longus

Flex.

Brevis

Exten.

Exten. Digitorum
Communis

Gluteus Maximus
& Medius

Adductor Magnus

Iliotibial Band

Biceps Femoris

Semitendinosus

Gracilis

Semimembranosus

Gastrocnemius

Soleus

Peroneus Longus and Brevis

Tendo Calcaneus

(Posterior View)

Figure 14-2. Posterior view of muscles of the body. (Reprinted by permission from *Anatomy and Physiology*, Unit 4, "The Muscular System." Bowie, Md.: Robert J. Brady Company)

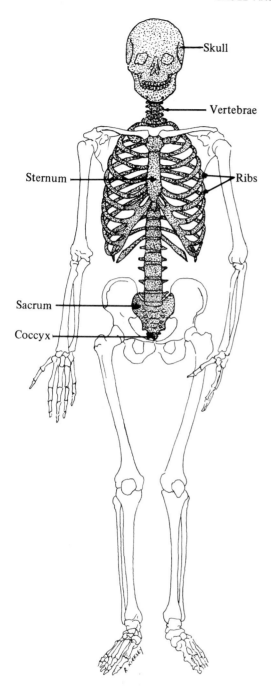

**Figure 14-3.** The axial skeleton (shaded area) is shown with the appendicular skeleton (white).

also contains sockets for the upper teeth. A maxillary sinus is contained within each maxilla.

The **mandible** (Figures 14-4 and 14-5) is the lower jaw bone. It is composed of one bone that articulates with each temporal bone. The central portion of the mandible is U-shaped and is called the body. It contains sockets for the lower teeth. Two projections, or rami, extend upward to the temporal bone. Each ramus articulates with the temporal bone by means of a condyle.

The two **lacrimal bones** (Figure 14-4) are very thin, small bones. They are located on the medial wall of the orbits. They can be identified easily by the lacrimal canal through which the tear duct passes from the orbit to the nasal cavity.

The **vomer** (Figure 14-5) forms the lower, posterior portion of the central septum or partition between the nasal cavities.

The two **palatine bones** (Figure 14-5) are shaped similar to the letter L. They form a small part of the hard palate, floor of the orbits, and floor of the nasal cavities.

The two **inferior nasal conchae** (Figure 14-5) are long, slightly curved bones that lie along the lateral sides of the nasal cavities. Superior and middle conchae processes of the ethmoid bone lie above the inferior conchae. The three conchae projections increase the surface area of the nasal cavity considerably. The large surface area is covered with ciliated mucous membrane, which acts to filter, warm, and moisten air as it passes upward in the nasal cavity.

The **hyoid bone** (Figure 14-6) is an isolated U-shaped bone that lies below the chin in the anterior part of the neck. Two projections, called cornu, extend upward from either side of the body. Ligaments connect the hyoid to the styloid process of the temporal bone. Muscles that move the tongue attach to the hyoid bone.

The six **ossicle bones,** three in each middle ear (malleus, incus, stapes), were discussed previously. They articulate with each other and extend across the middle ear from the **tympanic membrane** through the oval window into the inner ear.

### Air Sinuses

Previously we stated that a sinus is a cavity located within a bone that decreases the weight of a bone. Sinuses also act as resonance chambers, which influence the sound of the voice. The air sinuses are classified into two groups: **paranasal** and **mastoid.**

The **paranasal sinuses** (Figure 14-7) are located in the maxilla, ethmoid, sphenoid, and frontal bones. They communicate with the nasal cavity, and the ciliated mucous membrane that lines the nasal cavity continues into the paranasal sinuses. Sinusitis involves inflammation of the sinus mucous membranes, often accompanied by large production of mucus. The mucus drains from the paranasal sinuses into the nasal cavity.

The **mastoid bone** contains air cells that communi-

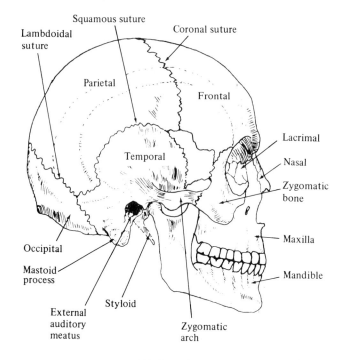

**(A)** Lateral view

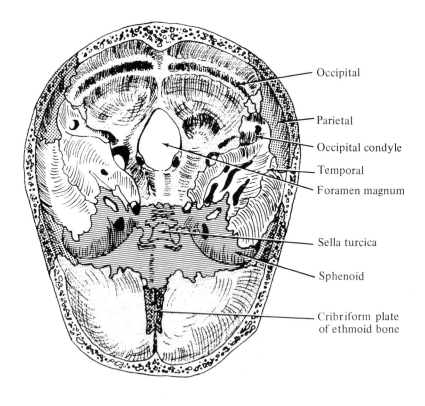

**(B)** Internal view

**Figure 14-4.** (A) Sutures and bones of the skull and face. (B) The top of the skull has been removed to show the bones from an internal view.

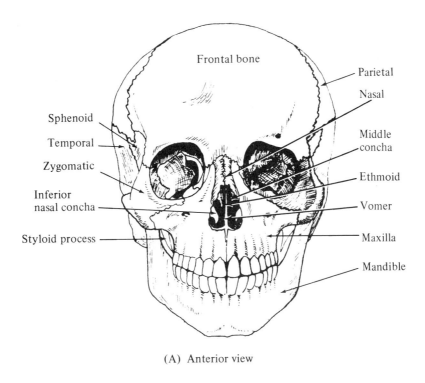

Frontal bone

Parietal

Nasal

Sphenoid

Temporal

Middle
concha

Zygomatic

Ethmoid

Inferior
nasal concha

Vomer

Styloid process

Maxilla

Mandible

(A) Anterior view

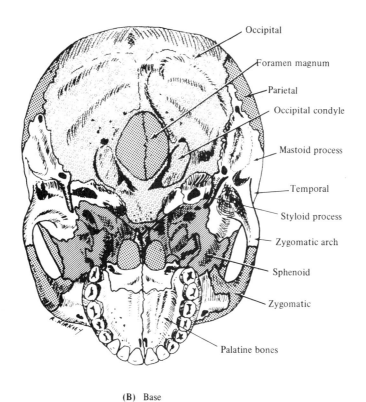

Occipital

Foramen magnum

Parietal

Occipital condyle

Mastoid process

Temporal

Styloid process

Zygomatic arch

Sphenoid

Zygomatic

Palatine bones

(B) Base

Figure 14–5. (A) Bones of the skull and face are shown from an anterior view. (B) The mandible has been removed to show the skull bones from below.

295

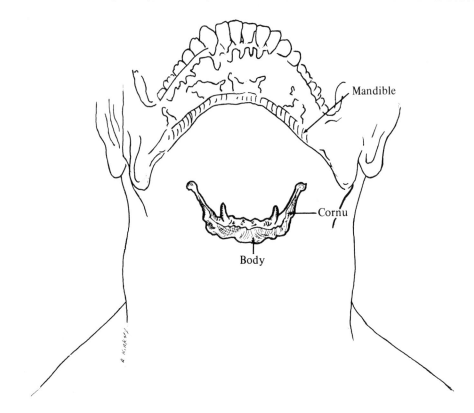

**Figure 14-6.**   The U-shaped hyoid bone is shown from an anterior view.

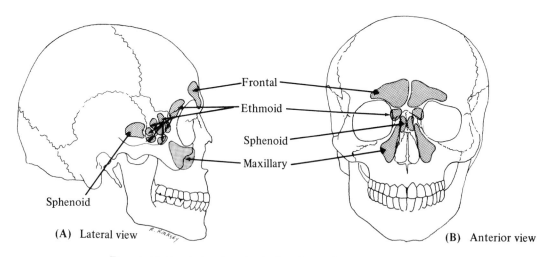

**Figure 14-7.**   Lateral and anterior views of paranasal sinuses.

cate with the middle ear. A mucous membrane lines the middle ear and is continuous into the mastoid air cells. Infections located in the throat and nose can spread through mucous membranes into the middle ear. This results in inflammation of the mastoid sinus, called mastoiditis.

## Fetal Skull

In a newborn child the cranial bones do not join with each other by sutures at all points. At six points the cranial bones are connected by membranous tissue. These six membranous areas are the **fontanels,** often

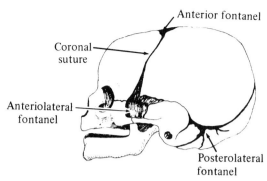

**(A) Lateral View**

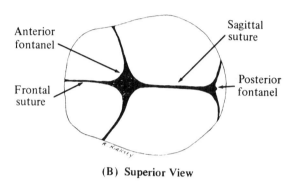

**(B) Superior View**

**Figure 14-8.** The fontanels of a fetal skull are shown from lateral and superior views.

called "soft spots." The anterior, posterior, and four lateral fontanels (two posterolateral and two anterolateral) (Figure 14-8) make up the six fontanels. They play an important role during childbirth. They permit the cranial bones to be moved and molded, so that the baby's head can pass through the mother's birth canal. They also allow the brain to rapidly increase in size after birth. After birth, these membranous areas gradually are closed as bone tissue replaces them. By the second year they are all closed.

## MOVEMENT OF THE HEAD

The head is moved for various reasons, one of which is to signify agreement or disagreement. The major movements of the head are flexion, extension, and rotation. The major muscles that move the head are sternocleidomastoid and semispinalis capitis. The origins, insertions, and actions of these muscles are given in Table 14-1.

The **sternocleidomastoid** (Figure 14-9) muscle is named for its two origins and one insertion. It originates on the sternum and clavicle (collar bone) on the right and left side, and inserts on the mastoid process (Table 14-1) on the same side. When one sternocleidomastoid muscle is contracted, the head is rotated toward the muscle that is contracting. If both of them contract simultaneously, the head is flexed or moved into a prayer position. The XI spinal accessory cranial nerve stimulates the sternocleidomastoid muscle to contract.

The **semispinalis capitis** (Figure 14-10) muscle is the antagonist of the sternocleidomastoid. It extends the head. After one has bowed the head, the right and left semispinalis capitis muscles act together to extend the head back to the normal upright position. Extension of the head beyond the normal upright position is an example of hyperextension.

The sternocleidomastoid muscle is innervated by the spinal accessory nerve (XI), and the semispinalis capitis is innervated by cervical nerves rather than cranial nerves.

## MASTICATION (CHEWING) MOVEMENTS

The chewing and swallowing of food results from the contraction of several muscles in a coordinated manner. The mandible is the only movable bone in the skull (ex-

### TABLE 14-1. *Movement of Head**

| BONE(LEVER) | MUSCLE | ORIGIN | INSERTION | ACTION |
|---|---|---|---|---|
| Head | Sternocleido-mastoid | Sternum and clavicle | Mastoid process of temporal bone | Rotates head—one muscle; flexes head—two muscles |
| | Semispinalis capitis | Last four cervical, upper five thoracic vertebrae | Occipital bone | Extends head |

*See Figs. 14-9 and 14-10.

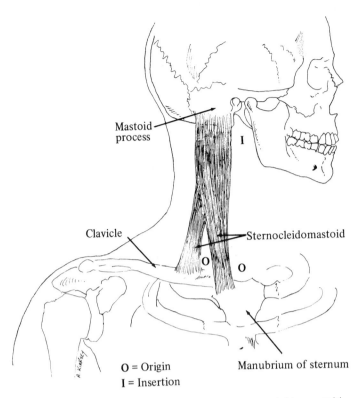

O = Origin
I = Insertion

**Figure 14-9.** A lateral view of the sternocleidomastoid muscle with the origin and insertion.

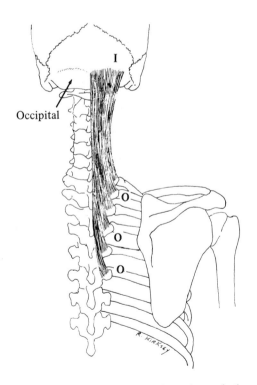

**Figure 14-10.** The origin and insertion of the right semispinalis capitis muscle.

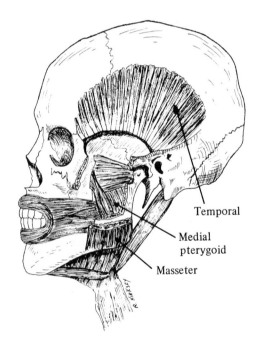

**Figure 14-11.** Three mastication muscles important for chewing.

298

### TABLE 14-2. *Muscles of Mastication**

| Bone (Lever) | Muscle | Origin | Insertion | Action |
|---|---|---|---|---|
| Mandible | Masseter | Zygomatic arch | Mandible | Pulls mandible up |
| | Temporal | Temporal bone | Mandible | Pulls mandible up |
| | Medial pterygoid | Maxilla bone | Angel of the mandible | Lowers mandible |

* See Fig. 14-11.

cept for the ossicles); four muscles attach to the mandible and move it up and down during chewing.

The **masseter** (Figure 14-11) muscle originates on the zygomatic arch and inserts on the ramus (Table 14-2) and angle of the mandible. The insertion contracts toward the origin, which pulls the mandible up, and the lower and upper teeth grind the food. It is innervated by the trigeminal nerve (V).

The **temporal** (Figure 14-11) muscle originates on the temporal bone and inserts on the coronoid process of the mandible bone. It helps to close the mandible. The trigeminal nerve (V) innervates this muscle.

The **medial pterygoid** (Figure 14-11) muscle originates on the maxilla bone and inserts on the angle of the mandible. These two muscles lower the mandible when they contract simultaneously. They grate the teeth when each one contracts alternately. The trigeminal nerve (V) innervates the medial pterygoid.

## 2 VERTEBRAL COLUMN

The vertebral column is made up of 26 bones:

| | |
|---|---|
| Cervical vertebrae | 7 |
| Thoracic vertebrae | 12 |
| Lumbar vertebrae | 5 |
| Sacrum | 1 |
| Coccyx | 1 |
| | 26 total |

The vertebral column (spine) (Figure 14-12) is a strong flexible column. It is located in the midline of the body and acts as an axial support for the body. It extends downward from the base of the skull to the coccyx (tail bone). The vertebral column houses the spinal cord, supports the skull, and serves as an attachment for both the posterior ends of ribs and the pelvic girdle. The vertebrae are attached to each other by ligaments and muscles, and cartilaginous discs (intervertebral discs) separate them. This type of attachment allows the vertebrae to move considerably without slipping out of place.

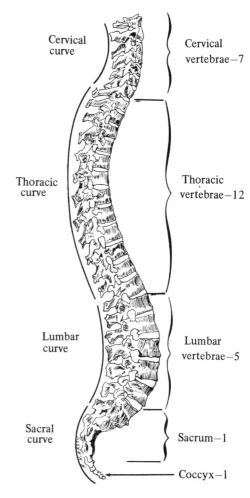

**Figure 14-12.** The regions of the vertebral column and the number of vertebrae in each are shown. The four curves of the vertebral column also are shown.

There are five regions to the vertebral column with a varying number of vertebrae in each: cervical (7), thoracic (12), lumbar (5), sacrum (1), and coccyx (1). The vertebrae in each region differ slightly in their anatomic characteristics. The vertebral column is curved rather than straight. These curvatures are important in that they allow one to hold the head upright and stand upright.

## Four Curves of Vertebral Column

From a lateral view one can see that there are four curves (Figure 14-12) of the vertebral column. The **cervical curve** gradually develops in a child and is totally developed when a child can hold his head erect. The **thoracic curve** is present at birth. The **lumbar curve** gradually develops in a child and is totally developed when a child can stand erect and walk. The **sacral curve** is present at birth. When a child is born, the entire vertebral column has a concave curve (from anterior view). The thoracic and sacral curves are called **primary curves** since they are present at birth. The cervical and lumbar curves are **secondary curves** since they develop after a child is born.

## Abnormal Curvatures of the Vertebral Column

Three major types of abnormal curvatures can affect the vertebral column. **Scoliosis** is a lateral curvature. **Kyphosis** is an exaggerated thoracic curve and frequently is called a "hunchback condition." **Lordosis** is an exaggerated lumbar curve and commonly is called a "swayback condition."

## General Anatomic Features of Vertebrae (sing. vertebra)

There are slight differences in the structure of the vertebrae in each region; however, they have some common features (Figure 14-13). The body is the weight-bearing portion and internally is composed of spongy bone. The vertebral foramen is an opening through which the spinal cord passes. The neural arch is formed by two lamina and pedicles that protect the spinal cord. Three processes project from the vertebrae: the spinous process and two transverse processes. These processes serve as points of attachment for muscles. The vertebrae articulate with each other at inferior and superior articular processes (Figures 14-13 and 14-14A).

## Anatomy of Vertebrae in Each Region

**Cervical vertebrae** (Figure 14-14A) are characterized by three foramina: a transverse foramen in each transverse process and the vertebral foramen. The first cervical vertebra, atlas, lacks a body. The atlas supports the head, and its name is derived from the mythical Greek god, who supported the world on his shoulders. Occipi-

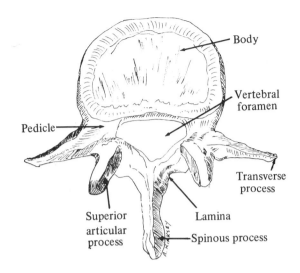

**Figure 14-13.** Parts of a typical vertebra.

tal condyles, from the occipital bone of the skull, articulate with the atlas. The second cervical vertebra, axis, has an odontoid process that extends up into the anterior portion of the vertebral foramen. When a person rotates the head to say "no," the atlas rotates around the odontoid process; when a person moves the head to say "yes," the occipital condyles glide on the articulating processes of the atlas.

One end of each **thoracic vertebra** (Figure 14-14B) articulates with a rib. The point at which the rib articulates with a vertebra is called an articular facet. It is a distinguishing feature of the thoracic vertebrae. There are two facets on each side of a thoracic vertebra: one on the body of the vertebra and one on the transverse process. The spinous processes are long, thin, and slope downward.

The five **lumbar vertebrae** (Figure 14-14C) have massive bodies and are the largest of all the vertebrae. They are well adapted to support an increasing amount of weight at the bottom of the lumbar region. Another distinguishing feature is a long, thin transverse process on each side. The second lumbar vertebra is the level at which the spinal cord ends. To perform a lumbar puncture the needle must be inserted between lumbar vertebrae 3, 4, or 5, into the subarachnoid space.

The **sacrum** (Figure 14-12) is composed of five fused vertebrae. It is easily identified by its triangular shape and anterior concave depression. The sacrum is wedged between the two iliac bones of the hip or pelvic girdle.

The **coccyx** (Figure 14-13) or tail bone is composed of three to five fused vertebrae. This triangular bone has no processes or foramina. The coccyx is slightly movable, which is important during childbirth.

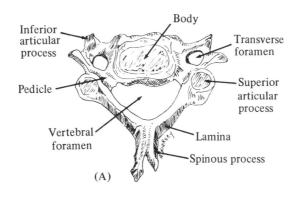

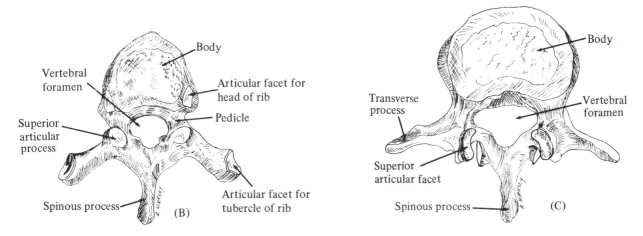

Figure 14-14.    (A) Cervical vertebra. (B) Thoracic vertebra. (C) Lumbar vertebra.

# 3  BONES OF THE THORAX

The thorax is composed of 25 bones:

| True ribs | 14 | |
|---|---|---|
| False ribs | 10 | |
| Sternum | 1 | |
| | 25 | total |

The thorax (Figure 14–15) resembles a bony cage. It is narrow at the top and broad at the bottom and is composed of ribs, cartilages, and the sternum. The bars of this cage are the ribs, and the floor is the diaphragm. This cage is different from others in that muscles are present between the bars of the cage. The thorax acts to protect the heart, lungs, and major blood vessels and is important in respiration.

## Sternum or Breast Bone

The sternum or breast bone (Figure 14–15) is a dagger-shaped bone in the midsagittal plane. It is composed of the manubrium, body, and xiphoid process. The first rib on each side attaches to the manubrium, and the next 11 on each side attach to the body either directly or indirectly. The sternum is located near the surface of the skin and is a favorite site for obtaining samples of bone marrow. The procedure for obtaining the bone marrow is called a **sternal puncture.** It involves inserting a needle into the bone marrow of the sternum and withdrawing a sample. The sample is analyzed to diagnose possible blood diseases, such as leukemia.

## Ribs

Twelve pairs of ribs attach to the sternum. A typical rib is shown in Figure 14–16. Each rib is composed of a head, neck, and shaft. The head articulates with an articular facet on the body of the thoracic vertebra. The tubercle articulates with a transverse process facet. The shaft is a flattened, curved portion of each rib.

Each member of the 12 pairs of ribs articulates with a thoracic vertebra. From the thoracic vertebrae the ribs curve upward, downward, and forward. The first seven

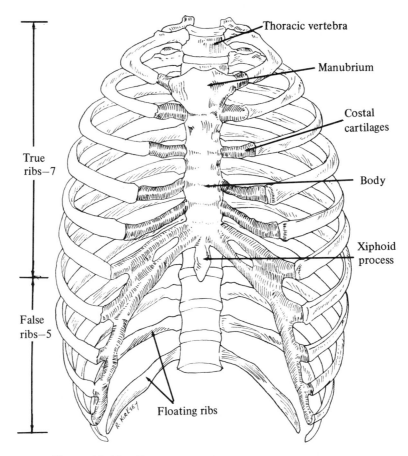

**Figure 14-15.**   The thorax and the various types of ribs.

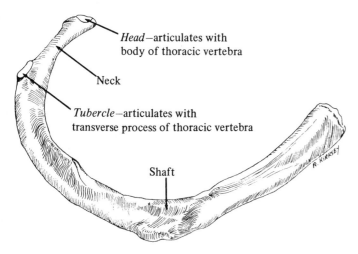

**Figure 14-16.**   A typical rib, showing the parts of a rib and what the head and tubercle articulate with.

pairs of ribs are called **true ribs** because costal cartilages attach their anterior ends to the sternum directly (Figure 14-15). The next five pairs (8 to 12) are called **false ribs** because they attach indirectly to the sternum.

The eighth, ninth, and tenth pairs of the false ribs attach anteriorly by costal cartilages to the ribs above them. The last two pairs of false ribs do not attach anteriorly to anything; therefore, they are called **floating ribs** (Figure 14-15).

The vertebral attachments of the ribs act as fulcrums, and the anterior ends move up and down. The ribs are levers, and they act to increase and decrease the size of the thoracic cavity. These changes in the size of the thoracic cavity are important in respiration, and they will be discussed in detail in Chapter 17. The main sources of power for these respiratory levers are the internal and external intercostal muscles.

## Muscles of Respiration

The external and internal intercostal muscles attach to the ribs and move them up and down. The **external intercostals** have their origin on the lower surface of the first 11 pairs of ribs. Their fibers extend downward and forward and insert on the ribs below them (Figure 14-17). Since muscle insertions contract toward origins,

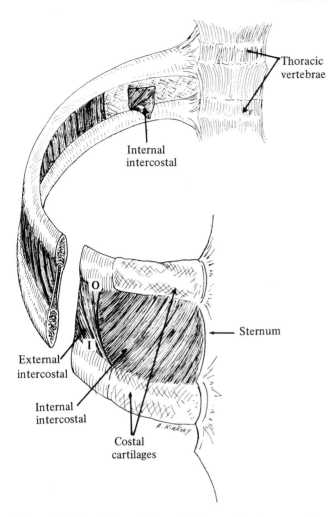

the external intercostal muscles contract upward and pull the ribs upward (Table 14–3). This action acts to increase the size of the thoracic cavity and occurs when one inspires.

The **diaphragm** is a dome-shaped muscle that forms the floor of the thorax. The origin of the diaphragm includes the costal cartilages of the lower six ribs, upper lumbar vertebrae, and xiphoid process of sternum (Figure 14–18). The fibers come together to insert on a central tendon. The diaphragm contracts downward until its normal dome shape is flattened out. This action

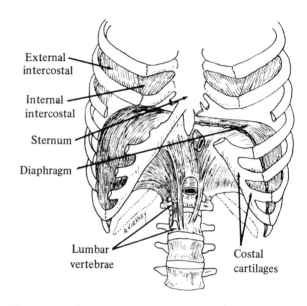

**Figure 14–17.** The position of the internal and external intercostal muscles between two ribs.

**Figure 14–18.** The diaphragm is shown in relation to the ribs, sternum, and vertebrae.

## TABLE 14–3. *Muscles of Respiration**

| BONE(LEVER) | MUSCLE | ORIGIN | INSERTION | ACTION |
|---|---|---|---|---|
| Ribs | External intercostals | Inferior surface of first 11 pairs of ribs | Superior surface of ribs below origin | Pulls ribs upward and increases size of thoracic cavity |
| | Internal intercostals | Superior surface of ribs | Inferior surface of ribs above origin | Pulls ribs downward and decreases size of thoracic cavity |
| | Diaphragm | Costal cartilage of lower 6 ribs; upper lumbar vertebrae; xiphoid process | Central tendon | Contracts to increase size of thoracic cavity |

* See Figs. 14–17 and 14–18.

acts to increase the size of the thoracic cavity. The diaphragm is the main respiratory muscle during quiet normal breathing. The external intercostals are used when one inspires deeper than normal. The **internal intercostal** muscles (Figure 14-17) have their origin and insertion (Table 4-3) in positions such that when they contract they pull ribs downward. The action is called expiration, and it reduces the size of the thoracic cavity. Actually, the internal intercostals are used only when a person forcibly expires. Normal quiet breathing involves passive expiration, and it occurs when the inspiratory muscles relax.

# SUMMARY

### Skull and Muscles That Move It

A. Adult skull bones: frontal, parietal, temporal, occipital, sphenoid, ethmoid, nasal, zygomatic, maxilla, mandible, lacrimal, vomer, palatine, inferior nasal conchae, hyoid, and mastoid.

B. Fetal skull: At six points the cranial bones do not join by sutures but rather by membranous fontanels (soft spots); permit cranial bones to be moved and skull to be molded.

C. Movement of head
   1. Sternocleidomastoid: Rotates head, one muscle; flexes head, two muscles.
   2. Semispinalis capitis: extends head.

D. Mastication (chewing) movements
   1. Masseter: pulls mandible up.
   2. Temporal: pulls mandible up.
   3. Medial pterygoid: lowers mandible.

### Vertebral Column

Composed of 26 bones or vertebrae; cervical (7), thoracic (12), lumbar (5), sacrum (1), coccyx (1).

A. Four curves: (1) cervical, totally developed when child can hold head erect; (2) thoracic, present at birth; (3) lumbar, totally developed when child can stand erect and walk; (4) sacral, present at birth.

B. Abnormal curvatures: (1) scoliosis, lateral curvature; (2) kyphosis, exaggerated thoracic curve; (3) lordosis, exaggerated lumbar curve.

### Bones of the Thorax

A. Sternum: composed of manubrium, body, and xiphoid process.

B. Ribs: 12 pair; true, the anterior ends of the first 7 pair attach directly to sternum; false, next 5 pair attach indirectly to sternum.

C. Muscles of respiration
   1. External intercostals: pulls ribs upward
   2. Internal intercostals: pulls ribs downward
   3. Diaphragm: increases and decreases size of thoracic cavity.

Levers (Bones), Muscles, and Movements of the Axial Skeletal System

1. Fontanels in a fetal skull are:
   1. Six in number
   2. Located at junctions of bones
   3. Membranous regions of skull bones
   4. Openings in skull bones
   (a) 1, 2, 3     (b) 1, 3     (c) 2, 4     (d) 4     (e) All of these

2. Which of the following is (are) correct for vertebrae of the vertebral column?
   1. Cervical (7)     3. Lumbar (5)
   2. Thoracic (12)     4. Sacrum (1)
   (a) 1, 2, 3     (b) 1, 3     (c) 2, 4     (d) 4     (e) All of these

3. Which one of the following is correct for curves of the vertebral column?
   (a) Cervical, coccyx, lumbar, thoracic
   (b) Cervical, brachial, lumbar, thoracic
   (c) Cervical, thoracic, lymbar, sacral
   (d) None of these

True (A) or false (B). Questions 4 to 8.

4. Sternocleidomastoid muscles contracting together flex the head.

5. When one chews foods, one uses the masseter, temporal, and medial pterygoid muscles.

6. When breathing inward or inhaling, the external intercostals assist by pulling ribs upward.

7. When exhaling, the internal intercostals assist by pulling ribs downward.

8. The diaphragm muscle aids both inhalation and exhalation.

# Chapter 15

# LEVERS (BONES), MUSCLES, AND MOVEMENTS OF THE APPENDICULAR SKELETAL SYSTEM

After reading and studying this chapter, a student should be able to:

1. Name the bones that compose the pectoral girdle.
2. Give the functions of the levator scapulae, pectoralis minor, and trapezius muscles.
3. Identify on a figure the major markings on the humerus bone.
4. Write the functions of the pectoralis major, latissimus dorsi, and deltoid muscles.
5. Recognize on a figure the major markings on the radius and ulna bones.
6. State the functions of the biceps brachii and triceps brachii muscles.
7. Give the name of the group of bones that compose the wrist and hand.
8. Write the functions of the flexor carpi radialis and extensor carpi radialis muscles.
9. Name and recognize the markings on the bones that compose the pelvic girdle.
10. Identify on a figure the markings on the femur bone.
11. Give the functions of the iliopsoas, gluteus maximus, gluteus medius, and adductor muscles.
12. Identify on a figure the markings on the tibia and fibula bones.
13. Give functions of the biceps femoris, semitendinosus, semimembranosus, and quadriceps femoris muscles.
14. Name the group of bones that composes the ankle and foot.
15. Give functions of the tibialis anterior, gastrocnemius, and soleus muscles.
16. Distinguish among synarthrosis, amphiarthrosis and diarthrosis joints.

*The appendicular division of the skeletal system consists of bones in the appendages plus the pectoral and pelvic girdles. Below are the names and numbers of each bone that composes the appendicular system.*

| *Upper Extremities* (64 bones) | | *Lower Extremities* (62 bones) | |
|---|---|---|---|
| clavicle | 2 | pelvic bone | 2 |
| scapulae | 2 | femur | 2 |
| humerus | 2 | patella | 2 |
| ulna | 2 | tibia | 2 |
| radius | 2 | fibula | 2 |
| carpals | 16 | tarsal bones | 14 |
| metacarpals | 10 | metatarsals | 10 |
| phalanges | 28 | phalanges | 28 |

# 1 UPPER EXTREMITIES (64 BONES) AND MUSCLES THAT MOVE THEM

## *SHOULDER*

The shoulder girdle (pectoral girdle) on each side is composed of two bones: **clavicle** and **scapula** (Figures 15–1 and 15–2). These two bones are attached to the axial skeleton. The two shoulder girdles attach bones of the upper extremities to the axial skeleton.

The **scapula** (Figure 15–1) or shoulder blade is a flattened, triangular-shaped bone located on the posterior (dorsal) side of the thorax. It has two prominent processes, **coracoid** and **acromion.** The **glenoid cavity,** located laterally, is the point at which the bone of the upper arm (humerus) articulates with the scapula. The acromion process is an extension of the spine of the scapula. Each scapula is attached to ribs 2 to 7 by muscles and tendons. The large surface area, processes, and spine of the scapula serve as excellent points for muscles to attach.

The **clavicle** or collar bone (Figure 15–2) is unusual in that it has a double curvature. Each clavicle is located

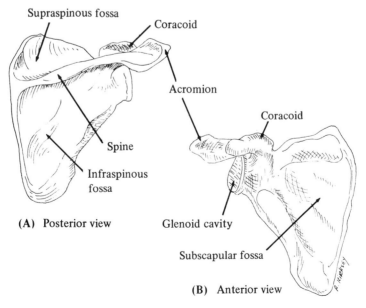

Supraspinous fossa

Coracoid

Acromion

Spine

Infraspinous fossa

**(A)** Posterior view

Coracoid

Glenoid cavity

Subscapular fossa

**(B)** Anterior view

Figure 15–1. Scapula.

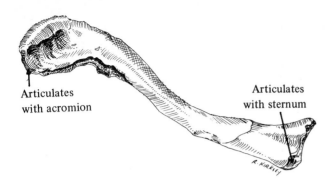

**Figure 15-2.** The clavicle has a double curvature and articulates with the sternum and acromion.

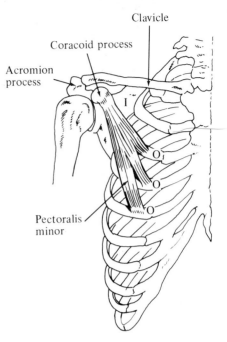

**Figure 15-4.** The origin and insertion of the pectoralis minor muscle.

on the anterior (ventral) surface of the thorax. The medial end of the clavicle articulates with the acromion process of the scapula. The clavicle acts as a rigid brace to hold the shoulder out from the body and allow the arms to swing freely. Since the clavicle is immovable, it does not give much when blows are received in the shoulder region; therefore, fractures to the clavicle are common for people who engage in contact sports.

The movements of the shoulder primarily involve the scapula. The **levator scapulae** muscle (Table 15–1) is responsible for elevating the shoulder (Figure 15–3). The origin of the levator scapulae is on the transverse processes of the first four cervical vertebrae (Table 15–1), and it inserts on the lateral border of the scapula. The antagonist of the levator scapulae is the **pectoralis minor** (Figure 15–4). The origin of the pectoralis minor

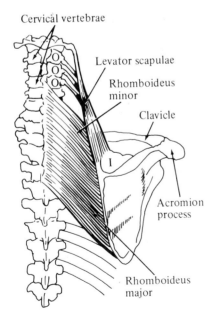

**Figure 15-3.** The origin and insertion of the levator scapulae muscle.

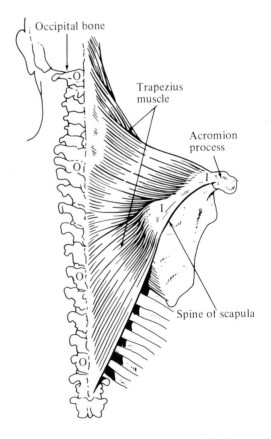

**Figure 15-5.** The origin and insertion of the trapezius muscle.

### TABLE 15-1.   Muscles That Move the Shoulders*

| Bone (Lever) | Muscle | Origin | Insertion | Action |
|---|---|---|---|---|
| Scapula | Levator scapulae | Transverse processes of C-1 through C-4 | Lateral border of scapula | Elevates shoulder |
| | Pectoralis minor | Anterior surface of ribs 2-5 | Coracoid process of scapula | Lowers the shoulder |
| | Trapezius muscle | Occipital bone, cervical and thoracic vertebrae | Spine of scapula and acromion | Elevates and shrugs shoulders |

*See Figs. 15-3, 15-4, and 15-5.

is the anterior surface of ribs 3 to 5, and it inserts on the coracoid process of the scapula. It is responsible for lowering the scapula. The **trapezius** muscle is responsible for elevating and shrugging the shoulders. The two trapezius muscles joined together have a trapezoid shape. The origin of each trapezius muscle extends from the occipital bone down through the cervical and thoracic vertebrae (Figure 15-5). It inserts on the spine of the scapula and the acromion process.

## ARM (UPPER ARM)

The only bone of the upper arm is the **humerus** (Figure 15-6). The rounded head of the humerus extends from the **proximal epiphysis,** and it articulates with the gle-

noid cavity of the scapula. The **greater** and **lesser tubercles** also extend from the proximal epiphysis. **Medial** and **lateral epicondyles** extend from the distal epiphysis of the humerus (Figure 15-6). The tubercles and epicondyles serve as points for muscles to attach. The **capitulum** and **trochlea** articulate with the bones of the forearm (lower arm). The **olecranon fossa** is on the posterior surface of the humerus, and it receives the olecranon process from the ulna bone.

The muscles that move the humerus illustrate quite well the first principle of skeletal muscle actions. The muscles that move this lever are located superior or inferior to the humerus, but they do not lie over it.

The **pectoralis major** muscle (Table 15-2) is a broad fan-shaped muscle. It originates on the clavicle and sternum and inserts on the **greater tubercle** of the humerus

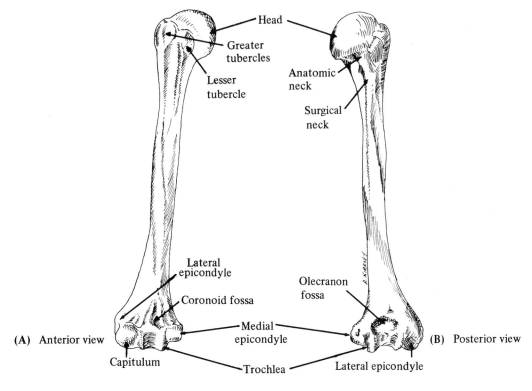

Figure 15-6.   Humerus.

**TABLE 15-2.   *Muscles That Move the Humerus*\***

| Bone (Lever) | Muscle | Origin | Insertion | Action |
|---|---|---|---|---|
| Humerus | Pectoralis major | Clavicle, sternum, and costal cartilages of true ribs | Greater tubercle of humerus | Adduction and flexion |
| | Latissimus dorsi | Lower thoracic, lumbar, and sacral vertebrae | Near head of humerus | Extension |
| | Deltoid | Spine of scapula, clavicle | Lateral side of humerus about halfway down | Abduction |

*See Fig. 15-7.

(Figure 15-7A). When the pectoralis major contracts, it adducts and flexes the humerus. Flexion of the humerus is essentially the movement of the arm across the chest. Adduction of the upper arm is movement of the humerus downward toward the side of the body.

The **latissimus dorsi** muscle (Figure 15-7B) is antag-

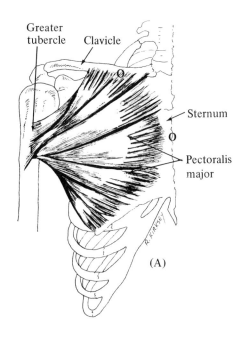

(A)

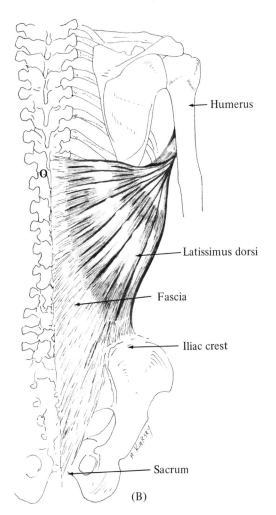

(B)

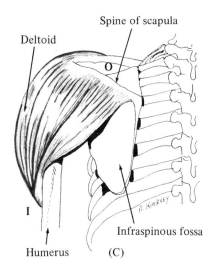

(C)

**Figure 15-7.**   (A) The origin and insertion of the pectoralis major muscle. (B) The origin and insertion of the latissimus dorsi muscle. (C) The origin and insertion of the deltoid muscle.

onistic to the pectoralis major, since it extends the humerus. The latissimus dorsi is a broad, flat triangular muscle that extends from the vertebral column laterally across the back and inserts on the humerus. Table 15–2 gives the origin, insertion, and action. The extension of the humerus is a third-class lever since the power, latissimus dorsi, is between the resistance and the fulcrum (Figure 15–7B).

The **deltoid muscle** (Figure 15–7C) also is antagonistic to the pectoralis major since it abducts the humerus. The triangular-shaped deltoid muscle extends across the shoulder joint. It originates on the spine of the scapula and inserts on the lateral surface of the humerus (deltoid tuberosity). Since the insertion end of the muscle moves toward the origin, the humerus is abducted (moved away from midline). The deltoid is often a site for injections because of its thickness and location. The abduction of the humerus is an example of a third-class lever since the power, deltoid muscle, is between the resistance and the fulcrum.

## FOREARM OR LOWER ARM

The forearm contains two bones, **radius** and **ulna.** The ulna (Figure 15–8) is on the medial side of the forearm. An unusual hook-shaped projection, the **olecranon process,** extends off the proximal end. This process forms the projection called the elbow. Slightly inferior and anterior to this process is a concave area called the **semilunar notch.** This notch articulates with the trochlea of the humerus. When the lower arm is held in an extended position, the olecranon process fits into the olecranon fossa of the humerus. The head of the ulna and the styloid process extend from the distal end of the ulna.

The **radius** bone (Figure 15–8) is on the lateral side of the forearm (or thumb side). The head is round and articulates with the round capitulum of the humerus. (One way to distinguish the radius bone is that the head is circular shaped, and half of the diameter of a circle is a radius.) The distal end of the radius has a large styloid process that articulates with two wrist bones and the ulna.

The articulation between the semilunar notch of the ulna and trochlea on the humerus is the elbow joint. Two movements can occur here, extension and flexion. The circular head of the radius permits medial and lateral rotation between the radius and the capitulum on the humerus. Lateral rotation is called **supination,** and medial rotation is called **pronation.** The muscles that move the forearm are extensors, flexors, pronators, and supinators.

**Biceps brachii** (Figure 15–9A) flexes the lower arm and lies superior to it. The biceps brachii has two heads of origin (Table 15–3) and inserts on the radius. The bi-

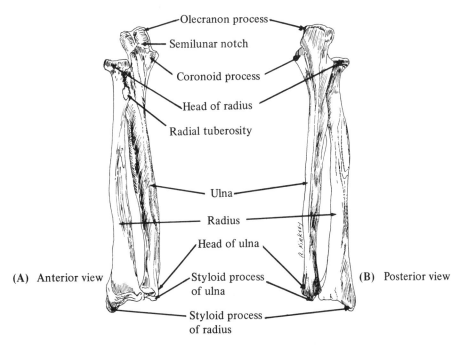

Olecranon process
Semilunar notch
Coronoid process
Head of radius
Radial tuberosity
Ulna
Radius
Head of ulna
Styloid process of ulna
Styloid process of radius

**(A)** Anterior view    **(B)** Posterior view

Figure 15–8. The radius and the ulna.

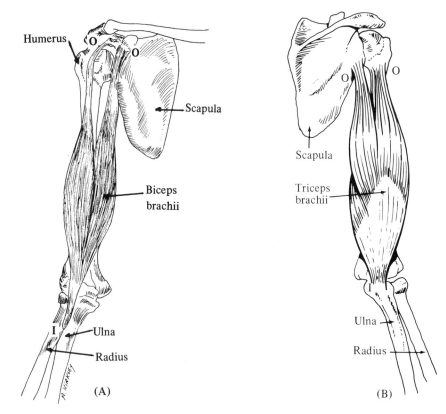

**Figure 15-9.** (A) The origin and insertion of the biceps brachii muscle; (B) the origin and insertion of the triceps brachii muscle.

ceps brachii also supinates the lower arm or turns the palm so that it is facing forward.

The **triceps brachii** (Figure 15-9B) extends the forearm (lower arm) and is antagonistic to the biceps brachii. It is located superior to the forearm and on the posterior surface of the humerus. The triceps brachii has three heads of origin (Table 15-3) and inserts on the olecranon process of the ulna.

## BONES OF THE WRIST AND HAND

The wrist is composed of eight short bones, carpals, that are arranged in two rows of four each (Figure 15-10).

The names of the bones are navicular, lunate, triquetral, pisiform, greater multangular, lesser multangular, capitate, and hamate. Ligaments hold the bones together tightly so there is little movement between them. The radius articulates with the navicular and lunate bones.

The bones of the hand are called **metacarpals** (Figure 15-10). There are five metacarpal bones that are numbered from the lateral side (thumb side). Proximally the metacarpals articulate with the carpals; distally they enlarge and articulate with the bones of the fingers, the **phalanges.** The distal ends of the metacarpals are large and form the knuckles located between the hand and the fingers. The phalanges are the bones of the fingers.

### TABLE 15-3.   Muscles That Move Forearm*

| BONE (LEVER) | MUSCLE | ORIGIN | INSERTION | ACTION |
|---|---|---|---|---|
| Radius and ulna | Biceps brachii | Long head, scapula; short head, scapula | Proximal end of radius | Flexion and supination |
|  | Triceps brachii | Long head, scapula; lateral head, humerus; medial head, humerus | Olecranon process of ulna | Extension |

*See Fig. 15-9.

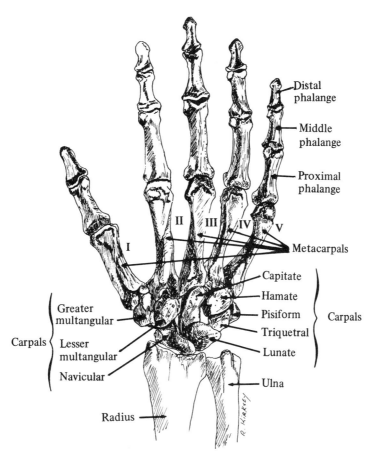

Figure 15-10.   Bones of the wrist and the hand, showing carpals, metacarpals, and phalanges.

There are three phalanges in each finger except the thumb, which has two. Each finger, except the thumb, has a proximal, middle, and distal phalange. The thumb has only a proximal and distal phalange.

The number of muscles that move the hand are numerous. We will discuss a representative of each group that flexes and extends the hand. The muscles are located in the forearm and extend ligaments into the wrist, hand, and fingers.

The **flexor carpi radialis** (Figure 15-11A) helps to flex the hand or draw the palm toward the wrist. The origin of this muscle is on the medial epicondyle of the humerus, and it inserts on the second and third medial epicondyle of the humerus, and it inserts on the second and third metacarpal bones. The other flexors originate on the medial epicondyle and insert on the metacarpals, as well as on tendons and ligaments attached to the metacarpals.

The **extensor carpi ulnaris** (Figure 15-11B), since it extends the hand, is antagonistic to the flexor carpi radialis. Table 15-4 gives origins, insertion, and actions for these muscles.

## TABLE 15-4.   *Muscles That Move Wrist and Hand**

| Bone (Lever) | Muscle | Origin | Insertion | Action |
|---|---|---|---|---|
| Carpals and metacarpals | Flexor carpi radialis | Medial epicondyle of humerus | Second and third metacarpals | Flexion |
| | Extensor carpi ulnaris | Upper portion of ulna | Proximal end of fifth metacarpal | Extension |

*See Fig. 15-11.

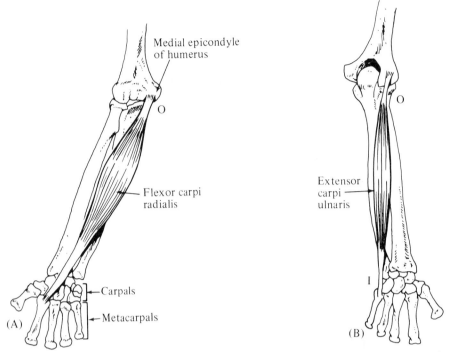

Figure 15-11.   (A) The origin and insertion of the flexor carpi radialis muscle (anterior view). (B) The origin and insertion of the extensor carpi ulnaris muscle (posterior view).

# 2   LOWER EXTREMITIES (62 BONES) AND MUSCLES THAT MOVE THEM

## PELVIC GIRDLE

The pelvic girdle is a ring that is composed of four bones: two hipbones, sacrum, and coccyx. The sacrum and coccyx are the last two bones of the vertebral column and are wedged between the two hipbones. The bones of the legs are attached to the pelvic girdle.

Each **hipbone** or **oscoxae** (Figure 15–12) is an irregular-shaped bone that is composed of three fused bones: ilium, ischium, and pubis. The **ilium** is the broadest flaring bone of the three. It has a prominent **iliac crest** referred to as the hipbone. Projecting from the ilium is the **anterior superior iliac spine,** which often is used as a reference point for surgery. The two ilium bones articulate with the sacrum, where they form the sacro-iliac joint.

The **ischium** bone (Figure 15–12) extends downward from the ilium and enlarges to form the ischial tuberosity, which supports the weight of the body when one is sitting. Superior to the ischial tuberosity is the ischial

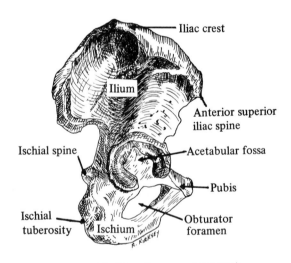

Figure 15-12.   Oscoxae (hipbone).

spine. The pubis extends anteriorly and curves downward to the ischium. Anteriorly it unites with the pubis from the other oscoxae to form the **symphysis pubis** joint. Two other features of each oscoxae are the **obturator foramen** and the **acetabulum.** The obturator foramen is a large foramen that is surrounded by the ischium and pubis bones. The acetabulum is a deep socket formed where the ilium, ischium, and pubis are fused. It articulates with the head of the femur.

## TRUE AND FALSE PELVIS

The middle, basinlike area between the oscoxae bones is divided into the true and false pelvis. The true pelvis is the area inferior to the pelvic brim (Figure 15-13). The entrance into the true pelvis is the inlet, followed by the cavity, and the exit point is the outlet (Figure 15-14). In a female, during childbirth, the measurements of these areas are critical if a baby is to pass through the true pelvis. The false pelvis is the area superior to the pelvic brim.

The female pelvis differs from the male pelvis (Figure 15-13) since it has to be adaptable for childbirth. The true pelvis in the female is larger in all directions, bones are smoother and lighter, and the coccyx is more movable. The male pelvis has a narrow true pelvis, bones are heavier and rougher, and the coccyx is rigid.

The pubic arch in the male is narrower and pointed compared to the wide pubic arch of the female.

## FEMUR

The **femur** or thigh bone (Figure 15-15) is the longest, strongest, and heaviest bone of the body. These characteristics enable the femur to transfer weight from the pelvic girdle to the lower leg. The proximal end of the femur is characterized by a large rounded head that articulates with the acetabulum. Inferior to the head and neck are the **greater** and **lesser trochanters,** to which muscles attach. The diaphysis (shaft) of the femur is thick and slightly curved anteriorly. The distal epiphysis of the femur is characterized by **lateral** and **medial condyles.** The condyles facilitate the articulation of the

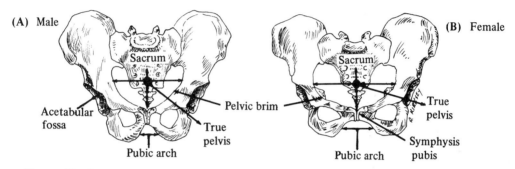

Figure 15-13.   The similarities and differences between (A) male and (B) female pelves.

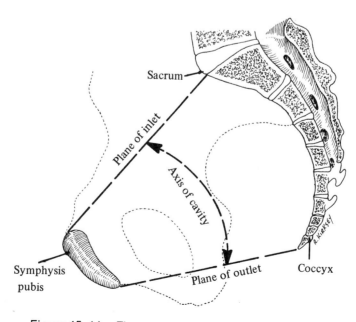

Figure 15-14.   Three measurements of the true pelvis.

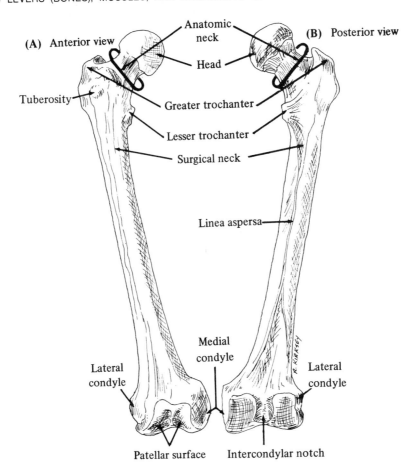

Figure 15-15.    Femur.

femur with the **tibia** of the lower leg. On the posterior surface of the femur is a ridge called the **linea aspersa,** to which muscles attach.

The femur is flexed and extended when one walks and climbs stairs. Adduction and abduction movements do not occur as often; however, the femur and thigh must be adducted when one rides a horse.

The **iliopsoas** (Figure 15-16) flexes the femur or pulls it toward the abdomen. It is composed of fibers from the iliacus and psoas major muscles, which insert on the lesser trochanter. The **gluteus maximus** (Figure 15-17) is the antagonist of the iliopsoas; therefore, it extends the femur. Extension of the femur involves moving it downward, backward, and upward. The gluteus maximus is the heaviest muscle in the body and forms the bulk of the buttocks. This muscle often is used as the site for injections of large quantities of medication. The size of the muscle is appropriate to receive large injections. Abduction of the femur is brought about by the other two gluteal muscles, **gluteus medius** and **gluteus minimus.** The antagonists of the gluteal muscles are the members of the adductor group (brevis,

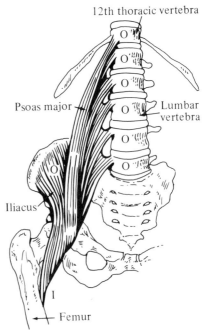

Figure 15-16.    The iliacus and psoas major muscles combine to form the iliopsoas muscle.

### TABLE 15-5.  Muscles That Move the Femur*

| Bone (Lever) | Muscle | Origin | Insertion | Action |
|---|---|---|---|---|
| Femur | Iliopsoas | Ilium and vertebrae (T-12 to L-5) | Small trochanter | Flexion |
| | Gluteus maximus | Ilium and sacrum | Femur, gluteal tuberosity | Extension |
| | Gluteus medius and minimus | Ilium | Great trochanter of femur | Abduction |
| | Adductor muscles | | | |
| | Brevis | Pubic bone | Linea aspersa of femur | Adduction |
| | Longus | Pubic bone | Linea aspersa of femur | Adduction |
| | Magnus | Pubic bone | Linea aspersa of femur | Adduction |

*See Figs. 15-16, 15-17, 15-18.

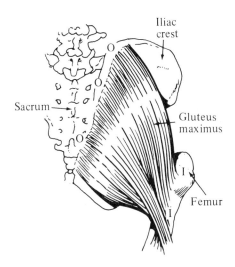

**Figure 15-17.** The origin and insertion of the gluteus maximus muscle.

longus, and magnus) (Figure 15-18). Table 15-5 gives details concerning the origin, insertion, and action of these muscles. The movements of the femur are examples of a third-class lever (power is between the resistance and the fulcrum).

## TIBIA AND FIBULA

The lower leg is composed of two bones, **tibia** and **fibula** (Figure 15-19). The tibia, or shinbone, is the largest of the two and is located more medially. The proximal epiphysis of the tibia is characterized by **medial** and **lateral condyles.** The condyles of the tibia are concave and articulate with the convex lateral and medial condyles of the femur. Inferior to the condyles is the large **tibial tuberosity.** The anterior surface of the shaft is a sharp ridge. The distal epiphysis is characterized by the **medial malleolus.** Distally, the tibia articulates with the talus ankle bone. The tibia is a weight-bearing bone and transfers body weight from the femur to the foot.

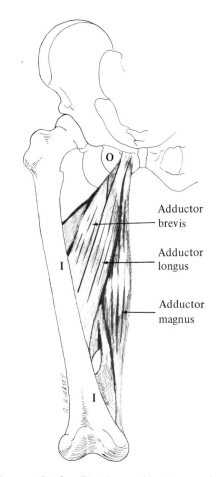

**Figure 15-18.** The three adductor muscles.

The **fibula** (Figure 15-19) is located lateral to the tibia and deeper within the tissues. The proximal end of the fibula is characterized by a head that articulates with the lateral condyle of the femur, but it does not help form the knee joint. The distal end of the fibula, **lateral malleolus,** is enlarged slightly. This enlargement forms the obvious lateral projection superior to the ankle. Slightly superior to the lateral malleolus, the

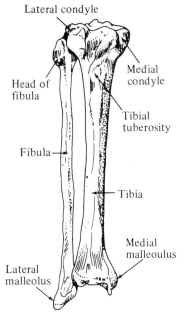

**Figure 15-19.** Tibia and fibula (anterior view).

fibula articulates with the tibia. The fibula is not a weight-bearing bone.

The patella or knee cap is a **sesamoid bone** (bones found in capsules of joints and tendons). It is a triangle-shaped bone that lies anterior to the knee joint (Figure 15–20). The patella is inserted into the tendon of the quadriceps femoris muscle, which extends from the thigh across the knee joint and inserts on the tibia. The patella floats or moves as the insertion tendon

moves, and it protects the tendons where it passes across the knee joint. The patella protects the tendon of the quadriceps femoris muscle and the anterior surface of the knee joint.

Only flexion and extension movements of the lower leg are possible between the femur and tibia. Flexion of the tibia and fibula is the movement of the lower leg posteriorly toward the buttocks. Extension is straightening the lower leg or returning it to its normal position. The muscles that move the lower leg are located superior to it and lie over the femur. The "hamstring" muscles primarily are responsible for flexing the lower leg. The hamstring group includes **biceps femoris, semitendinosus,** and **semimembranosus.** The **quadriceps femoris** muscle extends the lower leg and is the antagonist to the hamstring group.

The "hamstring" muscles are so named because of stringlike tendons that insert on the tibia and fibula. Each muscle name reflects its anatomy and location.

The **biceps femoris** (Figure 15–21A) is located on the posterior, lateral surface of the thigh (near the femoral artery and vein). It is composed of a short and long head. The **semitendinosus** (half-tendon) muscle is medial to the biceps femoris. It has a belly that extends distally about halfway down the thigh and then forms a tendon that continues to the tibia. The **semimembranosus** (half-membrane) is located deeper than the other two. As the name indicates, the semimembranosus extends about halfway as a membranous band (Figure 15–21B) before muscle fibers are evident. Table 15–6 gives details on the origin and insertion of these muscles.

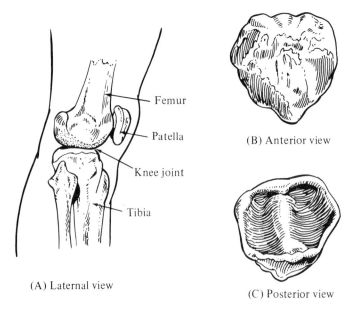

**Figure 15-20.** The patella is shown from a lateral view anterior to the knee joint. Individual, anterior, and posterior views of the patella are also shown.

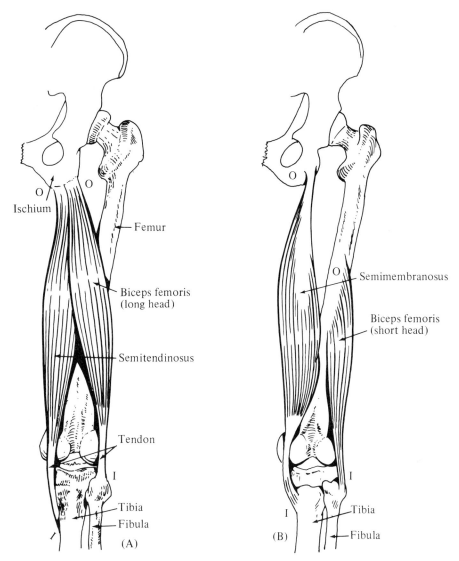

**Figure 15-21.** (A) The origin and insertion of the biceps femoris (long head) and semitendinosus muscles. (B) The origin and insertion of the semimembranosus and biceps femoris (short head) muscles.

## TABLE 15-6. *Muscles That Move Lower Leg (Tibia and Fibula)**

| Bone (Lever) | Muscle | Origin | Insertion | Action |
|---|---|---|---|---|
| Tibia and fibula | Biceps femoris | Ischial tuberosity | Fibula | Flexion |
| | | Linea aspersa of femur | Tibia | |
| | Semitendinosus | Ischial tuberosity | Tibia | Flexion |
| | Semimembranosus | Ischial tuberosity | Tibia | Flexion |
| | Rectus femoris | Ilium (inferior iliac spine) | Tibia | Extension |
| | Vastus lateralis | Femur (linea aspersa) | Tibia | Extension |
| | Vastus medialis | Femur | Tibia | Extension |
| | Vastus intermedius | Femur | Tibia | Extension |
| | Sartorius | Anterior superior iliac spine | Tibia | Crossing of legs |

*See Figs. 15-21 and 15-22.

The **quadriceps femoris** muscle forms the mass of the anterior and lateral surfaces of the thigh. Actually, it is four muscles: **rectus femoris, vastus lateralis, vastus medialis,** and **vastus intermedius.** The four names actually are the four heads of origin, and they all insert by a common tendon (quadriceps femoris tendon) on the tibial tuberosity of the tibia. The rectus femoris (Figure 15–22A) is anterior to the other three. The vastus lateralis is lateral and posterior to the rectus femoris. The **vastus medialis** is medial and posterior to the rectus femoris (Figure 15–22B). The **vastus intermedius** (Figure 15–22C) is deep and between the rectus femoris and vastus medialis. The contraction of these four parts of the quadriceps femoris extends the tibia and fibula. Table 15–6 gives details of their origin and insertion.

The **sartorius** (Figure 15–22C) muscle is long, nar-row, and extends across the thigh. It extends from the anterior superior iliac spine medially across the thigh and inserts on the tibia. The contractions of the sarto-rius muscles allow the legs to be crossed, much like tail-ors used to when they sat on the floor. The flexion and extension of the tibia and fibula are examples of third–class levers (power is between the resistance and the ful-crum).

## BONES OF THE ANKLE AND FOOT

The bony structure of the foot is similar to the hand; however, the structure of the foot is designed to sup-port the weight of the body and help one to walk and jump effectively.

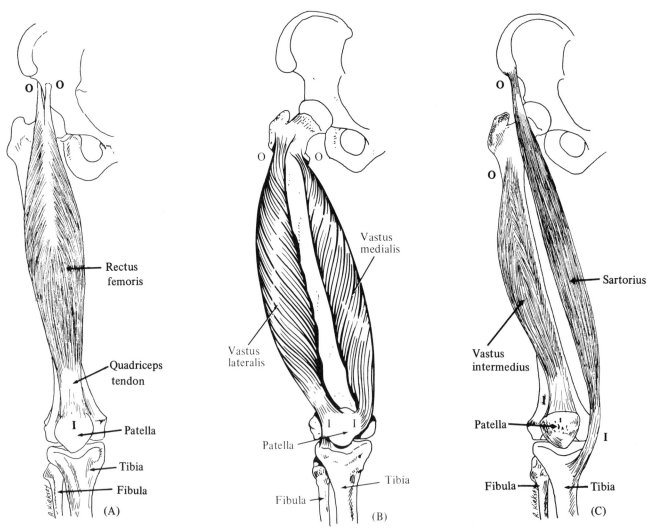

**Figure 15–22.** (A) The origin and insertion of the rectus femoris muscle. (B) The origin and insertion of the vastus lateralis and vastus medialis muscles. (C) The origin and insertion of the sartorius and vastus intermedius muscles.

The seven bones of the ankle are called tarsals: **calcaneus, talus , navicular, cuboid,** and **cuneiforms** (lateral, medial, and intermediate) (Figure 15-23). The calcaneus and talus support the weight of the body, which is transferred to them from the tibia. The talus articulates with the tibia. The calcaneus (heel bone) lies inferior to the talus and has a posterior projection that forms the heel.

The foot is composed of five **metatarsals,** which are numbered from medial to lateral (Figure 15-23). The distal end of each metatarsal is enlarged to form a head, and the heads as a group form the ball of the foot.

The bones of the toes are called **phalanges,** and each toe has three, except the large toe, which has only two phalanges (Figure 15-23). Like the phalanges of the fingers, these are referred to as proximal, middle, and distal phalanges; the large toe has only two phalanges, a proximal and a distal.

The foot supports the weight of the body and helps one to walk and jump. These functions are possible because of two springy arches, longitudinal and transverse. The longitudinal arch (Figure 15-24) extends from the calcaneus to the metatarsals. The transverse arch extends across the foot, at the point of the distal row of tarsals and the five metatarsals. Tendons and ligaments maintain both arches in such a way that each

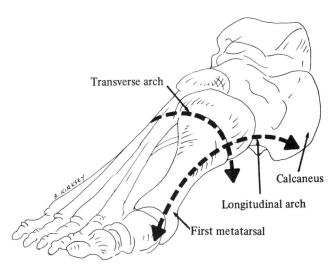

**Figure 15-24.** The position of the longitudinal and transverse arches of the foot.

arch has a certain degree of spring. When the tendons and ligaments weaken, fallen arches or flat feet result.

Like the knee joint, only flexion and extension movements are possible at the ankle joint; however, different terms are used to describe these movements. Flexion of the foot (upward movement) is called **dorsiflexion,** and extension of the foot (downward movement) is called **plantar flexion.** Inversion and eversion movements can be carried out by the foot; however, they actually result from movement of the tarsal bones.

The muscle primarily responsible for flexion (dorsiflexion) of the foot is the **tibialis anterior.** This muscle originates on the lateral condyle of the tibia and inserts on the first metatarsal and cuneiform bones. The tibialis anterior also inverts the foot.

The muscles primarily responsible for extension (plantar flexion) of the foot are the **gastrocnemius** (Figure 15-25A) (calf muscle) and soleus (Figure 15-25B). Both of these are on the posterior surface of the lower leg. The origins of the gastrocnemius are the medial and lateral condyles of the femur. It inserts by means of the **tendon of Achilles** on the calcaneus. The soleus originates at the upper ends of the tibia and fibula and also inserts on the calcaneus by the tendon of Achilles (Table 15-7). These two muscles are vital to walking, standing and jumping. The contraction of the gastrocnemius and soleus muscle enables a person to stand on his tiptoes. This movement at the joint of the talus and tibia is the controversial example of a second-degree lever (resistance is between power and fulcrum). The power is the soleus and gastrocnemius muscles; the resistance is the weight of the body; the fulcrum is the ball of the foot.

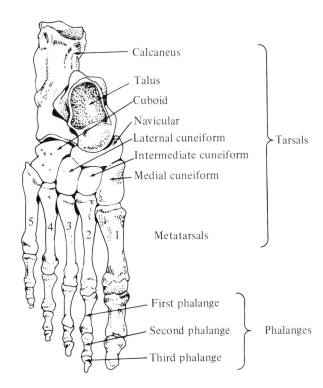

**Figure 15-23.** Bones of the ankle and the foot, showing the tarsals, metatarsals, and phalanges.

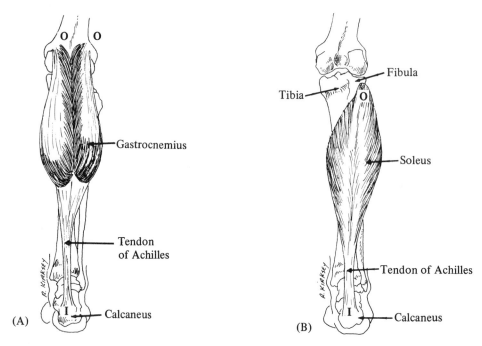

**Figure 15-25.**    (A) The origin and insertion of the gastrocnemius muscle. (B) The origin and insertion of the soleus muscle.

### TABLE 15-7.    *Muscles That Move Ankle and Foot\**

| Bone (Lever) | Muscle | Origin | Insertion | Action |
|---|---|---|---|---|
| Tarsals, metartarsals, phalanges | Tibialis anterior | Tibia | First tarsal and metarsal | Flexion = dorsiflexion |
| | Gastrocnemius | Medial and lateral condyles of femur | Calcaneus (by tendon of Achilles) | Extension = plantar flexion |
| | Soleus | Tibia, fibula | Calcaneus (by tendon of Achilles) | Extension = plantar flexion |

*See Fig. 15-25.

## 3 MUSCLES OF THE ABDOMEN

The muscles of the abdomen are important in forced breathing, and compressing internal organs. They also aid the processes of defecation, urination, childbirth, and movement of the vertebral column.

Four flat sheetlike muscles are located on each side of the midline. The **external** and **internal oblique, transverse abdominis,** and **rectus abdominis** muscles (Figure 15–26) join each other at midline by means of flat, broad, sheetlike tendons called **aponeuroses.** The aponeuroses join each other at midline from sternum to pubis to form a white seam, called the **linea alba.**

The muscles composing the lateral sides of the abdomen are arranged in three layers: **internal** and **external oblique** and **transverse abdominis.** The external oblique is the most superficial of the three. It arises from the lower eight ribs, and the fibers course downward and forward where they insert on the iliac crest by means of an inguinal ligament. The external oblique functions to compress the abdomen (aiding inspiration), draw the pelvis upward, and flex the vertebral column. The internal oblique (Figure 15–26) is below the external oblique and its fibers extend upward and forward. It originates on the iliac crest and inserts on the lower three ribs, pubic bone, and linea alba (Table 15–8). The internal oblique functions in the same way as the external oblique. The transverse abdominis muscle fibers extend transversely or around the body. It originates on the crest of the ilium and the lower six ribs. It extends forward around the body and inserts on the pubic bone,

# 4  HERNIA SITES IN THE ABDOMINAL WALL

The abdominal wall has several weak places that can rupture and give rise to a hernia. A **hernia** is defined as a protrusion or projection of an organ or a part of an organ through the wall of the cavity that normally contains it. A hernia can occur in many different places of the body; the most common type is a protrusion of an abdominal organ through a weak area of the abdominal wall. The weak places in the abdominal wall include openings that are not completely closed and spaces in which the wall is closed but is not reinforced. Undue pressure and lifting can tear and enlarge these points, resulting in protrusion of abdominal organs. These weak sites are inguinal canals, femoral rings, and umbilicus.

**Inguinal canals** are openings that lie above the inguinal ligaments (formed by external oblique in groove between abdomen and thigh). The inguinal canals connect the external inguinal ring (Figure 15–27) to the internal inguinal ring (opening). In the male the spermatic cord passes upward on each side, from the testicle, through the rings and canal to the urinary bladder. In the female the round ligaments, which help support the uterus, pass through these structures. Inguinal hernias are the most common site of hernias in males and laymen often refer to them simply as "hernias."

**Femoral rings** (Figure 15–27) are openings in the groin slightly lateral to the external inguinal ring, one on each side. These openings are about a half inch in size and slightly larger in females than in males. They serve as the passageway for the femoral artery and vein. A femoral hernia protrudes from the femoral ring and is seen on the inside of the thigh. Women tend to have more femoral hernias than men.

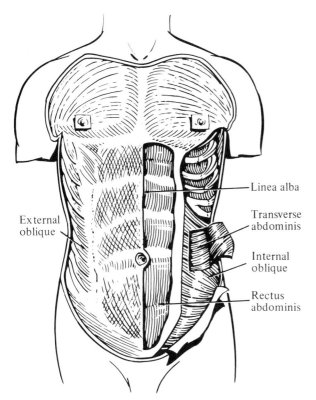

**Figure 15–26.**  The four layers of muscles located in the abdomen.

linea alba, and xiphoid process. The transverse abdominis has the same functions as the external and internal oblique. The anterior surface of the abdominal wall is composed of the **rectus abdominis** muscle. This muscle is similar to a long thin strap. It originates on the pubic bone and extends upward where it broadens before inserting on the costal cartilages of the fifth, sixth, and seventh ribs plus the xiphoid process of the sternum. The rectus abdominis functions to compress the abdomen and flex the vertebral column.

## TABLE 15–8.  Muscles of Abdominal Wall*

| Bone (Lever) | Muscle | Origin | Insertion | Action |
|---|---|---|---|---|
| Vertebral column and pelvis | External oblique | Lower eight ribs | Iliac crest and linea alba | Compress abdomen, flex vertebral column |
| | Internal oblique | Iliac crest | Lower three ribs, pubic bone | Compress abdomen, flex vertebral column |
| | Transverse abdominis | Iliac crest and lower six ribs | Pubic bone, linea alba | Compress abdomen, flex vertebral column |
| | Rectus abdominis | Pubic bone | Costal cartilages of fifth, sixth, and seventh ribs, xiphoid process | Compress abdomen, flex vertebral column |

*See Fig. 15–26.

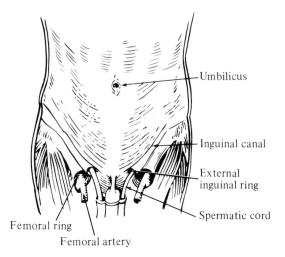

**Figure 15-27.** Hernia sites in the abdominal wall. The three weak spots in the abdominal wall—the umbilicus, inguinal rings, and femoral rings—are shown.

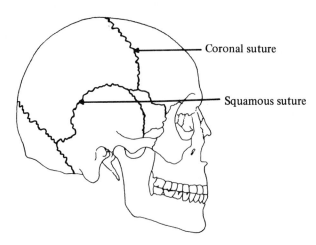

**Figure 15-28.** Lateral view of the synarthroses (immovable) joints.

The **umbilicus** (Figure 15–27) is the scar present in the umbilical region of the abdomen. The scar occurs when the umbilical cord finally is detached from a newborn child. This point is weak in a newborn child and an umbilical hernia can occur here.

# 5 CLASSES OF JOINTS (FULCRUMS)

A joint is the place at which bones articulate or the ends rub against each other. Where the bones function as levers, the joint also is a fulcrum. The amount and type of movements (angular, circumduction, rotation and special movements) that occur at each joint depend on the anatomy of the joint. Joints are classified, according to the amount of movement they allow, into three classes: **synarthroses** (immovable), **amphiarthroses** (slightly movable), and **diarthroses** (freely movable).

**Synarthroses** (immovable) joints do not allow movement because the ends of the bones are connected to each other by fibrous tissue, cartilage or bone tissue. For example, the bones of the skull (except mandible) are connected to each other by immovable joints (Figure 15–28) or sutures. The delicate brain tissue is protected effectively by suture joints between skull bones. If the skull bones moved freely, the size and shape of the skull would change constantly and brain tissue could be damaged easily.

**Amphiarthroses** (slightly movable) joints move

slightly since either fibrocartilaginous disks or fibrous tissue connects the bones. For example, intervertebral disks are located between each vertebra (Figure 15–29A) of the vertebral column. They permit slight articulation between each vertebra. A fibrocartilaginous disk is located in the joint between the pubis bones (Fig-

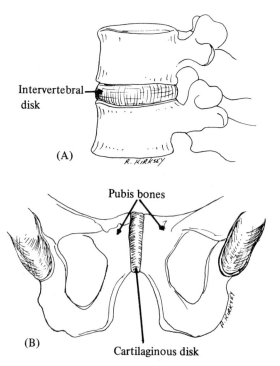

**Figure 15-29.** (A) An amphiarthrosis (slightly movable) joint between two vertebrae. (B) Amphiarthrosis joint. The symphis pubis joint is shown with the cartilaginous disk between pubis bones.

ure 15-29B) of the pelvic girdle and is called symphis pubis. The cartilaginous disk allows slight movement between the pubic bones and is especially important during childbirth. This action allows the pelvic bones to separate sightly; this separation slightly increases the size of the true pelvis and aids the passage of the child through the true pelvis.

**Diarthroses** (freely movable) joints permit a great amount of movement, due to the structure of each diarthrosis joint. A cavity is present between the ends of the bones that compose a diarthrosis joint, and a synovial membrane lines this joint cavity (Figure 15-30B). Synovial fluid is secreted by the membrane and acts to lubricate the articular surfaces of the bones. A sleevelike fibrous capsule surrounds the joint (Figure 15-30A), and connects the two bones together. The capsule helps to strengthen the joint; and ligaments, within some joints, give additional strength. The flexibility of the capsule and the shape of the articulating bone surfaces determine the amount of movement that can occur at a diarthrosis joint. Most of the joints in the body are in this class, and they are divided into subgroups:

1. **Ball and socket:** hip and shoulder joints are examples. This group permits all angular movements as well as rotation.
2. **Hinge joint:** the elbow, knee, and ankle are examples. Hinge joints permit movement only in one plane.
3. **Pivot joint:** the atlas vertebra rotating around the odontoid process of the axis is an example. Only rotation movement is possible at a pivot joint.
4. **Gliding joint:** the carpal and tarsal bones of the wrist and ankle, respectively, are examples. Gliding movement between bones occurs at this joint.
5. **Saddle joint:** the thumb joint is an example and many movements are possible at this joint.

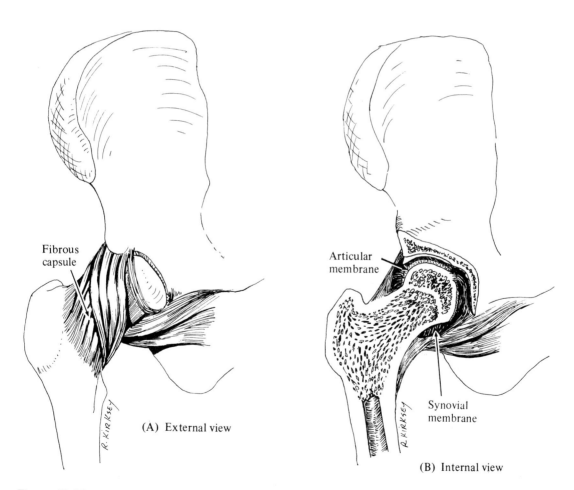

Figure 15-30. (A) The fibrous capsule of a diarthrosis joint. (B) The synovial membrane and articular membrane of a diarthrosis joint.

## 6  BURSAE

A **bursa** (singular) is a small synovial fluid sac. The outer wall of the bursa is composed of fibrous connective tissue and the inner wall is composed of loose areolar connective tissue. Bursae are lined with synovial fluid membranes, which secrete synovial fluid.

Bursae are found between structures that rub against each other. For example, the **prepatellar bursa** (Figure 15-31) is located between the skin and the patella or knee cap. The subdeltoid bursa is located between the deltoid muscle and the head of the humerus.

These sacs reduce the friction between two moving structures. Since they are slippery and contain fluid, they act as cushions to reduce friction that occurs between two moving parts. Large numbers of bursae are found around diarthrotic joints. The bursae enable the muscles and bones to work more smoothly and reduce friction, which otherwise could gradually remove layers of tissue.

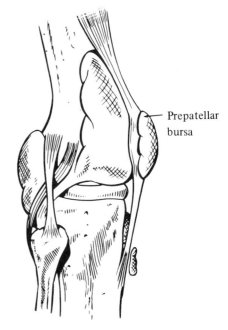

Prepatellar bursa

Figure 15-31.    Several bursae in the knee joint.

## SUMMARY

**Upper Extremities (64 bones) and Muscles That Move Them**

A. Shoulder girdle (pectoral girdle): composed of clavicle and scapula; muscles that move shoulder girdle:
1. Levator scapulae: elevates shoulder.
2. Pectoralis minor: lowers shoulder.
3. Trapezius: elevates and shrugs shoulders.
B. Arm (upper arm): composed of humerus; muscles that move arm:
1. Pectoralis major: adduction and flexion.
2. Latissimus dorsi: extension.
3. Deltoid: abduction.
C. Forearm or lower arm: composed of radius and ulna bones; muscles that move forearm:
1. Biceps brachii: flexion and supination.
2. Triceps brachii: extension.
D. Bones of wrist and hand: wrist is composed of eight carpal bones; hand is composed of five metacarpals; muscles that move wrist and hand:
1. Flexor carpi radialis: flexion.
2. Extensor carpi radialis: extension.

**Lower Extremities (62 bones) and Muscles That Move Them**

A. Pelvic girdle: composed of four bones: two hipbones, sacrum, and coccyx.
B. Femur: located in upper leg; longest and strongest bone in body; muscles that move femur:
1. Iliopsoas: flexion.
2. Gluteus maximus: extension.
3. Gluteus medius and minimus: abduction.
4. Adductor muscles: adduction.

C. Tibia and fibula: located in lower leg; muscles that move tibia and fibula:
    1. Biceps femoris: flexion.
    2. Semitendinosus: flexion.
    3. Semimembranosus: flexion.
    4. Quadriceps femoris: extension.
D. Bones of the ankle and foot: seven tarsal bones compose the ankle; the foot is composed of five metatarsals plus phalanges, which compose the toes; muscles that move ankle and foot:
    1. Tibialis anterior: flexion or dorsiflexion.
    2. Gastrocnemius: extension or plantar flexion.
    3. Soleus: extension or plantar flexion.

### Muscles of the Abdomen

Four muscles compose the abdominal wall: external oblique, internal oblique, transverse abdominis, and rectus abdominis.

### Hernia Sites in the Abdominal Wall

Three weak spots in the abdominal wall exist where a hernia (protrusion or projection of organs through wall of cavity) might occur: inguinal canals, femoral rings, and umbilicus.

### Classes of Joints (Fulcrums)

A bony joint is where bones rub against each other; three classes of joints:
A. Synarthroses (immovable): joints do not allow movement; *Ex.*—bones of skull.
B. Amphiarthroses (slightly movable): joints permit slight movement; *Ex.*—intervertebral disks.
C. Diarthroses (freely movable): joints permit a great amount of movement; joints lined with synovial fluid; subgroups:
    1. Ball and socket: hip and shoulder.
    2. Hinge: elbow and knee.
    3. Pivot: atlas and axis.
    4. Gliding: carpals and tarsals.
    5. Saddle: thumb joint.

### Bursae

A bursa is a small synovial fluid sac; located between structures that rub against each other; function, reduce friction between two moving structures.

## Levers (Bones), Muscles, and Movement
## of Appendicular Skeletal System

True (A) or false (B). Questions 1 to 6.

1.  The pectoral girdle is composed of the sternum and clavicle bones.

2.  The shoulder is elevated by the pectoralis minor muscles.

3.  The forearm is composed of radius and ulna bones and is flexed by the biceps brachii muscle.

4.  Wrist bones are called carpal bones and hand bones are called metacarpal bones.

5.  When one flexes the femur one utilizes the iliopsoas muscle.

6.  The extension of the femur involves the gluteus medius muscle.

7.  Which of the following are incorrectly paired in relation to movement of the lower leg?
    (a)  Biceps femoris—flexion
    (b)  Semitendinosus—flexion
    (c)  Semimembranosus—extension
    (d)  None of these

8.  The muscles of the abdomen include the:
    (a)  External and internal oblique
    (b)  Transverse abdominis and rectus abdominis
    (c)  None
    (d)  a and b

9.  Hernia sites in the abdominal wall include:
    (a)  Inguinal canals
    (b)  Umbilicus
    (c)  None of these
    (d)  All of these

# Chapter 16

# FLUIDS AND ELECTROLYTES

After reading and studying this chapter, a student should be able to:

1. State the two major types of body fluids, their location and percentage of body weight.
2. Describe blood hydrostatic pressure (BHP) and colloidal osmotic pressure (COP).
3. Give the basic BHP and COP values at arterial and venous ends of capillaries.
4. Describe whether fluids and materials move into or out of plasma compartment at arterial and venous ends of capillaries and which pressure is responsible for the movement.
5. Distinguish between hyperosmolar and hypoosmolar imbalances.
6. Distinguish between volume excess and deficit.
7. Discuss the role of the lymphatic system in fluid and electrolyte exchange.

*The internal environment of man is similar to the external environment that we live in. Two important components of the external environment are the air and water. The quality of these two components must be regulated if man is to function properly. Gases and fluids that circulate throughout the body are important components of man's internal environment.*

*The focal point of this unit will be to discuss how various organ systems integrate their functions to maintain and regulate man's internal environment. The organ systems that will be discussed are the cardiovascular, respiratory, and urinary. In addition, this unit will cover the types of body fluids and the processes involved in maintaining normal pH and electrolyte levels.*

# 1  FLUIDS OF THE BODY

All fluids in the human body are composed primarily of water. Water makes up approximately 65 to 75 percent of the total body weight and, depending on its location, is divided into extracellular and intracellular fluids.

## EXTRACELLULAR FLUIDS

Extracellular fluid (ECF) is found between or outside cells, in blood vessels and in tissue spaces (Figure 16–1). It is composed of water mixed with other compounds. Extracellular fluid is further divided into blood, interstitial fluid, and lymph. The extracellular fluid compartment and the percentage of total body weight is shown in Figure 16–1.

## INTRACELLULAR FLUID

Intracellular fluid (ICF) is a fluid found within cells (Figure 16–1). Intracellular fluid makes up 40 percent of the body weight and is found in the intracellular compartment. It is much the same from one cell to another, but the chemical composition of intracellular fluid differs considerably from extracellular fluid (Figure 16–2). Distribution of electrolytes in ICF and ECF fluids, Figure 16–2, shows some interesting things about the concentrations and distribution of electrolytes in ICF

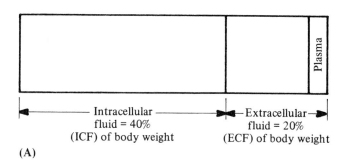

(A)

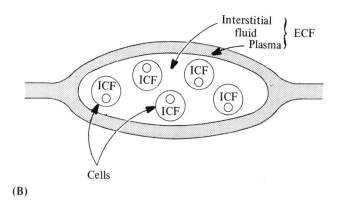

(B)

**Figure 16–1.** (A) The ICF and ECF compartments and the percentages of total body weight that water occupies in them. (B) Diagrammatic representation of the ICF and ECF compartments.

and ECF. In ECF the main cation is $Na^+$, generally about 140 mEq/l. As Figure 16–2 shows, the total cations in ECF are only 154 mEq/l; therefore, the concentration of $Na^+$ composes over 90 percent of the total cation concentration. The major anions are $Cl^-$, $HCO_3^-$

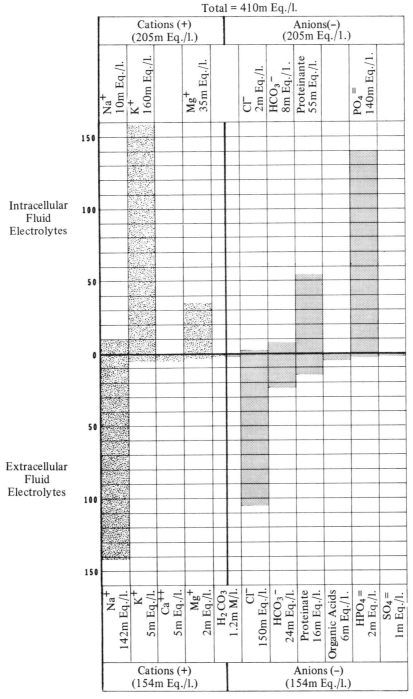

**Figure 16-2.** Distribution and concentrations of electrolytes in ECF and ICF.

(bicarbonate ions) and proteinate. Notice that the total cation concentration (154 mEq/l) equals the total anion concentration (154 mEq/l).

In ICF the major cations are K⁺ (potassium) and Mg⁺ (magnesium). The major anion is $PO_4^-$ (organic phosphate). Notice in Figure 16-2 that the total concentration of electrolytes in ICF is 410 mEq/l compared to 308 mEq/l in ECF.

## 2 MOVEMENT OF FLUIDS AND ELECTROLYTES BETWEEN COMPARTMENTS

Previously we discussed the fact that body fluids circulate in fluid compartments. One should not think that each fluid circulates only in a certain compartment. In reality, they continually move back and forth from one compartment to another (Figure 16–3). One of the most troublesome problems in working with seriously ill patients is the maintenance of both normal body fluid volumes and proper balance between extracellular and intracellular fluid volumes.

Before discussing the factors and mechanisms involved in regulating the levels of fluids, some terms and definitions must be presented.

### BLOOD HYDROSTATIC PRESSURE

**Blood hydrostatic pressure (BHP)** is pressure that results from a fluid being forced against a membrane or wall. Blood hydrostatic pressure results from the heart continually pumping blood through blood vessels and forcing the blood against blood vessel walls. This pressure will vary depending on how hard the heart is pumping and on the size of the vessels. The direction of hydrostatic or blood pressure is always out of blood vessels;

therefore, it is a **"pushing pressure."** It is always trying to push fluids out of the blood vessels. Fluids are exchanged from the plasma compartment through blood capillaries. The hydrostatic pressure varies throughout the length of a capillary.

### COLLOIDAL OSMOTIC PRESSURE

**Colloidal osmotic pressure (COP)** is pressure created by solutes not diffusing through a selectively permeable membrane. Normal living cell membranes are "selectively permeable" (semipermeable); that is, they allow water to freely move through the membrane, but prevent certain compounds (solutes) from passing through. The solutes that are prevented from moving through create a pressure on cell membranes. The pressure is determined by the concentration of solutes in a fluid.

Osmotic pressure tends to "attract" or "draw" water through a membrane; osmotic pressure also is important in movement of materials into and out of capillaries. Blood contains a greater concentration of solutes (especially proteins) than does interstitial fluid; therefore, the osmotic pressure in blood is higher than that of interstitial fluid. Normally, very few proteins leave the blood. This enables blood to maintain a high **"pulling pressure"** or osmotic pressure. Proteins are colloids (solute particles whose diameters range from about 1 to 100 millimicrons), and they primarily determine osmotic pressure; therefore, the name colloidal osmotic pressure is commonly used.

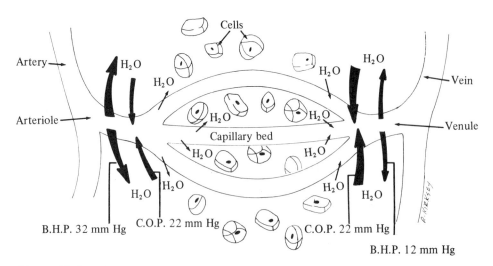

**Figure 16–3.** The relationship between hydrostatic and osmotic pressures is shown (by means of width and length of arrows) at the arteriole and venule ends of a capillary bed.

## Hydrostatic and Colloidal Osmotic Pressure Values in Capillaries

Blood hydrostatic pressure (BHP) is different at the arteriole end of a capillary vessel from what it is at the venule end (Figure 16-3). The BHP normally is about 32 mm Hg at the arterial end, whereas colloidal osmotic pressure (COP) normally is about 22 mm Hg. At the venous end, the BHP is about 12 mm Hg, and COP is about 22 mm Hg. BHP values are assigned a positive sign (+), whereas COP values are assigned a negative sign (−). The interaction of the BHP and COP pressures determines the **net effective pressure**. This is summarized below.

> Arterial end of capillary vessel
> + 32 mm Hg BHP
> − 22 mm Hg COP
> + 10 mm Hg Net effective pressure
> (BHP)
> Venous end of capillary vessel
> − 22 mm Hg COP
> + 12 mm Hg BHP
> − 10 mm Hg Net effective pressure
> (COP)

## MOVEMENT OF FLUIDS AND ELECTROLYTES BETWEEN PLASMA AND INTERSTITIAL FLUID COMPARTMENTS

At the arteriole end of the capillary vessel, the hydrostatic pressure (+ 32 mm Hg) is greater than colloidal osmotic pressure (− 22 mm Hg); therefore, the **net effective pressure** is + 10 mm Hg. Since the "pushing pressure" is the greatest at the arterial end of a capillary, fluids and materials are pushed out of capillaries (plasma compartment) by filtration into the interstitial compartment (Figure 16-3). At the venule end of a capillary vessel the colloidal osmotic pressure (− 22 mm Hg) is greater than the blood hydrostatic pressure (+ 12 mm Hg); therefore the net effective pressure is − 10 mm Hg. As a result of COP being higher and the negative (−) net effective pressure, fluids and materials are pulled from the interstitial compartment into the capillary bed (plasma compartment) at the venule end.

### Summary

The hydrostatic "pushing pressure" is the greatest pressure at the arteriole end of a capillary vessel; therefore, fluids and materials are pushed from the plasma into the interstitial compartment. The colloidal osmotic "pulling pressure" is the greatest pressure at the venule end of a capillary vessel; therefore, fluids and materials are pulled into capillaries at the venule end. Normally the amount of fluids and materials pushed out at the arterial end of a capillary vessel are approximately equal to the amount pulled in at the venous end. This means that normally there is no appreciable loss or gain of fluids and materials between the plasma and interstitial fluid compartments.

## PURPOSE OF FLUIDS AND MATERIALS BEING EXCHANGED BETWEEN PLASMA AND INTERSTITIAL COMPARTMENTS

The primary fluids and materials that move out of capillary vessels by filtration are nutrients ($O_2$, glucose, $H_2O$, $Na^+$, and $K^+$). These nutrients are pushed out of the capillaries, through the interstitial compartment and into the cells. Without these nutrients a cell cannot carry out its normal physiologic functions. Under normal physiologic conditions, cells produce waste products, $CO_2$, and ammonia, which must be removed from cells for them to function properly. Waste materials dissolved in water are the major substances that are pulled into the venous end of a capillary vessel. The blood carries these wastes to the proper organs where they are removed from the body.

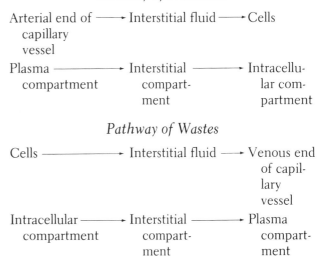

*Pathway of Nutrients*

Arterial end of ⟶ Interstitial fluid ⟶ Cells
capillary
vessel

Plasma ⟶ Interstitial ⟶ Intracellular
compartment compart- lar com-
ment partment

*Pathway of Wastes*

Cells ⟶ Interstitial fluid ⟶ Venous end
of capillary
lary
vessel

Intracellular ⟶ Interstitial ⟶ Plasma
compartment compart- compartment ment

There is a constant exchange of fluids and materials between the plasma and interstitial compartment. If the fluid level in one of the compartments drops below normal, fluids move into it from one of the other compartments to bring the level back to normal. Since the interstitial fluid volume is about three times greater than the plasma compartment, it acts as a reservoir to furnish fluids to the plasma and intracellular compartments.

## FLUID AND ELECTROLYTE EXCHANGE BETWEEN EXTRACELLULAR AND INTRACELLULAR COMPARTMENTS

Just as fluids constantly are exchanged between blood vessels and interstitial fluid, fluids also are exchanged between interstitial fluid and cells. The mechanisms that move water through cell membranes are similar to those that regulate water movement through capillary membranes. The concentrations of certain electrolytes and their transport across cell membranes are important in the exchange between extracellular and intracellular fluids. For example, the concentration of sodium ions ($Na^+$) in interstitial fluid and potassium ions ($K^+$) in intracellular fluid helps to regulate the exchange of fluids between the interstitial and intracellular fluid compartments. Sodium ions ($Na^+$) readily can diffuse across a cell membrane, but are actively transported (pumped) out of a cell as fast as they diffuse into it. Potassium ions are actively transported (pumped back) into a cell as fast as they diffuse out of it. This is the phenomenon of the **$Na^+$ and $K^+$ pump.** Osmotic pressure inside and outside a cell results greatly from potassium and sodium, respectively. A decrease or increase of sodium or potassium concentration will upset the osmotic pressure equilibrium between intracellular and extracellular fluids. The result will be a shifting of fluids into the compartment that has the highest concentration of electrolytes; this process is called **osmosis.** For example, if the concentration of sodium decreases in interstitial fluid, then the intracellular osmotic pressure temporarily is greater. This higher osmotic pressure pulls interstitial fluid into the cell. Likewise, fluid can be shifted out of a cell when the osmotic pressure outside is greater. If excessive amounts of fluids are shifted out of or into compartments a water–sodium imbalance results. The types of water–sodium imbalances are discussed next.

## TYPES OF WATER–SODIUM IMBALANCES

Water–sodium imbalances can be divided into the following subgroups:

1. Osmolar imbalances
   A. Hyperosmolar
   B. Hypoosmolar
2. Volume imbalances
   A. Volume excess
   B. Volume deficit

### Osmolar Imbalance

This imbalance involves disturbances in **osmolarity,** which results in disturbances in water distribution throughout the body's fluid compartments. Disturbances in osmolarity affect water distribution due to differences in osmotic pressures. This can be understood better as we discuss hyperosmolar and hypoosmolar imbalances.

**HYPEROSMOLAR IMBALANCE.** Notice in Figure 16–4A that this problem exists when the ECF osmotic pressure (OP) is greater than the ICF OP, since water is pulled from a lower OP to a higher OP. Then water is pulled out of cells. The ultimate result is that cells will shrink and therefore will be destroyed if the condition is not rapidly corrected. Also notice in Figure 16–4A that this problem can result either from (1) $H_2O$ decreasing [↓] in relation to $Na^+$ or (2) $Na^+$ increasing [↑] in relation to $H_2O$. In (1) the $Na^+$ level is within the normal range (133 to 146 mEq/l), but the $Na^+$ is dissolved in too little water; therefore, the osmotic pressure is increased. In (2) the normal range of $Na^+$ is exceeded and the amount of water stays the same. This also will result in increased osmotic pressure.

**HYPOOSMOLAR IMBALANCE.** Notice in Figure 16–4B that this problem occurs when the ICF OP is higher than the ECF OP. As a result more $H_2O$ is pulled into body cells than is pulled out. The ultimate result is that cells will swell and finally rupture if the condition is not rapidly corrected. Also notice in Figure 16–4B that this condition can result either from (1) $Na^+$ [↓] in relation to $H_2O$ or (2) $H_2O$ [↑] in relation to $Na^+$. In either case, the ultimate result is that ECF OP ↓ in relation to ICF OP.

The outstanding symptoms in osmolar imbalances are the results of **cerebral dysfunctions.** Examples are confusion, agitation, depression, and coma. These symptoms result from the shrinking of neurons and nerve tissue during hyperosmolar imbalances, also the swelling of neurons and nerve tissue during hypoosmolar imbalances. Table 16–1 gives some of the causative factors for hyperosmolar and hypoosmolar conditions.

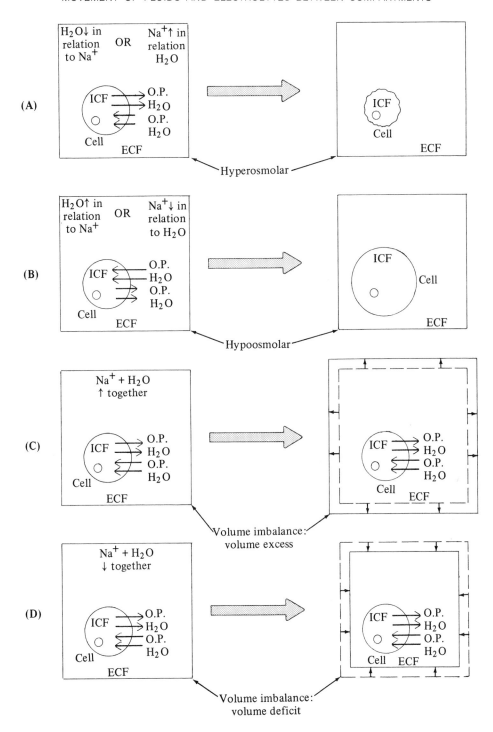

**Figure 16-4.** Diagrammatic representation of the types of water–sodium imbalances: (A) hyperosmolar; (B) hypoosmolar; (C) ECF volume excess; (D) ECF volume deficit. See text for description and discussion of these types.

## Volume Imbalances (Isotonic Imbalances)

This imbalance is characterized by Na⁺ and H₂O increasing or decreasing together in roughly the same proportions as found in ECF, rather than disproportionately as in osmolar imbalances.

Volume (isotonic) imbalances result in fluctuations in ECF volume. When ECF volume increases, circula-

**TABLE 16–1.** *Causative Factors for Hyperosmolar and Hypoosmolar Conditions*

| | $H_2O$ [↓] ɪɴ ʀᴇʟᴀᴛɪᴏɴ ᴛᴏ $Na^+$ | $Na^+$ [↑] ɪɴ ʀᴇʟᴀᴛɪᴏɴ ᴛᴏ $H_2O$ |
|---|---|---|
| **Hypoosmolar** | 1. Difficulty in swallowing<br>2. Impaired thirst (cerebral injury)<br>3. Coma<br>4. Watery diarrhea<br>5. Diabetes insipidus<br>6. Diabetic acidosis | 1. Excessive infusions of hypertonic solutions<br>2. Excessive intravenous feedings of glucose with $Na^+$ salts<br>3. Excessive tube feeding of protein |
| | $H_2O$ [↑] ɪɴ ʀᴇʟᴀᴛɪᴏɴ ᴛᴏ $Na^+$ | $Na^+$ [↓] ɪɴ ʀᴇʟᴀᴛɪᴏɴ ᴛᴏ $H_2O$ |
| **Hyperosmolar** | 1. Excessive fluid intake<br>2. Kidney disease and inability to excrete $H_2O$ excesses<br>3. Forcing fluids (IV or oral) on patients with increased ADH secretion<br>4. Excessive infusions of 5% dextrose in water | 1. Poor NaCl intake<br>2. Diuretics<br><br>3. Replacement of $H_2O$ and $Na^+$ losses with water only |

tory overload and edema result. When ECF volume decreases, dehydration and circulatory collapse result. These changes do not result in changes in osmolarity in the body fluids; therefore, cells neither swell nor shrink. Since the cells are not affected, there are no cerebral symptoms in volume imbalances as there are in osmolar imbalances.

**VOLUME EXCESS.** Figure 16–4C shows that this problem is characterized by $Na^+$ and $H_2O$ increasing together. Notice in the figure that the ECF and ICF osmotic pressures are equal and, therefore, the cell doesn't shrink or swell; however, notice that the ECF compartment does increase or **edema** occurs.

This condition is oftentimes referred to as a circulatory overload. Situations that can cause volume excess or edema are:

1. Patients who have received intravenous (IV) saline in excessive amounts
2. Patients with cardiac failure, chronic kidney failure, liver disease, or cerebral damage
3. Patients who receive cortisone injections often suffer from sodium and water retention

Even though the body cells are not affected by this condition some other problems associated with it are:

weight gain, edema, pulmonary edema, puffy eyelids, and **ascites** (an accumulation of fluid in the abdomen).

### Volume Deficit

Figure 16–4D shows that this problem is characterized by $Na^+$ and $H_2O$ decreasing together. Notice in the figure that these changes do not result in alterations of the ECF and ICF osmotic pressures; therefore, the cell doesn't shrink or swell. However, the ECF compartment does shrink or dehydration results. Situations that can cause a person to lose large amounts of $Na^+$ and $H_2O$ are hemorrhage, diarrhea, vomiting, kidney disease, excessive sweating, burns, fever, and decreased production of aldosterone.

The above situations can cause the following problems in a person's body: shock as a result of circulatory collapse, **oliguria** (decrease in urine elimination), and **anuria** (no urine formation) as a result of decreased blood flow to the kidneys.

### Summary of Water–Sodium Imbalances

As a result of osmolar and volume imbalances two major tissue conditions can result: **edema** and **dehydration** of tissues. Figure 16–5 shows some interrelated steps that can result in edema and Figure 16–6 shows some interrelated steps that can result in dehydration of tissues.

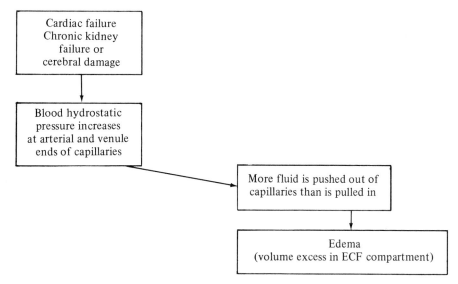

**Figure 16-5.** Interrelated steps that can result in edema (volume excess in ECF compartment).

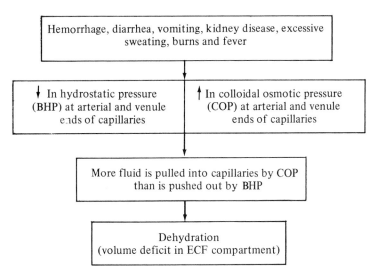

**Figure 16-6.** Interrelated steps that can result in dehydration (volume deficit in ECF compartment).

# 3 ROLE OF LYMPHATIC SYSTEM IN FLUID AND ELECTROLYTE EXCHANGE

If large quantities of fluids and materials move from the blood into tissue spaces (interstitial compartment), the lymphatic system absorbs the excess fluids and materials. A small amount of proteins constantly leaks from the blood into the interstitial fluid. Lymphatic vessels ultimately transport the fluids and proteins back to the blood and also pick up bacteria and other foreign material.

Lymphatic capillaries arise as open-ended vessels near blood capillaries and course through tissues to form larger vessels. Fluid, once absorbed by lymph vessels, is called **lymph.** Lymph vessels drain lymph through

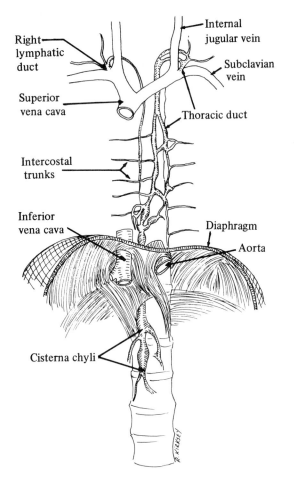

**Figure 16-7.** Origin and pathways of lymphatic vessels. Lymphatic ducts opening into subclavian veins also are shown.

the body into several collecting trunks. The collecting trunks ultimately drain lymph into two terminal vessels, the **thoracic duct** and **right lymphatic duct.** The right lymphatic duct (Figure 16–7) is formed by a combination of collecting ducts from the right side of the head, shoulder, and thoracic regions. The duct empties into the right subclavian vein where it joins with the right internal jugular vein.

The thoracic duct empties lymph into venous blood where the **left subclavian** and **left internal jugular** vein join. The thoracic duct originates as a dilated saclike region called cisterna chyli (Figure 16–7) at the level of the second lumbar vertebra. Lymph vessels draining lymph from the lower extremities, abdominal region, and pelvic region empty into the cisterna chyli. As the thoracic duct moves upward through the diaphragm, it receives lymph from intercostal lymph vessels. Just prior to joining the **left internal jugular** and **subclavian veins,** the thoracic duct combines with lymph vessels from the head, neck, and shoulder regions. Two valves at the entrance of the thoracic duct into the left subclavian vein prevent venous blood from entering the thoracic duct.

## FLOW OF LYMPH

The lymphatic system does not have a pump to move the lymph, like the heart in the cardiovascular system. There are three methods by which lymph is moved:

1. *Continuous inflow of new lymph:* as new lymph fluid is absorbed, it pushes the old lymph through the lymph vessels.
2. *Muscle contractions:* lymph vessels come in close contact with arteries and muscles, and as they contract, they tend to push on the lymph vessels. This force causes the lymph to move through the lymph vessels.
3. *Pressure changes in the thorax:* as a person inhales, a negative pressure (any pressure below atmospheric pressure, 760 mm Hg) is created in the thoracic cavity. This negative pressure acts on the thoracic and right lymphatic ducts to pull lymph from the lower parts of the body that have a positive pressure. In other words, the lymph moves upward from high–pressure regions to the negative-pressure areas in the lymphatic ducts.

---

# SUMMARY

---

**Fluids of the Body**
A. Extracellular fluids (ECF): fluid found between or outside cells; composed of water mixed with other compounds; divided into blood, interstitial fluid, and lymph; ECF fluid composes 20% of body weight; major cation is $Na^+$ (sodium), major anions are $Cl^-$ and $HCO_3^-$ (bicarbonate ions).

B. Intracellular fluid (ICF): fluid found within cells; composes 40% of body weight; major cations are $K^+$ (potassium) and $Mg^+$ (magnesium); major anions are organic phosphate.

## Movement of Fluids and Electrolytes between Compartments

Movement of fluids between compartments results from the interaction of two pressures: (1) blood hydrostatic pressure (BHP), pressure of blood; "pushing pressure" or pushes blood out of capillaries, (2) colloidal osmotic pressure (COP), pressure from solutes not diffusing through a membrane; "pulling pressure" or pulls fluids through membranes.

A. Hydrostatic and colloidal osmotic pressure values in capillaries:

| Arterial end of capillary | Venous end of capillary |
|---|---|
| + 32 mm Hg BHP | − 22 mm Hg COP |
| − 22 mm Hg COP | + 12 mm Hg BHP |
| + 10 mm Hg Net effective pressure (BHP) | − 10 mm Hg Net effective pressure (COP) |

B. Movement of fluids and electrolytes between plasma and interstitial fluid compartment.
   1. Fluids and materials pushed out of blood vessels into tissue spaces at arterial end of capillaries; results from BHP being greater than COP.
   2. Fluids and materials pulled into capillaries at venule end of capillaries; results from COP being greater than BHP.
C. Purpose of fluids and materials being exchanged between plasma and interstitial compartments
   1. Fluids containing nutrients are pushed out of blood into cells so that they can carry on normal functions.
   2. Fluids containing wastes are pulled into blood.
D. Fluid and electrolyte exchange between extracellular and intracellular compartments: osmosis interacts with $Na^+$–$K^+$ pump to move fluids into and out of cells.
E. Types of water–sodium imbalances
   1. Osmolar imbalance: involves disturbances in osmolarity that affect water distribution.
      a. Hyperosmolar imbalance: results from ECF osmotic pressure being greater than ICF osmotic pressure; results in water being pulled out of cells, which causes cells to shrink.
      b. Hypoosmolar imbalance: occurs when ICF osmotic pressure is higher than the ECF osmotic pressure; results in more water being pulled into body cells than pulled out and cells swell and rupture.
   2. Volume imbalance (isotonic imbalances): characterized by $Na^+$ and $H_2O$ increasing or decreasing together in roughly the same proportions as found in ECF.
      a. Volume excess: characterized by $Na^+$ and $H_2O$ increasing together; cells don't shrink or swell, but ECF compartment does increase or edema occurs.
      b. Volume deficit: characterized by $Na^+$ and $H_2O$ decreasing together; cells don't change, but ECF compartment does shrink.

## Role of Lymphatic System in Fluid and Electrolyte Exchange

A. Lymphatic capillaries absorb excess fluids and materials; capillaries transport fluid and proteins back to blood through either thoracic duct or right lymphatic duct.
B. Flow of lymph; lymph is moved by three methods:
   1. Continuous inflow of new lymph.
   2. Muscle contractions: muscles contracting push on walls of lymph vessels and move lymph along.
   3. Pressure changes in thorax: inspiration causes a negative pressure in the thorax to be created, which acts to help pull lymph upward into the thoracic and right lymphatic ducts.

## Fluids and Electrolytes

Matching. Questions 1 to 5.

| | | | |
|---|---|---|---|
| **1.** | extracellular fluids (ECF) | **A.** | pressure from solutes not diffusing through membrane |
| **2.** | intracellular fluids (ICF) | **B.** | fluid found outside cells |
| **3.** | blood hydrostatic pressure (BHP) | **C.** | results from interaction of BHP and COP |
| **4.** | colloidal osmotic pressure (COP) | **D.** | pressure in blood |
| **5.** | net effective pressure | **E.** | fluid found within cells |

True (A) or false (B). Questions 6 to 15.

6. Colloidal osmotic pressure (COP) is a "pushing pressure" or attempts to push fluids out of blood capillaries.

7. The net effective pressure at the arterial end of a capillary vessel is positive and forces fluids out.

8. At the venous end of a capillary vessel, COP normally is higher than BHP and pulls fluids into capillaries.

9. The major cation in ECF is potassium ($K^+$), and in ICF it is sodium.

10. The exchange of fluids and electrolytes between cells and tissue fluids results from osmosis and the $Na^+$–$K^+$ pump.

11. A hyperosmolar imbalance occurs when ECF osmotic pressure is higher than ICF and results in shrinkage of cells.

12. A volume excess is characterized by $Na^+$ and $H_2O$ decreasing together, but no changes to cells occur.

13. A volume deficit is characterized by $Na^+$ and $H_2O$ decreasing together, and the result is that cells shrink.

14. A blockage of lymphatic vessels would have no effect on fluid levels in the tissues.

15. The flow of lymph results from continuous inflow of new lymph, muscle contractions, and pressure changes in the thorax.

# Chapter 17

# THE RESPIRATORY SYSTEM

After reading and studying this chapter, a student should be able to:

1. Describe the anatomy and give the functions of the nose, pharynx, larynx, trachea, and bronchial tree.
2. Describe the anatomy and give the functions of the thoracic cavity.
3. Give respiratory functions of the diaphragm and external and internal intercostals.
4. Write a description of respiratory acidosis and alkalosis as to pH of blood and amount of $CO_2$ in blood in each case.
5. Define and give values for atmospheric, intrapulmonic, and intrapleural pressures.
6. Describe the steps involved in inspiration.
7. Describe the steps involved in expiration.
8. Give the location and function of the respiratory control center.
9. Discuss the function of the Hering–Breuer reflex.
10. Discuss the effects of carbonic acid, oxygen, and pH on control of respiration.
11. Define and give value for each lung volume.
12. Give partial pressure values for $O_2$ and $CO_2$ in air.
13. Describe exchange of gases at lungs and tissues with blood.
14. Discuss the effects of $O_2$, $CO_2$, and pH in dissociation of oxygen from hemoglobin.
15. Describe how carbon monoxide can cause death.

*The respiratory system primarily functions to bring oxygen into the body and remove carbon dioxide. In addition to these primary functions the respiratory system interrelates with other systems to help control body temperature, aid in production of sounds used in speech, and very importantly, it aids in regulation of blood pH.*

# 1 TYPES OF RESPIRATION

**External respiration** (breathing) involves oxygen being pulled into the lungs and diffusing into the blood. Carbon dioxide diffuses from the blood into the lungs and is exhaled out of the body. This is commonly called breathing.

**Internal respiration** involves the exchange of oxygen and carbon dioxide between the blood and cells. The oxygen diffuses into the cells where it oxidizes pyruvic acid in the mitochondria. The cellular reactions as a whole are called **cellular respiration.**

To understand how respiration works, one first has to be familiar with the anatomy and physiology of the respiratory system.

# 2 FUNCTIONAL ANATOMY OF THE RESPIRATORY SYSTEM

## NOSE

Air initially enters the body through openings in the nose called **external nares.** The interior of the nose is separated by a partition (nasal septum) into right and left cavities. The inner surface of the nose is lined with a ciliated mucous membrane containing goblet cells. The total surface of this membrane is increased by three plates of bone, called **turbinates** or **conchae,** which project from the nasal septum. These plates, are called **superior, middle,** and **inferior conchae** (Figure 17–1). The nasal membrane is well endowed with blood vessels that warm the air as it passes over the ciliated mucous membrane. The goblet cells produce about a quart of

mucous a day, which moistens the air and helps the cilia to trap and remove dust and foreign material from the air.

At the back of the nose the posterior nares open directly into the pharynx, the next region of this conducting passageway.

The nose essentially acts as a filter, removing dust and foreign material from the air we breathe. It also warms and moistens the air to prepare it for the deeper respiratory organs.

## PHARYNX

The pharynx is a muscular tube extending from the nose to the esophagus and larynx. The walls are composed of skeletal muscles and are lined with a mucous membrane. The pharynx can be divided into three regions, according to location (Figure 17–1).

The **nasopharynx** is the superior region and is located posterior to the nasal cavities and superior to the soft palate. It carries air downward from the nasal cavities to the soft palate in the mouth region.

The **oropharynx** is the middle region and extends from the soft palate downward to the hyoid bone. The oropharynx transports both food and air down to the entrance into the esophagus and larynx.

The **laryngopharynx** is the lowermost portion of the pharynx, continuing downward from the hyoid bone to the level of the larynx. At this point the laryngopharynx becomes continuous with the esophagus. The laryngopharynx lies behind the larynx, which is the continuation of the respiratory tract. This is the point at which the food passageway and the airway cross one another. Food is channeled backward into the esophagus; air moves forward to enter the larynx. The larynx is the next structure that air passes through on its way to the lungs.

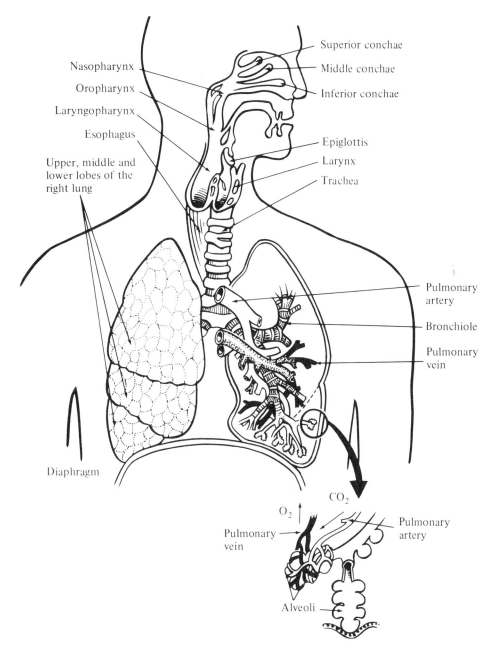

Figure 17-1. Respiratory structures and passageway. The structures along the respiratory passageway and an enlarged view of pulmonary alveoli are shown.

## LARYNX

The **larynx** is shaped like a triangular box and is located between the pharynx and trachea (windpipe). It is broad at its upper end and narrows at the lower end that joins the trachea. The larynx is composed of nine cartilages joined together by ligaments and controlled by skeletal muscles. Three of the nine cartilages will be discussed in more detail:

**Thyroid cartilage (Adam's apple)** (Figure 17-2) is the largest cartilage and is responsible for the shape of the larynx. It is more prominent in males than females.

**Epiglottis** (Figure 17-2) is a spoon-shaped cartilage that is attached along one edge of the thyroid cartilage, above the entrance to the larynx. The other edges are

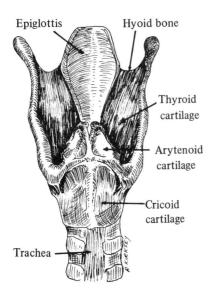

**Figure 17-2.** Three cartilages that compose the larynx along with other structures.

free, which allows the epiglottis to move up and down as a "lid" to prevent food and fluids from entering the larynx. During the act of swallowing the larynx moves up and forward, and the epiglottis moves downward. These actions close the opening into the larynx.

Occasionally food and water may "go down the wrong throat" or enter the larynx. This causes the muscles attached to the larynx to contract, and a cough reflex expels the particles.

**Arytenoid cartilages** furnish attachment for the vocal ligaments (Figure 17-2). The position and tension of the vocal ligaments are altered by changes in the position of the arytenoid cartilages, thereby changing the pitch of the voice.

TRUE AND FALSE VOCAL CORDS. The larynx is lined with a mucous membrane that forms two pairs of folds. The upper pair of folds are the **false vocal cords (ventricular folds)** and do not help create sounds. The lower pair of folds are the **vocal folds** or the **true vocal cords** (Figure 17-3).

Each vocal fold encloses a band of connective tissues called vocal ligaments. These ligaments stretch across the larynx opening from the vocal folds to arytenoid cartilages. The space between the vocal cords (when they are open or closed) is called the **glottis.**

Sounds are produced as air passes across the vocal ligaments, causing them to vibrate. **Pitch** (how high or low the tone is) of sound is determined by the length and tension of the vocal cords. Short, tense cords produce high-pitched sounds, and long, relaxed cords produce low-pitched sounds.

*Important Point*

The larynx is the organ of sound production, but not the organ of speech. Phonation or speech results from actions of the pharynx, tongue, lips, and palate on the sound produced by the vocal cords.

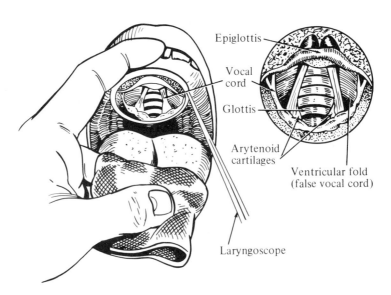

**Figure 17-3.** Internal view of larynx. The true and false vocal cords of a larynx are shown as seen through a laryngoscope. [Adapted from Philip Thorek, *Anatomy in Surgery,* 2nd edition. (Philadelphia: J. B. Lippincott Co., copyright 1962), Figure 165, p. 222]

**FUNCTIONS OF THE LARYNX.** The larynx has two basic functions. The epiglottis cartilage closes off the larynx and prevents the passage of solids and liquids into the air passages below. It also regulates the production of sound by the vocal cords.

## TRACHEA

The trachea is a rigid muscular tube about 10 to 13 cm long that extends downward from the larynx through the midline of the neck to the center of the chest behind the heart.

The rigidity of this tube is provided by 16 to 20 C-shaped cartilages. The open end of each cartilage is on the posterior surface and is bridged by connective and smooth muscle tissues. The cartilages keep the trachea open at all times, which is vital since air continually has to pass through the trachea to the lungs.

**TRACHEOTOMY OR TRACHEOSTOMY.** At times the passage of air through the trachea may be blocked by swelling, accumulation of secretions, or swallowing of a foreign object. If this occurs an opening must be made in the trachea below the obstruction to allow air to reach the lungs, or the person will die from **asphyxiation** (lack of oxygen). A **tracheotomy** is a surgical opening into the anterior surface of the trachea. A **tracheostomy** involves placing a tube in the surgical opening of the trachea. A tracheostomy is utilized to maintain an air pathway for a longer period of time, compared to a tracheotomy.

After a tracheostomy the patient requires special care to keep the tube free of mucus. A patient with a tracheostomy is much more susceptible to pulmonary infections since the air is not being conditioned (filtered, warmed and moistened) by the nasal cavities. This unconditioned air will bring in many organisms and compounds that can cause pulmonary infections.

## BRONCHIAL TREE

The trachea divides at its lower end into two smaller tubes, **primary bronchi** (Figure 17–4). Each primary bronchus enters the lung on its respective side. The right primary bronchus is more nearly vertical, shorter and wider than the left primary bronchus. Because of this structure, foreign compounds that may be inhaled are more likely to be found in the right primary bronchus or the right lung rather than on the left side. The bronchi are lined by a ciliated mucous membrane.

The bronchi contain C-shaped cartilages, like the trachea. Each primary bronchus enters its respective lung and divides into smaller or **secondary bronchi.** The secondary bronchi continue to branch and form smaller

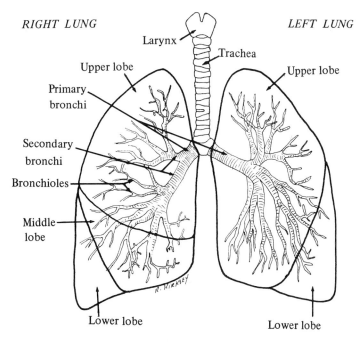

**Figure 17–4.** The divisions and branching of the bronchial tree. Also, the lobes of the right and left lungs are shown.

structures, **bronchioles** (Figure 17–4). At this point the amount of cartilage decreases, but the amount of smooth muscle increases. The smooth muscles of the bronchioles are innervated by sympathetic fibers that cause the bronchioles to dilate. Also, the smooth muscles are innervated by parasympathetic fibers that stimulate the muscles to contract and therefore narrow the bronchioles. The contraction and dilation of the bronchioles will be discussed in more detail later.

The bronchioles continue to form smaller and smaller branches, and at the diameter of about 1 mm (approximately 1/25 inch), the cartilage is gone. The bronchioles finally form microscopic branches called **alveolar ducts.** The alveolar ducts terminate in **alveolar sacs** (Figure 17–1). The alveolar sacs are found in clusters, called **alveoli,** that resemble a bunch of grapes. By the time the alveolar ducts finally give rise to alveoli, the walls are composed of a single layer of simple squamous epithelial tissue. Each alveolus is in contact with capillaries. The blood and alveoli readily exchange gases, with $CO_2$ diffusing from the blood into the alveoli and $O_2$ diffusing from the alveoli into the blood.

The term bronchial tree is quite appropriate since the primary bronchus (corresponds to trunk of tree) branches extensively until alveoli (corresponds to leaves of a tree) are formed. The total surface area available for exchange of gases between the lungs and blood is increased tremendously by the alveoli.

The bronchial tree has two important functions. First, the bronchi and bronchioles transport air to the alveoli, from the trachea. The size of the bronchioles can be regulated by nerve impulses, thereby regulating the amount of air flowing into and out of the alveoli. Second, the alveoli act as the functional units of the lungs. The exchange of gases occurs through the alveoli into and out of the blood. There are approximately 300 million alveoli per lung. The total surface area for exchange of gases is about 70 square meters.

# 3   THE THORACIC CAVITY (THORAX)

The thoracic or chest cavity is a closed cavity that contains the lungs, heart, and great vessels. The thorax is composed of 12 pairs of ribs and intercostal muscles between them, 12 thoracic vertebrae, sternum (breast bone) and the muscular diaphragm. It is lined by a serous membrane, the **pleura.** The pleura is composed of two layers: the **parietal layer** lining the thorax and the **visceral layer** covering the lungs. There are three subdivisions of the thorax:

1. The **pleural** subdivision containing the lungs.
2. The **mediastinum,** a subdivision located between the lungs and occupied by the esophagus, trachea and large blood vessels.
3. The **pericardial subdivision,** occupied by the heart and its surrounding sac, the pericardial sac.

## LUNGS

The lungs are cone-shaped organs that lie against the rib cage both anteriorly and posteriorly. The right lung is shorter and broader than the left lung. The right lung is divided by fissures into three lobes: **superior, middle,** and **inferior** (Figure 17–4). The left lung is divided into two lobes, upper and lower. The superior end or apex of the lungs extends about one inch above the first rib; the concave base of each lung rests on the diaphragm.

The lungs are light, porous, and spongy organs. An important characteristic of lung tissue is its great elasticity, which is important in the process of breathing. Within the spongy tissue are the secondary bronchi and bronchioles that carry air to and from the respiratory units, alveoli. The alveoli are well surrounded by capillaries, which connect pulmonary arteries to pulmonary veins.

*Function:* The lungs provide a place for the exchange of gases and furnish a tremendous area for approximately 300 million alveoli to rapidly exchange oxygen for carbon dioxide in the blood.

## MUSCLES USED PRIMARILY FOR BREATHING

The diaphragm and intercostal muscles are important in the breathing process. The **diaphragm** is a broad, arched skeletal muscular sheet extending across the body (Figure 17–5). It is arched toward the thoracic cavity and separates the abdominal and thoracic cavities. The base of each lung rests on the diaphragm. The **phrenic nerve** innervates the diaphragm. Contraction causes it to flatten out from the normal arched position, and relaxation involves the diaphragm moving back to its normal arched position. Contraction enlarges the size of the thoracic cavity, and relaxation decreases the size of the cavity.

**Intercostal muscles** are located in the spaces be-

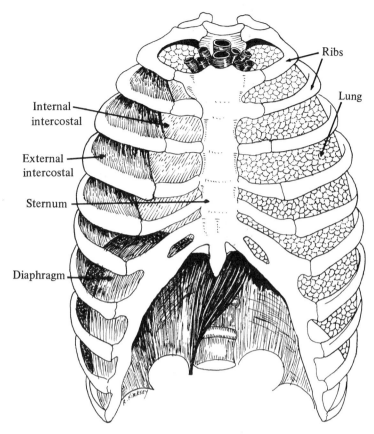

**Figure 17-5.** Thorax. The sternum, ribs, diaphragm, and intercostal muscles form a bony muscular cage that protects the lungs, heart, and blood vessels. The size of the thorax can increase and decrease during inspiration and expiration.

tween the ribs. There are two sets of intercostal muscles: the **external intercostals** and the **internal intercostals.** The external intercostals are located superficially. They contract during inspiration, elevating the ribs, which in turn enlarges the size of the thoracic cavity. The internal intercostals are located internal to the external intercostals (Figure 17-5). They are not important in ordinary respiration, but they do contract during forced expiration to depress the ribs or pull them down to their normal downward sloping position. This action decreases the size of the thoracic cavity, thereby forcing air out of the lungs.

## THE PLEURAL SPACE (CAVITY)

The **parietal pleura membrane** layer is separated from the **visceral pleura membrane** layer by the pleural space (Figure 17-6). The two pleural layers are in contact with each other under normal circumstances; therefore, this

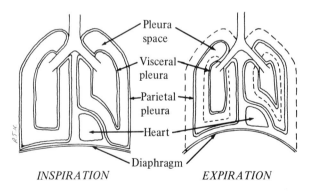

**Figure 17-6.** Pleural space, visceral pleura, and parietal pleura. The pleural space is located between the visceral and parietal pleurae.

is a potential space rather than an actual space. The pleural layers secrete a serous fluid that lubricates and prevents friction as the two pleural surfaces move against each other.

The pressure in the pleural space is always negative;

therefore, it is always slightly below atmospheric pressure (760 mm Hg). This negative pressure is important in respiration since it helps to pull lymph up from the lower parts of the body to the bloodstream near the heart. Also it helps to move venous blood back to the right atrium of the heart.

### Functions of the Thoracic Cavity

The thorax protects the vital respiratory organs, the heart, and the major blood vessels, with its bony and muscular structure. The thorax also plays a major role in respiration as a result of the contraction of the intercostal muscles and the diaphragm.

## 4  BLOOD GASES AND ACID–BASE TERMINOLOGY

Many diseases and disorders affect the normal levels of blood gases and therefore the acid–base balance of the blood. Table 17–1 gives the terms for these imbalances, pH values, and description.

**Respiratory acidosis** is more life threatening than **respiratory alkalosis.** The primary reason for this is the denaturation of vital enzymes. Notice in the last column the terms **uncompensated** and **compensated** in relation to pH values. Uncompensated refers to pH values of the blood that are above or below the normal pH range of 7.35 to 7.45. Compensated values are nor-

mal range values, and they imply that compensatory mechanisms by the blood buffers, respiratory and urinary systems have been successful in restoring homeostasis of blood pH. The compensatory mechanisms mentioned above will be discussed throughout the remainder of the unit.

## 5  RESPIRATORY MOVEMENTS AND ASSOCIATED PRESSURE CHANGES

To actually understand how oxygen moves into the body and carbon dioxide leaves, one must understand this basic principle: Gases travel from an area of higher pressure to an area of lower pressure or from an area of higher concentration to an area of lower concentration.

This principle applies not only to the movement of oxygen and carbon dioxide into and out of the body, but also to the exchange of these gases through blood capillaries. For the gases to be exchanged according to the above description, a high pressure followed by a low pressure is produced in the lungs. These pressure changes result from movements of the thorax. The contraction of the external and internal intercostal muscles plus the diaphragm cause the thorax to move up and down. Respiratory movements are divided into **inspiration (inhale)** and **expiration (exhale).** Before discussing inspiration and expiration the following pressures need to be defined:

### TABLE 17–1.  *Respiratory Acid–Base Disorders, Description, and pH values*

| Acid-Base Disorder | Terms in Common Usage | Description | pH Values |
|---|---|---|---|
| Respiratory acidosis | Primary $CO_2$ excess, carbon dioxide retention, hypercapnia or hypercarbia | An excessive amount of $CO_2$ in blood as a result of inadequate alveolar ventilation. *Ex.*—asthma or COPD | Uncompensated, 6.8–7.2; compensated, 7.3–7.5 |
| Respiratory alkalosis | Primary $CO_2$ deficiency | Deficit of $CO_2$ resulting from alveolar hyperventilation. A deficit of $CO_2$ means that there is less $CO_2$ + $H_2O \leftrightharpoons H_2CO_3 \leftrightharpoons$ H + $HCO_3^-$ and therefore fewer $H^+$. | Uncompensated 7.5–7.8; compensated 7.3–7.5 |

**Atmospheric pressure** is the pressure exerted by the air on all parts of our body. The average value, at sea level, is 760 mm Hg. This pressure will vary as you go above or below sea level. In discussions of atmospheric pressure, 760 mm Hg always is used as the standard pressure. This means that any pressure above 760 is positive, and anything below it is negative. An easy way to think of this is to visualize a scale in your mind. For example,

| | | |
|---|---|---|
| 763 | +3 | |
| 762 | +2 | Positive pressure |
| 761 | +1 | |
| 760 | 0 | ← Atmospheric pressure |
| 759 | −1 | |
| 758 | −2 | Negative pressure |
| 757 | −3 | |

**Intrapulmonic pressure** is the pressure within the bronchial tree and alveoli. This pressure will vary from positive to negative during inspiration and expiration. For example,

| | | |
|---|---|---|
| 764 | +4 | |
| 763 | +3 | Expiration |
| 762 | +2 | |
| 761 | +1 | During expiration and inspiration intrapulmonic pressure will vary from 764 (+4) to 756 (−4) mm Hg. |
| 760 | 0 | |
| 759 | −1 | |
| 758 | −2 | |
| 757 | −3 | |
| 756 | −4 | Inspiration |
| 755 | −5 | |
| 754 | −6 | |

**Intrapleural pressure** is the pressure within the pleural space, which is the potential space between the visceral and parietal layers of the pleura membrane. In other words, this is the pressure that exists in the space between the surface of the lungs and thorax wall. This pressure always is negative or below 760 mm Hg. For example,

| | | |
|---|---|---|
| 764 | +4 | |
| 763 | +3 | |
| 762 | +2 | |
| 761 | +1 | During inspiration and expiration the intrapleural pressure will vary from 752 (−8) to 756 (−4) mm Hg. This pressure is always negative. |
| 760 | 0 | |
| 759 | −1 | |
| 758 | −2 | |
| 757 | −3 | |
| 756 | −4 | |
| 755 | −5 | |
| 754 | −6 | Intrapleural pressure |
| 753 | −7 | |
| 752 | −8 | |

Since intrapleural pressure always is negative, the lungs are contained in a **partial vacuum** (area where constant negative pressure is present). This partial vacuum is important during inflation of the lungs.

Now that we have defined the pressures that are involved in inspiration and expiration, we are ready to discuss how these pressures change as the size of the thorax changes.

## INSPIRATION

This phase of respiration brings oxygen into the alveoli of the long. For oxygen to move into the alveoli, the intrapulmonic pressure must be lower or negative (in other words, below 760 mm Hg) compared to atmospheric pressure (Figure 17-7).

This has to be true because of the principle that gases move from an area of high pressure to an area of low pressure. The intrapulmonic pressure is lowered when the thorax increases in size. The events that increase the size of the thorax and lower the intrapulmonic pressure are the following:

**CONTRACTION OF DIAPHRAGM AND EXTERNAL INTERCOSTAL MUSCLES.** These two groups of muscles contract when they receive impulses from the phrenic and intercostal nerves. The diaphragm contracts and moves downward, which enlarges the size of the thorax from top to bottom. The external intercostals contract and elevate the ribs superiorly and laterally. This movement enlarges the size of the thorax laterally and anterior to posterior. The total size of the thorax is increased when the diaphragm and external intercostals contract.

**DECREASE IN INTRAPULMONIC AND INTRAPLEURAL PRESSURES.** Enlarging the size of the thorax lowers the intrapulmonic pressure from 760 mm Hg (0) to about 758 mm Hg (−2). Air now moves into the lungs since the atmospheric pressure 760 (0) is now greater than the negative intrapulmonic pressure 758 (−2). The intrapleural pressure decreases from 756 (−4) to 752 (−8) because the thorax wall pulls away from the lung surface, or the intrapleural space is increased slightly. This space does not increase much since the parietal and visceral pleural layers are in contact.

**AIR FLOWS INTO THE LUNGS.** As the air flows into the lungs, the intrapulmonic pressure rises gradually until it is equal to the atmospheric pressure. When

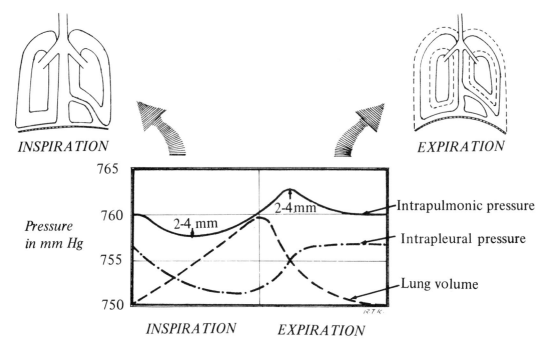

**Figure 17-7.** Pressure changes during inspiration and expiration. Inspiration and expiration result from increases and decreases in intrapulmonic and intrathoracic pressures. The relationship of lung volume to inspiration and expiration also is shown.

the atmospheric and intrapulmonic pressures are equal, no more air can enter the lungs. A person has completed inspiration at this point. During normal quiet inspirations, the diaphragm and external intercostals are the only muscles involved; but in deep forced expirations the scalenus, sternocleidomastoid and pectoralis minor muscles may be involved.

## EXPIRATION

This phase of respiration forces air out of the lungs. The intrapulmonic pressure increases above atmospheric pressure, and air moves from an area of high pressure to an area of low pressure (Figure 17-7). The thorax decreases in size, which increases the intrapulmonic pressure above atmospheric pressure. The decrease in the size of the thorax involves the following changes:

The **external intercostals** and **diaphragm** relax after nerve impulses from the intercostal and phrenic nerves cease. As the diaphragm relaxes, it moves upward to its normal position; the ribs return to their downward sloping position as the external intercostals relax.

The size of the thorax and lungs is decreased as the diaphragm and intercostals relax. Intrapulmonic pressure rises above 760 mm Hg as the thorax decreases in size. Air in the lungs is forced out until the in-

trapulmonic and atmospheric pressures are equal. The decrease in size of the thorax is passive during normal quiet breathing. In cases of deep forced expiration, the internal intercostals, along with abdominal muscles, contract to produce a greater amount of expiration.

Previously we stated that people who have emphysema have a hard time expiring because the intrapulmonic pressure remains negative when they expire. This occurs because the alveoli are broken down and they cannot create a positive intrapulmonic pressure.

## SUMMARY OF RESPIRATORY MOVEMENTS AND PRESSURE CHANGES

Oxygen moves into the lungs only when the intrapulmonic pressure decreases below atmospheric pressure or intrapulmonic pressure becomes negative (Figure 17-7). This decrease in pressure is produced when the contracting diaphragm and external intercostal muscles increase the size of the thorax. Air flows into the lungs until the atmospheric and intrapulmonic pressures are equal (760 mm Hg). Air flows out of the lungs when the intrapulmonic pressure rises above atmospheric pressure or intrapulmonic pressure becomes positive. The increase in intrapulmonic pressure occurs when the thorax decreases in size, which results from relaxation of the diaphragm and intercostal muscles.

# 6 NERVOUS CONTROL OF RESPIRATION

The respiratory rate of an average adult is about 16 to 18 respiratory cycles per minute. A respiratory cycle is one complete inspiration and expiration. The respiratory rate and depth will vary with age, body temperature, and exercise. If a person is quietly reading a book, his oxygen requirements and respiratory rate are completely different from a person who is vigorously mowing a lawn. A central control point in the body regulates the respiratory rate of a person to meet his immediate oxygen needs. The respiratory control center is located in the medulla and pons of the brain (Figure 17–8).

## RESPIRATORY CONTROL CENTER IN MEDULLA AND PONS

The respiratory control center is located primarily in the medulla and a small portion in the pons. This center includes the **inspiratory** and **expiratory** centers and **apneustic** and **pneumotaxic centers.**

The **inspiratory center** is a group of neurons in the lower part of the medulla (Figure 17–8). This center receives sensory impulses concerning the respiratory conditions in the body and sends out motor impulses that regulate inspiration.

The **expiratory center** is a group of neurons located superior and lateral to the inspiratory center. This center receives sensory impulses and sends out motor impulses causing the diaphragm and intercostals to relax.

**Pneumotaxic center** is located superior to the expiratory center in the pons. This area can inhibit the inspiratory and stimulate the expiratory center in emergency situations.

**Apneustic center** is located in the pons near the pneumotaxic center and can stimulate forceful inspirations in certain situations.

Notice in Figure 17–8 that these centers are paired and interconnected. This allows the centers to coordinate their actions with the activities on both sides of the chest. These centers send impulses through the phrenic nerve to the diaphragm and intercostal nerves to the intercostal muscles.

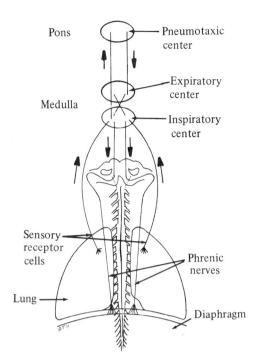

**Figure 17–8.** The respiratory control centers in the medulla and pons are interconnected so that they coordinate their nervous responses to the lungs and diaphragm. (Adapted from William F. Evans, *Anatomy and Physiology: The Basic Principles,* copyright 1971. Reprinted by permission of Prentice-Hall, Inc., Englewood Cliffs, N.J.)

## HERING–BREUER REFLEX

In normal breathing the respiratory rate and rhythm are determined by the Hering–Breuer reflex. Stretch receptor cells are located in the walls of the bronchioles and visceral pleurae. During inspiration and stretching of the bronchioles, a point is reached at which these stretch receptor cells are stimulated. Impulses move through the vagus nerve to the expiratory center and expiration follows. Notice that this is a reflex action; you are not even conscious of these actions.

# 7 CHEMICAL CONTROL OF RESPIRATION

The respiratory centers are affected by the chemical composition and temperature of the blood. Carbon dioxide, reacting with $H_2O$ to form carbonic acid ($H_2CO_3$), is the most important chemical in the blood, affecting respiration and acting directly upon the inspiratory center. Very small increases in blood $CO_2$ level increase the amount of $H_2CO_3$ formed (or respiratory acidosis) which stimulates the inspiratory center. These responses lower the level of $CO_2$ back to a normal range by increasing the rate at which a person expels $CO_2$. A drop in blood $CO_2$ slows respiration. Slight changes in the concentration of $O_2$ in blood normally have little effect on the respiratory rate. A severe increase of $CO_2$ or decrease of $O_2$ depresses the respiratory rate.

The pH of blood has the second most serious effect on respiration. Examples follow of how much pH can affect the rate of respiration: If respiratory alkalosis above pH 7.5 exists, respiratory rate is reduced by one-half, from 16 to 18 down to 8 to 9 respiratory cycles per minute. If respiratory acidosis exists below pH 7.2, respiratory rate quadruples, from 16 to 18 up to 64 to 72 cycles per minute.

## 8  LUNG VOLUMES

The depth of breathing is controlled by the requirements of the body under varying conditions. When a person is breathing normally, only about 12 percent of the lung capacity is being used. In cases where lung surgery is contemplated, it is often necessary to know the condition of the lungs. To learn about the condition of a patient's lungs, the patient breathes into a spiro-

meter. This device measures various aspects of lung capacity, such as the following:

**Tidal volume** is the volume of air that moves into and out of the lungs with each respiratory cycle (Figure 17–9). The average volume is about 500 ml or 0.5l.

**Inspiratory reserve volume** is the volume of air (in excess of the tidal) that can be inhaled by the deepest inspiration (Figure 17–9). This averages around 3000 ml or 3.0l.

**Expiratory reserve** is the amount of air that can be exhaled by the deepest possible expiration (Figure 17–9). This volume averages around 1000 ml or 1.0l.

**Vital capacity** is the volume that results from the addition of the tidal, inspiratory reserve, and expiratory reserve volumes:

Total vol + inspiratory + expiratory    = vital capacity
(500 ml)    reserve vol    reserve vol    (4500 ml)
              (3000 ml)      (1000 ml)

The vital capacity also can be determined by measuring the maximum amount of air that can be exhaled following a maximum inspiration. Vital capacity is an important clinical measurement in detecting heart and lung disease. A person afflicted with these diseases probably would have a vital capacity considerably less than 4500 ml.

**Residual air** is the volume of air remaining in the lungs even after the deepest possible expiration. The average volume is about 1500 ml or 1.5l (Figure 17–9). We have about 1000 ml or 1.0l of expiratory reserve volume, or a total of 2500 ml (2.5l) of air left in our lungs

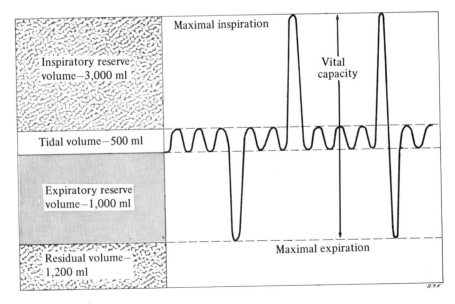

**Figure 17–9.**  A spirometer recording shows the respiratory volumes.

after a normal expiration. We breathe in about 500 ml of air with each normal breath, or we are renewing only one-fifth of the air in the lungs each time we take a breath.

# 9 GAS EXCHANGE BETWEEN BLOOD, LUNGS, AND TISSUES

The exchange of $O_2$ and $CO_2$ between the blood and alveoli and blood and tissues occurs because of pressure differences in these regions. In other words, the exchange of $O_2$ and $CO_2$ occurs essentially in the same way that air is inspired and expired, a movement of gases from a high-pressure region to a low-pressure region.

Previously, we discussed the fact that the pressure exerted by the air around the body is called atmospheric pressure and has a value of 760 mm Hg. Air primarily is composed of oxygen, carbon dioxide, and nitrogen gases in different quantities. Each of these gases exerts a pressure that is related to the amount of the gas in the air. The pressure of each of these gases is referred to as a **partial pressure** and is represented as $pO_2$ and $pCO_2$. Table 17–2 gives the quantities of each of these gases in air and their partial pressures. Notice that the partial pressure of each of the gases is the result of multiplying the percentage that gas occupies in the air times 760 mm Hg. For example, oxygen composes 20.93 percent of the air and $20.93 \times 760$ mm Hg = 159.1 mm Hg. In other words the $pO_2$ = 159 mm Hg in dry air. When the partial pressures of each of the gases are added up, $pO_2 + pCO_2 + pN_2$, the total is 760 mm Hg. This is an example of **Dalton's law of partial pressures**. This law, in effect, states that in a mixture of gases the pressure exerted by a gas is equal to the pressure that the same quantity of that gas would exert alone.

## TABLE 17–2. Concentrations and Pressures of Respiratory Gases in Dry Inspired Air

|  | PERCENTAGE | PARTIAL PRESSURES, MM Hg |
|---|---|---|
| Oxygen ($pO_2$) | 20.93 | 159.1 |
| Carbon dioxide ($pCO_2$) | 0.04 | 0.3 |
| Nitrogen ($pN_2$) | 79.03 | 600.6 |
|  | 100.00 | 760.0 |

## PARTIAL PRESSURES AND EXCHANGE OF GASES

Figure 17–10 shows the actual partial pressures and gas exchange between the cardiovascular system, lungs, and tissues. Notice in Figure 17–10A that $O_2$ diffuses into the blood as a result of the partial pressure being higher in the alveoli than in the blood. Likewise, in Figure 17–10A we see that $CO_2$ diffuses into the alveoli as a result of $CO_2$ partial pressure being higher in the blood.

Notice in Figure 17–10B that $O_2$ diffuses into the tissues as a result of $O_2$ partial pressure being higher in the blood. Likewise, $CO_2$ diffuses from tissues into blood as a result of the high $CO_2$ partial pressure in tissues.

# 10 FACTORS AFFECTING DISSOCIATION OF OXYGEN FROM HEMOGLOBIN

Figure 17–11 illustrates the unique property of hemoglobin to become saturated with (combine with) oxygen and then to dissociate from the oxygen as the hemoglobin reaches the tissues. Figure 17–11 shows that the oxygen-hemoglobin dissociation curve is an **S-shaped** or **sigmoid curve**. (Remember in Chapter 3 that the bacterial growth curve also was described as a sigmoid curve.) There are several important points about Figure 17–11 that should be carefully examined:

1. Figure 17–11A shows the normal $O_2 \cdot$ Hb dissociation curve. Notice that at $pO_2$ = 100 mm Hg hemoglobin is not 100 percent saturated with $O_2$, but rather about 97 percent saturated and 19.5 volumes percent. Notice that the physiologic dissociation curve shows that at $pO_2$ = 40 mm Hg that the percent $O_2$ saturation of hemoglobin begins to decrease rapidly. **What this means is that the amount of $O_2$ dissociating from hemoglobin and diffusing into tissues is increasing.** The **conclusion** from this then is that in a low $pO_2$ environment (which exists in systemic capillaries) **large amounts of $O_2$ dissociate from Hb and diffuse into tissues.**

2. Figure 17–11B shows the effect of $pCO_2$ on the $O_2 \cdot$ Hb dissociation curve. Notice that at $pO_2$ = 40 mm Hg how an increase in $pCO_2$ from 20 to 80 dra-

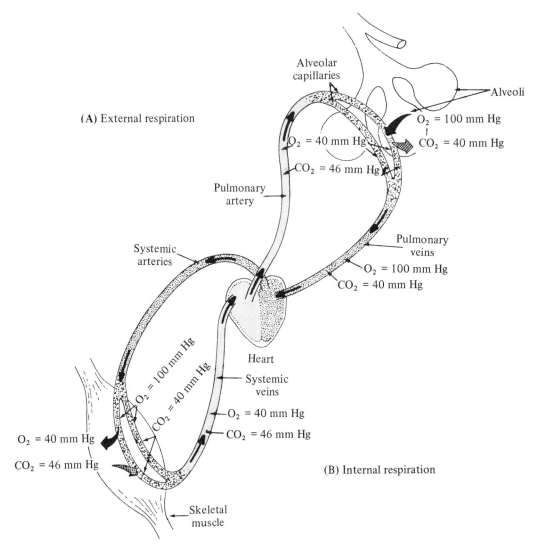

**(A) External respiration**

Alveolar
capillaries

Alveoli

$O_2 = 100$ mm Hg

$O_2 = 40$ mm Hg

$CO_2 = 40$ mm Hg

$CO_2 = 46$ mm Hg

Pulmonary
artery

Pulmonary
veins

$O_2 = 100$ mm Hg

$CO_2 = 40$ mm Hg

Systemic
arteries

$O_2 = 100$ mm Hg

$CO_2 = 40$ mm Hg

Heart

Systemic
veins

$O_2 = 40$ mm Hg

$CO_2 = 46$ mm Hg

$O_2 = 40$ mm Hg

$CO_2 = 46$ mm Hg

**(B) Internal respiration**

Skeletal
muscle

**Figure 17-10.**  Partial pressures and exchange of blood gases in (A) external and (B) internal respiration.

matically affects the amount of $O_2$ dissociating from Hb and diffusing into the tissues. The **conclusion** then is that **in a high p$CO_2$ environment** (which exists in systemic capillaries) **large amounts of $O_2$ dissociate from Hb and diffuse into tissues.**

3. Figure 17–11C shows the effect of pH on $O_2 \cdot$ Hb dissociation curve. Notice that at p$O_2$ = 40 mm Hg a decrease in pH from 7.6 to 7.4 to 7.2 increases considerably the amount of $O_2$ dissociating from Hb. The **conclusion** then is that **in a low pH** (increasing acidity) **environment** (which exists in systemic capillaries) **large amounts of $O_2$ dissociate from Hb and diffuse into tissues.** This effect of increasing acidity and increasing dissociation of $O_2$ from Hb is called the **Bohr effect.**

## 11  ANOXIA AND CARBON MONOXIDE POISONING

**Anoxia** (no oxygen) is a condition in which not enough oxygen reaches the tissues for normal tissue functions. The lack of oxygen reduces the oxidation of glucose and production of ATP. The lack of ATP inhibits the normal physiologic functions and the person will die, if the lack of ATP is not corrected.

Carbon monoxide (:C≡O) is an unstable gas that is found in automobile exhaust fumes. Normally each carbon monoxide molecule will combine with an oxygen atom to form a stable carbon dioxide (O≡C≡O) molecule; however, if a person is breathing carbon monoxide

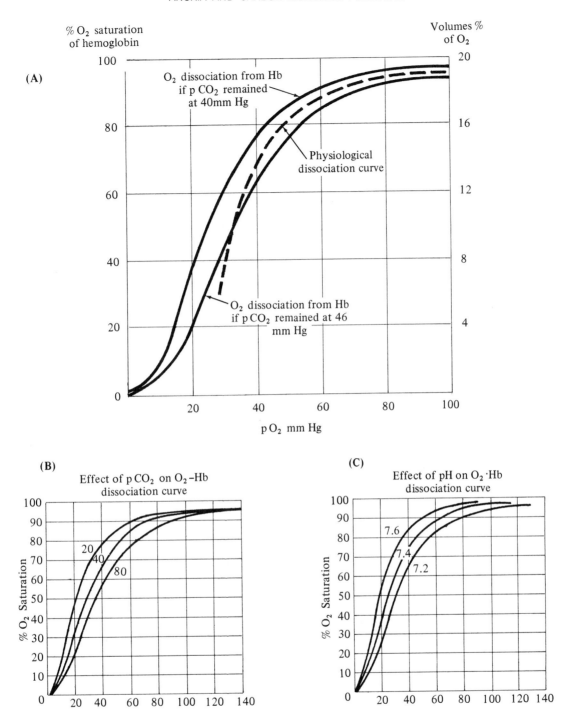

Figure 17-11.    Oxygen–hemoglobin dissociation curves: (A) normal $O_2 \cdot$ Hb dissociation curve; (B) effect of $pCO_2$ on $O_2 \cdot$ Hb dissociation curve; (C) effect of pH on $O_2 \cdot$ Hb dissociation curve.

in an unventilated garage, it can reach a lethal level. The reason it is lethal is because its affinity for hemoglobin is 200 times greater than that of oxygen. Carbon monoxide attaches with a greater affinity than oxygen to the $Fe^{2+}$ portion of hemoglobin. A 0.1 percent concentration of carbon monoxide attaches to half of all the hemoglobin molecules; therefore, only half as much oxygen can be transported to the tissues, resulting in anoxia. If the concentration of carbon monoxide rises above 0.2 percent, then all the hemoglobin is at-tached to carbon monoxide. No oxygen is transported to the tissues and death will follow.

# SUMMARY

### Types of Respiration
A. External (breathing): oxygen pulled into lungs and diffuses into blood; carbon dioxide diffuses into blood.
B. Internal: exchanges of oxygen and carbon dioxide between blood and cells.

### Functional Anatomy of the Respiratory System
A. Nose
  1. External nares: opening in nose.
  2. Turbinates (conchae): three plates of bone that project from lateral wall of nasal cavity. Function: increase surface area for filtering foreign material; warming and moistening air as it passes through nose.
B. Pharynx: muscular tube extending from nose to esophagus; divided into three regions: nasopharynx, oropharynx, and laryngopharynx.
C. Larynx
  1. Composed of nine cartilages joined together by ligaments and controlled by skeletal muscles.
  2. Contains true and false vocal cords.
  3. Functions: (1) epiglottis cartilage closes off larynx to prevent passage of solids and liquids; (2) regulates production of sound.
D. Trachea
  1. Rigid muscular tube; extends downward from larynx to center of chest behind heart.
  2. Rigidity provided by 16 to 20 C-shaped cartilages; help hold tube open for passage of air.
E. Bronchial tree: trachea divides into smaller tubes, which starts the bronchial tree:
  1. Primary bronchi: right and left primary bronchus enters the lung on its respective side.
  2. Secondary bronchi: branch off primary bronchi.
  3. Bronchioles: branch off secondary branchi; amount of cartilage decreases and smooth muscle increases; muscles innervated by sympathetic and parasympathetic fibers, which dilate and constrict them, respectively.
  4. Alveolar ducts: microscopic branches from bronchioles.
  5. Alveolar sacs: result from termination of alveolar ducts.
  6. Alveoli: clusters of alveolar sacs; composed of single layer of simple squamous epithelial tissue.
  7. Functions: (1) transport air to alveoli from trachea; (2) functional unit of lungs where exchange of gases between lungs and blood occurs.

### The Thoracic Cavity (Thorax)
A. Internally, it is composed of the lungs, heart, and great vessels; composed of three subdivisions:
  1. Pleural: subdivision containing lungs.
  2. Mediastinum: subdivision between lungs and contains esophagus, trachea, and large blood vessels.
  3. Pericardial: occupied by heart and pericardial sac.

B. Lungs
  1. Cone shaped; right lung divided into three lobes: superior, middle, and inferior; left lung divided into two lobes, upper and lower; light, porous, and spongy organs; great elasticity.
  2. Function: point of exchange for gases between blood and alveoli.
C. Muscles used primarily for breathing
  1. Diaphragm: broad, arched skeletal muscular sheet; extends across body. Function: enlarges and decreases size of thoracic cavity, thereby pulling air into and forcing air out of lungs.
  2. External intercostals: located superficially between ribs. Function: contract during inspiration, thereby elevating ribs and pulling air into lungs.
  3. Internal intercostals: located internal to external intercostals; function in forced expiration to pull down ribs.
D. The pleural space (cavity)
  Space between the visceral pleura (attached to lungs) and parietal pleura (lines thoracic cavity) membrane; pressure within cavity is always negative, which is important for pulling lymph up and moving venous blood back to heart.
E. Functions of thoracic cavity: (1) protects vital respiratory organs; (2) aids in inspiration and expiration by respectively increasing and decreasing size of thoracic cavity.

### Blood Gases and Acid–Base Terminology

A. Respiratory acidosis: pH of blood is in acid range (6.8 to 7.2) as a result of an excessive amount of $CO_2$ in blood; condition results in denaturation of enzymes, thereby can be life threatening; asthma or chronic obstructive pulmonary disease both can cause this problem.
B. Respiratory alkalosis: pH of blood is in the alkaline range (7.5 to 7.8) as a result of a $CO_2$ deficiency.

### Respiratory Movements and Associated Pressure Changes

A. Atmospheric pressure: pressure exerted by air on all parts of body; average value is 760 mm Hg.
B. Intrapulmonic pressure: pressure within bronchial tree; becomes positive (goes above 760 mm Hg) during expiration; becomes negative (goes below 760 mm Hg) during inspiration.
C. Intrapleural pressure: pressure within pleural space, space between visceral and parietal layers of the pleura membrane; partial vacuum.
D. Inspiration: to get air into lungs, intrapulmonic pressure must drop below 760 mm Hg; the events that bring this about are:
  1. Contraction of diaphragm and external intercostal muscles.
  2. Decrease in intrapulmonic and intrapleural pressures.
  3. Air flowing into lungs.
E. Expiration: to get air out of the lungs, the intrapulmonic pressure must rise above 760 mm Hg; the events that bring this about are:
  1. External intercostals relaxing.
  2. Diaphragm relaxing.
  3. Size of thorax decreasing.
  4. Intrapulmonic pressure increasing above 760 mm Hg.
  5. Air flowing out.

### Nervous Control of Respiration

A. Respiratory control center in medulla and pons; divided into inspiratory, expiratory, apneustic, and pneumotaxic centers.
  1. Inspiratory: receives sensory impulses concerning respiratory condition; sends out motor impulses that regulate inspiration.

2. Expiratory: receives sensory respiratory impulses; sends out motor impulses causing diaphragm and intercostals to relax.
3. Pneumotaxic: located superior to expiratory center in pons; inhibit inspiratory and stimulate expiratory center in pons.
4. Apneustic: located in pons near pneumotaxic center; can stimulate forceful inspirations in emergency conditions.

B. Hering–Breuer reflex: reflex response to stretching of bronchiole and alveolar walls; response results in regulating respiratory rate and rhythm.

### Chemical Control of Respiration

A. Carbonic acid ($H_2CO_3$): [↑] in $H_2CO_3$ = [↑] in respiration = [↓] in $CO_2$.
B. Oxygen ($O_2$): changes in $O_2$ have little effect on rate of respiration.
C. pH: increase in pH or respiratory alkalosis (pH above 7.5) results in reduction of respiratory rate; decrease in pH or respiratory acidosis results in increased respiratory rate.

### Lung Volumes

A. Tidal volume: volume of air that moves into and out lungs by inspiration; averages about 500 ml.
B. Inspiratory reserve volume: volume of air inspired by deepest inspiration; volume averages about 3000 ml.
C. Expiratory reserve: amount of air exhaled by deepest expiration; volume averages about 1000 ml.
D. Vital capacity: volume of air that results from addition of the tidal, inspiratory reserve, and expiratory reserve volumes.

### Gas Exchange between Blood, Lung, and Tissues

Each gas in the air exerts a pressure, which is referred to as a partial pressure; $pO_2$ = 159 mm Hg, $pCO_2$ = 0.3 mm Hg, $pN_2$ = 600.6 mm Hg; $pO_2$ + $pCO_2$ + $pN_2$ = 760 mm Hg. Dalton's law of partial pressures: in a mixture of gases the pressure exerted by a gas is equal to the pressure that the same amount of gas would exert alone.

A. Partial pressures and exchange of gases: due to principle of gases moving from a high-to a low-pressure region, $O_2$ diffuses into blood from alveoli; $CO_2$ diffuses from blood into alveoli; in tissues, due to same principle, $O_2$ diffuses from blood into tissues; $CO_2$ diffuses from tissues into blood.

### Factors Affecting Dissociation of Oxygen from Hemoglobin

A. Low $pO_2$ environment: tissues with low $pO_2$ stimulate the release of $O_2$ from hemoglobin.
B. High $pCO_2$: a high $pCO_2$, such as in tissues, stimulates release of $O_2$ from hemoglobin.
C. Low pH: a low pH or acidic condition increases dissociation of $O_2$ from hemoglobin.

### Anoxia and Carbon Monoxide Poisoning

A. Anoxia: lack of $O_2$ in tissues; reduces production of ATP and therefore death occurs.
B. Carbon monoxide poisoning: carbon monoxide (:C≡O) is an unstable gas that has a greater affinity for hemoglobin than does $O_2$. 0.2 percent of carbon monoxide attaches to all hemoglobin; therefore, no $O_2$ is transported and death occurs.

## The Respiratory System

Matching. Questions 1 to 5.

1. turbinates      **A.** cluster of alveolar sacs
2. larynx          **B.** composed of C-shaped cartilage
3. trachea         **C.** increase filtering surface area
4. bronchioles     **D.** pathway for air to alveolar ducts
5. alveoli         **E.** regulates production of sound

True (A) or false (B). Questions 6 to 11.

6. The diaphragm enlarges the size of the thoracic cavity, thereby pulling air into lungs when it relaxes.

7. External intercostals force air out of lungs when they contract.

8. Internal intercostals pull air into lungs when they contract.

9. The thoracic cavity functions to protect vital respiratory organs and aids in inspiration and expiration.

10. Respiratory acidosis results from an excessive amount of $CO_2$ in blood, and the condition can be fatal due to destruction of enzymes.

11. A $CO_2$ deficiency can result in an increase in pH and respiratory alkalosis.

12. Inspiration of air into lungs involves:

    1. Contraction of diaphragm          3. Decrease in intrapulmonic pressure
    2. Relaxation of external intercostals  4. Decrease in size of thoracic cavity

    (a)  1, 2, 3      (b)  1, 3      (c)  2, 4      (d)  4      (e)  All of these

13. Expiration of air out of lungs involves:

    1. Contraction of external intercostals
    2. Diaphragm relaxes
    3. Decrease in intrapulmonic pressure
    4. Decrease in size of thoracic cavity

    (a)  1, 2, 3      (b)  1, 3      (c)  2, 4      (d)  4      (e)  All of these

14. The nervous control center for respiration is in the _____.

    (a) Pons
    (b) Cerebellum
    (c) Medulla
    (d) a, b
    (e) a, c

15. Which of the following is (are) incorrectly paired?

    (a) Increase in carbonic acid — increase in respiratory rate
    (b) Tidal volume — volume of air inspired by deepest inspiration
    (c) Low pH — decreases dissociation of $O_2$ from hemoglobin
    (d) Carbon monoxide gas — strong affinity for hemoglobin molecule
    (e) b, c

# Chapter 18

# THE URINARY SYSTEM

After reading and studying this chapter, a student should be able to:

1. Describe the basic anatomy and functions of the kidneys, ureters, urinary bladder, and urethra.
2. Discuss filtration, reabsorption, and secretion processes in the formation of urine.
3. Describe the normal color, clarity, pH, specific gravity, and volume characteristics of urine.
4. Name five abnormal constituents found in urine and what each indicates.
5. Describe the steps involved in urination.
6. Name the intake and elimination sources of water.
7. Describe the roles of ADH, cortisone, glucocorticoid, and aldosterone hormones in regulating sodium ($Na^+$) in blood.

*The urinary system is of major importance in regulating the chemical composition of body fluids. The kidneys play a major role in regulating the chemical composition of blood by what they allow the body to retain and excrete.*

*In the previous area, we discussed how the lungs and respiratory tract acted as excretory organs in excreting the waste product $CO_2$. In this area we will discuss how the urinary system operates as the chief excretory system of the body. The activities of the body cells produce energy and needed products for the body, and in so doing produce waste products. These waste products are removed from the blood and excreted from the body by the urinary system as well as the respiratory system. The urinary system plays an important role in maintaining the internal environment of man in that it excretes waste products, and it adjusts the loss of water and electrolytes from body fluids.*

# 1  ORGANS OF THE URINARY SYSTEM

The urinary system consists of the kidneys, urinary bladder, urethra, and ureters (Figure 18–1). We will first discuss the anatomy and physiology of these organs and then discuss the process of urine formation by the nephrons, the functional units of the kidneys.

## KIDNEYS

The **kidneys** are shaped like kidney beans and are about 11.4 cm in length, 5 to 8 cm in width, and 2.5 in thickness. They lie against the posterior abdominal wall just above the waistline and behind the peritoneum, or they are **retroperitoneal** (Figure 18–1). The liver pushes the right kidney down slightly lower than the left. The kidneys are surrounded by adipose and connective tissue that connects them to the muscles in that area.

The medial surface of the kidney, near the center, has a deep fissure called the **hilum.** A tough fibrous layer of tissue called a **capsule** covers the kidney.

A coronal or longitudinal section of a kidney reveals the following regions:

The **cortex** (outer layer) is the outer layer of the kidney (Figure 18–2) and is composed of soft granular material, reddish-brown in color. It dips down forming **renal columns.**

The **medulla** (inner layer) is the inner layer of the kidney and is deep red in color and consists of triangular wedges, **renal pyramids** (Figure 18–2). The widest part, base, of each pyramid lies against the cortex. The pointed end, apex, of each pyramid is pointed toward the center of the kidney, and fits into cup-shaped structures called **calyces** (**calyx**—sing.).

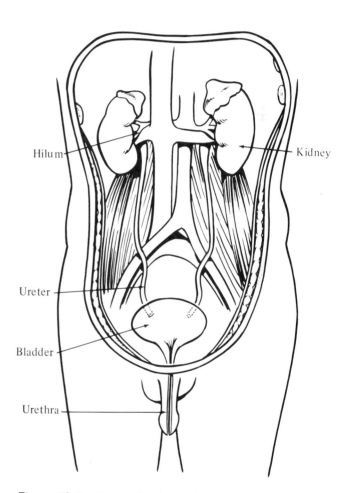

**Figure 18-1.** The abdominopelvic cavity is opened up to show the urinary organs.

*(Labels on figure: Hilum, Kidney, Ureter, Bladder, Urethra)*

The **renal pelvis** is the innermost region of the kidney and is a funnel-shaped cavity (Figure 18–2). The cup-shaped calyces are extensions of this cavity. The renal pelvis opens into the **ureter,** a tube that transports urine to the urinary bladder.

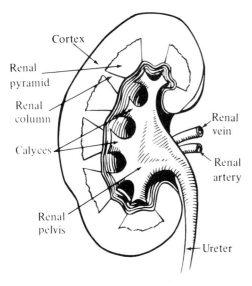

**Figure 18-2.** Longitudinal section of kidney.

## URETERS

One ureter from each kidney transports urine from the renal pelvis to the bladder (Figure 18–3). Each ureter is a smooth muscle tube about 25.4 cm to 30.5 cm long. It is lined with a mucous membrane that is continuous with the lining of the kidney and bladder. The ureters extend inferiorly from the kidneys and enter the posterior surface of the bladder. The mucous membrane forms a fold where the ureter enters the bladder, and this acts as a valve to prevent urine from flowing back up the ureter.

**FUNCTION OF URETERS.** The smooth muscle layers of the ureter contract causing peristaltic waves, which move urine to the bladder.

> **Kidney stones** or **renal calculi** generally are formed from uric acid and calcium salts in the renal pelvis. They can pass into the ureters, expanding the walls and causing pain and bleeding.

## URINARY BLADDER

The bladder is a hollow elastic smooth muscle sac that lies posterior to the pubic symphysis. The wall is composed of three layers of smooth muscle, forming the **detrusor musculature.** The middle layer of the muscular wall thickens near the entrance to the urethra (tube that

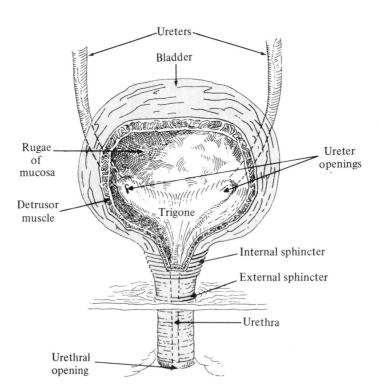

**Figure 18-3.** The urinary bladder and female urethra.

drains urine from bladder) forming an **internal sphincter valve** (Figure 18–3). An **external sphincter valve**, composed of striated muscle, surrounds the urethra and is under voluntary control.

The bladder is lined with a mucous membrane that forms folds or rugae when the bladder is empty. Rugae of the mucous membrane allow it to expand greatly as the bladder fills with urine.

**FUNCTION OF THE URINARY BLADDER.** The bladder functions as a reservoir for urine. Urine is stored here until it can be eliminated from the body. The bladder stretches greatly and holds a maximum of about 1000 ml of urine. The urge to urinate usually is experienced when approximately 300 to 400 ml of urine has accumulated in the bladder.

---

**Cystitis** is an inflammation of the mucous membrane lining the bladder and is most often caused by gram-negative rods, such as *Escherichia*, *Salmonella*, and *Klebsiella*. This condition often results from an endogenous infection of the urethra ascending to the bladder. Symptoms of this condition include a burning sensation in the bladder and urethra during urination and difficulty in urinating.

---

## URETHRA

The urethra is a small tube extending from the bladder to the outside. The male and female urethra differ in length and function.

**MALE URETHRA.** The male urethra consists of three portions, which will be described and discussed in Chapter 21. The male urethra is about 20 cm in length and extends through the penis and opens to the outside. The urethra is lined with a mucous membrane.

The main function of the urethra is to transport urine from the bladder to the outside of the body. The male urethra not only carries urine from the body but also transports **semen** (sperm and secretions) during ejaculation.

**FEMALE URETHRA.** The female urethra is only about 2.5 to 4.8 cm in length compared to about 20 cm in the male. The outer wall of the urethra is smooth muscle, and it is lined with a mucous membrane. It is at-

tached along its length to the anterior surface of the vagina. It opens to the outside through the urethra orifice, which is in front of the vaginal opening.

The function of the female urethra is to transport urine out of the body. Unlike the male urethra, the female urethra transports only urine.

---

## 2  NEPHRON: FUNCTIONAL UNIT OF THE KIDNEY

---

The functional unit of the kidney is the **nephron** (Figure 18–3); this is the structure in which urine is formed. Each kidney is composed of approximately two million microscopic nephrons. Most of the nephron is contained within the **cortex**, but a portion of it extends into the **medulla**. Each nephron looks like a tiny funnel with a long curved tube attached to it. It is composed of two major regions: **renal corpuscle** and **tubular system.**

### RENAL CORPUSCLE

The renal corpuscle is composed of a capsule called **Bowman's capsule (glomerular capsule)** (Figure 18–3). Bowman's capsule surrounds a tuft of capillaries, the **glomerulus.** The glomerulus receives blood from an afferent arteriole; an efferent arteriole carries blood away from the glomerulus. Notice that the efferent arteriole divides into peritubular capillaries, which surround the tubular system and finally converge to form a vein.

### TUBULAR SYSTEM

The Bowman's capsule is connected to a collecting tubule by a curved tube. The wall of the tube is composed of a single layer of epithelial cells. Each region of the tube has a special name.

**PROXIMAL CONVOLUTED TUBULE.** This is the first part of the tube (Figure 18–4) leaving Bowman's capsule. It is called convoluted because it loops and winds around rather than following a straight pathway.

**DESCENDING LIMB OF THE LOOP OF HENLE.** The proximal tubule winds around and finally extends

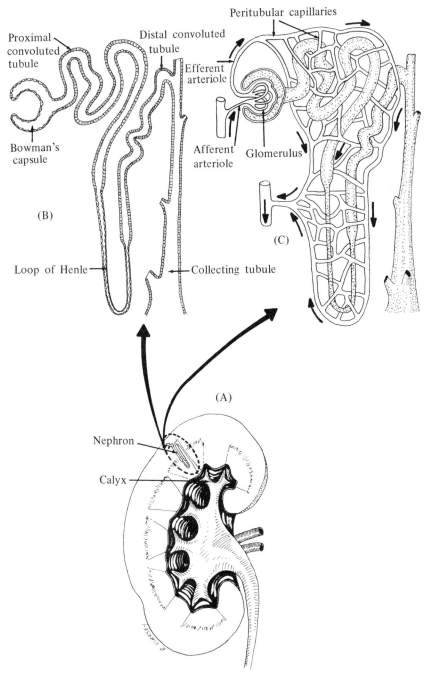

**Figure 18-4.** Parts of the kidney. (A) Sagittal section of a kidney shows a nephron. (B) Sagittal section of a nephron shows the regions. (C) A glomerulus within a Bowman's capsule and peritubular capillaries surrounding regions of nephron are shown.

downward into the renal medulla forming the descending limb of the loop of Henle (Figure 18–4).

**ASCENDING LIMB OF THE LOOP OF HENLE.** The ascending limb moves upward from the medulla back into the cortex.

**DISTAL CONVOLUTED TUBULE.** The distal convoluted tubule winds and loops around until it attaches to the collecting tubule.

**COLLECTING TUBULE.** The distal convoluted tubule connects to the collecting tubule which carries urine to a **calyx.**

*Important Point*
These tubular regions are extensively surrounded by the peritubular capillaries, which play an important role in the formation of urine. One may ask why is the tubular system so long, twisted, and convoluted? This provides an increased surface area for the exchange of fluids and materials between the pertibular capillaries and the tubular system.

# 3 FORMATION OF URINE

The formation of urine first starts with the renal artery (Figure 18-2) entering the hilum of the kidney. The renal artery carries waste products that were formed by various cellular and metabolic activities. The discussion that follows will consider how nutrient and waste materials are initially filtered out of the blood in the Bowman's capsule; then how some nutrient materials move back into the blood. The fluid that is excreted from the kidneys primarily contains waste products, and the nutrients needed by the body are retained.

The renal artery, after entering the kidney, divides into small branches, and finally afferent arterioles carry blood to glomeruli in Bowman's capsules. The formation of urine in the nephron involves three distinct processes: glomerular filtration, tubular reabsorption and tubular secretion.

## GLOMERULAR FILTRATION

The **afferent arteriole,** bringing blood to the glomerulus, is larger in diameter than the **efferent arteriole.** This difference in diameter helps to create a high blood pressure (**glomerular filtration pressure**) inside the glomerulus (Figure 18-5). This high pressure, combined with many pores in the walls of the glomerulus, forces fluids and dissolved substances through the glomerulus into the Bowman's capsule by the process of filtration. In other words the high filtration pressure and permeable walls filter fluids and dissolved crystalloid substances from the blood into the Bowman's capsule. Red blood cells, plasma proteins and other large particles (colloids) are too big to pass across the membrane and remain in the blood as it leaves the glomerulus and enters the efferent arteriole.

The fluid that enters Bowman's capsule is called **glomerular filtrate** and about 120 ml/min of filtrate are formed, or about 180 liters per 24-hour period. An average of about 1 to 1½ liters of urine is eliminated daily; therefore, approximately 179 liters are reabsorbed daily.

## *Glomerular Filtration Rate (GFR) and the Effects on It by the Juxtaglomerular Apparatus*

The GFR normally is about 120 ml/min. This rate is directly affected by the volume and pressure of blood circulating through the glomeruli. If the blood pressure drops, the GRF and all of the following processes could be hindered significantly. An apparatus, the **juxtaglomerular apparatus,** is an important structure in helping to maintain the normal pressure of blood entering the glomeruli. This apparatus is located near the point where the afferent arteriole enters a glomerulus. It is composed of modified cells in the walls of an afferent arteriole and an adjacent distal convoluted tubule. This apparatus is very sensitive to the pressure of blood that circulates through it into the glomerulus. Whenever the pressure drops below normal, the juxtaglomerular cells release a hormone called **renin.** Renin interacts with a plasma protein **angiotensin** and converts it ultimately to **angiotensin II.** This compound functions to raise blood pressure in two ways (Figure 18-6).

1. It causes constriction of arteries throughout the body. This increases the resistance which results in an elevation of blood pressure.
2. Angiotensin II stimulates the adrenal cortex to secrete large amounts of the hormone **aldosterone.** This hormone acts on the proximal tubules to increase their active transport of Na$^+$ back into the blood. This raises osmotic pressure and therefore the amount of water pulled into the blood. This increased water volume will raise blood pressure. These various steps are illustrated in Figure 18-6.

**The ultimate effect of the two angiotensin actions is that blood pressure is raised and therefore the normal glomerular filtration rate will be restored.**

*Important Point*
The filtration that occurs is not selective and therefore includes not only waste products but also many compounds needed by the body such as water, glucose, Na$^+$, and K$^+$. The blood must get these needed compounds back, or else blood leaving the kidney would be lacking many necessary nutrient compounds. The process by which the nutrients move back into the blood is discussed next.

## TUBULAR REABSORPTION

Previously it was mentioned that about 179 of 180 liters of glomerular filtrate are reabsorbed daily. This means that 124 ml out of the 125 ml/min are reabsorbed each

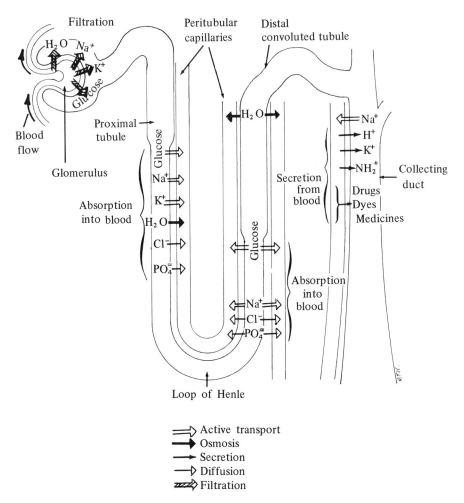

Figure 18–5.  The three processes involved in the formation of urine: filtration, absorption, and secretion. The methods by which materials are absorbed into the blood are indicated by the different arrows.

minute. Reabsorption of needed compounds into the peritubular capillaries occurs by three processes: active transport, diffusion, and osmosis.

**ACTIVE TRANSPORT.**   Active transport involves the movement of substances across a cell membrane from a low concentration to a high concentration and requires the expenditure of energy. Some of the substances reabsorbed into the blood by active transport, and the locations, are:

1. Glucose is absorbed through the proximal convoluted tubule (Figure 18–5). The amount of glucose reabsorbed depends on the concentration of glucose already present in the blood. If the blood has an adequate supply of glucose, and you eat a candy bar, the excess glucose would not be reabsorbed.

2. Potassium ($K^+$) is absorbed through the proximal convoluted tubule (Figure 18–5) and loop of Henle. Potassium seems to be reabsorbed regardless of its concentration in the blood. In fact all the potassium that is filtered is reabsorbed in the proximal tubule. Potassium found in urine is added by tubular secretion in the distal tubule. This is associated with the hydrogen ion exchange and will be discussed later.

3. Sodium ($Na^+$) is absorbed through the proximal convoluted tubule and loop of Henle (Figure 18–5). This compound is reabsorbed in greater quantities than any other compound, except water. It is reabsorbed in the forms of $Na^+Cl^-$ and $Na^+HCO_3^-$. Sodium, $Cl^-$, and $HCO_3^-$ are ions that play important roles in acid–base buffer systems and nerve impulse transmission.

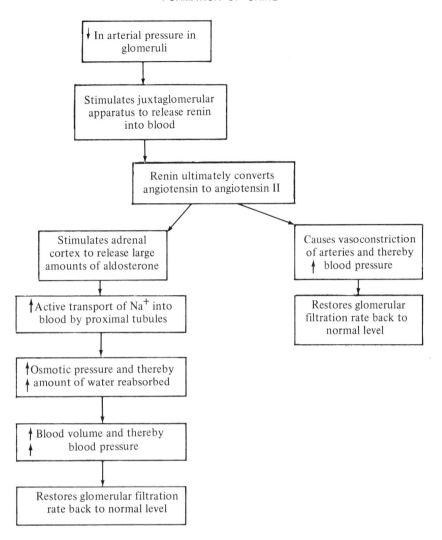

**Figure 18-6.**   Role of juxtaglomerular apparatus and renin in regulating blood pressure in kidneys.

**DIFFUSION.** As the $Na^+$ and $K^+$ cations are actively transported out of the nephron tubules they create a positively charged region in the peritubular capillaries and fluids surrounding the tubules. This positively charged region acts to attract negatively charged ions such as $Cl^-$ and $PO_4^{-2}$. The negatively charged ions diffuse from the nephron tubules into the peritubular capillaries.

**OSMOSIS.** Osmosis is a passive process that requires no expenditure of energy. Water is absorbed into the peritubular capillaries by osmosis, and the tubular sites of absorption are the proximal convoluted tubule, distal convoluted tubule, and collecting duct. The amount of water absorbed depends on the level of salt and other solutes in the blood.

**ROLE OF ANTIDIURETIC HORMONE (ADH) IN $H_2O$ ABSORPTION.** ADH hormone, produced by the hypothalamus region of the brain and released from the posterior pituitary, plays a role in water absorption in the tubules. The posterior pituitary is stimulated by the hypothalamus to release ADH when the salt concentration in the blood is high and therefore, the amount of water in the blood is low. ADH travels through the blood to the peritubular capillaries and increases the permeability of the tubular cells to water. The osmotic pressure of the peritubular blood is high because of the presence of proteins. This high "pulling pressure" pulls water into the peritubular capillaries until the salt concentration is lowered back into the normal range; as a result, the volume of urine excreted is less and it is more concentrated due to less water being excreted.

**Diabetes insipidus** is a disorder that is caused by a deficiency of ADH hormone (Figure 18–7). A person with this problem excretes large amounts of urine, from 6 to 40 liters daily. The urine is very dilute with a specific gravity of 1.001 to 1.005 due to large amounts of water compared to wastes. One cause of diabetes insipidus is tumors in the posterior pituitary area of the brain. These tumors prevent the proper receipt and release of ADH. Subcutaneous administration of posterior pituitary extracts can control diabetes insipidus.

## TUBULAR SECRETION (AUGMENTATION)

This is the third process involved in the formation of urine. Metabolic activities produce large quantities of various ions that upset the blood acid–base balance unless their level is adequately controlled. The concentration of these ions is controlled by secretion of the excessive amounts of them from the peritubular blood and cells of the distal convoluted tubule into the urine (Figures 18–5 and 18–8). These compounds are the following:

**HYDROGEN IONS (H⁺).** Remember that H⁺ (hydrogen ions) increase the acidity of the blood and body fluids. The concentration of H⁺ increases when the level of $CO_2$ increases, as shown by the following reaction:

$$CO_2 + H_2O \xrightarrow[\text{enzyme}]{\text{Carbonic anhydrase}} H_2CO_3 \rightarrow H^+ + HCO_3^-$$

As the level of $CO_2$ in the blood rises more carbonic acid is formed and moves into the epithelial cells of the distal convoluted tubule (Figure 18–8). The tubule cells secrete the H⁺ into the urine and, at the same time, Na⁺ move from the urine into the tubule cells where the following reaction occurs:

$$Na^+ + HCO_C^- \rightarrow Na^+HCO_3^-$$

The Na⁺ is from the urine; the sodium bicarbonate is formed in the tubule cells and moves into the blood. The movement of the sodium bicarbonate, which is a basic compound, into the blood along with the loss of H⁺ acts both to reduce the acid level and to restore the normal basic pH level of the blood.

**AMMONIA (NH₃).** NH₃ is formed from the breakdown of proteins. The concentration of ammonia in the blood must be regulated along with H⁺. As the concentration of NH₃ increases, it combines with H⁺ and

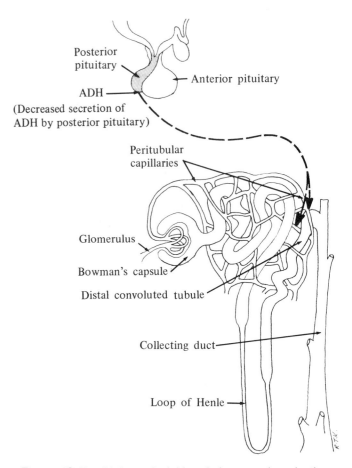

**Figure 18-7.** Diabetes insipidus. A decreased production of ADH hormone by the posterior pituitary results in a small amount of fluid being absorbed into the peritubular capillaries. The end result is that a person excretes large amounts of urine daily, and this condition is called diabetes insipidus.

moves from the blood into the tubule cells where the following reactions occur (Figure 18–8):

$$NH_3 + H^+ \rightarrow NH_4^+ + Na^+Cl^- \rightarrow Na^+ + NH_4^+Cl^-$$
$$\rightarrow \text{moves into the urine}$$

$$Na^+ \xrightarrow[\text{the tubules}]{\text{Moves into}} Na^+ + HCO_3^- \rightarrow Na^+HCO_3^-$$
$$\rightarrow \text{moves into the blood}$$

The elimination of NH₃ and H⁺ from the blood and simultaneously the movement of the basic compound Na⁺ HCO₃⁻ into the blood act to reduce the concentration of NH₃ and H⁺ and to increase the basic level of the blood.

**POTASSIUM (K⁺).** Potassium ions (K⁺) are absorbed into the blood from the proximal tubule, normally; however if the K⁺ level in the blood is too high, the excessive amounts are secreted from the peritubular capillaries into the epithelial cells of the distal convoluted tubule and collecting duct. The K⁺ then move into the

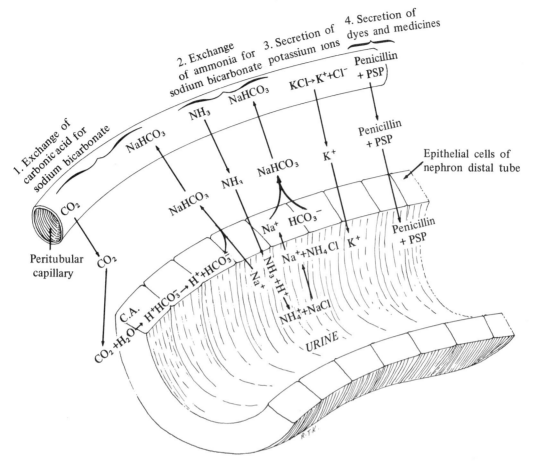

**Figure 18-8.** Secretion and exchange of materials between peritubular capillaries and nephron tubule.

urine. This tubular secretion of potassium usually does not fail until late in the development of chronic renal diseases.

**DRUGS AND DYES.** Whenever various drugs and dyes are present in the blood, they are secreted into the urine through the distal tubule cells. Penicillin is a common drug and it is secreted into the urine in the distal tubule area of the nephron (Figure 18-8).

# 4 CHARACTERISTICS AND COMPOSITION OF URINE

Laboratory examination of urine is called **urinalysis,** and it can be very useful in diagnosing problems. Urine has various constituents and characteristics that can readily be measured in a routine urinalysis examination. These constituents and characteristics are discussed below.

## Color

Normally urine is amber or yellowish in color. This color will vary depending on the amount eliminated and also somewhat on the diet. Urine dark in color is abnormal and could indicate the presence of blood or bile. Drugs may also color the urine. Strongly acidic urines have a pinkish color from the precipitation of uric acid salts.

## Clarity

Usually urine is a clear fluid, but it becomes cloudy on standing. It may be cloudy when first voided because of the presence of mucus and bacteria. Alkaline urines may be turbid from precipitated calcium phosphate.

## pH

The pH of urine varies from about 4.8 to 7.4 with an average pH value of 6.0. If a person is eating a normal mixed diet, the pH will probably be about 6.0; but if a person is eating predominantly a vegetable diet, urine pH will be basic.

### Specific Gravity

A specific gravity measurement of urine measures how heavy a certain volume of urine is compared to an equal volume of water. Dissolved solids in the urine make it heavier than water. The normal specific gravity range of urine is 1.002 to 1.040 with an average of about 1.020. If the reading is above 1.040, this indicates the presence of a large quantity of dissolved solids, which is abnormal. Urine of specific gravity below 1.002 indicates a low concentration of dissolved solids or the urine is almost pure water. This condition also is abnormal and is seen in cases of diabetes insipidus.

### Volume

The normal amount of urine eliminated daily is between 1000 and 1500 ml or 1 to 1½ liters. The quantity eliminated usually depends on the amount of water intake, the temperature, and the diet. Some important terms that refer to the elimination of abnormal volumes of urine are:

**Oliguria** is a decrease in the elimination of urine. One cause for this may be dehydration or water being pulled from the blood into the intracellular compartment.

**Polyuria** is a persistent increase in the amount of urine excreted. Diabetes insipidus is characterized by polyuria.

**Diuresis** is a temporary increase in the amount of urine excreted. This condition often occurs when a person has been retaining water and takes a diuretic to eliminate the water.

**Retention** of water occurs when a person has been retaining water and not eliminating the proper amounts. This can occur for many reasons, such as an enlarged prostate.

**Anuria** refers to no urine formation at all and indicates that the kidneys are totally malfunctioning or the blood pressure may be so low that no filtrate is formed.

### Normal Constituents of Urine

Ninety-five percent of the total volume of urine is water. The other 5 percent is solutes that result from cellular metabolism and any drugs that a person may be taking. Some of the various solutes, their concentrations and comments are given in Table 18–1.

## 5  ABNORMAL CONSTITUENTS OF URINE

Urine is 90 to 95 percent water. The other 5 to 10 percent is inorganic salts and organic substances. Approximately 60 g of solids are excreted daily. Some normal and abnormal constituents found in urine are:

1. *Glucose:* glucose normally is not present in urine or is present in very small quantities. If an appreciable amount of glucose is present, **glycosuria,** it is usually an indication of diabetes mellitus.

2. *Albumin and globulin:* albumin and globulin are proteins normally found in blood serum. Since they are too large to cross the capillary membrane, they are not filtered from the blood when glomerular filtrate is formed. If they are present, this can be an indication of a kidney malfunction probably in the glomeruli and Bowman's capsules. **Albuminuria** is the term that refers to albumin in the urine. Pregnancy often will be accompanied by albuminuria.

3. *Blood:* Blood in the urine indicates possible disease or injury of the kidney or urinary tract. This condition is called **hematuria.**

4. *Pus cells:* pus cells in the urine indicate an infection in the urinary system. This condition is called **pyuria.**

5. *Casts:* casts are tiny pieces of material that have solidified in the tubules and indicate injury.

## 6  MICTURITION, URINATION, OR VOIDING

The three terms **micturition, urination,** or **voiding** all refer to a person emptying his bladder. The bladder gradually fills with urine; and when it contains about 300 to 400 ml, stretch receptor cells are stimulated in the bladder wall, the **detrusor muscle.** The stretch receptor cells carry these stimuli to the brain, and the desire to urinate results. The parasympathetic nerve fibers carry efferent impulses to the detrusor muscle (smooth muscle tissue) causing it to contract rhythmically. The **internal sphincter muscle** at the entrance to the urethra relaxes, allowing urine to flow into the urethra. The **external sphincter muscle** (skeletal muscle tissue) is inferior to the internal sphincter muscle and surrounds

### TABLE 18-1. *Normal Constituents of Urine*

| Constituent | Amount* (g) | Comments |
|---|---|---|
| *Solutes* | | |
| Urea | 25–30 | The amount excreted varies with dietary intake; 60–90% of all nitrogen solutes excreted; origin is in liver (deamination of proteins). $(NH_3 + CO_2 \rightarrow NH_3 - \underset{\underset{O}{\|}}{C} - NH_3)$ Urea |
| Uric acid | 0.6–0.8 | Product of oxidation of the nucleic acid, purine. Sometimes its level builds up and is main component of kidney stones. |
| Creatinine | 1.0–2.0 | A derivative of creatine phosphate (high energy molecule stored in muscles). Produced by normal muscle metabolism during contraction. |
| Ammonia ketones | 0.6–0.8 0.04–0.06 | Produced in liver by deamination of proteins. Produced in liver by $\beta$-oxidation of fats. Very common in urine of individuals who are on low carbohydrate diets, pregnant women, and untreated cases of diabetes mellitus. |
| Hippuric acid | 0.7–1.0 | Compound that results from changes to benzoic acid (a toxic substance in fruits and vegetables). |
| *In organic Solutes* | | |
| NaCl | 13.0–15.0 | Most abundant and important inorganic salt. Composes approximately 44% of the urine solids. The amount excreted varies with dietary intake. |
| $K^+$ $Mg^{+2}$ $Ca^{+2}$ | 3.3 0.1 0.3 | These cations combine with the anions (chlorides, sulfates, and phosphates) to form salts that appear in the urine. |
| $SO_4^{-2}$ (Sulfate) | 2.0–2.5 | Results from catabolism of amino acids. |
| $PO_4^{-3}$ (Phosphate) | 2.2–2.5 | Appears in urine combined with sodium to form monosodium phosphate and disodium phosphate. These compounds are blood buffers. |
| $NH_4^+$ (Ammonium) | 0.7–1.0 | Appears in urine in combination with $Cl^-$, or ammonium salts. $NH_3$ results from protein catabolism; then as the $H^+$ ion concentraton in blood increases they combine with $NH_3$ to form $NH_4^+$, which is excreted by kidneys in large quantities as compensatory mechanism to correct for acidosis. |

\* Values are for 24 hr.

the urethra. The flow of urine through the urethra can be stopped by the external sphincter muscle.

# 7 MAINTENANCE OF FLUIDS AND ELECTROLYTES

Maintaining a normal balance of fluids and electrolytes and the pH range is critical to maintaining the internal environment of man. Fluids and electrolytes are utilized extensively in many different areas of the body.

Many systems utilize fluids and electrolytes, and when their concentrations are not maintained the systems tend to malfunction. Fluid balance and electrolyte balance are interdependent, and if one deviates from the normal, so does the other.

## FLUID BALANCE

During a 24-hour period a person takes in a certain amount of water and loses approximately the same amount. The body is able to maintain a normal fluid balance because the total fluid intake equals the total fluid output. A person takes in water from three sources:

| | |
|---|---|
| Fluid intake | 1500 ml |
| Water contained in the food eaten | 700 ml |
| Water formed by catabolism of foods eaten | 300 ml |
| Total fluid intake | 2500 ml |

You can see that a person takes in an average of about 2500 ml of fluid in a 24-hour period. To maintain fluid balance he must lose about this amount in the same period. A person eliminates water from four sources:

| | |
|---|---|
| Kidneys | 1500 ml |
| Lungs | 350 ml |
| Skin | 450 ml |
| Intestines | 200 ml |
| Total fluid output | 2500 ml |

As you can see from the above, the kidneys are the most important organs in regulating the loss of water. Previously, we said that the antidiuretic hormone (ADH) plays a major role in the amount of water that is absorbed into the blood; therefore, when the level of water in the blood is normal, the release of ADH is inhibited and more water passes out of the body.

## ELECTROLYTE BALANCE

Previously, we stated that $Na^+$ is the principal cation of extracellular fluid, and $K^+$ is the principal cation of intracellular fluid. These electrolytes are important in chemical reactions, muscle contractions, and nerve impulse conduction; therefore, the maintenance of a range of these ions is quite important.

SODIUM ($Na^+$) BALANCE. Four hormones act on the kidney renal tubule to regulate the balance of $Na^+$. **Antidiuretic hormone** regulates the absorption of water, but at the same time $Na^+$ are absorbed in the form of $NaCl$ and $NaHCO_3$. **Cortisone** and **glucocorticoid hormones**, secreted by the adrenal cortex, stimulate the kidney renal tubule to absorb $Na^+$. **Aldosterone** is a hormone secreted by the adrenal glands that stimulates the active transport of $Na^+$ from the urine into the peritubular capillaries. A high concentration of aldosterone stimulates large amounts of $Na^+$ to be reabsorbed, while at the same time large amounts of $K^+$ are eliminated from the body. Likewise, low concentrations of aldosterone, such as is seen in Addison's disease, cause retention of $K^+$ and elimination of large quantities of $Na^+$ and water. If the concentration of $Na^+$ drops considerably below normal levels, a person can experience cramps, apathy, headaches, weakness, nausea, and vomiting.

POTASSIUM ($K^+$) BALANCE. The kidneys play a major role in maintaining the balance of $K^+$. The proximal convoluted tubule is the site at which almost all of the $K^+$ that filters through Bowman's capsule is reabsorbed into the blood. The distal convoluted tubule is the site at which excessive $K^+$ in the blood are secreted into the tubule cells and on into the urine.

# SUMMARY

**Organs of the Urinary System**
A. Kidneys: shaped like kidney beans; located against posterior abdominal wall and behind peritoneum; internal regions of kidney include:
   1. Cortex: outer layer of kidney; composed of soft granular material.
   2. Medulla: inner layer; consists of wedges called renal pyramids.
   3. Pelvis: innermost funnel-shaped region of kidney; calyces are extensions; opens into ureter, which carries urine to bladder.
B. Ureters: smooth muscle tubes; connect kidneys to urinary bladder; transport urine from pelvis to urinary bladder.
C. Urinary bladder: hollow elastic smooth muscle sac; wall composed of three layers of smooth muscle tissue; middle layer thickens near urethra to form an internal sphincter valve; external sphincter valve, composed of striated muscle and surrounds urethra.

D. Urethra: small tube extending from bladder to outside.
  1. Male: composed of three parts; extends through penis and opens to outside; lined with mucous membrane; transports urine and semen out of body.
  2. Female: short compared to male; opens to outside through the urethra orifice; functions to transport only urine out of body.

## Nephron: Functional Unit of the Kidney

A. Renal corpuscle: composed of capsule called Bowman's capsule, which surrounds a tuft of capillaries, glomerulus.
B. Tubular system: curved tube connecting Bowman's capsule to a collecting tubule; regions of the tube are proximal convoluted tubule, descending limb of loop of Henle, ascending limb of loop of Henle, distal convoluted tubule, and collecting tubule.

## Formation of Urine

Three processes are involved in formation of urine:
A. Glomerular filtration: occurs in glomeruli; glomerular filtration pressure forces crystalloids out of blood into capsule; fluid is called glomerular filtrate and about 180 liters per 24 hours is formed; approximately 179 liters is reabsorbed daily.
  1. Glomerular filtration rate (GFR): drop in blood pressure results in release of renin from juxtaglomerular apparatus; renin results in formation of angiotensin II, which raises blood pressure in two ways: (a) constriction of arteries; (b) stimulates release of aldosterone, which raises blood pressure by increasing water volume.
B. Tubular reabsorption: fluids and needed crystaloids are reabsorbed into peritubular capillaries along length of tubular system; active transport, diffusion, and osmosis are involved in reabsorption; antidiuretic hormone (ADH), released from posterior pituitary, increases water absorption into blood in distal and collecting tubule regions.
C. Tubular secretion: some substances are secreted from peritubular capillaries into urine; one method for helping to control pH of blood; substances secreted are hydrogen, ions, ammonia, potassium, drugs, and dyes.

## Characteristics and Composition of Urine

Lab examination of urine is called urinalysis; constituent and characteristics of urine are:
A. Color: normally amber or yellowish; dark urine is abnormal.
B. Clarity: normally clear but becomes cloudy on standing.
C. pH: ranges from 4.8 to 7.4 with average being about 6.0.
D. Specific gravity: ranges from 1.002 to 1.040.
E. Volume: normal amount eliminated daily is 1000 to 1500 ml. Abnormal volumes of urine eliminated: (1) oliguria, decreased elimination of urine; (2) polyuria, increased amount eliminated; (3) diuresis, temporary increase in amount excreted; (4) retention, reduced elimination; (5) anuria, no urination formation.

## Abnormal Constituents of Urine

A. Glucose: presence of glucose in urine is glycosuria; possibly an indication of diabetes mellitus.
B. Albumin and globulin: proteins, if present in urine, are indicative of albuminuria; common problem in pregnancy.
C. Blood: presence of blood is called hematuria; indicative of urinary tract infection or injury.
D. Pus cells: indicative of a urinary tract infection.
E. Casts: tiny pieces of solidified material in tubules.

## Micturition, Urination, or Voiding

Emptying of bladder is stimulated when stretch receptor cells in bladder are stimulated; impulses transported from receptor cells to brain; parasympathetic efferent impulses cause bladder walls to contract; internal and external sphincter muscles relax, which allows passage of urine out of body.

## Maintenance of Fluids and Electrolytes

A. Fluid balance: normally the body eliminates the same amount of urine as it takes in; intake sources are fluids ingested, water in food eaten, and water released by catabolism reactions; four sources for elimination of water are kidneys, lungs, skin, and intestines.

B. Electrolyte balance: (1) sodium ($Na^+$); cortisone, glucocorticoid, and aldosterone hormones all affect absorption of $Na^+$. (2) Potassium ($K^+$); potassium is absorbed in proximal tubule and excessive $K^+$ are secreted from blood in distal tubule.

## The Urinary System

Matching. Questions 1 to 5.

1. cortex                      A.   transports urine and semen out of body
2. pelvis                      B.   location of kidneys
3. ureters                     C.   outer layer of kidney
4. urethra                     D.   innermost region of kidney
5. retroperitoneal             E.   transport urine from pelvis to urinary bladder

True (A) or false (B). Questions 6 to 12.

6. The first process involved in formation of urine is filtration and it occurs in the proximal convoluted tubule.

7. Glomerular filtration results in crystalloids being filtered out of blood and no large colloids.

8. Drop in blood pressure decreases glomerular filtration rate (GFR).

9. Angiotensin II raises blood pressure by (1) increasing heart rate, and (2) releasing antidiuretic hormone (ADH) and thereby increasing water volume.

10. The curved, twisted tubular system aids the reabsorption process.

11. Tubular secretion involves materials moving from urine into blood stream.

12. One important function of secretion is that it helps to control pH of blood.

13. Of the following characteristics of urine which is (are) incorrectly paired?

    1.   Color—amber or yellowish        3.   Specific gravity—1.002 to 1.040
    2.   Clarity—normally clear          4.   pH—7 to 12
    (a)   1,2,3,        (b)   1,3,        (c)   2,4        (d)   4

14. Which of the following is (are) incorrectly paired?

    (a) Glycosuria—glucose in urine
    (b) Albuminuria—albumin in urine
    (c) Hematuria—pus cells in urine
    (d) Casts—tiny pieces of solidified material in urine

15. Absorption of sodium (Na+) is influenced by which hormones.

    (a) Cortisone
    (b) Glucocorticoid        (d)   None of these
    (c) Aldosterone           (e)   a, b, c

# Chapter 19

# DIGESTIVE SYSTEM

After reading and studying this chapter, a student should be able to:

1. Name the five functions of the digestive system.
2. Name and locate the three salivary glands.
3. Name three functions of saliva.
4. Locate the fundus, body, and pyloric regions of the stomach.
5. Describe regulation of gastric juice production by the nervous system.
6. Describe regulation of gastric juice production by the endocrine system.
7. Discuss five functions of the stomach.
8. Name the three regions of the small intestine along with the layers of tissue (from the inside) that compose the small intestine wall.
9. Recognize the three functions of the small intestine.
10. Identify the regions of the large intestine from the cecum to the anal canal.
11. Discuss the three functions of the large intestine.
12. Describe the basic anatomy, location, and functions of the liver.
13. Describe the structure and function of liver lobules.
14. Discuss the anatomy, location, and functions of the gallbladder.
15. Discuss the anatomy, location, and functions of the pancreas.
16. Discuss chemical digestion of proteins as to enzymes and products produced.
17. Discuss chemical digestion of carbohydrates, lipids, and proteins in the small intestine.
18. Describe how the products of digestion are absorbed.

# 1 FUNCTIONS OF THE DIGESTIVE SYSTEM

The digestive system has five basic functions:

1. **Physically break food down:** the teeth and stomach physically break down large food particles into smaller ones, which facilitates the actions of the digestive enzymes.

2. **Transport food through the digestive tube:** the distance from the entrance to the digestive tube (mouth) and exit point (anus) along the outside of the body is a matter of a meter or less. However, in the body the digestive tube curls and coils around for a distance of 9 to 10 meters. The long, coiled digestive tube is functional since it provides a longer time for digestive reactions and absorption of the products. It also provides for reabsorption of the water, used in digestive reactions, into the blood before excretion of feces.

3. **Secretion of enzymes:** the digestive enzymes are secreted into the digestive tube. The enzymes are important in increasing the rate of digestive reactions.

4. **Absorption of digested products:** the small intestine is the longest part of the digestive tube. The long distance plus a good blood supply facilitates the absorption of digested products through the small intestine into the blood.

5. **Excretion of feces:** the final function of the digestive system is to excrete the unused materials, which are called feces. Water is reabsorbed from the waste material through the large intestine into the blood before the feces are excreted.

# 2 INGESTION AND PHYSICAL BREAKDOWN OF FOOD

Ingestion and physical breakdown of food involve the upper parts of the digestive tube (also called **gastrointestinal tract, alimentary canal,** and **gut**)—pharynx, esophagus, and stomach. Accessory digestive organs are structures that attach to the digestive tube. Accessory organs that play important roles in these digestive steps are the tongue, teeth, and salivary glands.

The digestive tube is a smooth muscular tube that extends for approximately 9 to 10 meters, from the mouth to the anus (Figure 19–1). It is lined with a mucous membrane. Each region of the tube contributes to the digestive process in a certain way: therefore, each region of the tube has its own specialized anatomic and physiologic characteristics.

## THE MOUTH AND ACCESSORY DIGESTIVE ORGANS

The mouth is the entrance point of food into the digestive tube. The accessory organs in the mouth play an important role in the physical breakdown of food.

The cheeks make up the side walls of the mouth; the hard and soft palates make up the roof and the tongue and other muscles make up the floor (Figure 19–2). All these accessory organs in the mouth are lined with a mucous membrane.

The accessory digestive organs include teeth, tongue, and salivary glands. The teeth that erupt beginning about six months of age are called "baby teeth" or "deciduous teeth." There are 20 deciduous teeth, which are gradually lost between the ages of 6 and 13 years. The deciduous teeth are replaced by "permanent

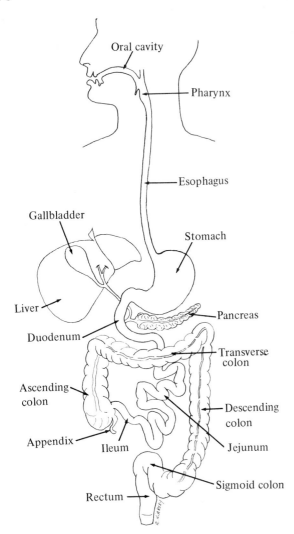

**Figure 19-1.** The regions of the digestive tube and the accessory organs attached to it.

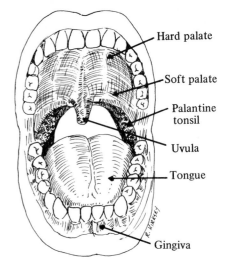

**Figure 19-2.** The mouth and internal structures.

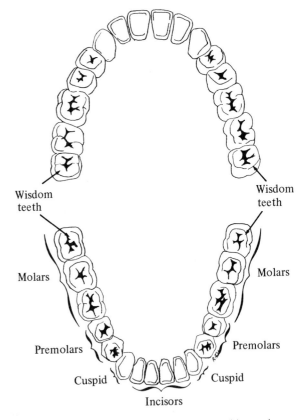

**Figure 19-3.** The teeth in the upper and lower jaws.

teeth," which number 28 plus 4 third molars (wisdom teeth), for a total of 32 teeth. The upper and lower jaws each contain 16 teeth. Starting at the midline, the teeth are (Figure 19-3): 4 incisors, 2 cuspids, 4 premolars, and 6 molars. The 4 backmost molars (two in the bottom jaw and two in the top) are called wisdom teeth and generally they are pulled. The wisdom teeth generally erupt between the ages of 17 to 25 years and sometimes not at all. Teeth function to tear and grind food into small pieces. This function increases the surface area of food, which facilitates the actions of the digestive enzymes.

### Structure of a Tooth

A tooth is divided into three regions (Figure 19-4). The **crown** protrudes into the mouth cavity; the **neck** is covered by gum tissue and the root is embedded into an al-

veolar cavity of the jaw bone. The crown is covered by an extremely hard substance called **enamel.** The enamel is composed of a calcium phosphate type compound. Beneath the enamel lies a layer of tissue called **dentine.** The composition of dentine is similar to bone tissue, and it surrounds the **pulp cavity.** The pulp cavity

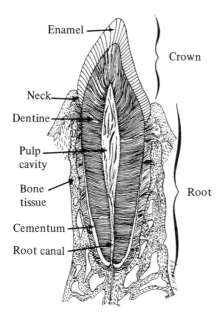

**Figure 19-4.** Longitudinal section of a tooth.

is composed of connective tissue, blood vessels, and nerves. These structures enter and leave a tooth through the **root canal** (Figure 19-4).

## Tongue

The tongue is composed of skeletal muscles and the root is anchored to the hyoid bone. A fold of mucous membrane called the **frenulum** attaches the tongue to the floor of the mouth. Taste buds that are sensitive to sour, salt, sweet, and bitter stimuli are located in the tongue. The tongue functions in taste, speech, swallowing, and chewing.

## Salivary Glands

The breakdown and swallowing of food are enhanced by the mixing of food with saliva. Three pairs of salivary glands, parotid, sublingual, and submandibular (Figure 19-5), are responsible for secreting saliva. The **parotid glands** are located slightly below the ears at the angle of the jaw. Stenson's duct carries saliva into the mouth close to the second molar in the upper jaw. Branches from the glossopharyngeal nerve (IX) stimulate secretion of saliva in the parotid gland.

Mumps is an acute, contagious viral infection of the parotid glands and is characterized by painful,

inflammatory swelling of one or both parotid glands. Generally mumps strike children between the ages of 5 to 15 years. The infection confers a lasting immunity and is usually not serious. If it occurs after a person is sexually mature, the viruses can descend into the testes and ovaries. Since the ovaries are not enclosed in a limited area, the viral infection usually does not result in permanent tissue damage in the female. However, in the male the tissue injury in the testes often is severe and permanent because of the limited membrane surrounding the testes. If both testes are affected, sterility may result.

The two **sublingual salivary glands** lie inferior to the tongue or under the anterior floor of the mouth (Figure 19-5). They have several ducts that open into the mouth on each side of the frenulum.

The two **submandibular salivary glands** lie inferior to the mandible (Figure 19-5) or under the posterior surface of the floor of the mouth. The **Wharton's ducts** open into the mouth on each side of the frenulum. Branches from the facial nerve (VII) innervate the sublingual and submandibular glands.

**CHEMICAL COMPOSITION OF SALIVA.** Saliva either can be thin or thick, depending upon the stimuli that initiate their secretion. A person secretes 1000–1500 ml of saliva per day, which has a pH of 6 to 7. Two important chemicals in saliva are **mucin** and **salivary amylase (ptyalin)**. Mucin is a protein that gives saliva its slippery consistency and aids the chewing and swallowing processes. Salivary amylase (ptyalin) is a starch-digesting enzyme that breaks polysaccharide starches into disaccharide maltose molecules. Saliva also contains lysozyme, which is a bacteriolytic enzyme.

**FUNCTIONS OF SALIVA.** Saliva has several functions:

1. **Helps hold food in a ball.** The chewing of food is aided by saliva, which helps to hold food in a ball form so teeth can grind it up.
2. **Aids swallowing of food.** Swallowing of food is aided by the mucin component of saliva.
3. **Initiates digestion of the polysaccharide, starch.** Salivary amylase is an enzyme that initiates the breakdown of starch into disaccharide maltose molecules.

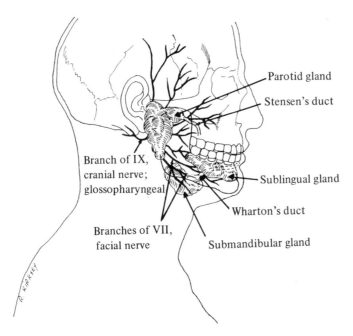

Parotid gland

Stensen's duct

Branch of IX,
cranial nerve;
glossopharyngeal

Sublingual gland

Wharton's duct

Branches of VII,
facial nerve

Submandibular gland

**Figure 19-5.** The three salivary glands along with their ducts. The cranial nerves that stimulate secretion of saliva by these glands also are shown.

## PHARYNX, ESOPHAGUS, AND SWALLOWING OF FOOD

After food has been chewed into small pieces and thoroughly mixed with saliva, it is in a round form called a **bolus.** As the bolus moves to the back of the tongue and pharynx it initiates sensory impulses that are carried to the swallowing reflex center in the medulla. The swallowing reflex center sends impulses to the pharynx, where skeletal muscles grip the bolus and move it into the esophagus. At the same time the bolus is passing backward, the soft palate moves upward to prevent the food from entering the nose. Simultaneously, the larynx is moved upward against the epiglottis, which prevents food from entering the larynx and trachea.

The esophagus is a collapsible smooth and skeletal muscle tube. It is located posterior to the trachea and extends downward 25 cm posterior to the heart to the stomach. The inner surface of the esophagus is lined with a mucous membrane that secretes mucus (Figure 19-6). The smooth muscles form a sphincterlike valve, the **cardiac valve** (Figure 19-7), where the esophagus joins the stomach. This valve is not a true sphincter valve, but functions to regulate passage of food into and out of the stomach. Rhythmic contractions of the esophageal muscles are called **peristalsis; peristaltic movements** (Figure 19-8) move food through the esophagus.

The cardiac valve opens to allow food to move into the stomach. Peristaltic movements also are responsible for moving food through the rest of the digestive tube.

## THE STOMACH

The stomach is a J-shaped smooth muscular sac (Figure 19-10). It is located inferior to the liver and diaphragm. The majority of the stomach is located in the **epigastric** and **left hypogastric** regions of the abdomen (Figure 19-9).

The superior region of the stomach is called the **fundus;** the middle region, the **body;** and the inferior region, the **pyloric** (Figure 19-10). The pyloric region joins the stomach to the **duodenum** (the first part of the small intestine). The walls of the stomach are composed of three layers of smooth muscles. The outer layer is called the longitudinal muscle layer, and the fibers run the length of the stomach. The circular layer is the middle muscle layer and the oblique layer is the inner muscle layer. The circular and oblique muscle fibers run in circular and oblique directions, respectively.

The entrance of food into the stomach and exit of food out of the stomach are regulated by two valves. The **cardiac valve** is located at the point where the esophagus joins the stomach. It opens to allow food to en-

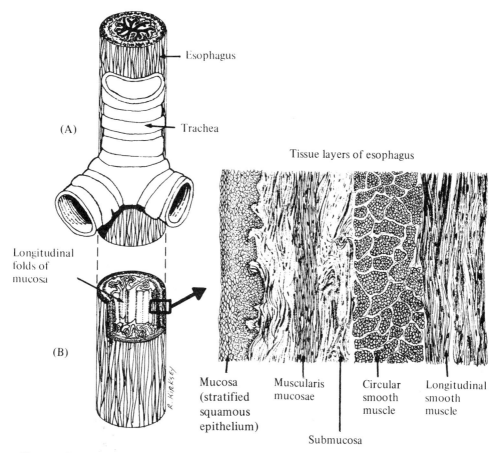

Esophagus

(A)

Trachea

Longitudinal
folds of
mucosa

(B)

Tissue layers of esophagus

Mucosa
(stratified
squamous
epithelium)

Muscularis
mucosae

Circular
smooth
muscle

Longitudinal
smooth
muscle

Submucosa

Figure 19-6.    (A) The position of the esophagus; (B) the layers of tissue that make up the walls of the esophagus.

ter, but closes to prevent food from moving up the esophagus. The **pyloric sphincter valve** is located at the point where the pyloric part of the stomach joins the duodenum. The pyloric sphincter valve regulates the passage of **chyme** (semiliquid form of digested food) from the stomach into the duodenum. The cardiac and pyloric sphincter valves are enlargements of the circular layer of smooth muscle. The autonomic nervous system regulates the opening and closing of the valves. Parasympathetic impulses carried by the vagus nerve stimulate the muscles of the valves to relax, causing the valves to open. Sympathetic impulses stimulate the muscles of the valves to contract, thereby closing the valves.

Male babies often are born with an abnormally small pyloric sphincter valve. This condition is called **pyloric stenosis,** and it prevents food from effectively moving into the duodenum so that it can be absorbed. The child vomits his food rather

than absorbing it properly. This condition can be corrected surgically. **Pylorospasm** is a condition in which the pyloric valve remains in a constricted or spastic state. It does not relax and allow the chyme to pass into the duodenum.

### Mucous Lining and Gastric Glands of the Stomach

The inner surface of the stomach is lined with a mucous membrane (**gastric mucosa**) that forms longitudinal folds called **rugae** (Figure 19-10) when the stomach is empty. These rugae allow for expansion of the inner surface of the stomach by flattening out when one eats a meal.

There are between 10 and 35 million gastric glands within the gastric mucosa of the stomach, and they secrete 1 to 2 liters of gastric juice per day. The glands in the fundus and body regions of the stomach secrete

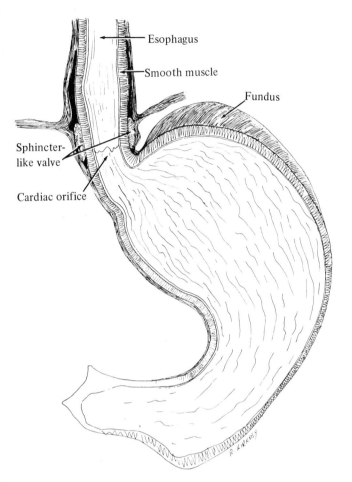

Figure 19-7. The esophagus and opening into the stomach. The smooth muscles of the esophagus that form a sphincterlike valve are shown, along with the cardiac orifice.

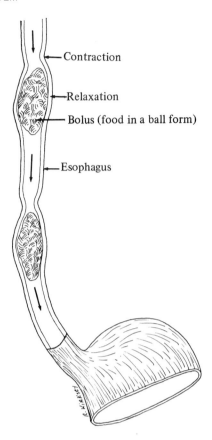

Figure 19-8. Peristaltic movements of food through the esophagus. Peristaltic movements involve alternate contraction and relaxation of smooth muscles.

most of the gastric juice. Figure 19–11 shows the rugae inside the stomach and the invaginations of the mucous membrane. Each invagination is called a **gastric pit.** Opening into each gastric pit are these cells that secrete mucus, enzymes, and hydrochloric acid. The **chief** or **zymogenic cells** secrete digestive enzymes (pepsinogen, rennin, and lipase). **Parietal cells** secrete hydrochloric acid (HCl) and **mucous cells** secrete mucus. These three cells compose a **gastric gland.** Secretions from these cells are poured into the gastric pit, and are carried up to the surface of the gastric mucosa. Let us now discuss the secretions of these three cells in greater detail.

**SECRETIONS OF CHIEF CELLS.** Several enzymes are secreted by chief cells, which are located in the body of a gastric gland (Figure 19–11). **Pepsinogen** is an inactive form of the enzyme **pepsin.** Pepsinogen is converted to the active form, pepsin, by hydrochloric acid. Pepsin breaks peptide bonds of proteins resulting in the formation of intermediate sized protein segments, **pro-**

**teoses** and **peptones.** If pepsin were present in large quantities at all times, it would digest the walls of the stomach since they are composed of proteins. Fortunately, pepsin is secreted in an inactive form, pepsinogen, which can be activated only by a concentrated amount of hydrochloric acid.

**SECRETION OF THE PARIETAL CELLS.** Hydrochloric acid (HCl) is secreted by the parietal cells (Figure 19–11) in the gastric glands. Enough HCl is secreted during digestion to give the gastric juice a pH = 1. When a person is not digesting food (fasting), the amount of hydrochloric acid in the gastric juice is considerably less, so that pH = 3.5. Hydrochloric acid functions to activate pepsinogen to pepsin and to destroy most bacteria that may enter the stomach.

**SECRETION OF THE MUCOUS CELLS.** Mucus is secreted by mucous cells located in the neck region of a gastric gland (Figure 19–11). The protein, **mucin,** also found in saliva, is an important constituent of mucus. The inner mucous membrane of the stomach is protected from the digestive enzymes by a layer of mucus.

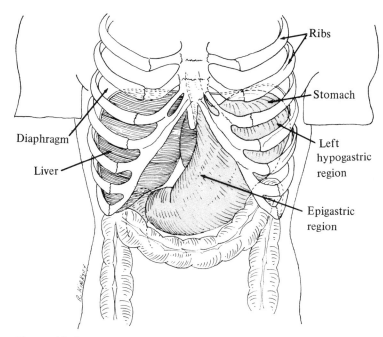

**Figure 19-9.** The stomach is located partly in the left hypogastric and epigastric regions. Also, it is located under the diaphragm and liver.

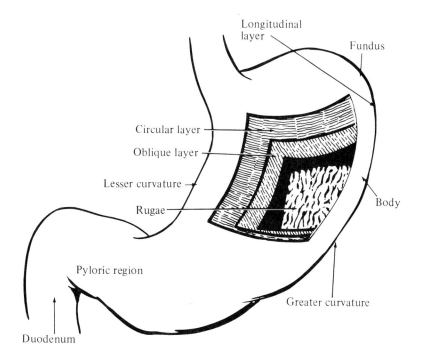

## Regulation of Gastric Juice Production

The nervous and endocrine systems stimulate the gastric glands to produce gastric juice. The nervous system is responsible for rapid production of gastric juice, whereas the endocrine system is responsible for slower, longer-lasting production of gastric juice.

**STIMULATION BY NERVOUS SYSTEM.** A person can stimulate the gastric glands by the sight, smell, thought, or taste of food. These stimuli are carried to the appropriate association areas of the cerebral cortex, the motor cortex, and the medulla oblongata. Nerve fibers of the parasympathetic division (vagus nerve) carry impulses rapidly to the gastric glands (Figure

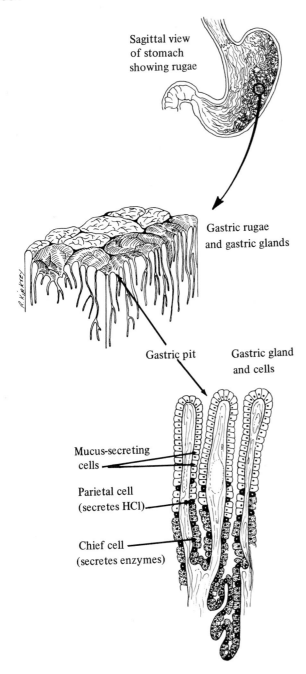

Sagittal view
of stomach
showing rugae

Gastric rugae
and gastric glands

Gastric pit

Gastric gland
and cells

Mucus-secreting
cells

Parietal cell
(secretes HCl)

Chief cell
(secretes enzymes)

Figure 19-11.  Gastric rugae and glands. The cells that compose each gastric gland and their secretions are shown.

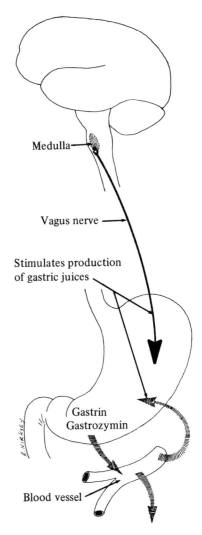

Medulla

Vagus nerve

Stimulates production
of gastric juices

Gastrin
Gastrozymin

Blood vessel

Figure 19-12.  Regulation of gastric juice production. Impulses carried by the vagus nerve rapidly stimulate the gastric glands to secrete gastric juices. Gastrin and gastrozymin hormones slowly stimulate the secretion of gastric juices.

19-12). This rapid stimulation of gastric glands insures that there will be a gastric juice present when food reaches the stomach.

Stretch receptor cells in the walls of the stomach are stimulated as the stomach stretches when it fills with food. Sensory impulses are carried to the medulla and motor impulses are carried back to the gastric glands by means of the vagus nerve.

## STIMULATION BY THE ENDOCRINE SYSTEM.

The pyloric region of the stomach secretes **gastrin** and **gastrozymin** hormones (Figure 19–12), when stimulated by products of protein digestion (polypeptides). The hormones are carried by the blood to the fundus and body regions of the stomach where the gastric glands are stimulated to produce gastric juice. Gastrin also is secreted from the duodenum when stimulated by polypeptides. **Enterogastrone** is released from the duodenum when stimulated by chyme, rich in lipids. Enterogastrone acts to inhibit production of gastric juice.

Some food may remain in the stomach for as long as three to four hours; therefore, a slow gradual release of gastric juice is needed to initiate digestion of these foods. Gastrin, gastrozymin, and enterogastrone are released slowly and regulate the release of gastric juice over a long period of time.

### Functions of the Stomach

1. **Reservoir for food:** the stomach can hold approximately 1000 ml of food while the food is prepared for further digestion.

2. **Secretion of gastric juices:** specialized cells in the gastric glands secrete 1000 to 2000 ml of gastric juice during a 24-hour period. The enzymes, primarily pepsin, act to initiate digestion of the food.

3. **Maintains acidic pH:** the gastric glands secrete a large amount of hydrochloric acid, so that the pH = 1 during digestion. An acidic pH is needed to activate the inactive pepsinogen to pepsin. The acidic pH also acts to destroy microbes that enter the stomach.

4. **Mixes and churns food to form chyme:** the peristaltic actions of the stomach plus the actions of the enzymes break down food particles into a semiliquid mass called chyme.

5. **Limited amount of absorption:** some water, alcohol, and chemical compounds are absorbed through the stomach into the blood.

## SMALL INTESTINE

The small intestine is the next part of the digestive tube, and it is about 2.5 cm in diameter (which is the reason it is called the small intestine). It winds and coils around for 6 to 7 meters from the stomach to the large intestine in the right inguinal region of the abdomen (Figure 19–13). The small intestine is composed of two layers of smooth muscle, compared to three for the stomach. A membrane, **mesentery,** attaches the small intestine to the posterior body wall.

### Parts of the Small Intestine

Starting at the stomach and moving to the large intestine, the parts of the small intestine are duodenum, jejunum, and ileum (Figure 19–13).

**DUODENUM.** The duodenum is the small intestine to which the pyloric region of the stomach attaches. It is C-shaped and is about 25 cm in length (Figure 19–13). Ducts from the gallbladder and pancreas joint the duodenum approximately 7.6 cm inferior to the pyloric sphincter valve.

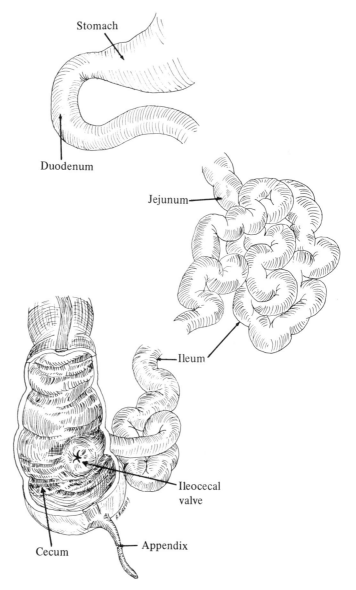

Figure 19-13. The three parts of the small intestine. Also shown is the ileocecal valve that regulates passage of materials from the ileum into the cecum.

Chyme gradually is moved through the pyloric sphincter valve into the duodenum. The ducts from the gallbladder and pancreas empty bile and digestive enzymes into the duodenum to act on the chyme.

**JEJUNUM.** The jejunum extends for approximately 2.4 meters, and then it gives rise to the ileum (Figure 19–13).

**ILEUM.** The ileum extends for about 3.6 meters until it connects to the large intestine. The **ileocecal valve** (Figure 19–13) opens from the ileum into the cecum part of the large intestine.

## Structural Features of the Small Intestine

The walls of the small intestine are composed of several layers of tissue (Figure 19-14). Starting with the inner layer and working outward, the layers are the mucosa, the submucosa, the circular smooth muscle, the longitudinal smooth muscle, and the serosa.

**MUCOSA.** The mucosa in the small intestine is composed of simple columnar tissue (Figure 19-14) with many mucus secreting **goblet cells** present. The simple columnar cells in the small intestine are specialized to absorb digested food in a liquid form. Even though the entire digestive tract is lined with a mucous membrane, the structure of the membrane varies from region to region. Figure 19-6 shows that the mucosa in the esophagus is composed of stratified squamous epithelial tissue. The mucosa in this area is specialized to resist friction of the solid ingested food. Figure 19-6 also shows that the mucosa in the esophagus is thrown into longitudinal folds, which allows it to expand as food passes through it during swallowing. The gastric mucosa in the stomach is thrown into **rugae** which allow the stomach to expand. Figure 19-14 shows that the intestinal mucosa is

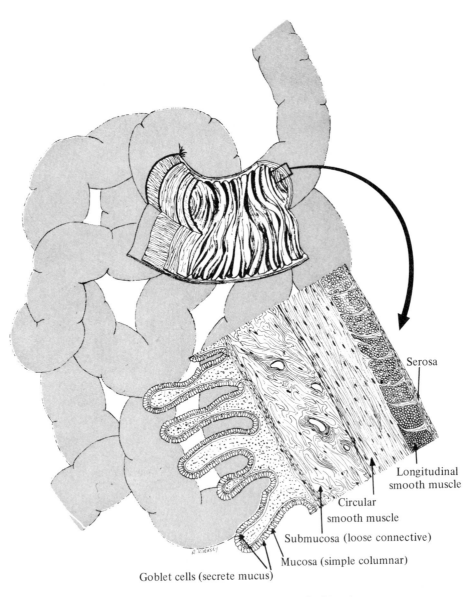

Serosa

Longitudinal smooth muscle

Circular smooth muscle

Submucosa (loose connective)

Mucosa (simple columnar)

Goblet cells (secrete mucus)

**Figure 19-14.** Layers of the intestinal tract.

thrown into fingerlike structures called **villi.** These structures increase the surface area for absorption many hundred times. Figure 19–15 shows a different view of the many thousands of villi that line the small intestine. Details concerning the blood supply and functions of the villi will be discussed later in the unit.

**SUBMUCOSA.** The submucosa is the next layer under the mucosa and is composed of loose connective tis-

sue (Figure 19–14). This layer connects the mucosa to the smooth muscle tissue.

**CIRCULAR AND LONGITUDINAL SMOOTH MUSCLE TISSUE.** These two layers of smooth muscle tissue contract slowly and rhythmically producing peristalsis (Figure 19–8) in the small intestine. The two layers of smooth muscle tissue are the same in the esophagus and small intestine; however, in the stomach there is a

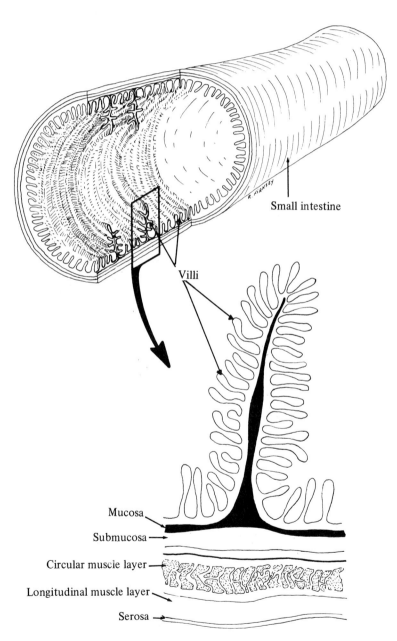

**Figure 19–15.** Structural features of the small intestine. The layers of the small intestine and villi are shown.

third layer of smooth muscle tissue, **oblique layer** (Figure 19–10).

**SEROSA.** The outer layer of the small intestine, **serosa,** is visceral peritoneum membrane. It secretes a serous fluid that reduces friction between the small intestine and other structures. This layer tends to join with the parietal peritoneum membrane to form the **abdominal mesentery** (Figure 19–14), which attaches the small intestine to the posterior abdominal wall.

### Intestinal Glands

The **crypts of Lieberkühn** are glands located between the villi. They secrete the intestinal juices, called **succus entericus,** which are slightly alkaline and contain all the enzymes necessary to digest carbohydrates, proteins, lipids, and nucleic acids.

**DUODENAL GLANDS. Brunner's glands,** located primarily in the duodenum, act to secrete mucus. The inner wall of the small intestine is protected from the digestive enzymes by a layer of mucus. Goblet cells, located along the entire length of the small intestine, also act to secrete mucus.

### Functions of the Small Intestine

**DIGESTION.** Digestive juices contain the enzymes necessary to complete the digestion or hydrolysis of food in chyme.

**ABSORPTION.** The basic chemical building blocks that result from digestion are absorbed through the villi into the bloodstream and lymphatic vessels.

**SECRETION OF HORMONES.** Gastrin and entero gastrone hormones regulate the production of gastric juices.

## LARGE INTESTINE (COLON)

The large intestine is approximately 6.3 cm in diameter, which is more than twice as large as the small intestine. It is approximately 1.4 to 1.8 meters in length.

### Regions of the Large Intestine

**CECUM.** The **cecum** is the pouchlike structure inferior to the **ileocecal valve** (Figure 19–16). The ileocecal valve opens from the ileum into the cecum. It opens to allow passage of feces from the ileum into the cecum, and closes to prevent their backflow into the ileum. Extending inferiorly from the cecum is a slender tube called the **vermiform appendix.** It is lined with lymphatic tissue. Due to its position, feces and bacteria frequently accumulate in the appendix, resulting in its inflammation (appendicitis) and possible rupture. Surgical removal of the appendix usually is necessary to correct the above problems. Two theories exist concerning the function of the appendix. One long-held theory is that the appendix is a nonfunctional structure, which only serves to cause appendicitis. A newer theory is that the lymphatic tissue in the appendix acts to filter out bacteria, like the Peyer's patches and other lymph nodes.

**ASCENDING COLON.** The **ascending colon** is the next part of the large intestine and it extends superiorly on the right side of the body from the cecum to the inferior surface of the liver. Here it turns abruptly to the left, forming the **hepatic flexure** (Figure 19–16).

**TRANSVERSE COLON.** The **transverse colon** extends from the ascending colon across the body from the right to left, inferior to the stomach (Figure 19–16). Near the spleen it turns downward, forming the splenic flexure.

**DESCENDING COLON.** The **descending colon** extends inferiorly from the splenic flexure to about the level of the iliac crest.

**SIGMOID COLON.** The **sigmoid colon** is an S-shaped portion of the colon (Figure 19–16) that extends from the descending colon, anterior to the rectum.

**RECTUM.** The **rectum** is the final few centimeters of the large intestine.

**ANAL CANAL.** The anal canal is the canal to the outside of the body. It is approximately 2.5 to 3.0 cm long. The mucous lining of the anal canal is in the form of folds called **rectal columns** (Figure 19–17), which contain arteries and veins. Inflammation of the veins is called **hemorrhoids** or **piles.** The opening to the outside of the body is called the anus. Two sphincters guard the anus. The **internal anal sphincter muscle** is composed of smooth muscle; therefore, it is not controlled voluntarily. Surrounding the outside of the anus is the **external anal sphincter muscle,** which is composed of skeletal muscle and is therefore under voluntary control.

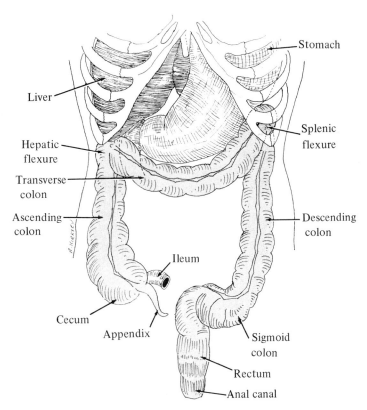

Figure 19-16.   The parts of the large intestine.

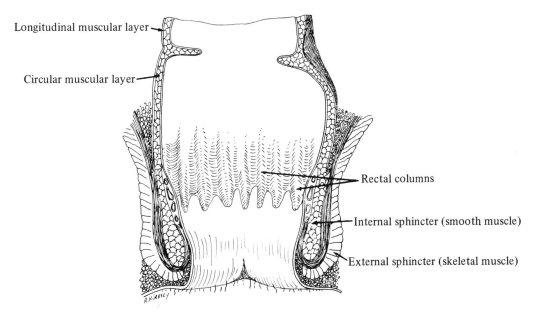

Figure 19-17.   The anal canal and sphincter muscles.

## Structural Characteristics
## of the Large Intestinal Wall

A mucous membrane lines the large intestine, but it is not arranged in folds and it lacks villi. The mucous membrane contains crypts of Lieberkühn glands that secrete large amounts of mucus, but no digestive enzymes. The circular muscle layer of the large intestine is the same as the rest of the digestive tube. However, the longitudinal muscle layer is incomplete. It is arranged in three flat layers, called **taeniae coli** (Figure 19–18). The layers are shorter than the large intestine itself; therefore, they produce bulges in the large intestine called **haustra.**

## Bacteria in the Large Intestine

A large number of bacteria are found in the large intestine. These intestinal bacteria are of nutritional value to humans. They function to produce the B-complex vitamins, vitamin K, and niacin, which are made available to the body. This function will be discussed later.

## Functions

**REABSORPTION OF WATER.** Large amounts of water are involved in the hydrolysis of food in the small intestine. The large intestine absorbs up to 6000 ml of this water per day into the blood. This is necessary to prevent dehydration.

**ELIMINATION OF WASTES (FECES).** Feces are the waste material that is left after the food and necessary water have been absorbed. The large intestine undergoes peristaltic contractions, thereby moving the feces to the anal canal. The internal and external anal sphincter muscles regulate excretion of the feces.

**SYNTHESIS OF VITAMINS.** The intestinal flora and bacteria produce B-complex vitamins, vitamin K, and niacin.

# LIVER, GALLBLADDER, AND PANCREAS

These organs attach to the intestinal portion of the digestive tube and actually are derivatives of the intestine. The liver, gallbladder, and pancreas contribute to the small intestine several chemical compounds important for digestion. Thus, these organs are designated as accessory digestive organs.

## Liver

The liver is inferior to the diaphragm, but in contact with it, and it occupies the right hypochondriac and a portion of the epigastric regions of the abdomen. It is somewhat arched since it is in contact with the diaphragm (Figure 19–19). The liver is the largest organ in the body and weighs approximately 2.7 to 3.6 kilograms (kg). It is dark reddish brown in color.

**ANATOMY OF THE LIVER.** The liver is divided into the right and left lobes. The **falciform ligament** (Figure 19–19) separates the larger right lobe from the smaller left lobe. The right lobe is composed of smaller

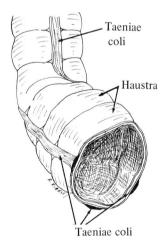

**Figure 19–18.** Structural characteristics of the large intestine.

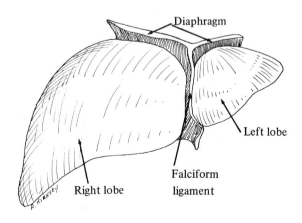

**Figure 19–19.** Basic external anatomy of the liver.

lobes. Each lobe is composed of many **liver lobules,** which are the **functional units** of the liver. The falciform ligament attaches the liver to the anterior body wall and inferior surface of the diaphragm.

**BLOOD SUPPLY TO THE LIVER.** The arteries and veins associated with the liver are vital for its many functions. The **hepatic artery** and **portal vein** both bring blood to the liver lobules. The hepatic artery (Figure 19–20) brings oxygenated blood to the liver tissue, and the portal vein brings blood rich in the products of digestion from the small intestine. The hepatic artery and portal vein branch numerous times to form **interlobular arteries** and **veins** (Figure 19–21). Blood flows from these vessels through sinusoid cavities into central veins located in the center of liver lobules. The central veins converge to form sublobular veins, which converge to form hepatic veins. The hepatic veins drain blood from the liver into the inferior vena cava. Figure 19–22 shows a summary of the blood supply to the liver.

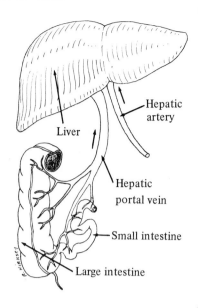

**Figure 19-20.** Arterial and venous blood supply to the liver.

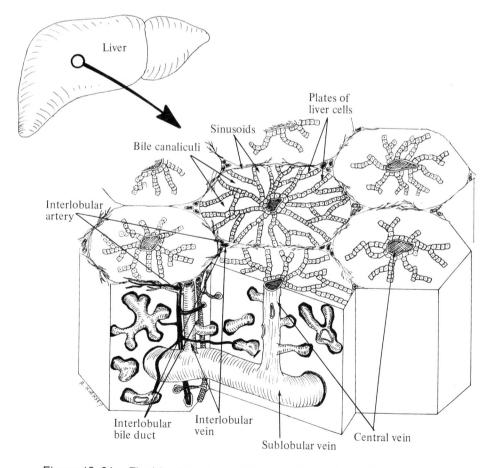

**Figure 19-21.** The blood supply and bile ducts that make up liver lobules.

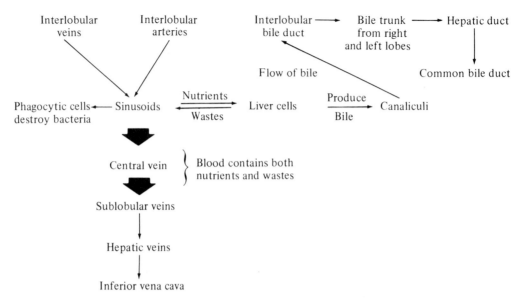

**Figure 19-22.** Flow of blood and bile through liver lobule.

The blood supply to the liver differs from the blood supply to most organs in the following ways:

1. The interlobular arteries and veins are not joined to each other by capillaries, but rather by sinusoids. The exchange of nutrients and wastes occurs as blood flows through the sinusoids.

2. Normally arteries bring nutrients to the tissues and veins remove the wastes; however, in the liver the hepatic artery delivers oxygenated blood but the portal vein brings the majority of nutrients to the liver tissue.

**LIVER LOBULES.** The liver is composed of many **lobules** (Figure 19-21), which are shaped like a six-sided (hexagonal) structure with a central vein in the center of each lobule. Radiating outward to the periphery of the lobule are plates of liver cells. Located around the periphery of a lobule are **interlobular arteries and veins** plus bile ducts. The interlobular artery and vein connect to the central vein by blood sinusoids. Phagocytic cells that are part of the reticuloendothelial system line the sinusoids. Blood passes from the interlobular arteries and veins through the sinusoids to the central vein. The sinusoids act as capillaries in that the exchange of nutrients and wastes between the blood and liver cells occurs here. The interlobular veins bring blood rich in digested product to the sinusoids where a certain amount are exchanged with the liver cells. Waste products move from the liver cells into the blood as it passes

through the sinusoids to the central vein. The phagocytic cells destroy any microorganisms that may be in the blood. The blood that drains into the central vein of a lobule has given off a certain amount of its nutrients to the liver cells and picked up waste products. The central veins from the lobules converge to form sublobular veins, which converge to form hepatic veins. The hepatic veins drain blood from the liver into the inferior vena cava.

**BILE STRUCTURES.** Around the periphery of each lobule are located **interlobular bile ducts.** Radiating out to these bile ducts are bile canaliculi (Figure 19–21) located between the plates of liver cells. Bile is produced by the liver cells and drains into the canaliculi, which drain bile into the interlobular bile ducts. The interlobular ducts combine repeatedly until a large duct drains bile from each lobe. Large bile trunks from the right and left lobes unite to form the hepatic bile duct (Figure 19–23). Figure 19–22 is a flow chart of the passage of blood and bile through liver lobules. The hepatic bile duct combines with a duct from the gallbladder to form the common bile duct. The liver cells are stimulated to secrete bile by the hormone secretin which is produced by the duodenum.

**FUNCTIONS OF THE LIVER.** The liver is an important organ because of the many functions it performs. Chemically it synthesizes, hydrolyzes, and stores compounds.

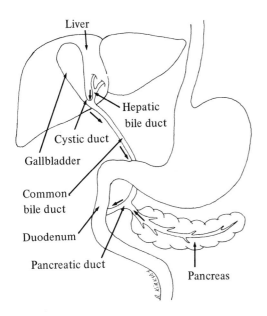

**Figure 19-23.** Bile ducts from the liver and gallbladder are shown as they join with the pancreatic duct just before entering the duodenum.

**PRODUCTION OF BILE.** The liver produces approximately 600 to 800 ml of bile per day. Bile contains various chemical compounds, one of which is **bile salts.** Bile acts to emulsify lipid molecules or increase their surface area, which facilitates the action of lipase (lipid enzyme). Bile salts also aid in the absorption of fatty acids into the bloodstream.

**METABOLISM OF ORGANIC COMPOUNDS.** The liver plays a major role in hydrolysis and synthesis of carbohydrates, lipids, and proteins. These functions will be discussed in greater detail later.

**DESTRUCTION OF WORN OUT RBCs.** The phagocytic cells in the blood sinusoids destroy worn out RBCs. Bile salts contain **bilirubin,** which is a waste product of RBC breakdown.

**REMOVAL OF BACTERIA AND OTHER HARMFUL MATERIALS.** The phagocytic cells in the sinusoids also destroy bacteria and other harmful substances.

**SYNTHESIS OF BLOOD PROTEINS.** **Fibrinogen** and **prothrombin** are proteins that are vital for the blood-clotting process. The natural anticlotting substance, **heparin,** also is produced by the liver.

**CLINICAL LIVER TESTS.** Since the liver is such an important organ, several clinical tests are performed to detect various liver malfunctions.

## Gallbladder

The gallbladder is a smooth muscular sac located on the inferior surface of the liver (Figure 19–23). It is about 7.5 to 10.0 cm in length and has a bile capacity of about 40 to 50 ml.

The **cystic duct** from the gallbladder joins the **hepatic bile duct** from the liver to form the **common bile duct.** The common bile duct joins the duodenum approximately 7.6 cm inferior to the pyloric valve. The **sphincter of Oddi** regulates the passage of bile into the duodenum.

**FUNCTIONS.** The gallbladder stores and concentrates bile by the removal of water. When lipids enter the duodenum, a hormone, **cholecystokinin,** is released, which causes the muscular walls of the gallbladder to contract and send bile into the duodenum.

## Pancreas

The pancreas is a narrow organ that extends from the duodenum to the spleen. The head of the pancreas lies in the "C" of the duodenum, and the tail comes in contact with the spleen (Figure 19–23). The pancreas functions both as an endocrine and exocrine gland.

**FUNCTIONAL UNITS.** The pancreas functions by secreting hormones and digestine enzymes.

1. Secretion of hormones. Irregular clumps of cells, called **Islets of Langerhans** (Figure 19–24), are scattered throughout the pancreas. The Islets of Langerhans surround capillaries, which carry hormones away from the pancreas. Two types of cells, **alpha** and **beta,** compose the Islets. The **alpha cells** secrete the hormone, **glucagon** (stimulates the liver to release glucose). The **beta cells** secrete **insulin,** (important for carbohydrate metabolism). The functions of these hormones were discussed previously.

2. Secretion of enzymes. An enzyme secreting region, **acinus,** is composed of a ring of epithelial tissue around the opening (lumen) to a duct (Figure 19–24). Each acinus secretes enzyme rich pancreatic juice into its duct. The enzymes are necessary for digestion of proteins, lipids, and carbohydrates. The ducts

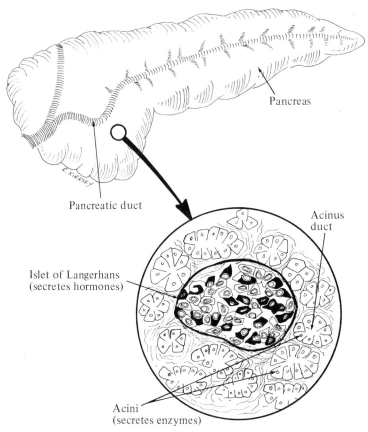

**Figure 19–24.**    Hormone and enzyme secreting areas of the pancreas.

from the acini join to form the main pancreatic duct, which joins the common bile duct just before entering the duodenum.

## PERITONEUM

The inner surface of the abdominal wall is lined by a double-layered membrane, the **peritoneum.** The layer lining the abdominal wall is called the **parietal peritoneum;** the innermost layer covering the surface of the abdominal organs is called the **visceral peritoneum** (Figure 19–25). The peritoneum is a serous membrane, and the serous fluid acts as a lubricant enabling the abdominal organs to move over each other and rub against the abdominal wall with very little friction.

### Mesentery

The **abdominal mesentery** (Figure 19–25) attaches the length of the small intestine and most of the large intestine to the posterior abdominal wall.

### Omenta

The **greater omentum** attaches to the greater curvature of the stomach (Figure 19–25) and the transverse colon. It contains a considerable amount of fat and hangs down in front of the intestine, much like an apron. The **lesser omentum** connects the stomach and duodenum to the liver.

## 3    CHEMICAL DIGESTION

Our discussions so far have concentrated on the ingestion and physical breakdown of food into small particles. The small particles increase the surface area for the action of the digestive enzymes. Digestion reactions or hydrolytic reactions break the bonds that connect the building blocks of carbohydrates, lipids, and proteins. The small chemical building blocks then will be absorbed through the small intestine into the blood.

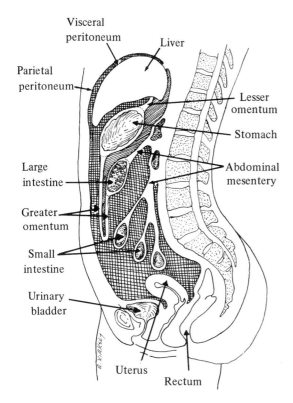

Figure 19-25. Sagittal view of the peritoneum and extensions.

Previously, we discussed the fact that enzymes are very specific as to the substrates with which they interact. For example, the disaccharide, maltose, is digested by the enzyme maltase.

We will discuss the secretion of enzymes and chemical reactions that involve carbohydrates, lipids, and proteins in each organ of the digestive tract. We will assume that a person is eating a meal that contains carbohydrates, lipids, and proteins.

## DIGESTION IN THE MOUTH

Saliva contains only one digestive enzyme, salivary amylase, which acts on starch molecules. Starch molecules are polysaccharides $(C_6H_{10}O_5)_n$ and **salivary amylase** plus water molecules break every other bond connecting the many glucose molecules. Dextrin and maltose (disaccharide) molecules result from the hydrolytic action of salivary amylase. The final digestion of dextrins and maltose to glucose occurs in the small intestine.

There is no digestion of proteins and lipids in the mouth. Most of the digestion in the mouth is the physical breakdown of food.

## DIGESTION IN THE STOMACH

When the bolus reaches the stomach, gastric juices are present that are secreted by the gastric glands. The hormone, **gastrin,** is released by the duodenum and is carried by the blood to the stomach (Figure 19-26) where it stimulates the gastric glands to release gastric juices.

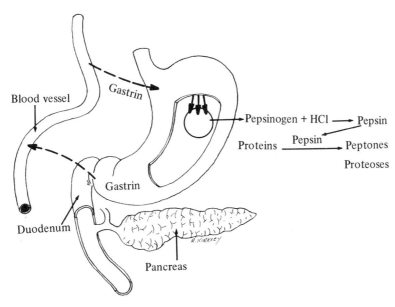

Figure 19-26. Actions of gastrin hormone and pepsin enzyme. Gastrin, released by the duodenum, stimulates the release of digestive enzymes in the stomach. The activation of pepsin and breakdown of proteins are shown.

There are various digestive enzymes in the gastric juices.

## Carbohydrate Digestion

The digestion of starch by salivary amylase and water is inhibited in the stomach because of the high concentration of hydrochloric acid. Very little, if any, **carbohydrase** (carbohydrate-splitting enzyme) is produced in gastric juices, therefore, there is little carbohydrate digestion in the stomach.

## Protein Digestion

The majority of digestion occurring in the stomach is protein digestion. The gastric glands secrete a large amount of **pepsinogen** and **hydrochloric acid.** Hydrochloric acid activates **pepsinogen** to **pepsin,** which catalyzes the hydrolysis (Figure 19–26) of the peptide bonds of proteins, forming peptones and proteoses. Pepsin is an unusual enzyme in that it is quite active in a highly acidic medium. Most enzymes are denatured and inactivated in an acidic medium.

## Lipid Digestion

The gastric glands secrete a very small amount of **lipase** (lipid-splitting enzyme) and, in addition, the high acidic level of the stomach inactivates lipase. A minimal amount of lipid digestion occurs in the stomach because of the small secretion and inactivation of lipase.

The peristaltic contractions of the stomach break the food into smaller pieces. Little breakdown of food by enzymes occurs in the stomach because of the small amount secreted and the high concentration of hydrochloric acid. The food in the stomach is gradually changed into a semifluid state, called **chyme.** The chyme gradually is passed through the pyloric sphincter valve into the duodenum, where the majority of digestion takes place.

## Intestinal and Pancreatic Enzymes

The crypts of Lieberkühn in the small intestine secrete the enzymes **enterokinase, proteases (erepsin), mal-** tase, **sucrase,** and **lactase.** The activities of these enzymes will be discussed shortly.

The **acini** in the pancreas secrete the following digestive enzymes: **pancreatic amylase (amylopsin), pancreatic lipase (steapsin), pancreatic proteases (trypsin, chymotrypsin,** and **carboxypeptidase).** The chemical activities of these enzymes will be discussed later along with those of the intestinal enzymes.

In addition to receiving digestive enzymes, the duodenum also receives bile from the gallbladder and liver. **Bile aids in the chemical digestion of lipids, but it is not classified as an enzyme.**

## Chemical Activity of Digestive Enzymes and Bile

The chyme that enters the duodenum contains partly digested carbohydrates, proteins, and intact lipid molecules. The pancreatic enzymes and the intestinal enzymes hydrolyze the molecules to their simplest chemical form, which can be absorbed into the bloodstream.

**DIGESTION OF CARBOHYDRATES.** The digestion of starch molecules begins in the mouth with **salivary amylase** breaking most starch molecules down to dextrins. **Pancreatic amylase** (Figure 19–27) breaks dextrins and starch molecules down to the disaccharide, maltose. The small intestine secretes the enzyme, **maltase,** which breaks maltose down to glucose molecules. The reaction is summarized below and also shown in Figure 19–27.

Disaccharides such as sucrose (table sugar), lactose (milk sugar), and maltose (malt sugar) that are ingested in the food are broken down by the appropriate intestinal enzymes to simple monosaccharides:

$$\text{Sucrose} \xrightarrow[\text{H}_2\text{O}]{\text{Intestinal sucrase}} \text{glucose} + \text{fructose}$$

$$\text{Maltose} \xrightarrow[\text{H}_2\text{O}]{\text{Intestinal maltase}} \text{glucose} + \text{glucose}$$

$$\text{Lactose} \xrightarrow[\text{H}_2\text{O}]{\text{Intestinal lactase}} \text{glucose} + \text{galactose}$$

These simple monosaccharides are ready to be absorbed into the bloodstream, which will be discussed shortly.

**DIGESTION OF LIPIDS (FATS).** Bile reacts with lipid molecules to emulsify them or increase their surface area. **Pancreatic lipase** reacts with emulsified fats to break them down to glycerol and fatty acids (Figure 19–27).

$$\left.\begin{array}{l}\text{Starch} \\ \text{Dextrins}\end{array}\right\} \xrightarrow[\text{H}_2\text{O}]{\text{Pancreatic amylase}} \text{maltose} \xrightarrow[\text{H}_2\text{O}]{\text{Intestinal maltase}} \text{Glucose}$$
$$\text{(polysaccharides)} \qquad\qquad \text{(disaccharide)} \qquad\qquad \text{(monosaccharide)}$$

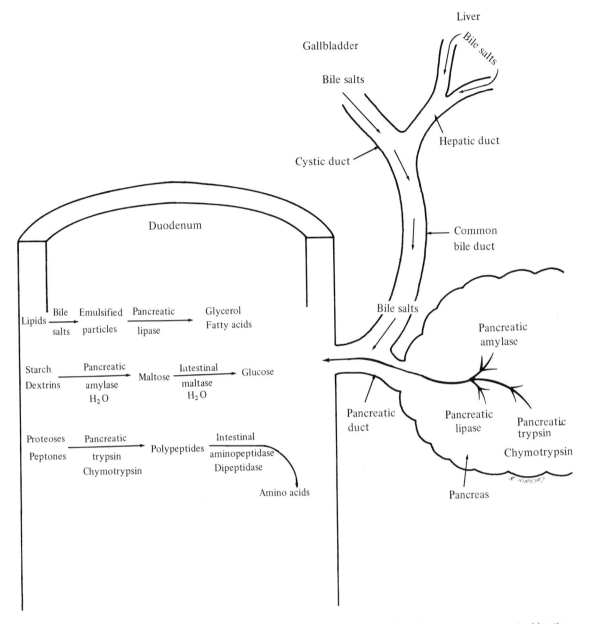

**Figure 19-27.** Chemical digestion in the duodenum. The reactions of digestive enzymes secreted by the pancreas and duodenum, plus bile salts, are shown.

$$\text{Lipids} \xrightarrow{\text{Bile salts}} \text{emulsified particles}$$
$$\text{emulsified particles} \xrightarrow[\text{lipase}]{\text{Pancreatic}} \text{glycerol} + \text{fatty acids}$$

**DIGESTION OF PROTEINS.** The breakdown of proteins begins in the stomach with pepsin breaking peptide bonds and forming proteoses and peptones. The pancreatic proteases (trypsin and chymotrypsin) break more peptide bonds of proteoses and peptones, resulting in polypeptides.

**Intestinal proteoses** (aminopeptidase and dipepti-

dase) break the remaining peptide bonds of polypeptides, resulting in amino acids (Figure 19-27). Trypsin and chymotrypsin are secreted in inactive forms, trypsinogen and chymotrypsinogen, from the pancreas. Trypsinogen is activated to trypsin by the enzyme, **enterokinase**. Trypsin then activates chymotrypsinogen to chymotrypsin.

$$\left.\begin{array}{c}\text{Proteoses} \\ \text{Peptones}\end{array}\right\} \xrightarrow{\text{Chymotrypsin}} \text{polypeptides} \xrightarrow{\text{Dipeptidase}} \begin{array}{c}\text{amino} \\ \text{acids}\end{array}$$

**TABLE 19–1.** *Digestive Enzymes*

| Enzymes | Source | Substrate | Products |
|---|---|---|---|
| *Carbohydrases* | | | |
| Salivary amylase | Salivary glands | Starch, glycogen, dextrins | Dextrins, maltose |
| Pancreatic amylase | Pancreas (acini cells) | Starch, glycogen, dextrins | Maltose |
| Maltase | | Maltose | Glucose |
| Sucrase | Intestinal glands | Sucrose | Glucose, fructose |
| Lactase | | Lactose | Glucose, galactose |
| *Lipases* | | | |
| Gastric lipase | Gastric glands (stomach) | Lipids | Fatty acids, glycerol |
| Pancreatic lipase (steapsin) | Pancreas (acini cells) | Emulsified fats | Fatty acids, glycerol |
| *Proteinases* | | | |
| Pepsin | Gastric glands | Protein | Proteoses, peptones |
| Enterokinase | Intestinal glands | Activates typsinogen | Trypsin |
| Trypsinogen (trypsin, active form) | Pancreas | Proteoses, peptones | Polypeptides |
| Chymotrypsinogen (chymotrypsin, active form) | Pancreas | Proteoses, peptones | Polypeptides |
| Amino peptidase, dipeptidase | Intestines | Polypeptides | Amino acids |

Table 19–1 lists all the digestive enzymes, their sources, and products.

# 4   ABSORPTION OF DIGESTED PRODUCTS

After the hydrolytic digestion of food occurs in the jejunum, the small chemical molecules are ready to be absorbed into the blood in the ileum region. There are anatomic and chemical reasons why the majority of absorption occurs in the small intestine:

1. The hydrolysis of the complex organic molecules into small chemical molecules is completed in the small intestine.
2. The surface area necessary for the absorption is increased considerably by the presence of **villi** and **microvilli.**
3. The blood and lymph supply to the villi is excellent.

## VILLI AND MICROVILLI

The mucosal membrane of the small intestine exhibits many folds. Along these folds, especially in the ileum region, are fingerlike extensions, called **villi** (Figure 19–28). Projecting from the surface of the **villi** are microscopic structures called **microvilli.** The outer surface of each villus is composed of columnar epithelium. The inner surface of each villus is characterized by a blood capillary network and a lymph capillary vessel, called a **lacteal.** The small chemical building blocks pass across the columnar epithelium into the blood and lymph vessels.

## METHODS BY WHICH MATERIALS MOVE INTO THE VILLI

The methods by which materials mope into the blood and lymph capillaries include diffusion, osmosis, and active transport. We will discuss how each group of chemical molecules is absorbed:

### Fatty Acids and Glycerol

Fatty acids and glycerol pass across the villi by diffusion. Bile salts help fatty acids diffuse through the villi, whereas glycerol diffuses across without any aid. Once inside the epithelial cells, the fatty acids and glycerol combine to form neutral fats, before passing into the **lymph capillary (lacteal)** (Figure 19–29).

### Monosaccharides

Glucose, fructose, and galactose are absorbed into the blood by active transport (Figure 19–29). One theory is that sodium ions (Na$^+$) combine with simple sugars and

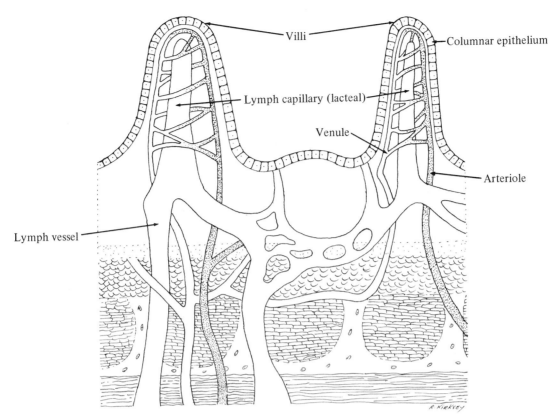

Figure 19-28. Blood and lymph supply to each intestinal villus.

aid their movement through epithelial cells into the blood. Active transport of the simple sugars requires energy. This method is the only one responsible for absorbing monosaccharides since the concentration of monosaccharides in the intestine generally is lower than that in the blood.

## Amino Acids

Amino acids are absorbed by active transport in the same manner as are monosaccharides. Again, one theory is that sodium ions (Na+) combine with amino acids and help to transport them through the epithelial tissue into the blood. (Figure 19-29).

## Water and Electrolytes

Water is absorbed by osmosis. As all of the nutrients and ions (solutes) are absorbed into the villi, the increased solute concentration increases the osmotic pressure inside the villi. The high osmotic pressure inside the villi acts to pull water through the epithelial tissue into the blood (Figure 19-29).

It is thought that the absorption of sodium, chloride, calcium, and potassium ions is by active transport. Most negative ions are absorbed by diffusion.

## Transport Pathway of Digested Materials

Blood containing digested nutrients leaves the villi in veins, which converge to join the portal vein of the hepatic portal system. The liver lobules destroy bacteria as well as remove a certain amount of nutrients from the blood, which has been carried to the lobules by branches of the portal vein. These actions of the liver act to remove foreign organisms from the blood as well as a certain amount of nutrients, before it empties into the inferior vena cava and the general circulation. Removal of a certain amount of nutrients is necessary to regulate blood sugar and various ions.

The lymph capillaries (lacteals) leave the villi with neutral fats and converge to form lymph vessels. The lymph drains through many lymph nodes in the mesentery membrane (especially the Peyer's patches in the ileum region), and the nodes filter out bacteria and secrete antibodies. The lymph moves through lymph vessels into the **cisterna chyli** and continues upward until the lymph passes through the thoracic duct into the left subclavian vein.

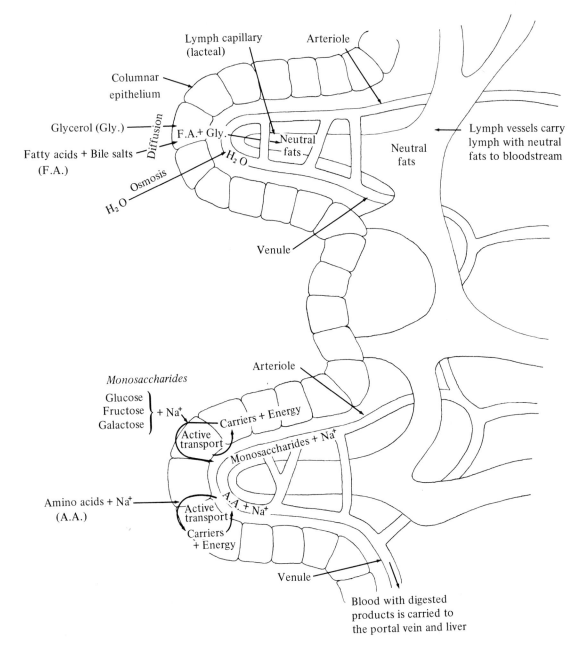

**Figure 19-29.** The absorption of digested products by diffusion, active transport, and osmosis.

---

# SUMMARY

---

### Functions of the Digestive System

Five functions of the digestive system are (1) physically breaks down food, (2) transports food through digestive tract, (3) secretion of enzymes, (4) absorption of digested products, (5) excretion of feces.

## Ingestion and Physical Breakdown of Food

A. Mouth and accessory digestive organs
   1. Mouth composed of cheeks and hard and soft palates.
   2. Accessory organs include teeth, tongue, and salivary glands.
B. Tongue: composed of skeletal muscles; anchored to hyoid bone; functions, taste, speech, swallowing, and chewing.
C. Salivary glands
   1. Three glands secrete saliva: (a) parotid, located at angle of jaw; Stenson's duct carries saliva into mouth; (b) sublingual, located under tongue; ducts carry saliva into mouth; (c) submandibular, inferior to mandible; Wharton's ducts open into lower floor of mouth.
   2. Chemical composition of saliva: (1) mucin, gives saliva slippery consistency; (2) salivary amylase (ptyalin), enzyme that breaks down the polysaccharide starch.
   3. Functions of saliva: (1) helps hold food in a ball, (2) aids swallowing of food, (3) initiates digestion of starch.
D. Pharynx, esophagus, and swallowing of food
   1. Pharynx: food moves from mouth into pharynx due to swallowing reflex center.
   2. Esophagus: smooth and skeletal muscle tube; located posterior to trachea; sphincter-like valve, cardiac valve, opens into stomach.
E. Stomach
   1. J-shaped and located in epigastric and left hypogastric regions of abdomen.
   2. Divided into (a) fundus, superior region; (b) body, middle region; (c) pyloric, joins stomach to the duodenum.
   3. Cardiac valve opens to allow food into stomach; pyloric sphincter valve regulates passage of chyme into duodenum.
   4. Mucous lining and gastric glands of stomach: inner lining is mucous membrane, which forms rugae; three different types of cells in lining: (a) chief, secretes pepsinogen; (b) parietal cells, secrete hydrochloric acid (HCl); (c) mucous, secrete mucus.
   5. Regulation of gastric juice production: (a) stimulation by nervous system; sight, smell, thought, or taste of food stimulates nerve responses to cells by vagus nerve; (b) stimulation by endocrine system; pyloric region secretes gastrin and gastrozymin hormones that stimulate production of gastric juice.
   6. Functions of the stomach: (a) reservior for food, (b) secretion of gastric juices, (c) maintains acidic pH, (d) mixes and churns food to form chyme, (e) limited amount of absorption.
F. Small intestine: about 2.5 cm in diameter; winds and coils around 6 to 7 meters from stomach to large intestine; parts of small intestine include duodenum, jejunum, and ileum.
   1. Structural features: layers of tissue composing the small intestine starting with the inside are (a) mucosa, arranged into rugae and villi; (b) submucosa, composed of loose connective tissue and functions to connect mucosa to smooth muscle layer; (c) circular and longitudinal smooth muscle tissue, contract slowly and rhythmically, thereby producing peristalsis; (d) serosa, visceral peritoneum that secretes serous fluid and reduces friction between small intestine and other organs.
   2. Intestinal glands: (a) crypts of Lieberkühn, located between villi and secrete intestinal juices that contain digestive juices; (b) Brunner's, located primarily in duodenum and secrete mucus.
   3. Functions: (a) digestion, completion of digestion occurs in small intestine; (2) absorption, basic chemical building blocks that result from digestion are absorbed; (3) secretion of hormones, gastrin and entrogastrone, regulate production of gastric juices.
G. Large intestine (colon)
   1. Regions: cecum, ascending, colon, transverse colon, descending colon, sigmoid colon, rectum, and anal canal.

2. Structural characteristics of large intestinal wall: lined with mucous membrane but not arranged into rugae and villi; longitudinal muscle layer is arranged in three flat layers, taeniae coli, which result in haustra.
3. Bacteria in large intestine: bacteria produce B-complex vitamins, vitamin K, and niacin.
4. Functions: (a) reabsorption of water, (b) elimination of wastes (feces), (c) synthesis of vitamins.

H. Liver, gallbladder, and pancreas
  1. Liver: inferior to diaphragm; located in right hypochondriac and epigastric regions of abdomen.
    a. Anatomy: divided into right and left lobes; each lobe composed of many lobules.
    b. Blood supply: hepatic artery brings oxygenated blood to the liver; hepatic portal vein brings blood rich in digested products to liver; interlobular arteries and veins branch off hepatic artery and portal vein; blood flows ultimately into central veins in the center of lobules, which converge to form hepatic veins.
    c. Liver lobules: six-sided (hexagonal) structure; central vein in center; interlobular arteries and veins around periphery of a lobule; sinusoids connect central veins to interlobular arteries, which act as capillaries in exchange of nutrients and waste.
    d. Bile structures: interlobular bile ducts around periphery of lobules; bile canaliculi, between plates of liver cells, carry bile to interlobular bile ducts.
    e. Functions: (1) production of bile, (2) metabolism of organic compounds, (3) destruction of worn out RBCs, (4) removal of bacteria and other harmful substances, (5) synthesis of blood proteins.

I. Gallbladder
  1. Anatomy and location: smooth muscular sac; located on inferior surface of liver; holds about 40 to 50 ml of bile; cystic duct from gallbladder joins hepatic duct to form common bile duct, which joins duodenum.
  2. Functions: storage of bile; bile is stored and concentrated in gallbladder; cholecystokinin hormone, released by duodenum when fat enters it, stimulates contraction of gallbladder.

J. Pancreas
  1. Anatomy and location: narrow, thin organ that extends from duodenum to spleen.
  2. Functions: (a) secretion of hormones, insulin and glucagon hormones are secreted, (b) secretion of enzymes, enzymes necessary for digestion of proteins, lipids, and carbohydrates are secreted.

K. Peritoneum
  1. Double-layered membrane; composed of visceral and parietal layers.
  2. Mesentery and omenta are extensions of peritoneum.

**Chemical Digestion**

A. Digestion in mouth: salivary amylase enzyme breaks starch molecules into dextrin and maltose.
B. Digestion in stomach
  1. Carbohydrate digestion: very little occurs due to hydrochloric acid denaturing enzymes.
  2. Protein digestion: pepsinogen is activated by hydrochloric acid to pepsin, which degrades proteins to peptones and proteoses.
  3. Lipid digestion: minimal amount occurs as a result of the acidic level.
C. Digestion in the small intestine
  1. Intestinal and pancreatic enzymes: the intestine secretes the following enzymes: enterokinase, proteoses (erepsin), maltase, sucrase, and lactase; enzymes secreted by the pancreas are pancreatic amylase, pancreatic lipase, and pancreatic proteoses.
  2. Chemical activity of digestive enzymes and bile
    a. Digestion of carbohydrates

21. The pancreas secretes digestive enzymes only.

22. Liver lobules are sites where exchange of nutrients occurs in the liver.

23. Osmosis is involved in absorption of water.

24. Veins transport nutrients from small intestine to lymph vessels.

25. Lacteals are lymph capillaries that transport fat from villi to lymph vessels, which carry them into blood.

## Chapter 20

# METABOLISM OF LIPIDS, CARBOHYDRATES, AND PROTEINS

After reading and studying this chapter, a student should be able to:

1. Discuss anabolism of carbohydrates in liver.
2. Describe three results of anaerobic respiration of glucose.
3. Describe four results of one citric acid cycle.
4. Discuss how many ATPs are synthesized by passage of a pair of electrons down the electron transport system.
5. Discuss beta oxidation of fatty acids as to the process and products produced.
6. Describe anabolism of lipids.
7. Distinguish between essential and nonessential amino acids.
8. Describe deamination of amino groups and synthesis of urea.
9. Differentiate between positive and negative nitrogen balance and give conditions that can cause each.

*After the complex lipids, carbohydrates and proteins are digested into their basic chemical building blocks and are transported to cells throughout the body. Inside the cells the basic chemical molecules undergo chemical reactions. The term **metabolism** refers to all the chemical reactions that absorbed chemical molecules undergo inside cells.*

# 1 ANABOLISM AND CATABOLISM

**Metabolism** is divided into two phases, **anabolism** and **catabolism. Anabolism** is a buildup phase or involves synthesis reactions. Each body cell converts the simple molecules into more complex molecules that are vital to maintain homeostasis of that cell. For example, the production of structural proteins inside a cell involves the synthesis or combining of various amino acids. **Catabolism** is a breakdown phase or involves the decomposition of complex molecules into more simple molecules (decomposition reaction). This phase is important since it furnishes the energy necessary for anabolism and other body functions.

We will discuss the anabolism and catabolism reactions of carbohydrates, lipids, and proteins. Also we will discuss the hormones that regulate the anabolic and catabolic reactions.

# 2 METABOLISM OF CARBOHYDRATES

The main function of carbohydrates is the release of energy as they are broken down by catabolic reactions. If a person digests and absorbs excessive quantities of monosaccharides, the excess is converted into polysaccharide (glycogen) and depot fat by anabolic reactions. The glycogen and depot fat are stored and will be used as reserve sources of energy when needed.

## *ANABOLISM*

The liver is a primary site of **anabolic reactions.** Monosaccharide molecules (glucose, fructose, and galactose)

are transported from the small intestine into the liver by the portal vein. The liver cells combine the monosaccharides to form glycogen (Figure 20–1). This synthesis of monosaccharides to form glycogen is called **glycogenesis;** and the hormone **insulin** aids this process (Figure 20–1):

$$\text{Many monosaccharides} + \text{many monosaccharides} \xrightarrow{\text{Insulin}} \text{glycogen}$$

If the blood glucose level is low, not all of the glucose carried to the liver will be converted to glycogen and stored; but rather some of it will pass through the liver directly into the general circulation. The normal concentration of glucose in the blood is 80 to 110 mg per 100 ml of blood. Glycogenesis helps to maintain this concentration. For example, if the level of blood glucose rises above 110 mg per 100 ml of blood, a person is in a **hyperglycemic** condition. The level of blood glucose is lowered by insulin and glycogenesis. Insulin helps to move glucose into the liver cells and helps to synthesize glycogen. The end result is that the excess glucose is removed from the blood, resulting in a restoration of the normal 80 to 110 mg per 100 ml of blood glucose. Simple carbohydrate molecules also can be converted to lipid molecules and stored in fat depots around the body.

Another anabolic reaction involving glucose is the formation of glycogen in skeletal muscles. Glucose is transported by blood to the skeletal muscles (Figure 20–2), where the hormone insulin aids in the combination of glucose molecules to form glycogen. When the muscle sarcomeres contract, glycogen undergoes catabolism and releases energy for the resynthesis of phosphocreatine.

## *CATABOLISM*

Previously, we discussed the fact that carbohydrates are the primary source of energy for the body. The pro-

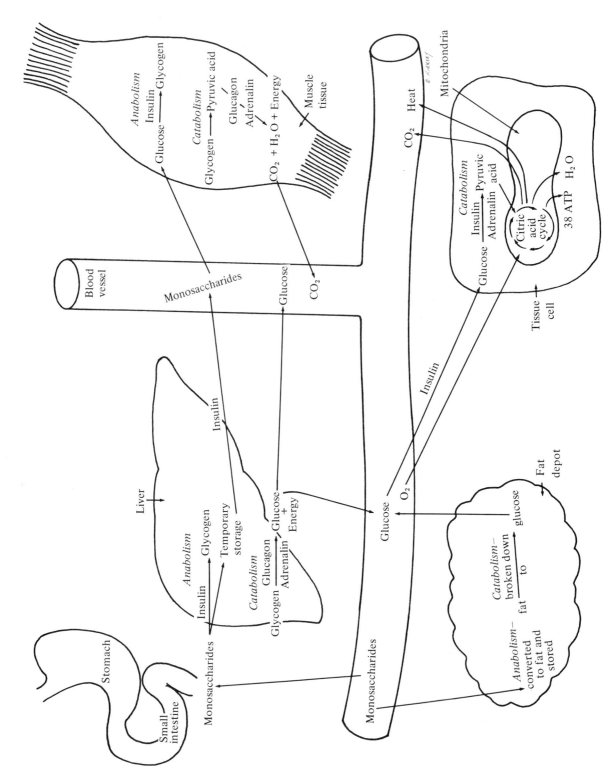

**Figure 20–1.** Metabolism of carbohydrates. The anabolism and catabolism of carbohydrates in the liver, muscle tissue, fat depot, and tissue cells are shown.

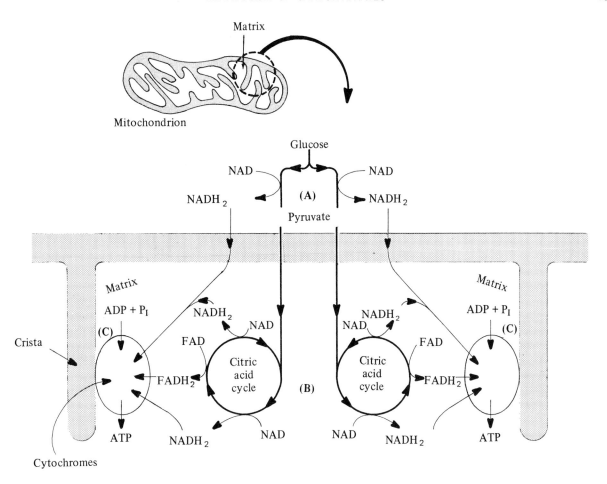

**Figure 20-2.** Location of glycolysis, citric acid cycle, and cytochrome system in a mitochondrion: (A) glycolysis in cytoplasm; (B) citric acid cycles in matrix of a mitochondrion; (C) cytochrome systems on crista in a mitochondrion.

cesses by which cells break down glucose to produce energy will be discussed next.

**SYNTHESIS OF ATP.** In Chapter 2, **ATP** was described as being a high-energy compound that is stored in cells. Each ATP molecule releases energy, when the high-energy bonds are broken, for cellular activities necessary to maintain homeostasis. The processes by which ATP molecules are formed, the chemical reactions involved, and the locations within the cytoplasm and mitochondria will be discussed now.

Two main processes are involved in the formation of ATP: **anaerobic respiration** or **glycolysis** and **aerobic respiration.** Figure 20–1 shows a summarization of these reactions and where they occur in cytoplasm and mitochondria. **Glycolysis** involves the breakdown (by oxidation reactions) of one glucose molecule to two **pyruvic acid (pyruvate)** molecules in the cytoplasm of cells. This process does not involve oxygen, and there-

fore is often referred to as **anaerobic respiration.** The end result of anaerobic respiration is that one glucose molecule has been oxidized to two pyruvic acid molecules. The two pyruvic acid molecules move into a mitochondrion where they become involved in the second process, **aerobic respiration** (Figure 20–1B). This process is called **aerobic** because oxygen is required to complete the formation of ATP. Aerobic respiration involves two smaller processes: **citric acid cycle** and **electron transport** through cytochromes. The citric acid cycle occurs in the liquid **matrix** of a mitochondrion because that is where the necessary enzymes for this process are located. The hydrogens that are removed from the compounds in the citric acid cycle are transported through cytochrome molecules which are attached to the **crista** of a mitochondrion. The **crista** greatly increase the internal surface area of a mitochondrion, thereby increasing the total number of cytochromes and enzymes that can attach to the crista. The localization of the citric acid cycle and electron transport in a mitochondrion has two main advantages:

- *The rate of interaction between the two is markedly increased.* Hydrogens removed from molecules in the citric cycle are transported through the cytochrome molecules, and ATP is produced as a result. Since the citric acid cycle and cytochromes are located near each other, the rate of interaction between them is increased.
- *The efficiency of ATP production is increased.* Each group of cytochrome molecules is confined to a small region on the surface of crista; however, many cytochrome groups are attached to the surface of one crista. This cytochrome confinement combined with the close proximity to the citric acid cycles increases the efficiency with which ATPs are produced.

Details concerning anaerobic respiration (glycolysis) and aerobic respiration will be discussed now.

# ANAEROBIC RESPIRATION (GLYCOLYSIS)

The term glycolysis means **glucose splitting** and that is exactly what happens. Figure 20–3A shows that glucose is a six-carbon molecule, and then is split into two three–carbon **PGAL (PhosphoGlycerALdehyde)** molecules. The splitting results from interaction of glucose with two ATP molecules that are broken down to ADP + $P_I$. The end result of glycolysis is two three-carbon pyruvate molecules. Three types of chemical reactions occur in the process of converting PGAL to pyruvate:

- *Rearrangement of bonds in each PGAL molecule.* This reaction involves some energy being released from **PGAL** which results in the next reaction.
- *Formation of two ATPs for each PGAL molecule.* The previous reaction furnishes energy necessary to combine ADP + $P_I$ to form ATP. Two ATPs per **PGAL** molecule are formed or a total of four ATPs (Figure 20–3A).
- *Removal of hydrogen with electrons.* Each PGAL molecule gives up two hydrogens with electrons. Remember (Chapter 2) that one type of **oxidation** involves atoms or molecules losing hydrogens with electrons. Also, one type of **reduction** involves atoms or molecules receiving hydrogens with electrons. Figure 20–3A shows that **PGAL** is oxidized and that NAD is

reduced to form $NADH_2$. **Nicotinamide Adenine Dinucleotide (NAD)** is a coenzyme that functions to accept hydrogens and transfer them to the cytochrome system. The portion of the **NAD** that accepts and releases hydrogen and electrons is the vitamin **nicotinamide** and **niacin**. This vitamin must be provided in the diet of a person or a deficiency can result in metabolic disorders.

## Summary of Anaerobic Respiration (Glycolysis)

This process in the ultimate formation of 38 ATPs includes the following results:

- One molecule of glucose (6C) split into two pyruvic acid (3C) molecules (Figure 20–3A).
- Two molecules of NAD are reduced to $NADH_2$.
- Four ATPs are produced or two for each PGAL molecule. Two ATPs are used up to split glucose to two PGAL molecules; therefore, **at the end of glycolysis a net gain of two ATPs results.**

# AEROBIC RESPIRATION

As mentioned earlier, this process in the formation of ATP requires oxygen, therefore, the name **aerobic**. This process is composed of the citric acid cycle and cytochrome transport system.

## Citric Acid Cycle

Figure 20–2A showed that this series of reactions occurs in the liquid **matrix** of a mitochondrion whereas glycolysis occurs in the cytoplasm of a cell. Figure 20–3A shows the details of this cycle. The two pyruvic acid molecules enter into a mitochrondrion and undergo a series of changes; however, we will describe the pathway of just one pyruvic acid molecule. After a pyruvic acid molecule enters a mitochondrion one of its carbons is lost in the form of $CO_2$ or **decarboxylation** occurs. The two-carbon molecule that results is called an **acetyl group.** Figure 20–3B shows that at the same time that decarboxylation occurred pyruvic acid was oxidized and NAD was reduced to $NADH_2$. The two–carbon acetyl group now attaches to a coenzyme called **coenzyme A (CoA)** now forming **acetyl CoA.** Acetyl CoA now enters the citric acid cycle by joining with **oxaloacetic acid** (4-carbon compound) to form **citric acid** (6-carbon compound). The CoA molecule is released and combines with another acetyl group. The citric acid molecule begins a series of reactions that are characterized by intermediate compounds being **oxidized** (losing hydrogens) and **decarboxylated** (losing $CO_2$). Some of the energy released by the oxidation of the intermediates is used to form the following:

- One ATP per cycle (Figure 20–3B).
- 3 NAD → 3 $NADH_2$ (Figure 20–3B). Three $NADH_2$ are formed per cycle, a total of 6 hydrogens with electrons are picked up by the 3 $NADH_2$.
- One FAD → $FADH_2$. **Flavin Adenine Dinucleotide (FAD)** is a coenzyme that functions as an electron acceptor and transport molecule like **NAD.** One FAD → $FADH_2$ is produced per cycle, or a total of 2 hydrogens with electrons are picked up by $FADH_2$.

This process is called the citric acid cycle because, as Figure 20–3B shows, the intermediates are oxidized and decarboxylated until oxaloacetic acid (4C) is reformed; it then combines with acetyl CoA to reform citric acid and complete the cycle.

### Summary of Important Points About Citric Acid Cycle

At the completion of the citric acid cycle the original glucose molecule has been totally oxidized. Each oxidation step involves the loss of two hydrogens with electrons along with energy. Some of the energy that is released by the oxidation steps is used to form one ATP. Most of the energy released, however, is in the electrons attached to the NAD and FAD carriers or $NADH_2$ and $FADH_2$. **The production of the three $NADH_2$ and one $FADH_2$ during each citric acid cycle is the most important function of the citric acid cycle. The total of eight or four pairs of electrons released by the citric acid cycle is very important in the total number of ATPs produced by the cytochrome system. One could say that the citric acid cycle generates the raw materials necessary to produce ATPs in the cytochrome system.**

### Cytochrome System

This is the final step in the production of ATPs that are so vital for the cell to maintain homeostasis. A cytochrome molecule is very similar to a hemoglobin molecule in that each one contains an atom of iron in a porphyrin ring. The ring is surrounded by a protein composed of about 100 amino acids. Each cytochrome differs from the others in the structure of the protein chain and also the energy level at which it holds the electrons. Notice Figure 20–3C that the cytochromes are arranged in such a way that the higher energy level cytochromes are at the top and the lower energy cytochromes are at the bottom (Cyt.b→ Cyt.c→ Cyt.a→ Cyt.$a_3$).

Figure 20–3C shows that the $NADH_2$ and $FADH_{2\,red}$ carry their hydrogens with electrons to the CoQ (coenzyme Q). Here the electrons are transferred from $NADH_2$ to CoQ. In other words, the $NADH_2$ becomes **oxidized** (lost electrons) and the CoQ becomes **reduced** (gained electrons). This oxidation-reduction reaction releases about 12.4 KCal/mole of energy, which is enough to join ADP + $P_i$ to form ATP. CoQ also is reduced by $FADH_2$. This transfer however does not release enough energy to form an ATP molecule. An interesting thing happens when $CoQ_{red}$ gives up its hydrogens with electrons to Cyt.$b_{ox}$. The iron atom will only accept electrons and not the two $H^+$ (hydrogen ions or protons). The two $H^+$ are released into the mitochondrial matrix fluid. Notice in Figure 20–3C that at the end of the cytochrome chain the hydrogen protons ($2H^+$) and electrons ($e^-$) are united together with the help of Cyt.$a_3$. From Cyt.b the two electrons are successively transferred through the other cytochromes. Each time the electrons are transferred an oxidation-reduction reaction is involved. The cytochrome that transfers is oxidized and the one that receives the electrons is reduced. Each transfer results in a loss of energy, however, unless it's at least 7 Kcal/mole ATP molecules will not be formed. The transfers from Cyt.b to Cyt.c and Cyt.a to Cyt.$a_3$ release enough energy to form ATP molecules (Figure 20–3C). In the final step Cyt.$a_3$ unites the two electrons with the two hydrogen protons ($H^+$) and also joins them with oxygen to form water. This final step is the reason the citric acid cycle and cytochrome system is called aerobic respiration. **Oxygen acts as the final hydrogen acceptor or it is reduced and that is why it is so critical to homeostasis and continuance of life. If oxygen were not present to finally receive the electrons, the successive transfer of electrons along the cytochrome molecules would be impossible. If the electrons are not transferred along the cytochromes, ATP molecules are not formed. Without ATPs homeostatic mechanisms are impossible and a person, therefore, will die shortly.**

### Summary of Cytochrome System

$NADH_2$ and $FADH_2$ carry electrons and hydrogen protons to the cytochrome system (located on the surface of cristae) from the citric acid cycle and glycolysis. The

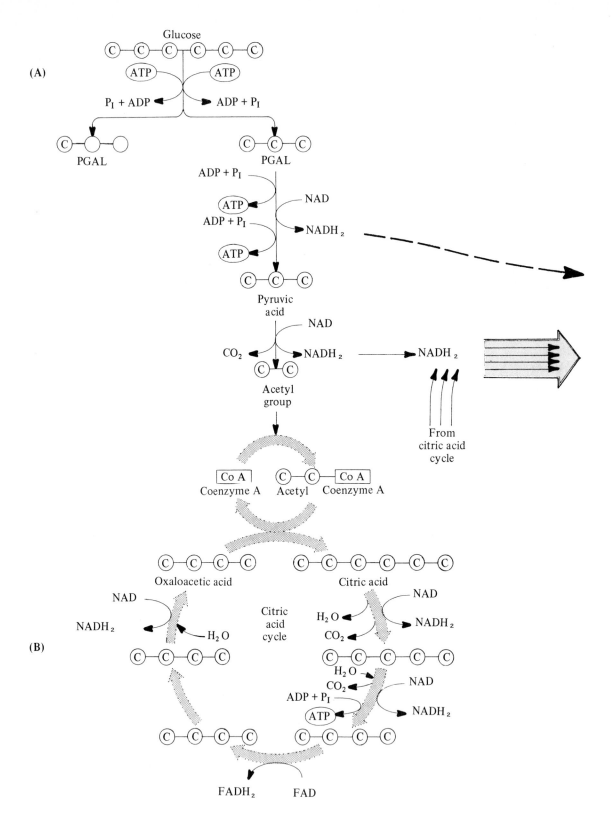

**Figure 20-3.** Interrelationship of glycosis, citric acid cycle, and cytochrome system: (A) glycolysis; (B) citric acid cycle; (C) cytochrome system.

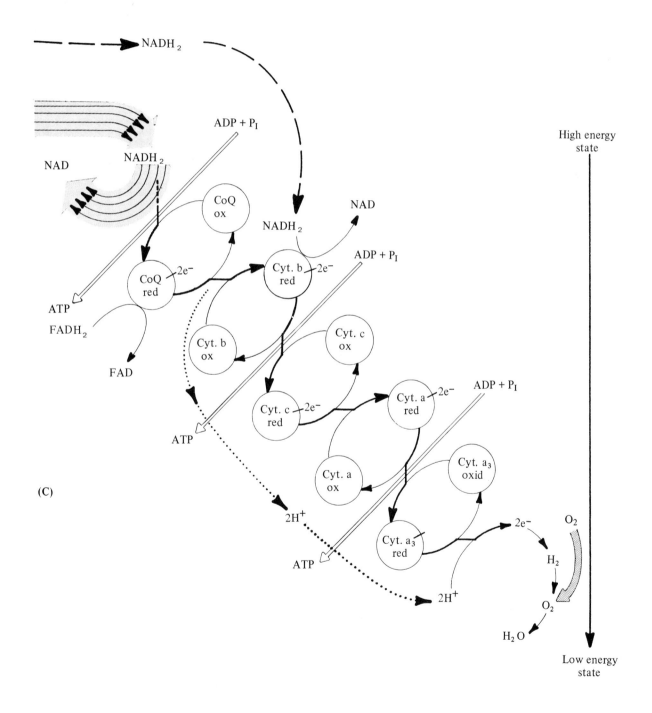

(C)

electrons are passed in pairs from one cytochrome to the next by oxidation-reduction reactions. For each pair of electrons transported through the cytochromes, three ATPs are produced (Figure 20–3C). Two exceptions to this are the electrons on $NADH_2$ which originated in the glycolysis step (Figure 20–3A) and electrons brought in by $FADH_2$. The **ultimate electron acceptor** is **oxygen,** without which the successive transfer of electrons would cease and no ATPs would be formed. Death would quickly follow. Notice in Figure 20–3C that the electrons are successively passed from a cytochrome molecule at a higher energy state to one at a lower energy state. This results from the fact that each transfer of electrons involves a loss of energy. If the loss is equal to at least 7 KCal/mole then ADP + $P_1$ to form ATP occurs.

From one molecule of glucose **a gross production of 38 ATPs is produced** (Table 20–1 shows how many are produced by each step). However, the net ATP gain is **36** since two ATPs were used during glycolysis.

## INTERACTION OF GLYCOGENESIS AND GLYCOLYSIS

The level of blood glucose is maintained by the interaction of glycogenesis and glycolysis. If the level of blood glucose is higher than 110 mg per 100 ml of blood, this condition is called **hyperglycemia.** Hyperglycemia is corrected by glycogenesis in the liver where insulin helps both to move the excess glucose out of the blood and to synthesize it into glycogen. If the level of blood glucose drops below 80 mg per 100 ml of blood, **hypoglycemia** results. **Glycolysis** (breakdown of glycogen to

glucose molecules) corrects hypoglycemia. The hormones, glucagon and epinephrine, stimulate the liver cells to undergo glycolysis or break down glycogen and release glucose into the blood. This release of glucose raises the level of blood glucose back into its normal range and corrects for hypoglycemia.

## 3  LIPID METABOLISM

After the neutral fats have been absorbed into the lymph vessels, they are emptied into the bloodstream and ultimately are carried to the liver. The liver carries out both catabolic and anabolic reactions on the lipid molecules.

### CATABOLISM

The liver breaks down the fatty acid molecules of neutral fats by **beta oxidation ($\beta$-oxidation).** The process is called beta oxidation because the beta carbon, second carbon (Figure 20–4), is oxidized, which results in the breaking off of a two-carbon segment. The two-carbon segment, acetic acid, combines with CoA to form acetyl CoA. Beta oxidation continues to break off two–carbon segments until an entire fatty acid is oxidized. Since fatty acids contain 14 to 20 carbons, then 7 to 10 acetyl CoA molecules result from the breakdown of one fatty acid. Each neutral fat molecule contains three fatty acids; therefore, the beta oxidation of one entire neutral fat molecule results in the formation of

**TABLE 20–1.**  *Summary of ATP Yield from One Molecule of Glucose*

| | Total | | | |
|---|---|---|---|---|
| Anaerobic respiration | | 2 ATP | | |
| (Glycolysis) | $NADH_2 \rightarrow$ 2 ATP | | (× 2) | → 8 ATP |
| Aerobic respiration: | $NADH_2 \rightarrow$ 3 ATP | | (× 2) | → 6 ATP |
| Pyruvic acid → acetyl CoA | | | | |
| Citric acid cycle | | 1 ATP | | |
| | 3 $NADH_2 \rightarrow$ 9 ATP | | (× 2) | → 24 ATP |
| | 1 $FADH_2 \rightarrow$ 2 ATP | | | |
| | Gross production | | | 38 ATP |
| | | | | − 2 ATP |
| | | | | (used in glycolysis) |
| | Net production | | | 36 ATP |

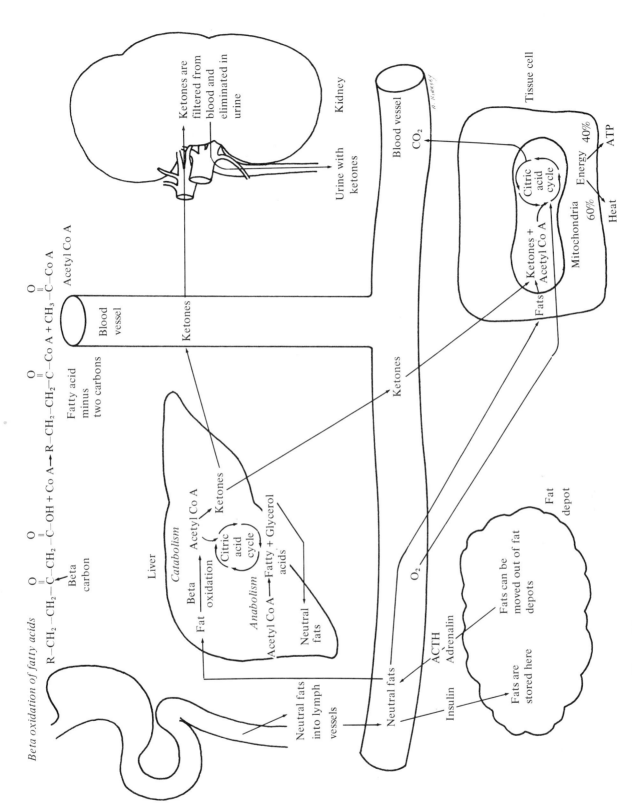

**Figure 20–4.** Lipid metabolism. The anabolism and catabolism of fat molecules in the fat depots, liver, and tissue cells are shown.

*Beta oxidation of fatty acids*

$$R-CH_2-CH_2-C-CH_2-C-OH+CoA \longrightarrow R-CH_2-CH_2-C-CoA+CH_3-C-CoA$$

Beta
carbon

Fatty acid
minus
two carbons

Acetyl Co A

Liver

*Catabolism*

Beta
oxidation

Acetyl Co A → Ketones

Fat

Citric
acid
cycle

*Anabolism*

Acetyl Co A → Fatty + Glycerol acids

Neutral
fats

Neutral fats
into lymph
vessels

Ketones

Ketones

Ketones are
filtered from
blood and
eliminated in
urine

Kidney

Urine with
ketones

Blood
vessel

Blood vessel

$CO_2$

$O_2$

Neutral fats

Insulin

ACTH
Adrenalin

Fats can be
moved out of fat
depots

Fats are
stored here

Fat
depot

Tissue cell

Fats

Ketones +
Acetyl Co A

Citric
acid
cycle

Mitochondria

Energy 40%

ATP

60%

Heat

415

21 to 30 acetyl CoA molecules. Remember that these acetyl CoA molecules enter into the citric acid cycle (Krebs cycle) resulting in the production of energy. The oxidation of pyruvic acid produces only two acetyl CoA, compared to 21 to 30 from a lipid molecule. This helps to explain why 1 g of lipids can produce more calories of energy (9 Cal/g) than 1 g of carbohydrates (4 Cal/g).

## FAT DEPOTS AND MOBILIZATION OF FAT

If the diet of an individual consists of excessive amounts of proteins, lipids, and carbohydrates, then the excess is converted to lipid molecules and stored in various regions of the body called **fat depots.** There is a continual inflow and outflow of lipids into the fat depots (Figure 20–4) depending upon the needs of the body. When the intake of carbohydrates is low the body must obtain energy by breaking down lipid molecules. The lipids in the fat depots are mobilized or they are transported from the fat depots to the liver, where they are oxidized. The decrease in the amount of fat in the fat depots is what losing weight is all about. The decrease in the quantity of fat results in weight loss and a change in the shape of various regions of the body.

The hormones ACTH (adrenal corticotrophic hormones) and epinephrine increase the mobilization of fat or remove fat from the depots.

## KETOGENESIS (FORMATION OF KETONES)

Beta oxidation of the fatty acids takes place in the liver, and the acetyl CoA molecules can enter into the citric acid cycle. Some of the acetyl CoA molecules do not enter into the citric acid cycle in the liver, but rather they are combined to form the ketone, **acetoacetic acid** (Figure 20–4). This ketone moves into the blood and is carried to cells, where it undergoes **ketolysis** (breakdown of ketones to stage where they enter citric acid cycle). Two other ketones, **beta hydroxybutyric acid** and **acetone,** result from the breakdown of acetoacetic acid. Normally the ketones are broken down rapidly so that the concentration of ketones in the blood usually is about 1 mg per 100 ml of blood (1 mg percent). Various conditions that result in the breakdown of large amounts of fat can cause an abnormal increase in the concentration of ketones in the blood. This abnormal concentration of ketones in the blood is called **ketonemia** and usually results in **ketonuria** (an increase in ketones in the urine). When ketonemia and ketonuria exist, a person is said to be in a state of **ketosis.** This state, over a period of time, can cause acidosis and dehydration. Ketones are acids; therefore an increase in ketones can cause a decrease in the blood pH into the acidic range. Dehydration also can accompany ketosis because sodium ions are excreted by the kidneys along with the ketones. Since water molecules always accompany the loss of sodium ions, the loss of sodium ions and ketones results in loss of water molecules.

## ANABOLISM OF LIPIDS

The synthesis of lipids occurs primarily in the liver and adipose tissue. The acetyl CoA molecules either can enter into the citric acid cycle or they can serve as the precursor for the synthesis of fatty acids (Figure 20–4). The acetyl CoA molecules are combined to gradually form fatty acids, cholesterol, and steroids. The fatty acids are combined with glycerol to form neutral fat or triglycerides.

The liver and adipose tissue have the ability to convert carbohydrates and proteins to fat molecules and to store then. If a person eats an excessive amount of proteins and carbohydrates, the excess will be converted to fat. The fat molecules are stored in the fat depots.

## HORMONAL REGULATION OF LIPID METABOLISM

The hormones of ACTH and epinephrine remove fat (or mobilize fat) from the fat depots to the liver. The hormone, **insulin,** increases the synthesis of lipids in the fat depots.

# 4    PROTEIN METABOLISM

The primary function of carbohydrates and lipids is the production of energy; however, amino acids and proteins function as tissue builders and components of enzymes and hormones. This means that the anabolism stage of protein metabolism, inside the various tissue cells, is more important than the catabolism of proteins.

## ANABOLISM

The proteins that you eat are broken down to amino acids that are absorbed into the bloodstream. The blood circulates the amino acids to all of the cells in the body. Each cell selects the amino acids it needs to synthesize specific proteins, enzymes, and hormones (Figure 20-5). DNA molecules in the nucleus of each cell contain the information that is necessary to combine the amino acids in the proper sequence. Messenger RNA (m-RNA), transfer RNA (t-RNA), and ribosomes play vital roles in the synthesis of proteins in each cell.

## ESSENTIAL AND NONESSENTIAL AMINO ACIDS

There are approximately 11 of 21 amino acids that can be synthesized by the body. These amino acids are classified as **nonessential amino acids,** in that it is not essential these amino acids be acquired in the diet. Approximately 10 of 21 amino acids cannot be synthesized by the body; therefore, it is essential that a person acquire these in his daily diet. These amino acids are classified as **essential amino acids.** It is important for one to understand that all of the 21 amino acids are needed to synthesize proteins; but the **nonessential** ones can be synthesized by the body and the essential ones cannot be synthesized. Therefore, it is essential to acquire them in your diet.

## CATABOLISM

Amino acids are broken down in the liver. The primary catabolic reaction involving amino acids is **deamination.** This process involves the removal of the amino group ($-NH_2$) from amino acids. As the amino group is removed, it picks up a hydrogen ion to form ammonia ($NH_3$). Ammonia is toxic if it accumulates; therefore, two ammonia molecules combine with $CO_2$ to form nontoxic urea.

$$CO_2 + 2\,NH_3 \xrightarrow{\text{Enzymes}} NH_2-\underset{\substack{\|\\O}}{C}-NH_2$$

Urea

Keto acids, such as pyruvic acid, also result from the deamination of amino acids (Figure 20-5). These keto acids can be converted to acetyl CoA, which enters the citric acid cycle. If the needs of the body are such that

the acetyl CoA is not needed, it can be converted to glycogen and lipids and then stored.

## HORMONES THAT REGULATE PROTEIN METABOLISM

The **somatotrophic hormone (SH)** produced by the anterior pituitary is important in that it accelerates protein synthesis. SH is quite important in regulating the production of new protoplasm and, therefore, in regulating the growth of the tissues. Insulin (produced by the pancreas) and thyroxine (produced by the thyroid) also accelerate protein synthesis.

## NITROGEN BALANCE

Nitrogen balance refers to the amount of nitrogen in the urine compared to the amount of nitrogen ingested in the food. The nitrogen excreted in the urine is in the form of urea that results from the deamination of amino acids in the liver. When the concentration of excreted nitrogen is equal to the amount ingested, a person is said to be in **nitrogen balance;** this is the normal state of an average adult. A **positive nitrogen balance** is a condition in which the intake of nitrogen is greater than the amount excreted. In other words there is very little deamination of amino acids taking place, and the body is synthesizing most of the amino acids into proteins. This condition is characteristic of growing children, pregnant women, and people recovering from operations. Each one of these people is either building or repairing damaged tissues. A **negative nitrogen balance** is a condition in which the amount of nitrogen excreted is greater than the amount ingested. This indicates that proteins, which compose the tissues, are being broken down. People in a state of starvation or suffering from metabolic disorders exhibit a negative nitrogen balance.

# 5   INTERCONVERSION BETWEEN CARBOHYDRATES, LIPIDS, AND PROTEINS

It is vital that the cells constantly channel chemical compounds into the citric acid cycle to produce energy. Also it is important that the cells be able to convert one

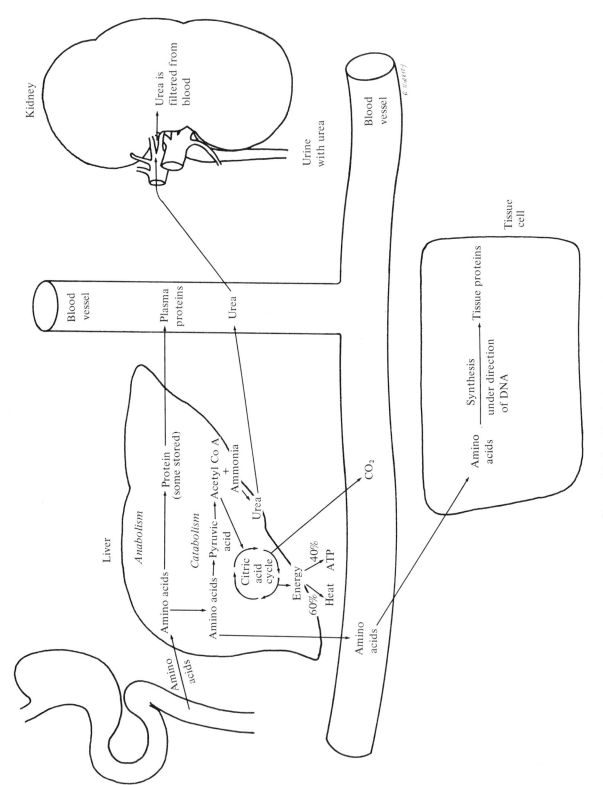

Figure 20-5. Metabolism of amino acids.

organic compound into another, depending upon the needs of the body. For example, if the body needs certain protein molecules, but they are not being ingested, then the cells have to be able to convert carbohydrates and fats to proteins. Likewise, if a person is on a low carbohydrate diet, then the cells have to be able to break down fats and proteins to the point that they can enter the citric acid cycle. The cells do have the ability to convert organic compounds from one form to another. The characteristic common to carbohydrates, lipids, and proteins is that they all are composed of carbon, hydrogen, and oxygen atoms. Since the basic components are the same for each compound, it is not too difficult to convert from one compound to another.

# SUMMARY

### Anabolism and Catabolism

Metabolism is divided into two phases:

A. Anabolism: buildup phase or involves synthesis reactions.
B. Catabolism: breakdown phase or involves decomposition of complex molecules into simple molecules.

### Metabolism of Carbohydrates

A. Anabolism
   1. Monosaccharides are joined together to form glycogen in liver.
   2. Insulin aids synthesis of glycogen.
   3. Helps to lower blood glucose if level is too high.
B. Catabolism
   1. Synthesis of ATP: involves two processes, anaerobic respiration (glycolysis) and aerobic respiration.
      a. Anaerobic respiration. Includes the following results:
         (1) Glucose is split into two pyruvic acid molecules.
         (2) Two molecules of NAD are reduced to $NADH_2$.
         (3) A net gain of 2 ATPs.
      b. Aerobic respiration. Composed of citric acid cycle and cytochrome transport system.
         (1) Citric acid cycle. One cycle includes the following results:
            (a) One ATP synthesized per cycle.
            (b) Three $NADH_2$ are formed by reduction reactions.
            (c) One $FADH_2$ is formed by reduction reaction.
            (d) Two $CO_2$ molecules are formed.
         (2) Cytochrome system. Passage of one pair of electrons down the cytochrome system results in the following:
            (a) Three ATPs synthesized.
            (b) $H_2O$ molecules synthesized from interaction of $O_2$ with $H_2$.

### Lipid Metabolism

A. Catabolism
   1. Beta oxidation breaks down fatty acid molecule, resulting in acetyl CoA molecules.
   2. Oxidation of a lipid molecule results in 21 to 30 acetyl CoA molecules; reason why 1 g of lipid releases 9 Kcal/g compared to 4 Kcal/g of carbohydrate.
B. Fat depots and mobilizing fat
   1. Intake of excess nutrients are converted to fat and stored in various regions of body.
   2. ACTH and epinephrine increase mobilization of fat from depots.
C. Ketogenesis (formation of ketones)
   1. Ketones formed from beta oxidation of fatty acids.

2. Some conditions result in buildup of ketones in blood (ketonemia) and urine (ketonuria); results in acidosis.

D. Anabolism of lipids
1. Synthesis of lipids occurs in liver and adipose tissue from fatty acids and glycerol.
2. Carbohydrates and fats can be converted to fat molecules.

## Protein Metabolism

A. Anabolism
1. Each cell selects amino acids needed to synthesize proteins for its own use.
2. DNA directs synthesis of proteins.
3. Essential and nonessential amino acids:
    a. Essential: amino acids that cannot by synthesized by body; must be acquired in diet.
    b. Nonessential: amino acids that can be synthesized by body.

B. Catabolism
1. Deamination involves removal of amino groups from amino acids.
2. Urea is formed in liver from amino groups.

C. Hormones that regulate protein metabolism: somatotrophic hormone (SH) and insulin accelerate protein synthesis.

D. Nitrogen balance
1. Nitrogen balance occurs when amount of nitrogen excreted in urine is equal to the amount ingested.
2. Positive nitrogen balance, intake of nitrogen is greater than the amount excreted; characteristic of growing children, pregnant women.
3. Negative nitrogen balance, amount of nitrogen excreted exceeds the amount ingested; characteristic of starvation and metabolic disorders.

## Interconversion between Carbohydrates, Lipids, and Proteins

Cells have ability to interconvert carbohydrates, lipids, and proteins, depending on the body's needs.

# CHAPTER 20 EXAM

## Metabolism of Lipids, Carbohydrates, and Proteins

Matching. Questions 1 to 5.

| | | | |
|---|---|---|---|
| **1.** glycogen | | **A.** | formed by synthesis of monosaccharides in liver |
| **2.** anaerobic respiration | | **B.** | passage of each pair of electrons results in synthesis of three ATPs |
| **3.** citric acid cycle | | **C.** | three $NADH_2$ and one $FADH_2$ are produced |
| **4.** cytochrome system | | **D.** | two molecules of pyruvic acid and ATPs are produced |
| **5.** oxygen molecules | | **E.** | final acceptor of hydrogen electrons |

6. Anaerobic respiration (glycolysis) produces:

    1. Two pyruvic acid molecules     3. A net gain of two ATPs
    2. Two $NADH_2$     4. $Co_2$ molecules
    (a) 1, 2, 3     (b) 1, 3     (c) 2, 4     (d) 4     (e) All of these

7. One citric acid cycle results in:

    1. Synthesis of 36 ATPs     3. Four $CO_2$ molecules
    2. Three $NADH_2$     4. One $FADH_2$
    (a) 1, 2, 3     (b) 1, 3     (c) 2, 4     (d) 4     (e) All of these

8. Passage of one pair of electrons down the entire length of a cytochrome system results in:

    1. Synthesis of three ATPs     3. Formation of $H_2O$ molecules
    2. Release of $CO_2$     4. Formation of $NADH_2$
    (a) 1, 2, 3     (b) 1, 3     (c) 2, 4     (d) 4     (e) All of these

True (A) or false (B). Questions 9 to 15.

9. Glycogenesis results in synthesis of glycogen and lowering of blood glucose.

10. Ketones result from anabolism of lipids.

11. Carbohydrates and fats can be converted to fat molecules.

12. Each cell in the body can synthesize essential amino acids.

13. Urea is formed in kidneys from uric acid.

14. A growing child is an example of a person who might be in a negative nitrogen balance.

15. Depending on the body's needs, cells have the ability to interconvert carbohydrates, lipids, and proteins.

# Chapter 21

# THE REPRODUCTIVE SYSTEM

After reading and studying this chapter, a student should be able to:

1. Name and give the function of the female secondary sex organs.
2. Describe the anatomy and function of clitoris, vestibular glands, and mammary glands.
3. Give two functions of seminiferous tubules in testes.
4. Describe the location and function of seminal vesicles, prostate gland, and Cowper's glands.
5. Describe the erection process of a penis.
6. Differentiate between spermatogenesis and oogenesis as to the final products and hormones that stimulate them.
7. Describe the structure, function, and hormone that influence development of the corpus luteum.
8. Describe the changes in the endometrium and development of secondary oocytes and corpus luteum that occur during the flow, follicular, and luteal phases of a menstrual cycle.
9. Describe the pathway that sperm follow to a secondary oocyte and what fertilization actually involves.
10. Describe how a sperm determines the sex of a child.
11. Distinguish between chorion and amnion membranes as to location and function.
12. Distinguish between the period of the embryo and the period of the fetus.
13. Trace the circulation of blood from the left ventricle to the placenta and back to heart within a fetus.
14. Discuss the roles of estrogen, oxytocin, and relaxin hormones in labor.
15. Discuss the roles of estrogen, progesterone, and prolactin hormones in the development and lactation of breasts.

*Male and female reproductive organs function to reproduce a new human being. In addition, they secrete some hormones that affect the secondary sexual characteristics of males and females. For example, the male hormone, testosterone, stimulates the development of deep voice and pubic, axillary, and facial hair. The female hormones, estrogen and progesterone, stimulate the development of breasts, axillary and pubic hair, and widening of the hips.*

*The production of a new human being is initiated when a male sex cell (sperm) combines with a female sex cell (oocyte). The male and female reproductive organs can be divided into primary and secondary sex organs, depending upon whether they produce, transport, or aid the transport of the sex cells.*

*Primary sex organs are male and female gonads that produce the sex cells (sperm and oocytes) and sex hormones. Secondary sex organs are male and female sex organs that transport or aid in the transport of sex cells. These organs include ducts, through which the cells travel, and accessory organs which aid the transport of sex cells. Hormones, produced by the anterior pituitary, regulate the production of sex cells by the primary sex organs.*

# 1   FEMALE REPRODUCTIVE SYSTEM

The primary sex organs of the female include two ovaries; the secondary sex organs include two fallopian tubes, uterus, vagina, and two mammary glands.

## OVARIES: PRIMARY SEX ORGANS

The female gonads, called **ovaries,** are shaped like almonds and are approximately 3 cm long. They are located on each side of the **uterus** against the posterior body wall (Figure 21–1). Each ovary is attached to the uterus by the **ovarian ligament.** The ovaries have an irregular scarred surface, which is the result of previous ovulations. The mechanism by which the ovaries produce ova will be discussed shortly.

## SECONDARY SEX ORGANS

### Fallopian Tubes

**Fallopian tubes** are approximately 10 cm long and extend from the uterus out to the ovaries (Figure 21–1). The distal end of each fallopian tube is characterized by many irregular, fingerlike structures, called **fimbriae,** which are in close contact with the ovaries. The wall of a fallopian tube is composed of circular and longitudinal layers of smooth muscle, and is lined with a ciliated mucous membrane. The actions of the cilia combined with contractions of the smooth muscles move the oocytes from the ovaries to the uterus.

### Uterus

The **uterus** is a hollow muscular organ that is approximately 7 to 8 cm in length and 5 to 6 cm in width (Figure 21–1). It lies superior to the urinary bladder and anterior to the rectum (Figure 21–2). The uterus is held in place by ligaments between the rectum and the bladder. The two most important pairs of ligaments are the **round** and **broad ligaments.** The round ligament (Figure 21–1) originates in the external genitalia, **labia majora,** and passes upward through the **inguinal canal** and finally joins the superior part of the uterus. The broad ligament extends from the lateral pelvic walls and floor to the lateral surface of the uterus. The peritoneum covers the broad and round ligaments.

The portion of the uterus superior to the fallopian tubes is called the **fundus** (Figure 21–1). The main portion of the uterus is called the **body** and the narrow inferior portion is called the **cervix.** Figure 21–2 shows that the walls of the uterus are composed of layers of smooth muscle tissue, which collectively are called **myometrium.** The inner surface of the uterus is lined with a mucous membrane called the **endometrium.** It is the endometrium that undergoes changes during the menstrual cycle and during pregnancy when a fertilized ovum implants and develops. The uterus has the capacity to stretch tremendously during pregnancy. For example, the uterus increases approximately 16 times during pregnancy as the fetus develops. This tremendous increase in the size of the uterus is made possible by an increase in the number of cells, an increase in the

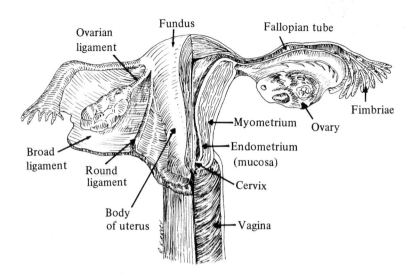

**Figure 21-1.** Internal female reproductive organs.

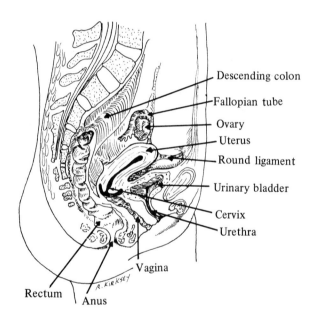

**Figure 21-2.** Sagittal section of internal sex organs.

size of the cells, and stretching of the fibrous and elastic fibers in the muscular myometrial wall.

## Vagina

The **vagina** is a collapsible muscular tube that extends from the vaginal opening to the cervix of the uterus (Figures 21-2 and 21-3). It is about 7 to 10 cm in length, but it can be extended to receive a **penis.** The walls of the vagina are composed of smooth muscle and fibrous

elastic connective tissues. The walls are lined with a mucous membrane that is thrown into folds called **rugae,** which can flatten out to allow the vagina to expand during sexual intercourse and childbirth.

A vascular fold of tissue, the **hymen,** partially blocks the entrance into the vagina. Rupturing or tearing of the hymen usually results in bleeding. Sometimes the hymen may totally block the vaginal opening, a condition known as **imperforate hymen.** This condition will not allow the proper flow of menstrual material, and surgery is required to correct imperforate hymen.

### Accessory Sex Organs

The accessory sex organs are classified as secondary sex organs and include labia majora, labia minora, vestibular glands, clitoris, and mammary glands.

**THE LABIA.** The **labia majora** are composed of two longitudinal folds of skin that extend from the **mons pubis** posteriorly toward the anus (Figure 21-4). Mons pubis is a rounded pad of fat lying over the pubic symphysis, which at sexual maturity is covered with pubic hair. The **labia minora** are two smaller folds of skin located medial to the labia majora, and they extend toward the anus. The **vestibule** is the area between the labia minora. The openings into the urethra and vagina are present in the vestibule.

**CLITORIS.** The **clitoris** is composed of erectile tissue and is located where the labia minora folds unite anteriorly (Figure 21-4). Nerves innervate the clitoris,

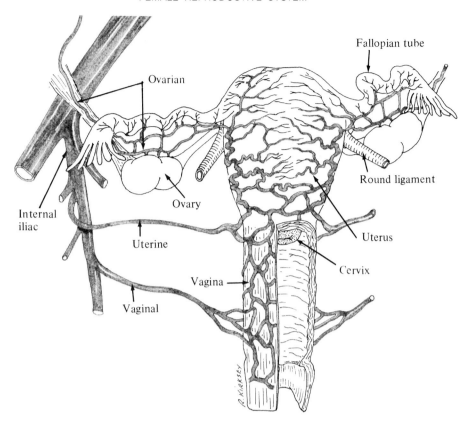

Figure 21-3. Arterial blood supply to female reproductive organs.

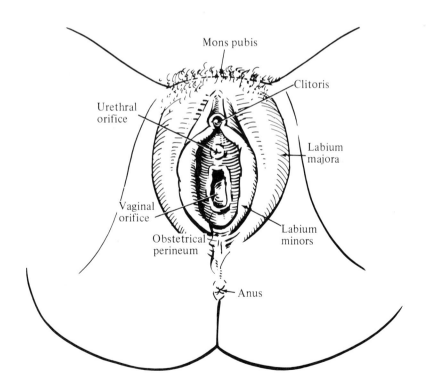

Figure 21-4. Female accessory sex organs.

making it quite sensitive to touch. During sexual intercourse it becomes erect from the stimulation by the penis. The clitoris plays an important role in the sexual arousal of a female because of the number of sensory nerve endings present. The clitoris corresponds in structure and origin to the penis of a male. The labia majora, labia minora, vestibule, and clitoris collectively are known as the **vulva.**

**VESTIBULAR GLANDS.**    On each side of the vaginal opening are the **Bartholin glands,** which secrete mucus. These glands are stimulated to secrete mucus during sexual intercourse, which acts as a lubricant to aid entrance of the penis into the vagina.

**PERINEUM.**    The **perineum** is the area between the pubic symphysis and the coccyx. It includes all of the deep muscles and fascia. The area between the vagina and anal opening is known as the **obstetrical perineum** (Figure 21–4). This area can be torn during childbirth if the head of the fetus is larger than the vaginal opening. To prevent tearing, an incision called **episiotomy** is made in the obstetrical perineum to enlarge the vaginal opening. An episiotomy is made prior to the delivery of the child, and it is easily closed after childbirth.

**MAMMARY GLANDS.**    The **mammary glands** actually are modified sweat glands. They are located on the anterior surface of the body between the second and sixth ribs. Each breast is composed of 15 to 20 lobes (Figure 21–5). A variable amount of adipose tissue is located between the lobes, and within each lobe are lobules that contain milk-producing glands. Milk is drained from the glands by small ducts that empty into one **lactiferous duct** that drains each lobe. The 15 to 20 lactiferous ducts open to the outside through the nipple. Surrounding the nipple is a pink pigmented area called the areola (Figure 21–5). During pregnancy the areola becomes dark brown in color.

The breasts begin to enlarge and develop at sexual maturity when estrogen and progesterone secretion begins. The lactation process (secretion of milk) and the hormones responsible for this will be discussed later.

# 2    MALE REPRODUCTIVE SYSTEM

The major functions of the male reproductive system are production and transport of sperm to the female for fertilization of an oocyte, and also the production of

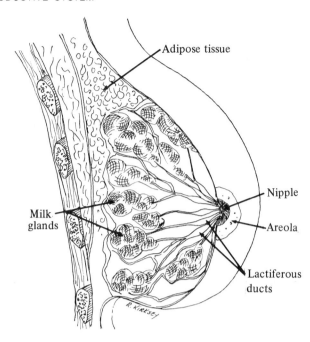

Figure 21-5.    Internal view of mammary glands.

male hormone, testosterone. The primary sex organs or gonads in the male are called **testes.** They produce the male sex cells called **sperm.** The secondary sex organs include the ducts—epididymis, ductus deferens, and ejaculatory ducts—that transport the sperm to the outside of the body. Accessory structures also are included as secondary sex organs, and they include seminal vesicles, prostate gland, Cowper's gland (bulbourethral gland), and the penis.

## TESTES: PRIMARY SEX ORGANS

**Testes** are enclosed in a double sac called the **scrotum** (Figure 21–6) suspended between the thighs. During embryonic development the testes are formed in the abdominal cavity near the kidneys. They gradually descend through the body cavity, as the fetus develops and, just prior to birth, they move through the inguinal canal into the scrotum. The testes cannot produce sperm at the normal body temperature of 37°C; therefore, the testes must descend into the scrotum where the temperature is 2 to 3 °C below normal body temperature. If the testes fail to descend into the scrotum a male cannot produce sperm and he is said to be sterile. Failure of the testes to descend into the **scrotum** is called cryptorchidism.

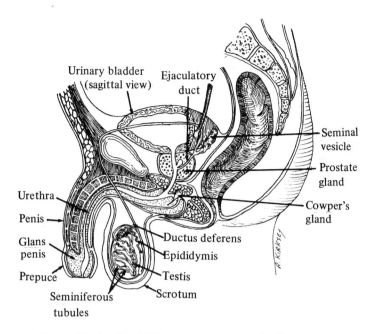

**Figure 21-6.** Sagittal view of male reproductive organs.

Each testis is divided internally into approximately 250 to 400 compartments, called **lobules** (Figure 21-7). One to three convoluted tubules called **seminiferous tubules** are contained within each lobule. The seminiferous tubules are important because they produce sperm. Scattered between the tubules are **interstitial cells,** which produce the male hormone, **testosterone.** The testes perform two important functions: (1) production of the male sex cells, sperm, and (2) production of the hormone, testosterone.

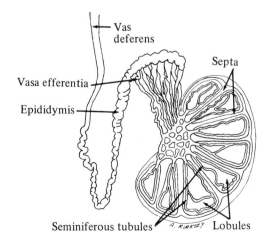

**Figure 21-7.** Internal view of testis.

## SECONDARY SEX ORGANS

The sperm are drained from the seminiferous tubules into the epididymis (Figure 21-7), which is a long coiled tubule on the posterior surface of each testis. The epididymis stores sperm after they are produced in the seminiferous tubules.

**Ductus deferens** or **vas deferens** is a duct (Figures 21-6 and 21-8) that carries sperm upward from the epididymis through the inguinal ring to the ejaculatory duct on the posterior surface of the urinary bladder. A spermatic artery, veins, nerves, and lymph vessels combine with the ductus deferens to form the spermatic cord. The outer covering of the spermatic cord is composed of fascia (connective tissue).

The ductus deferens carries sperm to the **ejaculatory duct** (Figure 21-6) which connects the seminal vesicle to the urethra. The ejaculatory duct is approximately 2.5 cm long and passes through the prostrate gland on its way to join the urethra.

## ACCESSORY STRUCTURES

The secondary sex organs are a series of ducts that transport sperm from the testes to the urethra, which will finally transport sperm out of the body. For the sperm to move through the vagina, uterus, and fallo-

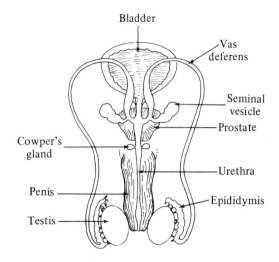

**Figure 21-8.** Front (anterior) view of male reproductive system.

pian tubes, they need secretions from the accessory structures. The accessory structures are glands that secrete alkaline materials that provide nourishment and aid movement of the sperm.

## Seminal Vesicles

The **seminal vesicles** are two elongated, coiled sacs on the posterior surface of the urinary bladder (Figures 21-6 and 21-8). The seminal vesicle ducts join with the **ductus deferens** to form the **ejaculatory ducts.** Sperm cells do not enter the seminal vesicles but rather pass on into the ejaculatory duct. The seminal vesicles secrete a viscous, alkaline fluid that aids the metabolism of the sperm cells. The alkaline fluid also aids the movement of sperm through acidic passageways of the urethra and vagina.

## Prostate Gland

The **prostate gland** is a muscular doughnut-shaped structure located just inferior to the bladder (Figures 21-6 and 21-8). It surrounds the proximal portion of the urethra. The prostate gland is composed of glandular, muscular, and connective tissues, and the glandular tissue secretes a thin alkaline fluid that mixes with sperm as they enter the urethra.

**FUNCTIONS OF PROSTATE GLAND.** The alkaline fluid secreted by the prostate gland neutralizes the acidic medium of the urethra, thereby aiding the movement of sperm. The smooth muscle tissue con-

tracts during ejaculation and thus aids the expulsion of the sperm and the secretions.

Cancer of the prostate is common in older men. It usually results in enlargement of the prostate so that the urethra is decreased in size. It is common for the prostate to become enlarged in men over the age of 60 years. Enlargement of the prostate gland, whether from cancer or old age, is characterized by **dysuria** (painful urination) as a result of a decrease in the size of the urethra. Dysuria causes a male to excessively contract the lower abdominal muscles, which can enlarge the inguinal canal, resulting in an **inguinal hernia.**

## Cowper's Glands

**Cowper's glands** (bulbourethral glands) are yellowish pea-shaped structures, one on each side of the urethra (Figures 21-6 and 21-8), immediately inferior to the prostate. Cowper's glands secrete a mucus-type substance into the urethra that apparently acts as a lubricant for the penis during sexual intercourse. The secretion also is alkaline, which helps to neutralize the acidic urethra.

Sperm plus secretions from the seminal vesicles and prostate and Cowper's glands make up the fluid called **semen,** which is ejaculated from the penis. The alkaline secretions from the three glands give nourishment to the sperm cells as well as neutralize the acidic passageways that sperm pass through on their way to fertilizing an oocyte in the female.

## Penis

The **penis** is an accessory organ that deposits semen near the **cervix** (entrance to the uterus). It is anchored to the pubic and ischial bones. Internally, the penis is composed of three masses of erectile tissue, with the urethra passing through one of the masses (Figure 21-9). Skin covers the outer surface of the penis. The dorsal half of the penis is composed of the **corpora cavernosa** masses of erectile tissue (Figure 21-9). The third mass, called **corpus spongiosum,** composes the ventral half of the penis. The urethra travels through the corpus spongiosum. The erectile tissue is composed of irregular spongy-type tissue. Sexual stimulation increases the flow of blood to the masses of erectile tissue, which results in the penis becoming erect and firm.

The distal end of the penis is expanded into a blunt structure called the **glans penis** (Figure 21-9). Skin

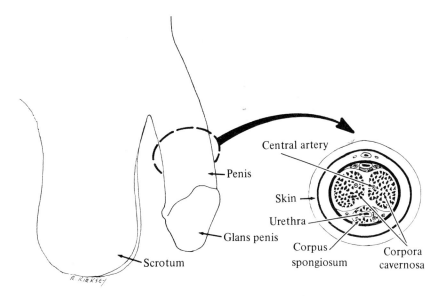

**Figure 21-9.** Cross-sectional view of penis showing the three masses of erectile tissue.

forms a loose flap over the glans, and it is known as the prepuce or **foreskin,** which is often removed by surgery shortly after birth to keep the glans penis area clearer. Removal of the prepuce is known as **circumcision.**

The most prevalent venereal disease today is *gonorrhea.* The causative organism is *Neisseria gonorrhoeae* (gonococcus), which is a gram–negative diplococcus. The point of entry in males is the **urethra,** and in females it is the **vagina.** In males *N. gonorrhoeae* react with the mucous lining of the urethra causing inflammation, production of a puslike discharge, and painful urination (dysuria). Usually gonorrhea is localized in the urethra; however, it can cause formation of fibrous tissue that can block the ductus deferens tubes. The *N. gonorrhoeae* organisms also can spread to the testes, causing inflammation and destruction of seminiferous tubules, finally resulting in sterility.

In females *N. gonorrhoeae* enter through the vagina and tend to spread up the cervix, uterus, and into the fallopian tubes. A woman usually is not aware of the initial stages of the disease; however, if scar tissue is formed in the fallopian tubes it can block the passage of the female sex cells (ova) resulting in sterility. Most women with gonorrhea exhibit no symptoms, and they unknowingly can harbor and transmit the organisms for many months.

# 3  GAMETOGENESIS

So far we have discussed the anatomy of the male and female primary and secondary sex organs. We will now discuss their function.

The primary sex organs produce **gametes** or **sex cells** and hormones. The term **gametogenesis** means origin of or production of gametes (*gameto*—gamete; *genesis* —origin or production of); therefore, we will discuss the production of male gametes or sex cells (sperm) and female gametes or sex cells (oocytes). These sex cells are vital for the production of a new human being, since they contain the genetic material (chromosomes and genes) that directs the synthesis and development of a new human being.

## *SPERMATOGENESIS (PRODUCTION OF SPERM)*

**Spermatogenesis** occurs in the seminiferous tubules of the testes. The **follicle stimulating hormone (FSH),** secreted by the anterior pituitary, stimulates the germinal epithelium in the seminiferous tubules to produce sperm (Figure 21-10). The secretion of FSH increases dramatically between the ages of 14 to 16, which is called puberty, and continues throughout a male's life. The **interstitial cell stimulating hormone (ICSH)** stimulates the interstitial cells between the seminifer-

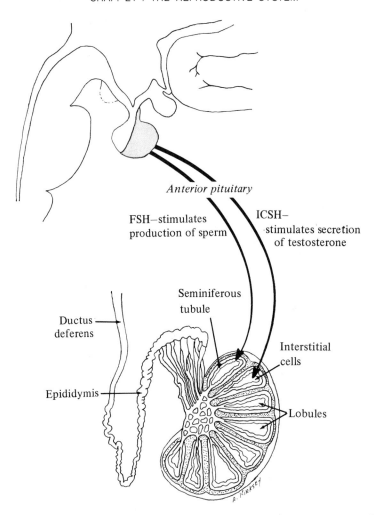

**Figure 21–10.** Hormonal influence of FSH (follicle stimulating hormone) and ICSH (interstitial cell stimulating hormone) on sperm production and testosterone secretion.

ous tubules to secrete testosterone, which is responsible for male secondary sex traits.

## Meiosis

The actual production of new sperm cells is not by mitosis, but rather by a process called **meiosis.** This process is responsible for producing four new cells, each with half the normal number of chromosomes (23). This reduction in the number of chromosomes to 23 (none of which is paired) also occurs in the formation of the female gametes (oocytes). The number of chromosomes in the gametes has to be reduced from 46 (2N or **diploid number**) to 23 (N or **haploid number**) so that when a sperm fertilizes an oocyte the normal number of 46 chromosomes will be reestablished. If 46 chromosomes

were maintained in the sperm and oocyte when they joined, the fertilized egg would have 92 chromosomes and would be an abnormal cell. This abnormal cell could then produce other abnormal cells, either resulting in an abnormal embryo or spontaneous abortion.

The steps involved in the formation of sperm cells are shown in Figure 21–11. Each cell that enters into meiosis is called a **primary spermatocyte,** and it is a diploid cell, which has a 2N number, or 46 chromosomes, in the nucleus. Twenty-two pairs or 44 chromosomes are called **autosomes,** and they contain genes that determine various traits (hair color, eye color, height, and others). The other pairs of chromosomes are designated as **sex chromosomes,** which determine the sex of an individual. A male will have X and Y chromosomes and a female will have X and X chromosomes (Figure 21–11).

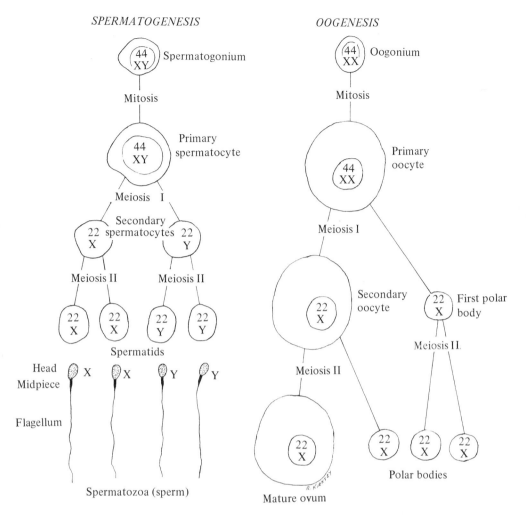

**Figure 21–11.** The mitotic and meiotic steps involved in spermatogenesis and oogenesis. The numbers in each cell represent autosomes. The X and Y letters represent sex chromosomes.

In the first stage of meiosis the reduction from 46 chromosomes to 23 takes place. Two secondary spermatocytes are formed each containing 22 autosomes plus an X chromosome or a Y chromosome but not both.

The second stage of meiosis is characterized by the secondary spermatocytes dividing by mitosis to form four spermatids. Two spermatids contain an X chromosome and two contain a Y chromosome. Half of all the millions of spermatids formed will contain a Y chromosome and half will contain an X chromosome.

### Transformation and Structure of Sperm Cells

The spermatids undergo a complex series of changes to form sperm cells, which are composed of a head, a midpiece, and a tail (flagellum) (Figure 21–12). The head contains the nucleus with 23 chromosomes. Covering the head like a cap is the **acrosome,** containing the enzyme **hyaluronidase.** The acrosome helps the sperm penetrate the membrane of an oocyte at fertilization.

The midpiece contains many mitochondria, arranged in a spiral manner. The mitochondria metabolize nutrients to furnish energy for the movement of the tail. Thrashing movements of the tail are responsible for moving the sperm. Once the sperm cells are formed they are stored in the epididymis until they are ejaculated.

### OOGENESIS (PRODUCTION OF OVA)

**Oogenesis** is similar to spermatogenesis in that one cell containing 46 chromosomes divides by meiosis to form four cells, each with 23 chromosomes. There are some

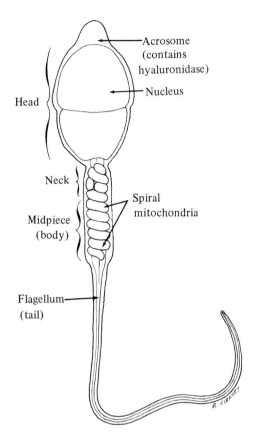

**Figure 21-12.**   Structure of a sperm cell.

differences between oogenesis and spermatogenesis, which will be discussed shortly.

## Follicle Development and Rupture

**Follicle stimulating hormone (FSH),** secreted by the anterior pituitary, stimulates several primary follicles to begin developing into **secondary follicles** within the ovaries. A follicle is simply a microscopic pocket within an ovary, and it contains an oogonium with 46 chromosomes. A primary follicle develops into a secondary follicle, and simultaneously the oogonium enlarges to form a **primary oocyte** (Figure 21-13). The cells forming the follicle secrete the hormone, estrogen, which is responsible for preparing the endometrium of the uterus for implantation of a fertilized ovum. The secondary follicle develops and moves toward the surface of an ovary, accumulating fluid within the follicle cavity. The secondary follicle develops into a **graafian follicle,** which bulges from the surface of the ovary. All the time that the graafian follicle is developing, the secretion of estrogen increases. The level of estrogen finally increases to a point that it inhibits the release of FSH

from the anterior pituitary, but stimulates it to release a large amount of luteinizing hormone (LH). The sudden increase of LH causes rupture of the graafian follicle and release of an oocyte into the pelvic cavity. Fimbriae act to guide the oocyte into the fallopian tube, which moves it toward the uterus.

As the follicle develops, the primary oocyte (Figure 21-11), with 46 chromosomes, divides by meiosis to form a **secondary oocyte** and the **first polar body,** each with 23 chromosomes. The secondary oocyte begins to divide by mitosis to form an ovum. This process is not completed unless the oocyte is fertilized by a sperm cell.

The primary oocyte is similar to a primary spermatocyte in that both contain 46 chromosomes; but the primary oocyte contains 44 autosomes and XX sex chromosomes. This means that following meiosis the secondary oocyte contains one X sex chromosome, whereas half the sperm cells contain a Y chromosome and half contain an X chromosome.

It takes approximately 13 days for FSH to stimulate development of the graafian follicle and secondary oocyte. On approximately the fourteenth day the graafian follicle ruptures and releases the secondary oocyte.

## Corpus Luteum

After the graafian follicle ruptures and releases the secondary oocyte, the cavity fills with blood. The luteinizing hormone (LH) stimulates the follicle cells surrounding the cavity to enlarge and to accumulate a yellowish substance called lutein in their cytoplasm. Gradually the yellowish colored cells enlarge to form a yellow structure called the **corpus luteum** (*corpus*—body; *luteum*—yellow). The corpus luteum secretes the hormone **progesterone** (Figure 21-13), which, like estrogen, prepares the endometrium for implantation of a fertilized ovum.

LH hormone continues to stimulate the corpus luteum to grow and secrete progesterone for about 10 to 12 days after ovulation. If the secondary oocyte that was released is not fertilized the concentration of LH drops and the corpus luteum degenerates and the secretion of progesterone ceases. A small white scar, called **corpus albicans,** results from degeneration of the corpus luteum. If the secondary oocyte is fertilized the LH hormone concentration remains high and the corpus luteum enlarges to the point where it occupies 30 to 50 percent of the entire ovary. The corpus luteum continues to secrete progesterone during approximately the first three months of pregnancy. Progesterone is essential during this time because it controls development of the placenta, which is a structure that helps the developing embryo receive nutrients from the mother.

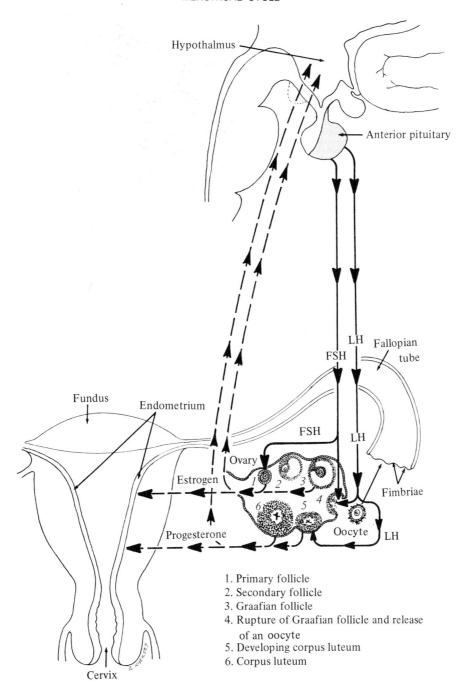

**Figure 21-13.** Hormonal influence on oogenesis and preparation of endometrium. The FSH and LH hormones influence the development of oocytes within follicles. The feedback of estrogen and progesterone hormones to the hypothalamus is shown. Release of estrogen and progesterone from follicles and corpus luteum also is shown.

1. Primary follicle
2. Secondary follicle
3. Graafian follicle
4. Rupture of Graafian follicle and release of an oocyte
5. Developing corpus luteum
6. Corpus luteum

# 4 MENSTRUAL CYCLE

In a female the development of an ovum takes place at the same time that the endometrium of the uterus is being prepared to receive a fertilized ovum. The simulta-neous changes in the uterus and ovaries are controlled by hormones. The overall changes are called the menstrual cycle. We have discussed the changes that occur in the ovaries and now we will discuss the hormones and changes that occur in the endometrium of the uterus.

The changes that the endometrium undergoes occur in cycles that last from 25 to 35 days but average about 28 days. A menstrual cycle can be divided into three phases that vary as to changes in the thickness of the endometrium and hormones controlling the changes. Figure 21-14 shows the relationship between development of the endometrium, level of hormones, days and development of an oocyte in the uterus.

## FLOW PHASE (MENSTRUAL PHASE)

The flow phase is characterized by the superficial layer of the endometrial wall being sloughed off (Figure 21-14). Blood, tissue fluid, and remnants of the endometrium flow through the uterus and vagina out of the body. The flow of materials lasts from four to six days.

The superficial layer of the endometrium is sloughed off when a secondary oocyte is not fertilized. Estrogen and progesterone hormones cause the endometrium to become quite thick and vascularized to receive a fertilized ovum. The superficial layer of the endometrium is sloughed off when the concentration of estrogen and progesterone hormones drops to a low level (Figure 21-14). The flow of materials stops after four to six days because of an increase in the concentrations of estrogen and progesterone. During the flow phase several follicles in an ovary begin to develop as the result of an increased concentration of FSH.

## FOLLICULAR PHASE (PROLIFERATIVE PHASE)

The follicular phase lasts from about the fifth day to the fourteenth day of the menstrual cycle. The superficial layer of the endometrium is reestablished during this phase due to stimulation from estrogen. The layer becomes quite thick and the size and number of blood vessels increase.

While the endometrial layer is developing or proliferating, a follicle continues to develop until a **graafian follicle,** containing an **oocyte,** is formed. The graafian follicle ruptures and releases its oocyte when stimulated by a high concentration of LH (Figure 21-14). Rupturing or ovulation of an oocyte occurs on about the fourteenth day of the menstrual cycle.

The developing follicle continues to release estrogen, which stimulates the endometrium to grow and develop. The proliferation and development of the endometrium is necessary so that it can properly receive and develop the ovum if it is fertilized.

## LUTEAL PHASE (POSTOVULATORY)

The luteal phase lasts from about the fourteenth to the twenty-eighth day of the menstrual cycle. This phase is characterized by the endometrium thickening even more. The corpus luteum is now formed in the ovary,

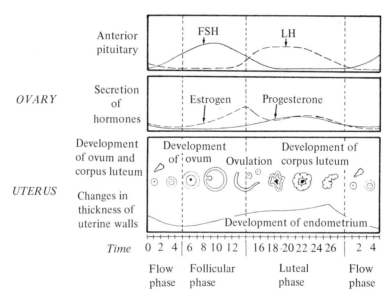

**Figure 21-14.** Human menstrual cycle. The interrelationship between the level of pituitary hormones and the development of oocytes is shown. Also, the level of ovarian hormones and the development of the endometrium are shown in relation to the phases.

and it begins to secrete progesterone (Figure 21-14), which stimulates arteries in the endometrium to become coiled and increased in length. Also, the amount of tissue fluid in the endometrium increases considerably during this phase. This is the final preparation of the endometrium for a fertilized ovum.

If the oocyte is not fertilized the corpus luteum degenerates and, therefore, the level of progesterone drops rapidly. When progesterone reaches a certain level the superficial layer of the endometrium begins to slough off. This is the end of one menstrual cycle and the beginning of the next.

If the oocyte is fertilized the corpus luteum does not degenerate and the level of progesterone remains high. This means that the endometrium does not slough off during the term of pregnancy; therefore, a woman normally does not have a period or a menstrual cycle during the time she is pregnant.

# 5 MENARCHE AND MENOPAUSE

The ovaries really do not begin to grow and develop until a female reaches puberty, which is between 10 and 14 years. Puberty is characterized by development of the female secondary sex characteristics, such as enlargement of the breasts, maturation of the uterus and vagina, growth of pubic and axillary hair, and development of the "female curves" or rounding of the body.

## MENARCHE

**Menarche** is the first menstrual cycle that a female has and usually it occurs between the ages of 12 and 15 years. At the time of menarche the ovaries contain over 200,000 primary follicles; however, only about 400 follicles develop totally during the lifetime of a female. Many of the 200,000 primary follicles start developing, but then stop and never reach maturity. A woman continues to develop oocytes and have a menstrual cycle approximately every 28 days until she reaches menopause at 45 to 50 years of age.

## MENOPAUSE

Menopause is the climax of the period when the ovaries, fallopian tubes, uterus, vagina, and breasts atrophy or degenerate. At menopause the ovaries no

longer produce oocytes and secrete hormones; therefore, the woman no longer menstruates and she no longer can bear children.

# 6 SEXUAL INTERCOURSE

Normally, sexual intercourse is necessary to deposit semen in the female near the entrance of the uterus. This has to occur before sperm and the seminal fluid secretions can move through the uterus to the fallopian tubes and fertilize an ovum.

## ERECTION OF THE PENIS

Prior to sexual intercourse the penis must change from the normal flaccid state into an enlarged, erect state. Many different stimuli can cause the penis to become erect, such as touch, visual stimuli, and even erotic thoughts. The stimuli initiate parasympathetic impulses that are sent to arteries that supply the erectile tissue in **corpora cavernosa** and **corpus spongiosum** (Figure 21-9). The arteries dilate, thereby carrying a large amount of blood into the spongelike spaces of the erectile tissue. Simultaneously, the drainage of blood from the erectile tissue by veins is restricted, which retains the blood within the erectile tissue. The increased flow of blood into the erectile tissue causes the penis to become erect; it remains erect until the stimuli cease and the veins drain blood away from the erectile tissue.

## EJACULATION

During sexual intercourse the glans of the penis is stimulated by touch so that an autonomic reflex response follows, called **ejaculation**. During ejaculation, sympathetic nerve impulses cause contractions of the smooth muscles of the epididymis, ductus deferens, and prostate gland. These contractions carry semen into the urethra. Skeletal muscles at the base of the penis then contract and force the semen out the end of the urethra. The semen is deposited in the vagina just below the cervix.

The average amount of semen that is ejaculated is between 3 to 5 ml. Each ml of semen contains approximately 100 million sperm, or in each ejaculation there is a total of 300 million to 500 million sperm. If the amount of sperm drops to 35 million per ml, a male may not be able to fertilize an oocyte; that is, he is sterile.

# 7  FERTILIZATION

The 3 to 5 ml of semen that is ejaculated contains nutrients and alkaline secretions that are important if the sperm are to reach and fertilize an oocyte. The nutrients are used as a source of energy for the sperm cells as they move toward an oocyte. The alkaline secretions help to neutralize the high acidity of the vagina, pH = 4. Sperm cannot survive or move through an acidic medium without help; therefore, the alkaline secretions and nutrients maintain viability of the sperm and aid their movement.

The sperm, by means of their tails, move through the cervix, uterus, and into the distal one-third of the fallopian tubes (Figure 21–15). It takes the sperm approximately 30 minutes to make this trip. When they reach the distal one-third of the fallopian tube (or the area nearest the ovary), fertilization of a viable secondary oocyte occurs, if one is present. Fertilization actually involves the nucleus of a sperm cell combining with the nucleus of the secondary oocyte. Usually only one sperm penetrates the membrane surrounding the oocyte. Sperm cells contain the enzyme **hyaluronidase** (within the acrosome), which enables them to break through the gellike membrane of the oocyte. Only one sperm penetrates a secondary oocyte, but the other sperm aid the one by contributing their hyaluronidase to the breakdown of the membrane of the secondary oocyte (Figure 21–15). The reason that only one sperm is able to penetrate the oocyte is because immediately after it enters, the membrane repairs the hole and becomes impenetrable to any other sperm. This prevents more than one sperm nucleus from combining with the oocyte nucleus; thus it allows only one set of 23 chromosomes to combine with the 23 chromosomes in the oocyte, reestablishing the normal number of 46 chromosomes. Once the sperm nucleus has united with

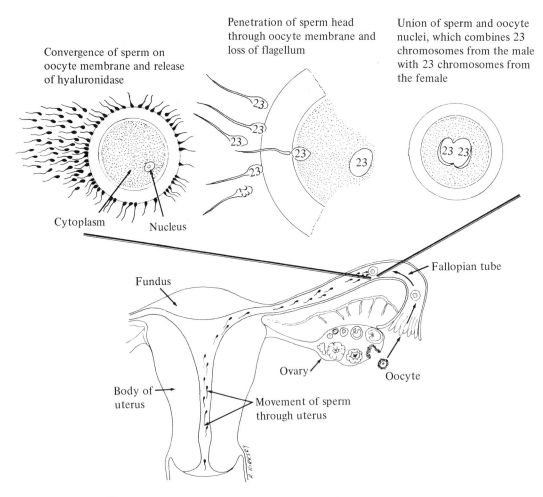

**Figure 21-15.**  Movement of sperm and stages of fertilization.

the nucleus of the secondary oocyte, development of the secondary oocyte into an **ovum** is completed.

Normally, fertilization occurs in the distal one-third of the fallopian tube because the oocyte is dead after it moves past this point. It takes approximately three to four days for an oocyte to be moved down the fallopian tube into the uterus. If it encounters sperm in the uterus fertilization will probably not occur because the oocyte is dead.

Only the head of the sperm with its nucleus containing 23 chromosomes penetrates the oocyte and unites with its nucleus containing 23 chromosomes. Since only one sperm is involved in fertilization, one might wonder why approximately 100 million sperm per ml of semen are ejaculated. Many things can happen to the sperm on their journey to the oocyte. Many of them do not survive the acidity of the vagina or the high temperature of the uterus; and many will go down the wrong fallopian tube since normally only one oocyte is released into one of the fallopian tubes.

# 8  RESTORATION OF 46 CHROMOSOMES AND DETERMINATION OF SEX

Union of the sperm nucleus containing 23 chromosomes with the nucleus of the oocyte containing 23 chromosomes first produces an ovum, then a zygote containing 46 chromosomes. Previously, we said that two chromosomes, X and Y, are responsible for deter-

mining the sex of an individual. An oocyte always contains an X chromosome, whereas the fertilizing sperm either contains an X or Y chromosome. If the fertilizing sperm contains an X chromosome, the union produces a female (XX) (Figure 21–16). If the fertilizing sperm contains a Y chromosome, the union produces a male (XY). Thus, it is the sperm cell that determines the sex of a child.

Normally, only one secondary oocyte is released each 28 day period; however, if more than one is released then multiple fertilization and multiple births can result. For example, if two secondary oocytes are released and fertilized, twins will be born. The infants are classified as **fraternal twins,** and they will not necessarily be of the same sex or have the exact same genetic traits (Figure 21–17). The differences result because the oocytes are fertilized by different sperm. **Identical twins** are born when one secondary oocyte is fertilized, and then it splits into two cells (Figure 21–17). The infants will be of the same sex and will inherit the same basic genetic traits.

# 9  DEVELOPMENT OF THE FERTILIZED ZYGOTE AND IMPLANTATION

Immediately after fertilization the zygote, with 46 chromosomes, begins to divide by mitosis. It quickly goes through a two-, four-, and eight-cell stage (Figure 21–18). The individual cells are called **blastomeres** and

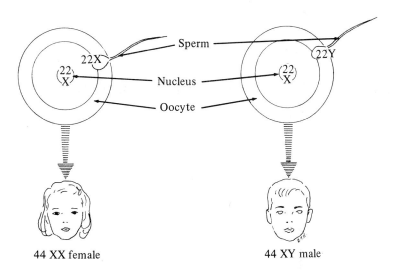

**44 XX female**                    **44 XY male**

Figure 21-16.   The determination of the sex of a child is dependent upon whether an X or a Y sperm fertilizes an ovum.

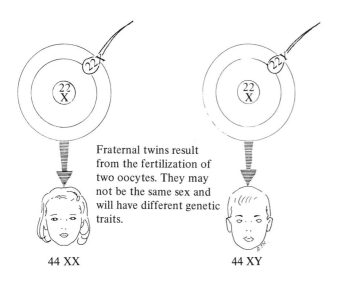

Fraternal twins result from the fertilization of two oocytes. They may not be the same sex and will have different genetic traits.

44 XX                    44 XY

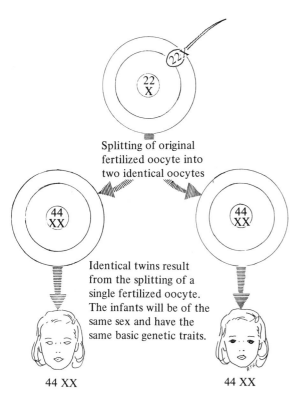

Splitting of original fertilized oocyte into two identical oocytes

Identical twins result from the splitting of a single fertilized oocyte. The infants will be of the same sex and have the same basic genetic traits.

44 XX                    44 XX

Figure 21-17.   Fraternal twins and identical twins.

the mitotic divisions that the zygote undergoes are called **cleavage.** During the time that the zygote is undergoing cleavage, it is moving down the fallopian tube toward the uterus. It takes approximately three to four days for the ball of blastomeres to reach the uterus. At that time it is a solid ball of cells called a **morula.** Gradually a central fluid-filled cavity, surrounded by an

inner cell mass, is formed with an outer layer of cells called **trophoblast.** This structure is called a **blastocyst** and the chorionic layer of cells will attach the blastocyst to the endometrium. The inner cell mass will develop into the embryo.

Approximately seven to ten days after fertilization the blastocyst begins to burrow into the thick vascularized endometrium. The chorionic layer secretes enzymes that make a hole in the endometrium and allow the blastocyst to embed. The point at which the blastocyst enters the endometrium is called the **decidua basalis.**

## DEVELOPMENT OF MEMBRANES AND PLACENTA

Two membranes develop around the embryo about the time that it implants. The outer membrane is called the **chorion,** and it is highly vascularized. The chorion forms **chorionic villi** (Figure 21-19), each of which is richly endowed with blood vessels. The innermost membrane is the **amnion,** which forms a loose-fitting sac around the developing embryo. Clear-colored **amniotic fluid** is located between the embryo and the amnion. The developing embryo is protected from jolts during its nine-month development by the amnion and amniotic fluid. These structures are similar to the cranial meninges and CSF as far as their locations and functions are concerned. The embryo is connected to the chorion by the body stalk, which eventually helps form the umbilical cord.

The chorionic villi grow into the **decidua basalis** area of the endometrium, where they come in close contact with endometrial blood vessels. Small lakes or lacunae, filled with maternal blood, develop around the ends of the villi. Exchange of nutrients and wastes occurs between the maternal blood in the lacunae and the embryo's blood in the chorionic villi. The maternal blood supply to this area continues to develop and the **chorion** develops until the **placenta** (Figure 21-20) is formed. When the placenta is totally developed it is about 8 inches in diameter and 1 inch thick. It is highly vascular because of the blood vessels in the endometrium and chorion; however, the maternal and embryonic blood do not mix.

The blood vessels in the chorion and body stalk converge to form two umbilical arteries and an umbilical vein. These blood vessels constitute the **umbilical cord** (Figure 21-20), which carries nutrients and wastes between the placenta and the developing embryo.

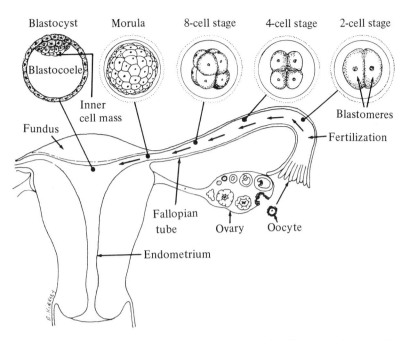

**Figure 21-18.** Development and passage of a fertilized zygote along the fallopian tube.

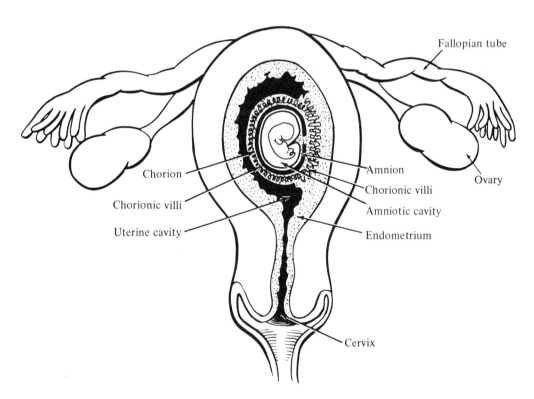

**Figure 21-19.** Embryonic and fetal membranes. The amnion and chorion membranes that surround an embryo and fetus are shown.

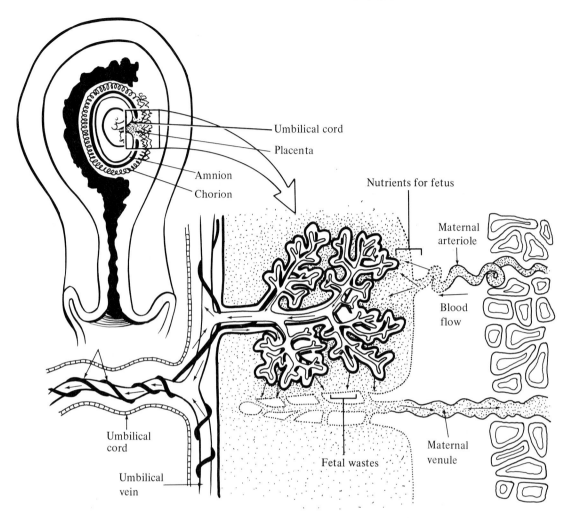

**Figure 21-20.** The umbilical cord and placenta are shown above. The detailed structure of the umbilical cord and placenta is shown below with the exchange of blood between the mother and the fetus indicated.

## FUNCTIONS OF THE PLACENTA

The placenta is a vital structure during the development of the embryo and fetus, and has several functions.

### Acts as a Lung and a Kidney

The lungs in the embryo and fetus are not functioning prior to birth; therefore, the placenta acts as a lung in that the exchange of oxygen and carbon dioxide occurs through the placenta. The umbilical vein (Figure 21-20) carries nutrients from the placenta to the tissues of the embryo. The kidneys in the embryo and the fetus also are not functioning prior to birth; therefore, waste materials are removed from the embryo's blood by the placenta. The umbilical arteries carry waste materials from the tissues of the embryo to the placenta. The waste materials move into the maternal blood and nutrients move into the umbilical vein.

### Acts as an Endocrine Organ

The placenta secretes **chorionic gonadotropins,** which stimulate the corpus luteum to secrete estrogen and progesterone. The presence of **chorionic gonadotropins** in the urine is a positive test indicating that a woman is pregnant. The placenta also secretes estrogen and progesterone, which help to maintain the endometrial tissue during pregnancy.

## Filters out Bacteria and Some Viruses

Most bacteria cannot pass across the placenta into the fetal blood. However the spirochete, **Treponema pallidum,** can penetrate the placenta. This is how a fetus can be infected by syphilis, causing congenital syphilis.

The placenta is not as effective against viruses, especially the rubella virus that causes German measles. This particular form of measles is not very severe in its effects on a woman, but it can be quite dangerous to a developing fetus during the first three months of pregnancy. If contracted during this time the rubella virus can do permanent damage to the heart, ears, and brain of the fetus.

Antibodies in the mother's blood can pass through the placenta into the fetal blood. This can be both good and bad for the fetus. If the antibodies protect the child against infections following birth they are beneficial; however, if a mother is Rh negative and the fetus is Rh positive, the mother's blood will form Rh antibodies that can move through the placenta into the fetal blood and destroy the RBCs. This condition is called **erythroblastosis fetalis.**

# 10 EMBRYOLOGIC DEVELOPMENT

Many changes take place from the time of fertilization until an infant is born. This period of time is called the **gestation period** and lasts approximately 270 days. To discuss these various changes we will subdivide the gestation period into the period of the ovum, the period of the embryo, and the period of the fetus.

## PERIOD OF THE OVUM OR PREEMBRYONIC PERIOD

The period of the ovum extends from fertilization through the second week. Following fertilization the ovum undergoes cleavage as it moves down the fallopian tube to the uterus. Generally by about the tenth day following fertilization the blastocyst implants in the endometrium. The formation of the amnion and chorion membranes occurs during this time, as does development of the chorionic villi.

During the second week of development some very important changes occur that are the prelude to the de-velopment of the tissues, organs, and systems. The inner cell mass of the blastocyst begins to change so that there is the formation of three distinct primary germ layers. From outside inward these layers are known as **ectoderm** (outer), **mesoderm** (middle), and **endoderm** (inner) (Figure 21-21). These layers are called germ layers because from them germinate or originate all the tissues of the body that in turn form the body's organs. The **ectoderm** or outer germ layer gives rise to the epidermis of the skin, hair, nails, the nervous system, lens of the eye, and enamel of the teeth (Figure 21-21). The **mesoderm** or middle layer gives rise to the three types of muscle tissue (cardiac, smooth, and skeletal), bones, peritoneum, and the lining of portions of the urinary and reproductive systems, and connective tissues. The **endoderm** or inner layer gives rise to the lining of the digestive tract and accessory organs; lining of the trachea and bronchi; and lining of portions of the urinary and reproductive systems. These germ layers will begin to germinate or produce these tissues during the period of the embryo.

## PERIOD OF THE EMBRYO OR EMBRYONIC PERIOD

From the beginning of the third week to the end of the eighth week is the duration of the embryonic period. Figure 21-22 shows that at the beginning of this period the embryo is about the size of a large dot and during this period it changes into a structure weighing about one ounce and measuring about one inch in length. By the end of the embryonic period the maternal circulation to the placenta is functioning and the chorionic villi are formed and functioning. Now that the maternal circulation to the placenta and the circulation to the embryo are functioning, development of tissues and organs from the germ layers begins to take place.

The visceral organs develop during this period as well as the face around a prominent nose (Figure 21-22). The limbs begin to develop with separation of the fingers and toes (Figure 21-22). The external genital organs are present but it is difficult to determine the sex.

## PERIOD OF THE FETUS

The period of the fetus lasts from the beginning of the ninth week through the fortieth week or birth. This period is characterized by the growth and development

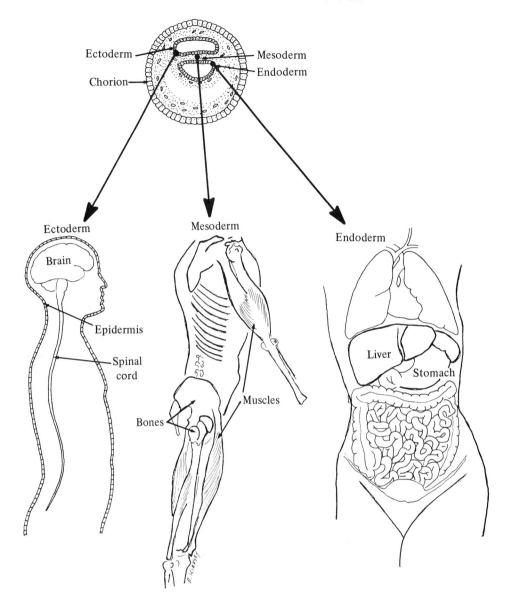

**Figure 21-21.** Derivatives of the embryonic germ layers. The organs and tissues that develop from ectoderm, mesoderm, and endoderm germ layers are shown.

of the previously formed structures (Figure 21-22). Some of the highlights of this period are the following:

### Ninth to Twelfth Week (Third Month)

Blood is now being pumped through the fetus by a heart that can be heard by a stethoscope. Teeth begin to develop and vocal cords are formed. Sexual development of a male proceeds rapidly with development of testes and some ducts.

### Thirteenth to Sixteenth Week (Fourth Month)

At the beginning of the fourth month, the fetus weighs about an ounce and is approximately 7.6 cm long. By the end of this month it will be about 15 to 20 cm long and will weigh some 170 to 227 g.

Fetal movements which possibly can be felt by the mother begin to occur during this time. Eyebrows and eyelashes appear now, as do fingerprints and footprints. Sexual development of the female proceeds rapidly now with formation of the vagina and uterus.

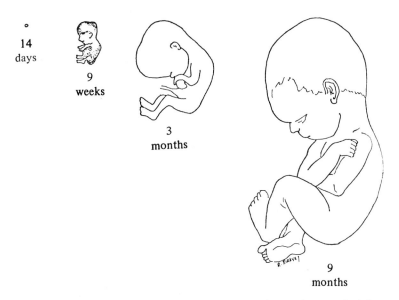

14
days

9
weeks

3
months

9
months

Figure 21-22.    The stages in the development of an embryo and a fetus are shown.

### Seventeenth to Twentieth Week (Fifth Month)

During the fifth month the growth of the fetus causes it to straighten out from a curved position. Bone marrow is now developed and forming blood. Structures derived from the skin, such as the fingernails, toenails, and hair, grow extensively. The oil glands become quite active and secrete an oily protective covering over the body that gives the fetus and newborn a creamy look. This coat is called **vernix caseosa.**

### Twenty-First to Twenty-Fourth Week (Sixth Month)

By the end of the sixth month the fetus weighs about 600 g. The skin is wrinkled and the deposition of fat beneath the skin is beginning. The eyes are well developed and open.

### Twenty-Fifth to Twenty-Eighth Week (Seventh Month)

By the end of the seventh month the weight of the fetus has increased to 1200 to 1300 g, and it is approximately 41 cm long.

### Twenty-Ninth to Thirty-Second Week (Eighth Month)

During the eighth month the testes descend from near the kidneys into the scrotum in a male fetus. Fat deposits continue and now the skin begins to lose some of its wrinkles. The extremities now are being moved about quite strenuously. If the fetus is born at this point, probably it could survive. The fetus weighs about 2500 g at the end of the eighth month.

### Thirty-Third to Thirty-Sixth Week (Ninth Month)

The weight of the fetus increases now to approximately 2700 to 3600 g and is about 51 cm in length. The fetus now is ready to be born, and normally the head is positioned downward in the uterus and the arms and legs are drawn up.

An interesting point about the development of the fetus is that normally the fetus gains over 50 percent of its weight during the last two months. In relation to this point, the size of an infant is determined primarily by heredity and not the amount of food a mother eats. A mother who eats large quantities of food, with the assumption that it is healthy for her and the child, will find that the extra food is not utilized by the baby but rather stored in her own body as fat.

## 11 CIRCULATION OF BLOOD IN THE FETUS

The circulation of blood in the unborn fetus is different in several respects, compared to the circulation in an infant after it is born. Previously, we discussed the fact that the lungs do not function in a developing fetus. The placenta functions as the exchange point for nutrients and wastes between the fetal and maternal blood, even though the bloods do not mix. Several circulatory structures are present in the fetus that bypass the lungs and liver as well as carry blood to and from the placenta. These structures are **ductus venosus, ductus arteriosus, foramen ovale,** the **two umbilical arteries,** and an **umbilical vein.**

Figure 21-23 shows these structures. We will trace the flow of deoxygenated blood from the fetus to the placenta, and then the flow of oxygenated blood from the placenta throughout the body of a fetus.

Two **umbilical arteries** branch off the internal iliac arteries (Figure 21-23) and carry deoxygenated blood through the umbilical cord to the placenta of the mother. Nutrients are picked up and wastes given off through capillaries in the placenta. Oxygenated blood rich in nutrients is carried by the umbilical vein from the placenta within the umbilical cord into the abdomen of the fetus and then courses upward. Near the liver the vein splits into two branches. One branch joins the portal vein and enters the liver; the other branch, the **ductus venosus,** bypasses the liver and joins the inferior vena cava. The ductus venosus acts as a bypass so that some blood is shunted away from the liver. This bypass is important since the liver is not functioning and the waste removal functions are performed by the placenta prior to birth.

The inferior vena cava carries both oxygenated blood from the umbilical vein and deoxygenated blood from the lower parts of the body. This mixed blood has a purplish color and is carried to the right atrium of the

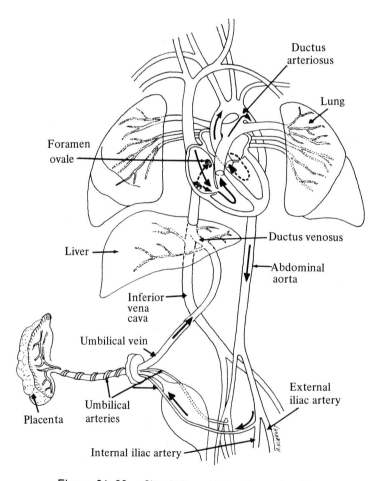

**Figure 21-23.**  Circulation of blood through a fetus.

heart, where blood also is brought in by the superior vena cava. A large amount of blood in the right atrium is channeled through an opening, **foramen ovale** (Figure 21-23), into the left atrium. The foramen ovale functions to shunt blood away from the right ventricle, which pumps blood to the lungs to be oxygenated. Fetal blood coming into the right atrium is deoxygenated and the lungs are not functioning; therefore, most of the blood is shunted away from the lungs. The blood that does move into the right ventricle is pumped into the pulmonary aorta where another bypass, the **ductus arteriosus,** connects the pulmonary aorta to the arch of the aorta (Figure 21-23). Most of the blood in the pulmonary aorta is channeled through the **ductus arteriosus;** however, enough blood is carried to the lung tissues to maintain their development.

The mixed blood is carried to the tissues of the body by the various branches of the aorta where the oxygen and nutrients move through capillaries into the tissues and waste materials move into the blood. When the blood reaches the internal iliac arteries, it passes into the umbilical arteries, which move through the umbilical cord to the placenta.

At birth the infant's lungs begin to function; he is separated from the placenta and the liver begins to remove wastes. This means that the specialized structures are no longer needed and they immediately begin to atrophy. The ductus arteriosus constricts so that blood now flows through the pulmonary arteries to the lungs. A flap of skin begins to cover over the **foramen ovale** and by the end of the first month most blood flow through the foramen has stopped. Generally by the end of the first year the foramen ovale is totally closed and a scar, **fossa ovalis,** is all that is left. The umbilical arteries, umbilical vein and ductus venosus all are changed into ligaments that connect to the liver and anterior body wall.

If the **foramen ovale** fails to close, the oxygenated blood in the left atrium and ventricle is mixed with the deoxygenated blood in the right atrium and ventricle. The result is that the blood and the skin have a bluish color and the child is said to be a "blue baby." Surgery is necessary to close the foramen ovale.

# 12  LABOR (PARTURITION)

At the end of the ninth month, or about 280 days since the last menstrual period, the gestation period is complete and the infant is ready to be born. The birth process involves labor, rhythmical contractions of the uterus, which force the infant through the birth canal.

## HORMONES INVOLVED IN LABOR

The muscles of the uterus are stimulated to start contracting by **estrogen** and **oxytocin** hormones. During the gestation period the placenta secretes little estrogen since it stimulates the uterine muscles; however, a few weeks prior to labor the concentration of estrogen increases considerably. Labor also is initiated by secretion of oxytocin from the posterior pituitary, which initiates forceful contractions of the uterus. At the same time the hormone, **relaxin,** acts to soften and relax the pubic symphysis ligament and other ligaments along the birth canal. Relaxin is released from the placenta and ovaries and it plays an important role in labor. If the fetus were forced down the birth canal prior to softening and relaxing of the ligaments, it could be damaged.

The process of labor can be divided into three phases or stages.

## LABOR

### The First Stage of Labor

This stage begins when the uterine contractions start and ends when the cervix is completely dilated. Uterine contractions force the amniotic sac into the cervix, which helps to dilate the cervix. The cervix usually is considered to be completely dilated when it is 10 centimeters in diameter. Generally, the amniotic sac ruptures and releases its fluids at the end of this stage (Figure 21-24).

### The Second Stage of Labor

The second stage of labor extends from the time the cervix is completely dilated until the fetus is born. Uterine contractions gradually force the fetus down the birth canal, generally head first (Figure 21-24). Sometimes the fetus may enter the canal feet or buttocks first, which is called a breech presentation. It is during this stage that tearing of the **obstetric perineum** can occur; therefore, an incision or **episiotomy** may be made. The incision is easily closed after the infant is born.

### The Third Stage of Labor

Expulsion of the placenta or afterbirth characterizes this stage. Thirty minutes to hours after an infant is born the placenta is expelled by strong contractions of the **myometrium** of the uterus (Figure 21-24). When

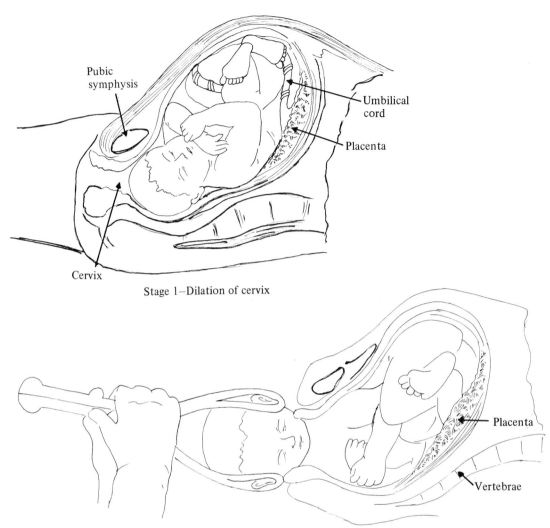

Stage 1–Dilation of cervix

Stage 2–Passage through cervix and birth canal

Stage 3–Expulsion of
placenta (afterbirth)

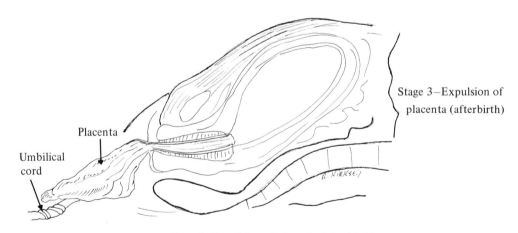

Stage 3–Expulsion of placenta (afterbirth)

Figure 21-24. Stages of labor.

the placenta is expelled, the large number of blood vessels that supplied it are now exposed and excessive hemorrhaging can occur. Normally, strong contractions of the myometrium act to constrict and shut off the blood vessels so that little hemorrhaging takes place.

# 13 DEVELOPMENT AND LACTATION OF THE BREASTS

During pregnancy the breasts enlarge and develop to the point that they can secrete milk (lactation) if stimulated. This process is controlled by several hormones. Estrogen, produced by the placenta, stimulates

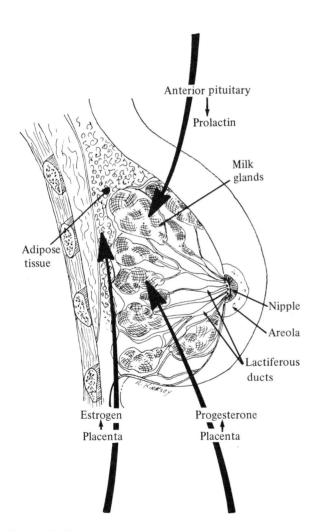

**Figure 21-25.** Hormones that stimulate development and lactation of the breasts.

development of the ducts and deposition of adipose tissue in the breasts (Figure 21-25). Progesterone, produced by the placenta, stimulates development of milk producing glands and prepares them to secrete milk.

Estrogen and progesterone stimulate development and enlargement of the breasts prior to birth; however, secretion of milk is controlled by the lactogenic hormone **prolactin.** The anterior pituitary secretes large amounts of prolactin immediately following birth of an infant. Prolactin also maintains the breasts and secretion of milk for six to nine months after an infant is born; breast feeding, or suckling, reflexly stimulates the release of **prolactin.** If a child is not breast-fed, the secretion of milk will cease and the breasts will decrease in size.

# 14 CONTRACEPTIVES AND BIRTH CONTROL

Birth control techniques and devices can be divided into four categories.

## PREVENT PRODUCTION OF OOCYTES AND SPERM

The "pill" can be taken by women to prevent the production of a viable oocyte, but they do not prevent the woman from having a menstrual cycle. Birth control pills contain synthetic **estrogen** and **progesterone** which inhibit secretion of FSH and LH. The estrogen and progesterone, in effect, "fool" the hypothalamus and anterior pituitary into thinking that a woman is pregnant, thereby inhibiting secretion of FSH and LH, which are responsible for the development and secretion of an oocyte. The outer surface of the endometrium in the uterus thickens and prepares for implantation of a fertilized ovum because of the estrogen and progesterone. When a woman stops taking the pills for seven to eight days, the estrogen and progesterone levels drop and the outer endometrial layer is sloughed off or she menstruates. At the end of seven or eight days she then resumes taking the pills and the inhibition of FSH and LH begins again.

The "pill" is 99 to 100 percent effective in preventing pregnancy when it is taken properly. The disadvantages of taking the pill include complaints of weight gain, headaches, bloatedness, nausea, and cramps. Evidence indicates that the pill may increase cases of

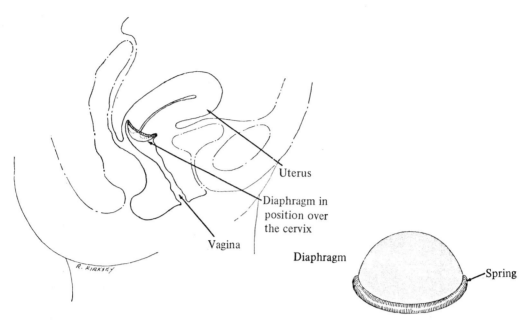

Figure 21-26.   The structure and normal position of a diaphragm.

pulmonary embolism (blood clot in pulmonary vessels) and thrombophlebitis (inflammation of veins and formation of clots).

The production of a male birth control pill, without serious side effects, has not been perfected at this time. There are several possible candidates, but they have serious side effects.

## PREVENT FERTILIZATION BY SPERM OR OOCYTE

Various chemical and mechanical devices can be used to prevent fertilization of an oocyte by a sperm. The most common mechanical devices are a **condom** and a **diaphragm.** A condom is a rubber sheath that fits over the penis and collects semen after ejaculation. It also helps to protect the male against veneral disease. A diaphragm is a rubber dome structure (Figure 21-26), with a spring located around the base. It is inserted in the vagina and positioned over the cervix so that it prevents sperm from entering the uterus. When the diaphragm is used with spermacidal cream, it can be quite effective in preventing pregnancy.

Various chemical foams, jellies, tablets, and suppositories (that are inserted into the vagina) are used to prevent sperm from entering the uterus. A combination of a condom or diaphragm and the chemicals can be quite effective in preventing fertilization.

Permanent steps can be taken to prevent fertilization, which involve sterilization operations. The male sterilization operation is called **vasectomy.** This operation involves exposing the spermatic cord on each side by an incision in the top of the scrotum. The ductus deferens is cut and tied (Figure 21-27), which prevents sperm from moving past this point. A vasectomy does not prevent the production of sperm; however, after they are produced they gradually die and are broken down by phagocytosis. A male who has had a vasectomy can still ejaculate semen (minus sperm) and experience an orgasm. The female sterilization operation is called **tubal ligation.** This operation involves an incision in

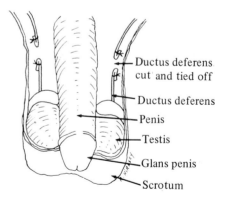

Figure 21-27.   A vasectomy involves the cutting and tying off of the ductus deferens tubes.

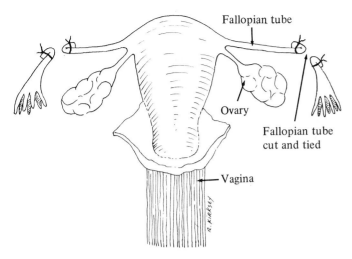

**Figure 21-28.** A tubal ligation involves the cutting and tying off of the fallopian tubes.

the abdomen or the wall of the vagina and insertion of a special instrument that allows a surgeon to locate the fallopian tubes. The fallopian tubes then are cut and

tied (Figure 21-28), or **cauterized** (close the tubes by burning them with an electric current). Tubal ligation does not affect the production of FSH and LH; therefore, a woman still produces oocytes and experiences normal menstrual cycles, but oocytes cannot move past the tied fallopian tubes.

## PREVENT IMPLANTATION OF A FERTILIZED BLASTOCYST

This type of birth control involves implantation of an intrauterine device (IUD) into the uterus. These structures are shaped like loops, spirals, rings, T's, and other shapes (Figure 21-29), and they have a thread or tail that extends from the bottom. An IUD is inserted by a physician through the cervix into the uterus, with the thread or tail hanging into the vagina. In the uterus the IUD implants into the endometrium where it prevents a blastocyst from implanting. How it prevents implantation is not fully understood. One theory is that it ir-

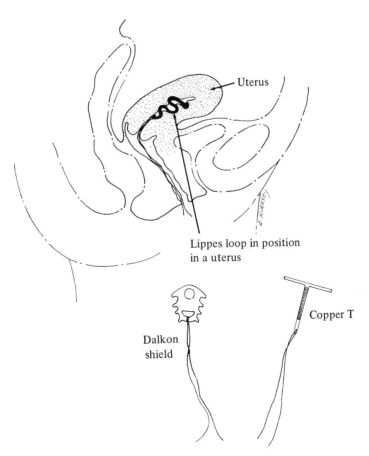

**Figure 21-29.** An IUD is shown in position in a uterus. Two other IUDs are shown at the right.

ritates the endometrium and stimulates white blood cells (WBCs) to enter the uterine tissues. The WBCs create an unfavorable environment for the implantation and development of a blastocyst.

## REMOVAL OF DEVELOPING EMBRYO

**Abortion** is the removal of a developing embryo. Abortion can be induced or spontaneous. Spontaneous abortions or miscarriages occur in approximately 15 percent of all pregnancies; they are not considered as a means of birth control.

Induced abortion is termination of pregnancy prior to the twenty-eighth week of gestation. When an abortion is performed during the first three months of pregnancy, there are two techniques mainly used—dilation and curettage (D and C) and uterine aspiration. Dilation and curettage involves dilation of the cervix and insertion of forceps to remove the embryo or fetus. The uterine lining then is scraped with a curette tool to remove the placenta. Uterine aspiration involves dilation of the cervix and insertion of a hollow curette connected to a suction pump. The embryo or fetus, placenta, and membranes are sucked out. If an abortion is done during the second three months of pregnancy, the process is much more involved.

# SUMMARY

### Female Reproductive System
A. Ovaries: primary sex organs
   Shaped like almonds; attached to uterus by ovarian ligaments. Function: produce secondary oocytes, estrogen, and progesterone hormones.
B. Secondary sex organs
   1. Fallopian tubes: extend from uterus out to ovaries; lined with ciliated mucous membrane. Function: transport oocytes from ovaries to uterus.
   2. Uterus: superior to urinary bladder and anterior to rectum; held in place by ligaments; composed of fundus, body, and cervix regions; wall composed of myometrium (smooth muscle) and endometrium (mucous membrane).
   3. Vagina: collapsible muscular tube; extends from vaginal opening to cervix; can be extended to receive a penis.
C. Accessory sex organs
   1. Labia majora and minora: two longitudinal folds of skin that extend from mons pubis toward anus; labia minora are two smaller folds of skin located medial to labia majora.
   2. Clitoris: erectile tissue; located where labia minora folds unite anteriorly; sensitive to touch and becomes erect from stimulation of penis; important to sexual arousal of female.
   3. Vestibular glands: Bartholin glands on each side of vaginal opening; secrete mucus that lubricates vagina.
   4. Perineum: area between pubic symphysis and coccyx; site where episiotomy is performed to prevent tearing of tissue during childbirth.
   5. Mammary glands: composed of 15 to 20 lobes; lobules with milk glands are contained in lobes; lactiferous ducts drain milk to nipple.

### Male Reproductive System
A. Testes: primary sex organs. Located within scrotum sac; divided into 250 to 400 compartments called lobules; seminiferous tubules within lobules secrete testosterone and produce sperm.
B. Secondary sex organs
   1. Ductus deferens (vas deferens). Transports sperm from testes to ejaculatory duct on posterior surface of bladder.

C. Accessory structures
 1. Seminal vesicles: elongated sacs on posterior surface of bladder. Function: secrete alkaline fluid that aids metabolism and movement of sperm.
 2. Prostate gland: muscular doughnut-shaped gland that surrounds urethra inferior to bladder. Functions: (1) secretes alkaline fluid that neutralizes acidity of urethra, (2) contractions aid ejaculation of sperm.
 3. Cowper's glands: pea-shaped structures; inferior to prostate. Function: secrete mucous substance that lubricates vagina.
 4. Penis: composed of erectile tissue that fills with blood and causes erection; urethra transports sperm and urine to outside.

## Gametogenesis

Gametogenesis produces gametes (sex cells).
A. Spermatogenesis (production of sperm): occurs in seminiferous tubules; stimulated by FSH hormone.
 1. Meiosis: process by which sperm cells are formed and chromosome number reduced from 46 to 23.
B. Oogenesis (production of ova): process by which egg cell is formed with 23 chromosomes.
 1. Follicle development and rupture: follicle-stimulating hormone (FSH) stimulates development of secondary oocyte; takes approximately 13 days.
 2. Corpus luteum: yellowish structure; develops after rupture of graafian follicle and release of secondary oocyte; stimulated by luteinizing hormone (LH); function, secretes progesterone that prepares endometrium for implantation of ovum.

## Menstrual Cycle

Changes in development of endometrium in uterus and secondary oocyte in ovaries.
A. Flow phase (menstrual phase): characterized by superficial layer of endometrial wall being sloughed off; lasts 4 to 6 days; results from drop in estrogen and progesterone hormones.
B. Follicular phase (proliferative phase): characterized by thickening of superficial layer of endometrium; lasts from day 5 to day 14 of cycle; graafian follicle develops and ruptures, thereby releasing secondary oocytes; developing follicle releases estrogen.
C. Luteal phase (postovulatory): lasts from about day 15 to day 28 of menstrual cycle; characterized by endometrium thickening even more than follicular phase; corpus luteum formed and secretes progesterone; if oocyte not fertilized, then corpus luteum degenerates and progesterone level decreases, which results in sloughing off of endometrium.

## Menarche and menopause

A. Menarche: first menstrual cycle of female and usually occurs between ages 12 and 15.
B. Menopause: ovaries no longer produce oocytes and secrete hormones; woman no longer menstruates.

## Sexual Intercourse

A. Erection of penis: corpora cavernosa and corpus spongiosum fill with blood and cause penis to become erect; more blood flows in than flows out, due to constriction of veins.
B. Ejaculation: nerve impulses cause contraction of smooth muscles of epididymis, ductus deferens, and prostate gland; result is that semen is transported into urethra; skeletal muscles at base of penis contract and force semen out of penis; average amount of semen ejaculated is 3 to 5 ml or about 300 to 500 million sperm.

## Fertilization

Sperm swim through uterus to fallopian tubes; fertilization actually occurs in approximately the distal one-third of fallopian tubes; involves nucleus of sperm uniting with nucleus of secondary oocyte, thereby restoring 46 chromosome number.

### Restoration of 46 Chromosomes and Determination of Sex

A. Oocyte and sperm each contribute 23 chromosomes at fertilization; therefore, restoration of 46 chromosomes.

B. Since every egg contains an X chromosome, then a sperm determines sex at fertilization; if sperm is X, then XX and female; if sperm is Y, then XY and male.

### Development of the Fertilized Zygote and Implantation

After fertilization, the zygote undergoes many changes until a blastocyst is formed, which implants into the endometrium.

A. Development of membranes and placenta: two membranes develop around embryo:
   1. Chorion: outer, highly vascularized membrane; function, exchanges nutrients and wastes between embryo and mother's blood.
   2. Amnion: loose-fitting sac around embryo; amniotic fluid is contained within sac and protects embryo against jolts and blows.
   3. Placenta develops from chorion; when developed it is about 8 inches in diameter and 1 inch thick; highly vascular. Functions (1) acts as a lung and a kidney, (2) acts as an endocrine organ, (3) filters out bacteria and some viruses.

### Embryologic Development

A. Period of the ovum or preembryonic period. Extends from fertilization through second week; at the end of the period the primary germ layers—ectoderm, mesoderm, and endoderm—have formed.

B. Period of the embryo or embryonic period. Extends from third week to the end of the eighth week; at end of period the visceral organs, face, limbs, and external genitalia have developed.

C. Period of fetus: extends from ninth week to birth; during this period the organs and structures complete their development; fetus gains over 50 percent of its weight during the last two months.

### Circulation of Blood in the Fetus

Circulation of blood in unborn fetus is different from in infant after birth in several ways: (1) blood bypasses lungs, (2) blood bypasses liver, (3) several structures are present that disappear after birth: ductus venosus, ductus arteriosus, foramen ovale, two umbilical arteries, and an umbilical vein.

### Labor (Parturition)

A. Hormones involved in labor
   1. Estrogen: level is low during pregnancy; level begins to increase a few weeks prior to birth; stimulates uterine muscles to contract and initiate labor.
   2. Oxytocin: secreted by posterior pituitary; initiates forceful contractions of uterus and labor.
   3. Relaxin: secreted by placenta and ovaries and softens pubic symphysis ligament and others along birth canal.

B. Labor
   1. First stage: begins with contractions of uterus; ends with cervix completely dilated.
   2. Second stage: extends from dilation of cervix until fetus is born.
   3. Third stage: expulsion of placenta or afterbirth characterizes this stage; excessive hemorrhaging can occur if myometrium does not forcefully contract.

## Development and Lactation of the Breasts

A. Lactation
1. Development of breasts to secrete milk as a result of estrogen and progesterone hormones.
2. Actual secretion of milk results from prolactin hormone.

## Contraceptives and Birth Control

A. Prevent production of oocytes and sperm: birth-control pills contain estrogen and progesterone, which inhibit secretion of FSH and LH; end result is that an oocyte is not released.
B. Prevent fertilization by sperm of oocyte
1. Condom: rubber sheath fits over penis and collects semen.
2. Diaphragm: a rubber dome structure that fits over cervix and prevents sperm from entering the uterus.
3. Vasectomy: ductus deferens on each side of male testes are cut and tied off; sperm cannot be ejaculated but rest of semen can be.
4. Tubal ligation: fallopian tubes are cut and tied off; does not affect ability of woman to produce FSH and LH.
C. Prevent implantation of a fertilized blastocyst: implantation of an intrauterine device (IUD) into uterus; prevents implantation of blastocyst into endometrium.
D. Removal of a developing embryo: abortion is removal of embryo; can be induced or spontaneous; dilation and curettage (D and C) of uterus and aspiration are two common methods.

## The Reproductive System

Matching. Questions 1 to 15.

1. fallopian tubes    **A.** produce secondary oocytes
2. uterus    **B.** transport oocytes from ovaries to uterus
3. clitoris    **C.** composed of myometrium and endometrium
4. ovaries    **D.** important to sexual arousal for female
5. mammary glands    **E.** composed of milk glands

6. testes    **A.** inferior to prostate and secrete mucus for lubrication
7. seminal vesicles    **B.** composed of erectile tissue
8. prostate gland    **C.** secrete testosterone
9. Cowper's glands    **D.** aids ejaculation
10. penis    **E.** secretes alkaline fluid that aids motility of sperm

11. FSH    **A.** stimulates development of female secondary sex characteristics
12. LH    **B.** secreted by corpus luteum
13. estrogen    **C.** stimulates development of secondary oocytes
14. progesterone    **D.** stimulates development of corpus luteum
15. oxytocin    **E.** initiates labor contractions

True (A) or false (B). Questions 16 to 27.

16. Spermatogenesis is stimulated by FSH and results in sperm with 46 chromosomes.
17. Oogenesis results in four secondary oocytes with 23 chromosomes in each.
18. A corpus luteum secretes LH hormone that prepares endometrium for implantation of fertilized egg.
19. Semen is composed of sperm plus fluid secretions from seminal vesicles, prostate gland, and Cowper's gland.
20. Fertilization actually occurs when nuclei of sperm and secondary oocyte unite.
21. If a sperm carrying an X chromosome fertilizes an egg, then the sex of the infant will be male.
22. The chorion membrane fits loosely around an embryo and protects it against jolts and blows.
23. A placenta functions as a kidney and lung, secretes hormones, and filters out bacteria and some viruses.
24. Circulation of blood in a fetus bypasses the lungs as a result of the ductus venosus and foramen ovale.
25. An increase in estrogen and decrease in oxytocin initiate labor contractions.
26. Prolactin hormone stimulates the development of milk glands and ducts.
27. A vasectomy and tubal ligation prevent fertilization by inhibiting production of sperm and secondary oocytes.

# Glossary

**Abdominal mesentery** A fold of peritoneum that attaches the length of the small intestine and most of the large intestine to the posterior abdominal wall.

**Abduction** Angular movement of a body part away from the midsagittal plane of the body.

**Accommodation** The change in shape of lens and iris as the eyes focus on near and distant objects.

**Acellular organisms** Organisms lacking a cellular organization, e.g., viruses.

**Acetyl CoA** An intermediate compound in the metabolism of carbohydrates and fats; enters the citric acid cycle.

**Acid** A substance that forms hydrogen ions ($H^+$) in water solutions. Conversely, an acid can also be defined as a substance that gives up protons ($H^2$) in a water solution.

**Acid oxyhemoglobin ($HHbO_2$)** Hemoglobin that has combined with $O_2$ at the level of alveoli; major transport form of $O_2$.

**Acidosis** A condition in which the level of $H^+$ in body tissues and fluids is above normal. Blood acidosis is indicated when the blood pH drops below 7.3. If the blood pH drops to 6.8, death will occur.

**Acinus** Exocrine secreting unit of the pancreas; secretes digestive enzymes.

**Acromegaly** Hypersecretion of growth hormone during adult years.

**Adduction** Angular movement of a body part toward the midsagittal plane of the body or a body part.

**Adenohypophysis** (adeno—gland, hypo—under) Anterior lobe of pituitary gland; releases hormones that regulate a whole range of bodily activities.

**Aerobic respiration** Stage of cell respiration wherein pyruvic acid is oxidized completely and oxygen is needed.

**Afferent** Carrying toward; e.g., afferent neurons carry nerve impulses toward the central nervous system; opposite of efferent.

**Afferent arteriole** Blood vessel that carries blood to a Bowman's capsule in a nephron.

**Agglutinin** Protein located in blood plasma. There are two types, a and b, which have complementary shapes for A and B agglutinogens.

**Agglutinogen** Protein attached to RBC membrane. Three types A, B, and Rh, can attach to complementary agglutinin, resulting in agglutination or clumping.

**Albuminuria** Refers to albumin in the urine.

**Aldosterone** Adrenal cortex hormone that stimulates kidneys to absorb more $Na^+$ and water and excrete more $K^+$.

**Alkalosis** A condition in which the concentration of $H^+$ decreases and $OH^-$ increases. Alkalosis of the blood is characterized by an increase in pH above 7.5. At 7.8, death occurs.

**Alveoli** Clusters of simple squamous epithelium sacs in lungs; function as gas exchange point, since pulmonary capillaries surround them.

**Amenorrhea** Absence of menstrual flow.

**Amnion** The innermost of two membranes that enclose the fetus.

**Amniotic fluid** Fluid located between embryo and amnion membrane; protects embryo against jolts.

**Amoebic dysentery** An intestinal disorder caused by the protozoan *Entamoeba histolytica*.

**Amphetamines** A group of synthetic drugs that function as stimulants and include Benzedrine® (bennies), Dexedrine® (oranges), Methedrine® (speed), and Diphetamine® (footballs).

**Amphiarthrosis** Slightly movable joint.

**Amphitrichous bacteria** Bacteria with one flagellum from each pole.

**Anabolism**   A buildup phase of metabolism; involves synthesis reactions.

**Anaerobes**   (an—without, aero—air) Microbes that cannot exist in the presence of atmospheric oxygen.

**Anaerobic respiration**   Stage of cell respiration wherein glucose is oxidized to pyruvic acid. Oxygen is not needed.

**Analgesis(ic)**   Relief of pain or a drug that relieves pain.

**Anaphylaxis**   A state of hypersensitivity to certain antigens; exposure to them results in various physiological disorders and can lead to shock.

**Anemia**   1. Abnormal decrease in RBCs and hemoglobin; decrease in $O_2$-carrying capacity. 2. A condition in which the number of RBCs or hemoglobin is below normal.

**Anesthetic**   An agent that produces anesthesia (loss of feeling or sensation).

**Aneurysm**   A sac or bulged out section of the wall of an artery or a vein.

**Angina pectoris**   Pain in the heart resulting from a lack of oxygen to the cardiac muscles.

**Angiotensin II**   Plasma protein that functions to raise blood pressure by constricting arteries and stimulating release of aldosterone.

**Angular movement**   Movement that changes the angle between bones by decreasing or increasing the angle between them.

**Anion**   A negatively (−) charged atom or molecule. Example: $Cl^-$.

**Ankylosis**   Immobilization of a joint by pathological or surgical process; an example is ankylosis condition in rheumatoid arthritis.

**Anoxia**   A condition in which normal tissue functions are impaired due to lack of oxygen.

**Antagonist**   An agent (muscle, drug) that exerts an action opposite to that of another. An example is triceps brachii's antagonism to biceps brachii.

**Anticodon**   A triplet of nucleotides on the t-RNA molecule.

**Antigen**   Any foreign substance that stimulates the tissues to produce antibodies. With few exceptions (polysaccharides, lipids, and nucleic acids), antigens are proteins or substances that contain proteins.

**Antiserum**   Blood serum that contains specific antibodies and is used to give a person artificial passive immunity. Antisera are often used in the treatment of gas, gangrene, rabies, and botulism.

**Antithrombin**   Normal anticlotting substance.

**Anuria**   No urine formation; indicates that the kidneys are totally malfunctioning.

**Apnea**   Cessation of breathing.

**Apneustic center**   A group of neurons located in the pons near the pneumotaxic center; can stimulate forceful inspirations in certain situations.

**Aponeurosis**   Flat sheet of white fibrous tissue or tendon that serves to attach muscles to bones or other structures.

**Aqueduct**   A passage that conducts fluids; example: cerebral aqueduct.

**Arteriole**   Small artery that connects to a capillary network.

**Arteriosclerosis**   Hardening of the arteries. Results from calcium salts and scar tissue reacting with the elastic tissue of the middle layer—tunica media—of arteries.

**Artery**   Vessel that transports blood away from the heart to the capillaries in tissues.

**Arthritis**   Inflammation of a joint; example: rheumatoid arthritis.

**Articular cartilage**   Cartilage that covers the articular surface of the epiphyses of long bones.

**Ascites**   Accumulation of fluid in the abdomen.

**Asphyxiation**   Lack of oxygen.

**Asthma**   An allergic disorder characterized by violent breathing and inflammation of bronchi.

**Atelectasis**   Incomplete expansion of lung alveoli at birth or the collapse of previously aerated alveoli.

**Atherosclerosis**   A disease of the inner lining of arteries. Large deposits or plaques of fat decrease the size of lumen.

**Athetosis**   Repetitive and involuntary slow gross movements.

**Atmospheric pressure**   The pressure exerted by the air on all parts of the body. The average value, at sea level, is 760 mm Hg.

**Atomic mass number**   The total number of protons and neutrons in an atom.

**Atomic number**   The number of protons in the nucleus of an atom.

**Atomic weight**   The relative weight of an atom compared to a standard, carbon 12.

**Atrichous bacteria**   Bacteria that lack flagella.

**Atrium**   A small chamber or cavity. Example: atria of the heart.

**Atrophic**   Derivative of atrophy or the wasting away of tissue.

**Autoimmune disease** A body's production of antibodies against its own proteins. Rheumatoid arthritis is possibly an example.

**Autonomic nervous system (ANS)** Controls the activity of all smooth (visceral) and cardiac muscles.

**Autosomes** Twenty-two pairs (44 individual) of chromosomes that contain genes, which determine various traits.

**Autotrophic bacteria** Bacteria that are able to use $CO_2$ as their sole carbon source for synthesizing organic compounds.

**Axilla** Armpit region.

**B cells** *See* Humoral immunity.

**Bacillary dysentery** Intestinal disorder caused by bacterial organisms of the genus *Shigella.*

**Base** A substance that gives up hydroxide ions ($OH^-$) or accepts hydrogen ions ($H^+$) in water solutions.

**Belly (body)** The thickest part of a muscle; part that shortens when muscle contracts.

**Benign tumor** A neoplasm or tumor that does not metastasize (spread).

**Bile sale** A steroid compound secreted from the liver into the small intestine that aids in the digestion and absorption of fats.

**Bilirubin** A pigment formed from the breakdown of hemoglobin and secreted into bile by the liver.

**Blastocyst** Early stage of embryonic development; a hollow ball of cells.

**Blood pressure** Pressure of blood as it pushes outward on blood vessels and chambers of the heart. Results from contractions of the heart.

**Bolus** Round mass of chewed food that is swallowed.

**Botulism** An example of food poisoning; causative organism is *Clostridium botulinium,* a gram-positive rod.

**Bowel** Intestines.

**Brain stem** The diencephalon (thalamus and hypothalamus), midbrain, pons, and medulla oblongata.

**Brittle** Likely to break; fragile.

**Bronchi** Two small cartilaginous tubes that branch off the trachea and enter their respective lung.

**Bronchioles** Branches off secondary bronchi; composed of little cartilage and primarily smooth muscle.

**Bronchitis** Inflammation of the mucosa membrane lining the bronchi; a staphylococcal infection.

**Brunner's glands** Glands located primarily in the duodenum that act to secrete mucus.

**Buffer system** A pair of compounds that resist changes in pH with the addition of acids or bases. A buffer system is composed of a weak acid and salt of the weak acid.

**Bursa** A small synovial fluid sac located between structures that rub against each other.

**Bursitis** Inflammation of bursa sacs.

**Calcification** Deposition of calcium salts in the matrix.

**Calcitonin** A hormone that functions to lower the level of blood calcium.

**Calcium citrate** Artificial anticlotting substance.

**Calcium oxalate** Artificial anticlotting substance.

**Callus** An area of hardened and thickened skin; fibrous tissue formed by condensation of granulation tissue at the site of a bone fracture.

**Canaliculi** Small canals that radiate from the haversian canals and connect to the lacunae in bone tissue.

**Cancer** A cellular disease characterized by malignant growth.

**Carbaminohemoglobin (HHbCO$_2$)** Hemoglobin that has combined with $CO_2$.

**Carbohydrase** Carbohydrate-splitting enzyme.

**Carbohydrates** Organic compounds composed of carbon, hydrogen, and oxygen with a 2:1 ratio of hydrogen to oxygen atoms.

**Carbonic acid** ($H_2CO_3$) A very important acid formed by $CO_2$ reacting with $H_2O$; a transport form of $CO_2$.

**Carbuncles** Deeper abesses, compared to furuncles, usually found in the subcutaneous tissue. They generally result from *S. aureus.*

**Carcinoma** A cancer that arises from ectodermal or endodermal tissue.

**Caseation** Transformation of tubercles in lungs into cheesy mass.

**Castration** Accidental or intentional removal of the testes.

**Catabolism** Breakdown phase of metabolism; involves the conversion of complex molecules into more simple molecules.

**Catalyst** A compound that changes the speed of a chemical reaction without itself being changed. Within the body, catalysts are called enzymes.

**Cataract** Condition characterized by opaqueness of the lens of the eye.

**Cations** Positively ($+$) charged atoms or molecules. Example: $Na^+$.

**Cauterize** To burn or sear as with a caustic drug or with an electric current. Cauterization of fallopian tubes involves closing them off using an electric current.

**Cell**   The smallest and simplest unit of living matter that is capable of maintaining and reproducing itself. Simplest structural and functional unit of the body that can sustain life.

**Cell-mediated immunity (T cells)**   Immunity that results from lymphocyte cells called T cells. The T cells are located in certain tissues and directly attack antigens, providing immunity.

**Cellular immunity**   Immunity produced by T cells in lymph nodes.

**Cerebral dysfunction**   Absence of complete normal cerebral function.

**Cerebrospinal fluid (CSF)**   Fluid produced in brain ventricles; circulates through spinal cord and brain to function as a shock absorber and circulate nutrients and wastes.

**Ceruminous glands**   (Derivative of skin) Located in the dermis along the length of the canal leading into the middle ear; secrete a waxy substance (cerumen) that commonly is called ear wax.

**Cervical**   Pertaining to the female cervix; pertains to neck region of an individual. Example: cervical vertebrae, cervical nodes.

**Cervical curve**   A secondary curve of the vertebral column in the cervical region; develops after birth and allows a child to hold his head erect.

**Chemical change (chemical reaction)**   Produces new substances with different chemical properties than the original substance.

**Cheyne–Stokes respiration**   A condition of breathing in which a period of apnea is followed by hyperpnea.

**Chickenpox (Varicella)**   Skin disease caused by a virus in the herpes group; spherical, enveloped DNA-containing virus.

**Cholecystitis**   Infection and inflammation of the gallbladder.

**Cholecystokinin**   Hormone that causes the muscular walls of the gallbladder to contract and send bile into the duodenum.

**Cholelithiasis**   Formation of gallstones (calculi) in the gallbladder.

**Cholesterol**   A structural component of cell membranes; a steroid.

**Chondroblasts**   Cartilage-forming cells.

**Chondrocytes**   Connective tissue cells located in cartilage; secrete cartilage intercellular material.

**Chorion**   Outermost of two fetal membranes that enclose the fetus.

**Chromatin material**   Granular, dark-staining DNA and proteins in the nucleus of a cell.

**Chyme**   Semifluid mass of food that passes from stomach into duodenum.

**Circumduction**   Movement of a body part through each angular movement in succession to complete a circle.

**Citric acid cycle**   A series of chemical reactions in the mitochondria that generate the raw materials to produce ATPs in the cytochrome system.

**Codon**   Triplet of nucleotides on a m-RNA molecule.

**Collagen fiber**   Protein fiber found in matrix of various connective tissues; when stretched, it does not resume its original shape.

**Colloid**   Large solute molecules not capable of passing through a selectively permeable membrane. Example: most plasma proteins such as albumin.

**Colloidal osmotic pressure (COP)**   Pressure created by colloidal solutes not capable of diffusing through a selectively permeable membrane.

**Coma**   A state of deep unconsciousness brought on by disease or injury.

**Compound**   A substance made up of two or more elements chemically bonded together. Examples: NaCl, $H_2O$, $C_6H_{12}O_6$.

**Congenital**   A condition that exists at birth and usually occurred earlier in the development of the fetus or embryo; example: cleft palate.

**Congenital syphilis**   Syphilis infection in a newborn child; the disease is transmitted from the mother to the developing child.

**Conjunctiva**   A mucous membrane that lines the eyelids and covers the anterior surface of the eyeball.

**Consolidation**   The process of becoming solidified or more dense, as of a lung with pneumonia.

**Convulsion**   Involuntary spasm or contraction of groups of muscles.

**Cornea**   The anterior transparent region of the sclera of the eye; refracts light rays.

**Corpus**   Body.

**Corpus albicans**   White body; white scar that results from degenerating corpus luteum in an ovary.

**Corpus luteum**   Yellow body; structure formed after Graafian follicle in an ovary ruptures and secretes the hormone progesterone.

**Cortex**   The outer or peripheral portion of an organ. Example: cerebral cortex.

**Cowper's glands (bulbourethral glands)**   Yellowish pea-shaped structures, one on each side of the urethra immediately below the prostate gland in a male; secrete a mucus-type substance into the urethra that apparently acts as a lubricant for the penis during sexual intercourse.

**Cranial nerves**   Twelve pairs of nerves that attach directly to the inferior surface of the brain.

**Cretin**   A dwarf, mentally retarded child; condition caused by hyposecretion of thyroxin hormone.

**Crypts of Lieberkühn**   Intestinal glands located between the villi; secrete the intestinal juices, called succus entericus.

**Cusp**   A pointed projection, such as on the crown of a tooth.

**Cutaneous mycoses**   Common fungal diseases on the skin. Examples: ringworm, athlete's foot.

**Cystic duct**   Duct that carries bile from the gallbladder to the hepatic bile duct.

**Cystitis**   Inflammation of the mucous membrane lining the bladder. It is most often caused by gram-negative rods, such as *Escherichia, Salmonella,* and *Klebsiella.*

**Cytochrome**   A respiratory assembly molecule; composed of an iron atom in a porphyrin ring which is surrounded by a protein; transfer electrons from one molecule to another, resulting in production of ATP molecules.

**Cytochrome system**   A series of four cytochrome molecules, arranged with the higher energy cytochromes above the lower energy ones; transfer electrons from high-energy cytochromes to low-energy ones with production of three ATP molecules.

**Deamination**   A process that involves the removal of the amino group ($-NH_2$) from amino acids.

**Decarboxylation**   Loss of carbon, in the form of $CO_2$, from a molecule.

**Decomposition reaction**   Breakdown of a compound into the elements that make it up, or into simpler compounds. Example: $NaCl \xrightarrow{H_2O} Na^+ + Cl^-$.

**Decubitis ulcers (bedsores)**   Skin ulcers that result from interference with the blood supply to various regions of the dermis.

**Dehydrogenation**   Loss of hydrogen atoms from a compound.

**Denaturation**   Destruction of a substance; example: Denaturation of a protein which results in changes in the native structure of the protein.

**Density**   The mass (quantity) of a substance contained in a certain volume.

**Dermis**   The layer under the epidermis. It is considered the true skin, and is firmly attached to the epidermis.

**Detrusor musculature**   Three layers of smooth muscle that compose the walls of the urinary bladder.

**Diabetes**   Excessive and persistent increase in urinary secretions, e.g., diabetes mellitus and diabetes insipidus.

**Diabetes insipidus**   Disorder caused by a deficiency of ADH hormone; large amounts of dilute urine are excreted.

**Diapedesis**   Movement of WBCs through pores in capillaries into tissues; WBCs phagocytize bacteria.

**Diaphysis (shaft)**   The central portion of a long bone.

**Diarrhea**   An intestinal disorder characterized by frequent watery bowel movements.

**Diarthrosis**   Freely movable joint; examples: knee, elbow, and sholder joints.

**Diastole**   Phase of cardiac cycle when heart chambers are relaxed.

**Diencephalon**   "Tween brain"; region of the brain between the midbrain and telencephalon.

**Diphtheria**   Upper respiratory infection; caused by gram-positive rods which secrete an exotoxin.

**Diploid number**   The "2N" number of chromosomes in cells, or 46; N stands for the number of chromosomes in one set, or 23.

**Disease**   A condition of the body that results in tissue damage or alteration of bodily functions, producing symptoms noticeable by laboratory or physical examination. Most diseases result from an infection of pathogenic or opportunistic microbes, but they also can result from imbalance of hormones, genetic defects, and nutritional deficiencies.

**Dislocation**   Displacement of the bones of a joint.

**Diuresis**   A temporary increase in the amount of urine excreted.

**Drug**   A substance used as medicine in the treatment of disease; a narcotic, especially one that is addictive.

**Dynamic equilibrium**   Maintenance of body position (mainly the head) in response to sudden movements.

**Dysentery**   Intestinal disorder characterized by fluids containing mucus, pus, and blood.

**Dysfunction**   Absence of complete normal functions.

**Dysmenorrhea**   Painful menstruation.

**Dyspnea**   Difficult or labored breathing.

**Ectoderm**   Outer germ layer which gives rise to the epidermis of the skin, hair, nails, nervous system, lens of the eye, and enamel of the teeth.

**Effectors**   Muscles and glands that carry out the commands from the CNS.

**Efferent**  Leading away from, e.g., efferent neurons carry nerve impulses away from central nervous system; opposite of afferent.

**Efferent arteriole**  Blood vessel that carries blood from Bowman's capsule to peritubular capillaries.

**Elastic fiber**  Protein fiber found in matrix of various connective tissues; can be stretched and then resume its original shape.

**Element**  Matter that is composed of only one type of atom.

**Embolus**  A substance (clot), carried from its origin by blood to a new site, that causes obstruction.

**Endemic**  Constantly present at a low level of incidence. Example: Ascariasis.

**Endergonic reaction (endothermic reaction)**  An energy-absorbing reaction. At the completion of an endergonic reaction, the amount of free energy in the solution is greater than it was at the beginning. This increase in free energy is represented by $+\Delta G$.

**Endocardium**  Innermost tissue layer of the heart; same as endothelium.

**Endochondral ossification**  Process by which the majority of bones are formed; process originates in the hyaline cartilage.

**Endoderm**  Inner germinative layer which gives rise to the lining of the digestive tract and accessory organs, lining of the trachea and bronchi, and lining of portions of the urinary and reproductive systems.

**Endolymph**  Fluid contained within the membranous labyrinth of the inner ear.

**Endometrium**  Mucous membrane lining the uterus.

**Endospore**  A cell unique in that it has very thick spore coats, a dehydrated cytoplasm, unusual cytoplasmic chemicals, and no metabolic activity. Formed by certain bacteria when conditions are not suitable for normal life.

**Endosteum membrane**  Membrane lining the medullary cavity of long bones; contains osteoclasts.

**Endothelium**  Simple squamous tissue that lines blood vessels and heart; same as endocardium.

**Endotoxins**  Poisonous compounds that are part of the gram-negative cell wall of a bacterium and are not released until the bacterium dies.

**Energy**  The capacity for doing work.

**Energy of activation ($E_a$)**  Energy needed to cause chemical reactions.

**Enzymes**  Catalysts within the body.

**Epicardium (visceral pericardium)**  The outermost membrane of the heart.

**Epidermis**  The outer layer of the skin; composed of strata or layers of keratinized stratified epithelial tissue.

**Epidural space**  Space between the surface of the dura mater and the walls of the vertebral cavity.

**Epinephrine**  A hormone that prepares the body to meet stress situations by stimulating certain systems and activities of the body and inhibiting others.

**Epiphyseal cartilage**  Located in the epiphyses of long bones; produces cartilage cells that ossify into bone tissue.

**Epiphysis**  The flared end of a long bone.

**Episiotomy**  Incision made in the obstetrical perineum of the female to enlarge the vaginal opening prior to the birth of a child.

**Erythroblastosis fetalis**  Condition wherein Rh negative maternal blood forms antibodies against Rh positive blood of a fetus; antibodies destroy RBCs in the fetus.

**Erythrocytosis**  An increase in the number of RBCs; can result from a lack of oxygen to the tissues.

**Erythropoiesis**  Production and maturation of RBCs.

**Estrogen**  A female hormone that affects development of secondary female characteristics (breasts, hips, etc); a steroid.

**Eucaryotic cells**  Cells that contain a true nucleus and defined cellular organelles such as the mitochondria and lysosomes.

**Eupnea**  Normal, resting breathing.

**Exergonic reaction (exothermic reaction)**  An energy-releasing reaction. At the completion of an exergonic reaction, there is less free energy in the solution than there was at the beginning. This decrease in free energy is represented by $-\Delta G$.

**Exophthalmos**  Protrusion of the eyeballs.

**Exotoxins**  Poisonous metabolic products of certain species of gram-positive and a few gram-negative bacteria.

**Expiratory center**  A group of neurons located superior and lateral to the inspiratory center in medulla oblongata; regulates expiration.

**Expiratory reserve**  The amount of air that can be exhaled during the deepest possible expiration.

**Extension**  Movement that increases the angle between two body parts by moving them farther apart.

**Extracellular fluid (ECF)**  Fluid found between or outside cells, in blood vessels and in tissue spaces.

**Extrinsic muscles**  Muscles attached to the outer surface of the eye.

**Exudate** Fluid that has oozed from a space or blood vessels; may contain serum, pus, and cellular debris.

**Facultative bacteria** Bacteria that grow with or without atmospheric oxygen.

**False pelvis** The area superior to the pelvic brim.

**Fats** Organic compounds that contain carbon, hydrogen, and oxygen with a ratio greater than 2:1 of hydrogen to oxygen atoms.

**Fetus** Developing offspring in uterus from ninth through fortieth week or birth.

**Fibrillation** Abnormal contraction of a muscle; fibers contract in an uncoordinated manner.

**Filariasis (elephantiasis)** Disorder that results from filarial worms blocking the flow of lymph in lymph vessels, resulting in massive edema; often occurs in the extremities, where edema causes gross stretching of the skin.

**Fissure** Deep groove that separates the various areas of the brain.

**Flaccid** Limp or soft.

**Flagella** Thin hairlike appendages that protrude through the cell wall of bacteria and propel the bacteria through fluids.

**Flavin adenine dinucleotide (FAD)** A coenzyme that transports hydrogens from citric acid cycle and glycolysis to electron transport system.

**Flexion** Movement that decreases the angle between two body parts by moving them closer together.

**Flexor reflexes** Three-neuron protective reflex; allows one to quickly flex an extremity away from a painful stimulus.

**Floating ribs** Last two pairs of false ribs, which do not attach to the sternum either directly or indirectly.

**Flu (influenza)** Viral respiratory infection.

**Follicle-stimulating hormone (FSH)** Hormone secreted by the anterior pituitary. Stimulates the germinal epithelium in the seminiferous tubules to produce sperm.

**Fontanel (soft spot)** Membranous tissue that connects cranial bones.

**Foramen** An opening in a bone through which structures pass.

**Force (power)** The muscles that contract and move a lever (bone).

**Fossa** A shallow concave depression that can articulate with the head or condyle of another bone.

**Friable** Easily broken into small pieces.

**Fulcrum** The joint at which movement of bones takes place.

**Fundus** Part of a hollow organ farthest from the opening.

**Furuncle (boil)** Abscess localized in hair follicles and caused by staphylococcal organisms, usually *Staphylococcus aureus*.

**Gamete** Haploid (N) sex cell, e.g., sperm and oocytes.

**Gametogenesis** Process by which gametes are formed by meiosis.

**Ganglion** A mass of neuron cell bodies, generally outside of the central nervous system. Synapses occur in autonomic ganglia.

**Gas gangrene** Bacterial infection caused by anaerobic *Clostridium* bacteria; results in death of the affected tissues.

**Gastrin** Hormone secreted by pyloric region of stomach and duodenum; stimulates production of gastric juices.

**Gastroenteritis** Inflammation of the lining of the stomach and small intestine.

**Germ layers** Cell layers that germinate all the tissues of the body.

**German measles (rubella)** Skin disease found fairly frequently in adults; caused by a Toga virus.

**Glaucoma** Above normal intraocular pressure of eye; due to buildup of aqueous humor.

**Globular protein** Protein that consists of one or more alpha helical chains that have folded and wrapped themselves into a compact spherical or globular shape.

**Glomerular filtrate** Fluid forced out of glomerulus into Bowman's capsule due to blood pressure.

**Glottis** The space between the vocal cords in larynx.

**Glucocorticoid hormones** Secreted by the adrenal cortex; stimulate the kidney renal tubule to absorb $Na^+$.

**Glycogenesis** Synthesis of monosaccharides to form glycogen.

**Glycolysis** The breakdown (by oxidation reactions) of one glucose molecule into two pyruvic acid molecules in the cytoplasm.

**Glycosuria** Glucose in the urine.

**Goblet cells** Inverted cells that secrete mucus; located in simple and ciliated columnar epithelial tissue.

**Goiter** Abnormal enlargement of the thyroid gland.

**Gonorrhea** A disease of the mucous membranes that line the reproductive tracts. It is the most prevalent venereal disease and is caused by *Neisseria gonorrhoeae*, a gram-negative diplococcus.

**Graafian follicle** A follicle cavity in an ovary in which a secondary oocyte completes development and is released into the fallopian tubes.

**Gram calorie**   The amount of heat required to raise the temperature of one gram of water one degree Celsius.

**Granular leukocytes (Granulocytes)**   Group of WBCs that contain granules in the cytoplasm of the cells, and whose nuclei are lobed or branched; neutrophils, eosinophils, basophils.

**Gyrus (convolution)**   A fold of tissue. Example: Gyri in cerebral cortex.

**Hallucinogen**   Drug that stimulates the sensory excitatory pathways to the brain and depresses inhibitory nerve impulses; a person often experiences hallucinations (false perceptions of the stimuli actually being received).

**Haploid number**   The "N" number of chromosomes in cells, or 23; this number is achieved by meiosis (division) of "2N" cells.

**Haustra**   Bulges in the large intestine.

**Haversian canal**   The central canal of an Haversian system, running lengthwise through compact bone.

**Haversian system**   A series of components in compact bone that transports blood to and from osteocytes.

**Hay fever**   A seasonal allergic reaction to foreign antigens such as pollens, grasses or plants, ragweed, and dust.

**Helminths**   Parasitic multicellular worms that are visible without the aid of magnifying lenses.

**Hematocrit**   The percentage of formed elements in the blood.

**Hematuria**   Blood in the urine.

**Heme**   Iron-containing pigment portion of hemoglobin; $O_2$ attaches to this portion.

**Hemocytoblasts**   Cells that give rise to blood cells.

**Hemoglobin**   A complex protein composed of four subunits; chemically attaches to oxygen and carbon dioxide.

**Hemorrhage**   Loss of blood vessels; bleeding.

**Hemorrhoids (piles)**   Inflammation of veins in the rectal columns of the anal canal.

**Heparin**   1. A natural anticoagulant which prevents blood from clotting within blood vessels. 2. Normal anticlotting substance produced by the liver.

**Hepatic portal system**   Veins that transport partly deoxygenated blood and end products of digestion from digestive organs to the liver.

**Hepatitis**   Inflammation of the liver.

**Hering–Breuer reflex**   A reflex response that regulates normal respiratory rate and rhythm; initiated by stretch receptor cells in walls of bronchioles and visceral pleura.

**Hermaphroditic**   Refers to presence of both male and female sex-cell-producing structures in one organism.

**Hernia**   Protrusion or projection of an organ or part of an organ through the wall of the cavity that normally contains it.

**Herniated disc (slipped disc)**   Rupture of an intervertebral disc and protrusion of the inner contents (nucleus pulposus) through the walls.

**Heterotrophic bacteria**   Bacteria that require a preformed organic carbon source. This means they must utilize organic material that has already been synthesized by others.

**Histamine**   Chemical released from mast cells in loose (alveolar) connective tissue. Functions to dilate blood vessels and increase their permeability to loss of fluids.

**Hodgkin's disease**   Chronic, progressive enlargement of the lymph nodes, spleen, and other lymphatic tissues.

**Homeostasis (steady state)**   A dynamic state of equilibrium of bodily processes.

**Hormone**   A chemical messenger secreted into the blood that coordinates the physiologic activities of effectors distant from the point of secretion.

**Humoral immunity (B cells)**   Immunity that results from antibodies in the blood neutralizing antigens.

**Hyaline membrane disease (respiratory distress syndrome)**   A disorder in which a newborn's lungs do not expand and contract properly, due to lack of pulmonary surfactant.

**Hyaluronidase**   Enzyme contained within acrosome of sperm cells; breaks down gel-like membrane of oocyte.

**Hydrolytic reaction**   A decomposition reaction that involves water. *See* Decomposition.

**Hydrophilic**   Water-loving; the property of attracting water molecules; polar (charged) end of fatty acid and phospholipid molecules.

**Hydrophobic**   Water-hating; the property of not attracting water molecules; nonpolar (noncharged) end of fatty acid and phospholipid molecules.

**Hydrostatic pressure (HP)**   Pressure that results from a fluid being forced against a membrane or wall.

**Hypercalcemia**   Excessive concentration of blood calcium; can result in spastic heart contractions.

**Hyperglycemia**   High level of blood glucose.

**Hyperkalemia**   Excessive concentration of blood potassium ($K^+$); can result in cardiac arrhythmia (irregular heart rhythm).

**Hyperopia (farsightedness)** Condition wherein objects at a distance are clear but close objects appear blurry due to shortened eyeball.

**Hyperosmolar (hypertonic)** A solution that has a greater osmotic pressure than an adjacent solution.

**Hyperosmolar imbalance** ECF osmotic pressure is greater than ICF osmotic pressure; results in water being pulled out of cells.

**Hyperpnea** Excessively deep breathing.

**Hypervolemia** Elevated blood volume.

**Hypoglycemia** Low level of blood glucose.

**Hypoosmolar (hypotonic)** A solution that has a lower osmotic pressure than an adjacent solution.

**Hypoosmolar imbalance** ICF osmotic pressure is greater than ECF osmotic pressure. As a result more water is pulled into body cells than is pulled out.

**Immunity** The state of being resistant to injury by poisons, foreign proteins, and invading pathogens. Immunity is in reality, therefore, resistance.

**Immunoglobulins, Ig** Antibodies that circulate in the blood. Five classes exist: IgA, IgD, IgE, IgG and IgM.

**Incontinence** Inability to restrain defecation or urination.

**Incubation period** Time between the entrance of microbes and the appearance of disease symptoms.

**Infarct** A region of dead tissue resulting from a deficiency of blood to that area.

**Infection** The invasion and growth of microbes in the body. An infection does not always result in damage or disruption of the physiologic processes in the body as in the case of the microorganisms that normally live on and in the body.

**Infectious hepatitis** Inflammation of the liver caused by IH viruses.

**Infectious mononucleosis** A viral infection that affects primarily people between the ages of 15 and 24 years; causes an enlargement of the spleen and lymph nodes, as well as fever, sore throat, and general lack of energy.

**Inflammation** Tissue response to stress; characterized by dilation of blood vessels and an accumulation of fluid in the affected region.

**Inguinal** Pertaining to the groin region.

**Insertion** The most movable end of a skeletal muscle, which also is attached to a bone.

**Insipid** Lacking flavor or zest. Example: In diabetes insipidus, the urine has no sweet taste due to lack of sugar and high level of water.

**Inspiratory center** A group of neurons in the lower part of the medulla oblongata that regulate inspiration.

**Inspiratory reserve volume** The volume of air (in excess of the tidal) that can be inhaled during the deepest possible inspiration.

**Integument** A covering. Example: skin.

**Interstitial cell stimulating hormone (ICSH)** Hormone that stimulates the interstitial cells between the seminiferous tubules in a testis to secrete testosterone, which is responsible for male secondary sex traits.

**Intracellular fluid** Fluid found within cells.

**Intramembranous ossification** Process by which face, flat bones of skull, hyoid, and clavicle bones are formed in membranes.

**Intrapleural pressure** Pressure within the pleural space of lungs.

**Intrapulmonic pressure** Pressure within the bronchial tree and alveoli of lungs.

**Ion** An atom or molecule that has either a positive or a negative charge. *See* Cation, Anion.

**Ischemia** Lack of blood flow to a part of the body.

**Isotope** Atoms of the same element that have a different number of neutrons but whose number of protons and electrons remain the same.

**Juxtaglomerular apparatus** Structure located where the afferent arteriole enters the glomerulus. Releases the hormone renin when blood pressure drops.

**Keratin** A water-resistant protein located in epidermis of skin.

**Ketogenesis** Formation of ketones.

**Ketonemia** Abnormal concentration of ketones in the blood.

**Ketonuria** Increase in the number of ketones in the urine.

**Ketosis** State of high level of ketones in the body.

**Kilocalorie** The amount of heat required to raise the temperature of 1000 grams of water one degree on the Celsius scale; abbreviated Cal (with a capital C). Used when measuring heat energy of body and nutritional values of foods.

**Krebs cycle** A series of chemical reactions in the mitochondria that generate the raw materials to produce ATPs in the cytochrome system.

**Kyphosis** An exaggerated thoracic curve of the vertebral column.

**Labia (lips)** Labia majora and labia minora are lip-like folds of skin in females between the mons pubis and the anus.

**Labile** Not fixed; cells that retain the ability to divide.

**Labor** Rhythmical contractions of the smooth muscles in the uterus leading to childbirth.

**Labyrinth** A complicated series of canals; example: cochlea in inner ear.

**Lacrimal apparatus** A series of structures that secrete tears and drain them from the eye.

**Lacteal** Lymph capillary in small intestine that absorbs neutral fats.

**Lacunae** Hollow cavities in bone and cartilage tissue, containing osteocyte and chondrocyte cells respectively.

**Laryngopharynx** Lowermost portion of pharynx continuing downward from the hyoid bone to the level of the larynx.

**Leukemia** A cancerous condition of the bone marrow. The cancerous cells cause excessive production of white blood cells.

**Leukocytosis** 1. Excessive number of white blood cells. 2. An increase in the number of white blood cells to more than 10,000 per cubic millimeter; a characteristic response to most infections such as leukemia, appendicitis, and infectious mononucleosis.

**Lever** A rodlike structure that consists of a fulcrum, resistance (weight), and power (force) that is applied to some point on the lever; used to help perform work; in body bones are levers.

**Ligation** Constriction of a vessel accomplished by tying it off.

**Liver lobules** Six-sided (hexagonal) structures that are functional units of the liver.

**Lobar pneumonia** Bacterial or viral infection of lung alveoli; results in inflammation of alveoli and accumulation of exudate in alveoli.

**Lophotrichous bacteria** Bacteria with a tuft of flagella from one or both poles.

**Lordosis** An exaggerated lumbar curve of the vertebral column; "swayback."

**Lumbar curve** A secondary curve of the vertebral column; develops after birth and allows the child to stand up.

**Lumen** Inner open space in a tube. Example: blood vessels and intestine.

**Lymph** Watery fluid in the lymphatic vessels.

**Lymphadentitis** Inflammation of the lymph nodes.

**Lymphangitis** Inflammation of lymphatic vessels.

**Lymphoma** A benign or malignant tumor in lymphatic tissue.

**Lysozome** Bacteria-killing enzyme; found in tears and other tissue fluids.

**Macules** Discolored spots on the skin that are not elevated.

**Malignant** Refers to neoplasm (tumor) that has the ability to spread (metastasize) from its original location.

**Mass** Quantity of matter.

**Matrix** Intercellular (between cells) material located in connective tissue.

**Matter** Anything that occupies space and has weight.

**Medulla** The middle or central core of an organ or other structure.

**Medullary cavity** Elongated hollow space extending the length of the diaphysis of a long bone; contains yellow marrow.

**Megakaryocytes** Cells produced in red bone marrow that break apart into fragments called platelets (thrombocytes).

**Melanin** Skin pigment located in stratum germinativum cells of the epidermis. The coloration of skin depends upon the amount of melanin present.

**Mellitus** Sweet or sugary in taste.

**Menarche** The first menstrual cycle that a female has, usually occurring between the ages of 12 and 15 years.

**Meninges** Connective tissue membranes that enclose the spinal cord and brain.

**Meningocele** (mening—membrane, ocele—hernia) A hernia of the meninges which protrudes through an opening in the skull or spinal column.

**Menopause** The permanent cessation of menstruation, when the ovaries, fallopian tubes, uterus, vagina, and breasts atrophy or degenerate.

**Mesentery** Fold of peritoneum that attaches the intestine to the posterior body wall.

**Mesoderm** Middle germ layer which gives rise to the three types of muscle tissue (cardiac, smooth, and skeletal), bones, peritoneum, and lining of portions of the urinary and reproductive systems.

**Metabolic acidosis** Excessive amount of carbonic acid in plasma; e.g., excess production of organic acids.

**Metabolic alkalosis** Excessive amount of sodium bicarbonate or loss of carbonic acid, e.g., vomiting can cause this condition.

**Metabolism** The sum total of chemical reactions that occur in the body.

**Metacarpals** Bones of the hand, five in number, and numbered from the lateral side.

**Metastasis** A secondary malignant tumor that originated from a primary malignant tumor.

**Mitosis** A series of stages during which a parent cell

divides, forming two genetically identical daughter cells.

**Mixture** Substance containing two or more elements or compounds not chemically combined.

**Molecule** The smallest particle of a compound that exhibits the chemical characteristics of that compound.

**Monotrichous bacteria** Bacteria with one polar flagellum.

**Morula** Early stage of embryonic development; solid ball of cells.

**Motor unit** Composed of one motor neuron and all the muscle fibers supplied by its branches.

**Mucin** A protein that gives saliva its slippery consistency and aids the chewing and swallowing processes.

**Muscular dystrophy** A disease characterized by a gradual atrophying of muscular tissue, which is replaced by fat deposits.

**Mycosis** A fungal disease. Examples: athlete's foot, jock itch, ringworm.

**Myocardium** The middle layer of heart tissue.

**Myofibrils** Fine fibers running lengthwise through muscle fibers.

**Myometrium** Smooth muscle walls of the uterus.

**Myopia (nearsightedness)** Condition wherein objects close up are clear but those at a distance appear blurry because the eyeball has lengthened.

**Myxedema** Hyposecretion of thyroxin. Results in edema, low body temperature, and elevated blood volume.

**Narcosis** Sedation.

**Narcotic** Addictive drug that can produce sedation and relieve pain. Examples: morphine, codeine, and heroin.

**Nasopharynx** Region of the pharynx posterior to the nasal cavities and superior to the soft palate.

**Nausea** A distressing feeling or signal that vomiting may occur.

**Negative feedback** A mechanism that is activated by an imbalance; the mechanism results in a reversal of physiological responses back toward the normal range; helps keep a system in equilibrium.

**Neoplasm** A mass of new, abnormal, or tumor tissue.

**Nephron** Functional unit of kidney; composed of renal corpuscle and tubular system.

**Nerve** A structure composed of many bundles of nerve fibers.

**Nerve fiber** A single neuron.

**Neuroeffector junction** Junction between muscle and nerve.

**Neuron** The basic cell making up nerve tissue.

**Neurotoxin** An exotoxin that affects the nervous system.

**Nicotinamide adenine dinucleotide (NAD)** Coenzyme that transports hydrogens from the citric acid cycle and glycolysis to the electron transport system.

**Node** A swelling, knot, or protuberance. Examples: lymph node, sinoatrial node.

**Nongranular leukocytes (agranulocytes)** Group of WBCs that lack granules in the cytoplasm and whose nuclei are not branched; lymphocytes and monocytes.

**Normal flora** Microorganisms normally found on and in the body.

**Oblique** Exhibiting a slanting or sloping direction, course, or position.

**Occlusion** A structure that obstructs the passage of material through a tube. Examples: embolus and thrombus.

**Oliguria** Decreased urine output.

**Oogenesis** Process by which haploid (N) oocytes are formed in ovaries.

**Opiates** Drugs derived from opium; include codeine, heroin, and morphine.

**Orchitis** Inflammation of the testes.

**Oropharynx** Middle region of pharynx; extends from the soft palate down to the hyoid bone.

**Osmolar (isotonic)** Refers to body fluids (ECF) and fluids within cells (ICF) having equal osmolarities and equal osmotic pressures.

**Osmolar imbalance** A disturbance in water distribution throughout the body's fluid compartments.

**Osmolarity** The total number of dissolved particles (solute) per liter of solution.

**Osmosis** The movement of water from a region of low solute concentration to high solute concentration through a membrane permeable only to water.

**Osmotic pressure** Pressure that results from dissolved solutes that cannot pass through a membrane. This pressure varies directly with the amount of dissolved solute.

**Ossicles** Three small bones (malleus, incus, stapes) that articulate with each other and extend from the tympanic membrane across the middle ear to the inner ear.

**Ossification** Bone formation; synthesis of organic bone matrix by bone-forming cells (osteoblasts).

**Osteoarthritis** Gradual degeneration of the tissues in a joint.

**Osteoblasts** Bone-forming cells.

**Osteoclasts** Bone-destroying cells; located in endosteum.

**Osteocytes** Mature osteoblasts which have lost their ability to produce bone tissue; produce matrix material; located in bone lacunae.

**Otoliths** Particles of calcium carbonate ($CaCO_3$) in the utricle, saccule, and semicircular canals of the inner ear.

**Ovum** Haploid mature female sex cell.

**Oxidation** The loss of electrons or acceptance of oxygen by atoms or molecules.

**Oxidizing agent** A substance that causes the oxidation of another substance.

**Oxyhemoglobin** Molecule formed when oxygen attaches to hemoglobin in pulmonary capillaries; transports $O_2$ from lungs to tissues of body.

**Oxytocin (pitocin)** A hormone from posterior pituitary that stimulates myometrium of uterus to contract at childbirth.

**Pancreozymin** A hormone released by the duodenum which stimulates the pancreas glands to release a viscous fluid low in bicarbonate but high in enzyme content.

**Papules** Solid, elevated lesions of the skin.

**Paraplegia** Paralysis of a person's lower extremities and possibly the lower part of the trunk.

**Parasympathetic division** Division of autonomic nervous system.

**Parathormone** A hormone released by the parathyroid gland; stimulates osteoclasts to release an enzyme that breaks down the bone matrix.

**Partial vacuum** Area where constant negative pressure is present.

**Pathogen** Any organism capable of producing a disease.

**Pathogenic** Disease causing.

**Pathogenicity** The ability of an organism to cause disease or disrupt normal physiologic activities.

**Peduncle** A stemlike part; applied to collections of nerve fibers coursing between different regions in the central nervous system.

**Pepsin** Enzyme that breaks peptide bonds of proteins.

**Pepsinogen** Inactive form of the protein-splitting enzyme pepsin.

**Peptic ulcer** An open sore in the mucosal lining of the stomach and duodenum.

**Peptones** Intermediate-sized protein segments.

**Perfusion** Passage of blood through vessels of particular organs or tissues.

**Perichondrium** A fibrous membrane that surrounds cartilage.

**Perilymph** Fluid contained in the space between the membranous and osseous labyrinths of the inner ear.

**Perineum** Space between anus and vulva in female and between anus and scrotum in male.

**Periosteum membrane** Fibrous connective tissue membrane that covers the surface of bones except at joints.

**Peripheral** Away from the center of a structure; outer, external, distal.

**Peripheral resistance** Resistance to the flow of blood in the arterioles.

**Peristalsis** Rhythmic waves of smooth muscle contractions that occur in the walls of certain tubular organs.

**Peritonitis** Inflammation of the peritoneal membrane that lines the walls of the abdominopelvic cavity.

**Peritrichous bacteria** Bacteria with flagella covering their entire surface.

**Peritubular capillaries** The capillary bed that surrounds the tubular system of a nephron.

**Peyer's patches** Solitary nodules of lymphatic tissue under the intestinal mucosa; function to filter out bacteria.

**pH** -log ($H^+$). A unit used to measure the concentration of $H^+$ in a solution. *See* pH scale.

**pH scale** Numerical scale used to measure the degree of acidity and alkalinity. The scale runs from 0 to 14. The numbers below 7 refer to acid solutions; those above 7 refer to alkaline solutions.

**Phalanges** Bones composing the fingers and toes; each individual bone is a phalanx.

**Phlebitis** Inflammation of the walls of veins; may be accompanied by edema and pain.

**Phosphoglyceraldehyde (PGAL)** Three-carbon sugar that is produced by splitting a six-carbon glucose molecule.

**Phospholipids** Lipids that contain a phosphate group and a nitrogen-containing base in place of one of three fatty acids.

**Physical change** One that changes the form of matter but does not change its chemical properties.

**Physiological solutions** Solutions that are identical in osmotic pressure to those of body fluids.

**Pitch** The tone of a sound.

**Pleomorphic** Exhibiting many forms. Pleuropneumonia-like organisms (PPLO) are an example.

**Pleura** Two-layered serous membrane lining and covering organs in the thoracic cavity.

**Pleurisy** Inflammation of pleural membrane; often occurs with lobar pneumonia.

**Plexus** A complicated network of nerves or blood vessels.

**Pneumotaxic center** A group of neurons located superior to the expiratory center in the pons; can inhibit the inspiratory and stimulate the expiratory center in emergency situations.

**Polar** Any chemical molecule that has positive and negative molecular regions. Example:

$$\overset{\displaystyle \overline{O}}{\underset{+\quad\quad+}{H\quad\quad H}}$$

**Polarization** A condition wherein + and − charged ions are separated from each other, e.g., nerves.

**Poliomyelitis** A disease of the nervous system that causes paralysis of muscles; viruses localize in ventral roots and prevent motor impulses from reaching muscles.

**Polycythemia** Excessive number of red blood cells.

**Polyuria** A persistent increase in the amount of urine excreted.

**Pons** Bridge; the bridge between the hindbrain and midbrain.

**Portal system** Veins that carry partly deoxygenated blood from one capillary bed to another. Example: Hepatic portal vein carries deoxygenated blood from intestinal capillaries in liver.

**Positive feedback** An abnormal state in which a change in a system in one direction serves as a command for continued change in that same direction; results in physiological responses moving farther and farther from normal range; destroys equilibrium.

**Postsynaptic neuron** Neuron that conducts an impulse away from a synapse.

**Precocious** Unusually early in development.

**Precocious puberty** Premature development of secondary sexual characteristics in young children.

**Precursors** Substances from which another substance is formed.

**Prepuce (foreskin)** Skin over the glans penis.

**Presbyopia** A condition in which the lens loses fluid and, therefore, some of its elasticity. The result is farsightedness or decreased ability to focus on near objects.

**Presynaptic neuron** A neuron that conducts an impulse to a synapse.

**Prime mover** The muscle responsible for the particular movement that a lever undergoes.

**Procaryotic cells** Cells that lack a true nucleus and other internal cellular compartments. This simple cell type is seen only in the bacteria and blue-green algae.

**Pronation** Movement of the forearm so that the palm is facing downward with the radius crossed over the ulna bone.

**Proprioceptors** Receptors located in muscles, tendons and joints that are sensitive to changes in movement of these structures.

**Proteoses** Intermediate-sized protein segments.

**Pseudomembrane** Thick, tough membrane formed on tonsils and soft palate in diphtheria.

**Psychosomatic** Pertaining to the interrelations of mind and body; e.g., psychosomatic illness can be traced to an emotional cause.

**Puberty** Stage of bodily development in which reproductive organs become functional.

**Pulmonary emphysema** A disorder characterized by the walls of the alveoli being dilated, atrophied, and thin; results in difficult respiration.

**Pulmonary surfactant** Fluid secreted by simple squamous cells of alveoli in lungs; reduces surface tension between inner surfaces of alveoli.

**Pulmonary system** Blood vessels that carry unoxygenated blood, rich in $CO_2$, from the heart to the lungs; exchange $CO_2$ for $O_2$; and return the oxygenated blood to the heart.

**Purkinje fibers** Specialized myocardium fibers that conduct nerve impulses from the AV bundle into the ventricles, resulting in their contraction.

**Pustules** Pus-containing lesions.

**Pyelitis** Inflammation of the renal basin.

**Pyelonephritis** Kidney disease located in the medulla region.

**Pyemia** A condition in which pyogenic bacteria spread throughout the body and produce pus.

**Pyloric stenosis** An abnormally small pyloric sphincter valve.

**Pylorospasm** A condition in which the pyloric valve remains in a constricted or spastic state.

**Pyogenic bacteria** Bacteria that spread to new parts of the body and produce pus.

**Pyuria** Presence of pus cells in the urine.

**Quadraplegia** Paralysis of all four extremities and the trunk.

**Ramus**   Nerve branch. Example: anterior and posterior rami of spinal nerves.

**Receptor cells**   Those which initiate nerve impulses and, therefore, detect changes in our external and internal environments.

**Red marrow**   Connective tissue found in spongy bone of certain bones; produces all of the various blood cells.

**Red measles (rubeola)**   Common childhood skin disease; caused by enveloped spherical RNA virus.

**Reduced hemoglobin**   Hemoglobin that has released $O_2$ to the alveoli.

**Reducing agent**   A substance that causes the reduction of another substance.

**Reduction**   Gain of electrons or loss of oxygen by atoms or molecules.

**Reflex**   An automatic act; does not require any conscious help.

**Reflux**   A return flow of fluid, e.g., movement of urine from bladder into kidneys.

**Refractrion**   Bending. Example: refraction of light rays as they pass through the eye.

**Renal calculi (kidney stones)**   Structures composed of uric acid and calcium salts.

**Renal corpuscle**   Composed of Bowman's capsule and tuft of capillaries (glomerulus) inside it.

**Reservoir**   Place where microbes normally reside.

**Resident flora**   Microorganisms normally found on and in the body.

**Residual air**   The volume of air remaining in the lungs even after the deepest possible expiration.

**Resistance**   The weight of the body part that is moved by a lever, plus any weight that the part may be supporting.

**Respiratory acidosis**   State wherein the acid content of blood is higher than normal, pH below 7.3, due to inability to exhale enough $CO_2$.

**Respiratory alkalosis**   State wherein the base content of blood is higher than normal, pH above 7.5, due to body exhaling too much $CO_2$.

**Reticuloendothelial system**   A widespread system of macrophage cells that keeps tissues free of foreign materials.

**Retina**   The innermost layer of the eye. Contains the receptors (rods and cones) for vision.

**Rheumatic fever**   Bacterial infection of joints; results in inflammation of synovial membrane and tendons.

**Rhodopsin**   A visual purple pigment in the rods of the retina that is very sensitive to light.

**Rotation**   Movement of a body part around a longitudinal axis with no change in position of the part. Example: shaking the head no.

**Rugae**   Folds of mucosa in the stomach, urinary bladder, and vagina that permit internal expansion of the above organs.

**Salivary amylase (ptyalin)**   A starch-digesting enzyme that breaks polysaccharide starches into disaccharide maltose molecules.

**Salt**   A compound often formed by the reaction of an acid with a base. A salt does not have a common ion like the $H^+$ and $OH^-$ of acids and bases; rather, it contains the negative ion of an acid linked to the positive ion of a base. Example: NaCl.

**Saprophytes**   Bacteria that break down the tissue material of dead plants and animals.

**Sarcolemma**   The membrane covering each muscle fiber.

**Sarcoma**   A cancer that arises from mesodermal tissue.

**Sarcomere**   The structural unit of a skeletal muscle; also the functional unit since contraction occurs here.

**Sclera**   The outer layer (white) of the eye.

**Scoliosis**   An abnormal lateral curvature of the vertebral column.

**Sedative**   A drug that produces effects like relaxation, depression of inhibitions, euphoria (a sense of good feeling), depression, relief of anxiety, loss of coordination, and decreased alertness. Examples: barbiturates and alcohol.

**Semen**   Sperm plus secretions from the seminal vesicles, prostate, and Cowper's glands.

**Semilunar**   Half-circle or half-moon shape.

**Septicemia**   An infection of the bloodstream caused by the invasion of bacteria. *Also called* blood poisoning.

**Serum hepatitis**   Inflammation of the liver caused by a virus termed SH.

**Sesamoid bone**   Bone that forms in tendons. Example: patella.

**Sex chromosomes**   Chromosomes that determine the sex of an individual.

**Sheath**   A structure that envelops another, e.g., neurilemma and myelin sheaths.

**Shock**   Inadequate circulation of blood to tissues.

**Sinoatrial (SA) node**   A modified knot of tissue located at the junction of the right atrium with the right ventricle. It receives nerve impulses from the atria and conducts them to the ventricles through the atrioventricular bundle (bundle of His).

**Sinus**   A cavity located within a bone that serves to decrease the weight of a bone.

**Sinusoids**  A space in certain organs that conducts blood. Similar to capillaries.

**Smallpox (variola)**  Skin disease, now rare, caused by pox virus.

**Solute**  A substance that dissolves in a solvent.

**Solution**  Homogeneous mixture of two or more elements or compounds.

**Solvent**  A fluid that causes a compound (solute) to dissolve, forming a solution. Water serves as the solvent for most chemical reactions in the body.

**Spastic paralysis**  Uncoordinated muscular twitchings to vigorous muscular reflexes.

**Specific gravity**  A measurement that expresses the relative mass of one liquid compared to that of another.

**Spermatogenesis**  Process by which sperm are formed by meiosis.

**Sphincter**  A circular muscle that narrows the lumen of a tubular structure when it contracts.

**Sprain**  Stretching or tearing of the ligaments, tendons, or capsule of a joint without the dislocation of bones.

**Stable cells**  Cells that have the ability to reproduce but do not do so unless cells are damaged.

**Stasis**  Stoppage of fluid flow; e.g., a pregnant uterus reduces urine flow.

**Static equilibrium**  The position of the body (mainly the head) in relation to the ground.

**Stenosis**  An abnormal constriction or narrowing of a passageway.

**Strep throat**  Streptococcal sore throat; caused by beta hemolytic streptococci.

**Stretch (extensor) reflex**  Two-neuron reflex initiated by stretch receptor cells; results in extension contraction of stimulated muscle(s).

**Stroke**  Sudden decrease in blood flow to brain. Results in cessation of certain bodily functions. Same as cerebrovascular accident.

**Substrate**  The substance acted upon by an enzyme.

**Sudoriferous glands (sweat glands)**  Exocrine glands that secrete sweat and regulate body temperature.

**Sulcus**  Shallow grooves. Example: sulci separating convolutions in cerebral cortex.

**Supination**  Movement of the forearm so that the palm is facing anteriorly and the radius and ulna bones of the forearm are parallel.

**Sympathetic division**  Division of autonomic nervous system that prepares the body to respond to fear, anger, worry, and strenuous activity; nerves exit from thorax and lumbar regions.

**Synarthrosis**  An immovable joint.

**Syndrome**  A group of symptoms that together characterize a disease condition.

**Synthesis reaction**  Two atoms, two elements, or an element and a compound chemically bonding together to form a more complex single compound.

**Syphilis**  A venereal disease; causative organism is *Treponema pallidum*, a spirochete type of bacteria.

**Systemic**  Affecting the entire body. Example: systemic circulatory unit.

**Systole**  Phase of cardiac cycle when heart chambers are contracted.

**T cells**  *See* Cell-mediated immunity.

**Tachypnea**  Shallow, rapid breathing.

**Taeniae coli**  Longitudinal muscle layer of large intestine; arranged in three flat layers.

**Target organ**  Organ that is stimulated by a hormone.

**Telencephalon**  Most anterior region of the forebrain, composed of two cerebral hemispheres.

**Testosterone**  A male hormone secreted from the testes; a steroid. It is responsible for development of secondary sex characteristics (beard and muscle configuration); the male sex drive and behvior are also dependent upon testosterone.

**Tetanus**  A bacterial disease caused by *Clostridium tetani*; results in spasms of certain muscles.

**Tetany**  Intermittent muscular contractions, tremors, and muscular pain.

**Thermophiles**  Organisms that grow at temperatures above 45–50°C.

**Thoracic duct**  Lymph duct that originates at the second lumbar vertebra; drains lymph from this level all the way up to the left subclavian vein, where lymph drains into venous blood.

**Thrombus**  A blood clot that forms and remains stationary.

**Thyroxin ($T_4$)**  A thyroid hormone that regulates the production of heat and energy or metabolism of tissues.

**Tidal volume**  The volume of air that moves into and out of the lungs with each respiratory cycle.

**Tinea (ringworm)**  Infections that occur on the skin at many different locations on the body.

**Tinea capitis**  Ringworm of the scalp.

**Tinea pedis**  Ringworm of the feet; athlete's foot.

**Tinnitus**  A condition of the ear characterized by abnormal buzzing, ringing, whistling, and other unusual noises in the ear.

**Tonic contraction**  Involves contraction of only a few

muscle fibers rather than all the fibers within a muscle; no movement of a body part results from contractions.

**Tonsils**   Three patches of lymphoid tissue located in the pharynx; they filter out microorganisms that enter the respiratory tract.

**Toxigenicity**   The ability of microbes to produce poisons called toxins.

**Toxins**   Poisonous chemicals that can damage the tissues of the body.

**Toxoid**   A chemically modified exotoxin. It is still an antigen and can stimulate the production of antibodies. It is injected like a vaccine and is used to prevent infection with *Clostridium tetani* (tetanus) and *Corynebacterium diphtheriae* (diphtheria).

**Trachea**   A rigid cartilaginous muscular tube that extends downward from the larynx to the center of the chest; conducts air.

**Tracheostomy**   Placing of a tube into a tracheotomy opening.

**Tracheotomy**   A surgical opening into the anterior surface of the trachea.

**Transient flora**   Organisms present on the body for a short time only.

**Trophic**   Having to do with growth and development.

**True pelvis**   The area inferior to the pelvic brim.

**Tubercules**   Firm, round lumps in the lungs, formed in response to TB organisms.

**Tuberculosis (TB)**   Respiratory infection caused by acid-fast bacillus organisms; they cause formation of tubercules and eventually caseation.

**Tumor**   A mass of new, abnormal tissue.

**Tunica**   A layer of tissue.

**Ulcer**   An open lesion of the skin or a mucous membrane of the body with loss of substance and necrosis (death) of the tissue.

**Uremia**   Buildup of wastes in the blood.

**Ureter**   A tube that carries urine to the urinary bladder from the kidney.

**Urethra**   A small tube extending from the bladder to the outside.

**Vaccine**   A chemical compound composed of antigens in the form of bacteria, viruses or rickettsiae, used to achieve artificial active immunity.

**Vagina (sheath)**   A collapsible muscular tube that extends from the vaginal opening to the cervix of the uterus.

**Valence (bonding capacity)**   The number of electrons an atom needs to share, acquire, or give up to have a stable outer orbit. Also, the number of bonds that an atom can form with other atoms.

**Varicose**   Abnormally swollen or enlarged, e.g., varicose veins.

**Vasectomy**   A male sterilization operation.

**Vectors**   Transmitters of pathogenic organisms. They are not a reservoir of the pathogen.

**Vegetation**   A plantlike neoplasm or growth.

**Vegetative form**   Actively growing form of bacteria.

**Veins**   Vessels that transport blood away from capillary beds to the heart.

**Venereal disease**   An infection transmitted by sexual contact.

**Ventricle**   1. A small cavity or chamber, as in the brain or heart. 2. Elongated fluid-filled cavity. Example: ventricles in the heart and brain.

**Venule**   A small vein that carries venous blood to a larger vein.

**Vesicles**   Small blisters or fluid-containing cavities.

**Virulence**   The ability of microbes to damage the body and produce disease.

**Viscosity**   Thickness or stickiness of a fluid.

**Vital capacity**   The volume of air that results from the addition of the tidal inspiratory reserve volumes.

**Vitreous humor (body)**   A thick fluid that has the consistency of gelatin.

**Volume imbalance (isotonic imbalance)**   An imbalance characterized by $Na^+$ and $H_2O$ increasing or decreasing together in roughly the same proportions as found in ECF, rather than disproportionately as in osmolar imbalances.

**Vulva**   External female reproductive organs that surround the opening of the vagina.

**Weight**   The degree of attraction between two objects. It varies with the position of the two objects.

**White matter**   Myelinated neurons that conduct nerve impulses.

**Whooping cough (Pertussis)**   An upper respiratory infection caused by gram-negative rods.

**Yellow marrow**   Adipose tissue in the medullary cavity of long bones.

**Zygote**   A fertilized ovum; results from the union of haploid (N) sperm and ovum (N).

# Answers to Chapter Exam Questions

**Chapter 1**  *Units and Methods of Measurement*

| | |
|---|---|
| 1. e | 8. b |
| 2. d | 9. b |
| 3. b | 10. a |
| 4. a | 11. d |
| 5. c | 12. c |
| 6. c | 13. a |
| 7. e | 14. d |

**Chapter 2**  *Chemistry of the Body*

| | | | |
|---|---|---|---|
| 1. b | 12. a | 23. a | 34. b |
| 2. b | 13. b | 24. d | 35. a |
| 3. a | 14. a | 25. c | |
| 4. b | 15. a | 26. b | |
| 5. b | 16. a | 27. d | |
| 6. c | 17. a | 28. c | |
| 7. a | 18. b | 29. b | |
| 8. e | 19. b | 30. a | |
| 9. d | 20. b | 31. a | |
| 10. a | 21. d | 32. a | |
| 11. b | 22. e | 33. b | |

**Chapter 3**  *Microbiology*

| | |
|---|---|
| 1. b | 8. b |
| 2. a | 9. a |
| 3. b | 10. a |
| 4. a | 11. b |
| 5. a | 12. a |
| 6. b | 13. a |
| 7. b | 14. a |

**Chapter 4**  *Introduction to Anatomy Physiology of the Body*

| | |
|---|---|
| 1. c | 10. b |
| 2. d | 11. d |
| 3. a | 12. c |
| 4. b | 13. b |
| 5. e | 14. a |
| 6. b | 15. b |
| 7. c | 16. b |
| 8. e | 17. a |
| 9. a | 18. a |

**Chapter 5**  *Nervous System*

| | |
|---|---|
| 1. d | 8. e |
| 2. a | 9. c |
| 3. b | 10. e |
| 4. a | 11. a |
| 5. a | 12. d |
| 6. b | 13. b |
| 7. a | |

**Chapter 6**  *Endocrine System*

| | |
|---|---|
| 1. e | 8. b |
| 2. d | 9. a |
| 3. c | 10. a |
| 4. b | 11. a |
| 5. a | 12. a |
| 6. a | 13. a |
| 7. b | 14. b |

**Chapter 7**  *The Blood*

| | |
|---|---|
| 1. a | 7. b |
| 2. d | 8. a |
| 3. c | 9. a |
| 4. e | 10. b |
| 5. b | 11. e |
| 6. a | |

**Chapter 8**  *The Cardiovascular System*

| | |
|---|---|
| 1. a | 7. a |
| 2. a | 8. c |
| 3. b | 9. e |
| 4. a | 10. b |
| 5. b | 11. a |
| 6. a | 12. d |

**Chapter 9**  *The Skin*

| | |
|---|---|
| 1. c | 7. b |
| 2. e | 8. a |
| 3. d | 9. a |
| 4. b | 10. b |
| 5. a | 11. c |
| 6. b | |

**Chapter 10**  *Lymphatic System*

| | |
|---|---|
| 1. c | 4. a |
| 2. a | 5. d |
| 3. c | 6. a |

**Chapter 11**  *Sensory Receptors and Sense Organs*

| | |
|---|---|
| 1. e | 6. b |
| 2. c | 7. b |
| 3. c | 8. a |
| 4. a | 9. a |
| 5. b | 10. a |

**Chapter 12**  *Bones and the Skeletal System*

| | |
|---|---|
| 1. d | 8. b |
| 2. b | 9. a |
| 3. e | 10. a |
| 4. c | 11. d |
| 5. a | 12. b |
| 6. a | 13. e |
| 7. b | |

**Chapter 13**  *Muscles and Muscular System*

1. b     8. a
2. c     9. b
3. e     10. b
4. a     11. a
5. d     12. b
6. a     13. b
7. b     14. a

**Chapter 14**  *Levers (bones), Muscles, and Movements
of the Axial Skeletal System*

1. a     5. a
2. e     6. a
3. c     7. a
4. a     8. a

**Chapter 15**  *Levers (bones), Muscles, and Movement
of Appendicular Skeletal System*

1. b
2. b
3. a
4. a
5. a
6. b
7. c
8. d
9. d

**Chapter 16**  *Fluids and Electrolytes*

1. b     9. b
2. e     10. a
3. d     11. a
4. a     12. a
5. c     13. b
6. b     14. b
7. a     15. a
8. a

**Chapter 17**  *The Respiratory System*

1. c     9. a
2. e     10. a
3. b     11. a
4. d     12. b
5. a     13. c
6. b     14. e
7. b     15. e
8. b

**Chapter 18**  *The Urinary System*

1. c     8. a
2. d     9. b
3. e     10. a
4. a     11. b
5. b     12. a
6. b     13. d
7. a     14. c
         15. e

**Chapter 19**  *Digestive System*

1. e     14. b
2. e     15. a
3. a     16. a
4. d     17. a
5. e     18. a
6. c     19. a
7. b     20. b
8. b     21. b
9. b     22. a
10. b    23. a
11. b    24. b
12. b    25. a
13. a

**Chapter 20**  *Metabolism of Lipids, Carbohydrates,
and Proteins*

1. a     9. a
2. d     10. b
3. c     11. a
4. b     12. b
5. e     13. b
6. a     14. b
7. c     15. a
8. b

**Chapter 21**  *The Reproductive System*

1. b     15. e
2. c     16. b
3. d     17. a
4. a     18. b
5. e     19. a
6. c     20. a
7. e     21. b
8. d     22. b
9. a     23. a
10. b    24. a
11. c    25. b
12. d    26. b
13. a    27. b
14. b

# INDEX

Electrovalent bonds (*see* Ionic bonds)
Elements
  definition of, 13, 17, 43, 460
  found in human body, 13
  properties of, 17
Embolus, 195, 465
  definition of, 460
Embryo
  development of, 441–43, 452
  development of membrane and placenta
    around, 438, 439
Emmetropic, 247, 248, 257
Emphysema, 350
Endergonic reactions, 22, 23
  definition of, 22, 43, 460
Endocardium, 184, 186, 209
  definition of, 460
  infection of, 188
Endochondral ossification, 265–66, 271
  definition of, 460
Endocrine glands, 97, 108, 154–65, 171
Endocrine system, 74, 153–67
  characteristics of, 153
  regulation of hormone secretion, 153
  role in gastric juice production, 383, 384–85,
    401
Endoderm, 96
  definition of, 460
Endolymph, 251, 252, 254, 255
  definition of, 460
Endometrium, 423, 432, 438, 451
  changes in (*see* Menstrual cycle)
  definition of, 460
Endoplasmic reticulum, 77–78, 107, 275
Endospores, 55, 56, 58
  definition of, 55, 65, 460
Endosteum membrane, 261, 262, 269, 270, 271
  definition of, 460
Endothelium, 186, 192, 193
  definition of, 460
Endothermic reactions (*see* Endergonic reactions)
Endotoxin, 53
  definition of, 460
Energy, 14–17
  conservation of, 16, 42
  definition of, 15, 42, 460
  forms of, 15–16, 42
  kinds of, 15, 42
  measurement of, 16, 43
  transformation of, 16, 42
Energy of activation, definition of, 38, 460
*Entamoeba coli*, 62
*Entamoeba histolytica*, 62, 66
Enterogastrone, 384, 388, 401
Enzymes, 25, 31, 89, 90, 171, 180
  definition of, 38, 460
  denaturation of, 348, 357
  digestive, 80–81, 107, 398
  effect on chemical reactions, 26, 38, 39, 52
  examples and naming of, 38, 40
  functions of, 38
  hydrolytic, 80–81, 107
  intestinal, 396, 398
  lock and key theory, 38, 39
  oxidative, 79, 80, 81
  pancreatic, 396, 398
  proteolytic, 80
Eosinophils, 174, 175, 180
Epicardium, 184, 209
  definition of, 460
Epidermis, 194, 214, 215, 217, 218, 221
  definition of, 460
Epidural space, 120, 123
  definition of, 460
Epiglottis, 100, 109, 343–44, 345, 356
Epinephrine, 132, 153, 162–63, 166, 414, 416, 419
  definition of, 460
Epiphyseal cartilage, 261, 262, 266, 271
  definition of, 460
Epiphyses, 261, 265, 271
  definition of, 460
Episiotomy, 426, 445
  definition of, 460

Epithelial tissue, 96, 97–98, 104, 109, 215, 217,
    220, 221, 222, 393
  anatomic features of, 97, 108
  maintaining homeostasis, 104
  types of, 97–98, 108
Equilibrium, 248, 251, 256, 258, 264
  dynamic, 254–56
  static, 254, 258
Erythroblastosis fetalis, 179, 181, 441
  definition of, 460
Erythrocytes (*see* Red blood corpuscles)
Erythropoiesis, 172, 180
  definition of, 172, 460
Erythropoietin, 172, 180
*Escherichia coli*, 64
Esophagus, 98, 342, 343, 356, 377, 380, 381, 382,
    386, 387, 401
Estrogen, 35, 162, 165, 423, 426, 432, 433, 434,
    445, 447, 452
  definition of, 35, 460
Ethmoid bone, 290, 293, 294, 295, 304
Eucaryotic cells, 50, 51
  definition of, 65, 460
Eustachian tube, 249, 250, 251
Exchange reactions, definition of, 24, 43
Excretory organs, 99, 108, 361
Exergonic reactions, 22, 23, 24, 25
  definition of, 23, 43, 460
Exocrine gland, 163
Exophthalmic goiter, 160, 166
Exophthalmos, 159, 160
  definition of, 460
Exothermic reactions (*see* Exergonic reactions)
Expiration, 304, 348, 349, 350, 351, 357
Extension, 311
  definition of, 284, 287, 460
Extensor carpi ulnaris muscle, 313, 314, 326
Extensor muscles, 126, 127
External acoustic meatus, 249, 250, 258
External auditory meatus, 217, 222
External ear, 100, 109, 249, 250, 258
External oblique muscle, 322, 323
Extracellular fluid, 330
  definition of, 330, 338, 460
  electrolyte distribution and concentration in,
    330–31
Eye, 36, 114, 141, 142–43, 147, 238–49
  abnormal vision conditions, 247–48
  cornea (*see* Cornea)
  iris (*see* Iris)
  layers of tissue, 239–43, 257
  lens (*see* Lens)
  movement of, 239, 240, 257
  normal vision with, 247
  physiology of vision (*see* Vision, physiology of)
  protective structures, of, 238–39, 257
  pupil (*see* Pupil)
  retina, 241–43, 245, 247
  retinal examination, 248–49
  rods and cones, 241–43
  sclera of, 105, 109, 239, 240, 468
  white of (*see* Sclera)

Facial muscles, 144
Facial nerves, 142, 143, 144, 256, 258, 379
Facultative bacteria, 59
  definition of, 461
FAD, 411
FADH$_2$, 411, 414, 419
Fahrenheit temperature scale
  conversion to Celsius, 5–6
  freezing and boiling point values, 5, 7
Fallen arches, 321
Fallopian tube, 423, 424, 427, 429, 450
False ribs, 302
Fascial membranes, 104, 105, 109
Fat (*see* Adipose tissue)
Fat depots, 414, 419
Fats
  breakdown of, 35–36
  definition of, 34, 461
Fatty acids, 34, 36, 45, 171, 180, 393, 398, 403,
    419, 420

Fatty acids (*cont.*)
  breaking down of, 414, 415
  essential, 35
Female reproductive system, 423–26, 450
  accessory organs, 424, 425, 426, 450
  clitoris, 163, 424, 425, 426, 450
  fallopian tube, 423, 424, 425, 429, 450
  labia, 424, 450
  mammary glands, 426, 450
  ovaries, 97, 108, 156, 157, 165, 379, 423, 435,
    450
  perineum, 426, 445, 450
  uterus, (*see* Uterus)
  vagina, 424, 425, 427, 450
  vestibular glands, 426, 450
Femoral rings, 323, 324
Femur bone, 314, 315–16
  muscles moving, 316–17
Fertilization, 436–37, 451
Fetus, 100
  circulation of blood in, 444–45
  definition of, 461
  development of, 441–43, 452
Fibrillation, 280, 286
  definition of, 461
Fibrin, 176, 177, 181
Fibrinogen, 171, 176, 177, 180, 181, 393
Fibroblasts, 100, 101, 221
Fibrocartilaginous callus, 270, 272
Fibroma, 96, 108
Fibrosarcoma, 96
Fibrous cartilage, 100, 101, 103, 109
Fibrous membranes, 104, 105, 109
Fibula bone, 317–18, 319, 320, 321
  muscles that move, 318, 319
Filtration, 90, 97, 104, 140, 171, 332
  definition of, 90, 107
  by lymph nodes, 226–27, 230
Fingers
  bones of the, 312–13
Fissure of Rolando, 133
Fissure of Sylvius, 133
Flagella, 53, 54
  definition of, 53, 65, 461
Flagellates, 63, 66
Flagellin, 53
Flat feet, 321
Flexion movement, 297, 311
  definition of, 283, 287, 461
Flexor carpi radialis muscle, 313, 314, 326
Flexor muscles, 122, 127
Flexor reflexes, 126–27, 149
  definition of, 461
Floating ribs, 302
  definition of, 461
Fluids
  balance of, 371–72, 374
  calculating density of, 4, 5
  calculating specific gravity of, 4–5
  changes in osmolality and osmotic pressure of,
    86–88, 89
  two major types of, 330–31
  water-sodium imbalances, 334–37, 339
Fluids, movement of, 332–37
  between plasma and interstitial fluid compart-
    ments, 333–34, 339
  exchange between extracellular and intracellu-
    lar compartments, 334, 339
  maintenance of, 371–72, 374
  two pressures involved, 332–33, 339
Follicle, definition of, 432
Follicle-stimulating hormone, 157, 429, 432, 433,
    434, 447, 451
  definition of, 461
Fontanels, 296–97, 304
  definition of, 461
Foot
  bones of the, 321, 327
  muscles that move, 321–22, 327
Foramen, definition of, 263, 461
Foramen magnum, 119, 120, 129, 148, 263, 290
Foramen of Monro, 139
Forearm (*see* Arm, lower)